Fetal Diagnosis and Therapy

Fetal Diagnosis and Therapy:
Science, Ethics and the Law

Edited by

Mark I. Evans, M.D.
Director of Reproductive Genetics, Hutzel Hospital, and Associate Professor of Obstetrics and Gynecology and Molecular Biology and Genetics and Center for Molecular Biology, Wayne State University School of Medicine, Detroit, Michigan

Alan O. Dixler, J.D., LL.M.
Member, New York Bar, Florham Park, New Jersey

John C. Fletcher, Ph.D.
Professor of Religious Studies and Biomedical Ethics in Internal Medicine, University of Virginia, and Hospital Ethicist, UVA Health Sciences Center, Charlottesville, Virginia

Joseph D. Schulman, M.D.
Director, Genetics and IVF Institute, and Attending Physician, Fairfax Hospital, Fairfax, Virginia; Professor of Human Genetics, Obstetrics and Gynecology, and Pediatrics, Medical College of Virginia, Richmond, Virginia

with 68 contributors

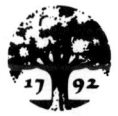

J. B. Lippincott Company
Philadelphia
Cambridge   London
New York   Singapore
St. Louis   Sydney
San Francisco   Tokyo

Acquisitions Editor: Lisa Biello
Manuscript Editor: Anna M. Avery
Indexer: Maria Coughlin
Design Coordinator: Michelle Gerdes
Cover Designer: Wendy Cummiskey
Production Coordinator: Barney Fernandes
Production Manager: Carol A. Florence
Compositor: Bi-Comp Inc.
Printer/Binder: R. R. Donnelley & Sons Co.

Copyright © 1989, by J. B. Lippincott Company. All rights reserved. No part of this book may be used or reproduced in any manner whatsoever without written permission except for brief quotations embodied in critical articles and reviews. Printed in the United States of America. For information write J. B. Lippincott Company, East Washington Square, Philadelphia, Pennsylvania 19105.

1 3 5 6 4 2

Fetal diagnosis and therapy : science, ethics, and the law / [edited by] Mark I. Evans . . . [et al.] ; with 65 contributors.
    p.   cm.
  Includes bibliographies and index.
  ISBN 0-397-50869-7
  1. Perinatology. 2. Perinatology—Moral and ethical aspects. 3. Human reproduction—Technological innovations—Moral and ethical aspects. 4. Fetus—Research—Law and legislation—United States. 5. Obstetrics—Law and legislation—United States. I. Evans, Mark I.
  [DNLM: 1. Ethics, Medical. 2. Fetal Distress—therapy. 3. Obstetrics—United States—legislation. 4. Prenatal Diagnosis. 5. Reproductive Technics—trends. WQ 209 F4193]
RG627.F47 1989
362.1'9832'0973—dc19
DNLM/DLC
for Library of Congress
                                                                88-9485
                                                                   CIP

The authors and publisher have exerted every effort to ensure that drug selection and dosage set forth in this text are in accord with current recommendations and practice at the time of publication. However, in view of ongoing research, changes in government regulations, and the constant flow of information relating to drug therapy and drug reactions, the reader is urged to check the package insert for each drug for any change in indications and dosage and for added warnings and precautions. This is particularly important when the recommended agent is a new or infrequently employed drug.

To our children:

*Kiera, Shara, Rufus, Harry,
Caldwell, Page, Adele,
Scott, Hillary,
Erica, and Julie*

Contributors

Ernest L. Abel, Ph.D.
Professor of Obstetrics and Gynecology
Wayne State University School of Medicine
Director of Operations
C.S. Mott Center, Hutzel Hospital
Detroit, Michigan

Duane Alexander, M.D.
Director
National Institute of Child Health and Human Development
Bethesda, Maryland

Robert L. Anderson, M.D.
Associate Clinical Professor
Department of Obstetrics, Gynecology, and Reproductive Services
School of Medicine
University of California, San Francisco
San Francisco, California

W. French Anderson, M.D.
Chief, Laboratory of Molecular Hematology
Chairman, Department of Medicine and Physiology
National Institutes of Health Graduate Program
National Heart, Lung and Blood Institute
National Institutes of Health
Bethesda, Maryland
Adjunct Professor, Graduate Genetics Program
George Washington University
Washington, D.C.

James H. Beeson, M.D.
Associate Professor and Chairman
Department of Obstetrics and Gynecology
Medical Center
University of Oklahoma, Tulsa
Tulsa, Oklahoma

Kåre Berg, M.D., Ph.D.
Institute of Medical Genetics
University of Oslo
Oslo, Norway

Contributors

Joan E. Bertin, J.D.
Associate Director of the Women's Rights Program
American Civil Liberties Union
New York, New York

Richard A. Bronsteen, M.D.
Assistant Professor
Department of Obstetrics and Gynecology
Wayne State University School of Medicine
Associate Director
Antenatal Diagnostic Unit
Grace Hospital
Detroit, Michigan

María Bustillo, M.D.
Clinical Assistant Professor
Department of Obstetrics and Gynecology
Medical College of Virginia
Richmond, Virginia
Reproductive Endocrinologist
Genetics and IVF Institute
Fairfax, Virginia

Alexander Morgan Capron, J.D.
Topping Professor of Law, Medicine, and Public Policy
University of Southern California Law Center
Los Angeles, California

Frank A. Chervenak, M.D.
Director of Obstetrical Ultrasound and Ethics
Associate Professor, Department of Obstetrics and Gynecology
New York Hospital—Cornell Medical Center
New York, New York

Nancy Clementino, M.P.H.
Formerly of the Division of Reproductive Genetics
Hutzel Hospital
Detroit, Michigan
Currently medical student at Wayne State University School of Medicine
Detroit, Michigan

Joshua A. Copel, M.D.
Assistant Professor
Director of Resident Education for Obstetrics and Gynecology
Department of Obstetrics and Gynecology
Yale University School of Medicine
New Haven, Connecticut

Alan O. Dixler, J.D., LL.M.
Member, New York Bar
Florham Park, New Jersey

Arie Drugan, M.D.
Assistant Professor
Department of Obstetrics and Gynecology
Wayne State University School of Medicine
Division of Reproductive Genetics
Hutzel Hospital
Detroit, Michigan

Thomas E. Elkins, M.D.
Associate Professor and Director of Gynecology
Department of Obstetrics and Gynecology
University of Michigan Medical Center
Ann Arbor, Michigan

Mark I. Evans, M.D.
Director of Reproductive Genetics
Hutzel Hospital
Associate Professor
Departments of Obstetrics and Gynecology and Molecular Biology and Genetics and Center for Molecular Biology
Wayne State University School of Medicine
Detroit, Michigan

Wendy J. Evans, M.P.H.
West Bloomfield, Michigan

David R. Field, M.D.
Director of Perinatal Services
Kaiser Permanante Medical Center
San Francisco, California

Lynn D. Fleisher, J.D., Ph.D.
Attorney, Sidney & Austin
Chicago, Illinois

Anne B. Fletcher, M.D.
Professor, Child Health and Development
George Washington University School of Health Sciences
Medical Director of the Neonatal Intensive Care Unit
Children's Hospital National Medical Center
Washington, DC

John C. Fletcher, Ph.D.
Professor of Religious Studies and Professor of Biomedical Ethics in Internal Medicine
University of Virginia
Hospital Ethicist, UVA Health Sciences Center
Director, Center for Biomedical Ethics
Charlottesville, Virginia

Martin L. Gimovsky, M.D., F.A.C.O.G.
Associate Clinical Professor of Obstetrics and Gynecology
University of Southern California School of Medicine
Director of Maternal-Fetal Medicine and Chief of Obstetrics
White Memorial Medical Center
Los Angeles, California

Leonard H. Glantz, J.D.
Professor of Health Law
Boston University Schools of Medicine and Public Health
Boston, Massachusetts

Gregory L. Glover, M.D.
Chief, Department of Obstetrics and Gynecology
Edge Regional Medical Center
Troy, Alabama

Mitchell Golbus, M.D.
Professor
Department of Obstetrics and Gynecology and Reproductive Services and Department of Pediatrics
School of Medicine
University of California, San Francisco
San Francisco, California

Robin Belsky Gold, M.S.
Genetic Counselor
Department of Obstetrics and Gynecology
Sinai Hospital of Detoit
Detroit, Michigan

Gregory L. Goyert, M.D.
Assistant Professor
Department of Obstetrics and Gynecology
Wayne State University School of Medicine
Assistant Director
Maternal-Fetal Medicine
Sinai Hospital of Detroit
Detroit, Michigan

Anne Greb
Genetics Coordinator
Division of Reproductive Genetics
Hutzel Hospital
Detroit, Michigan

Ruth S. Hanft, M.A.
Research Professor and Consultant
Department of Health Services Administration
George Washington University
Washington, DC

Michael R. Harrison, M.D.
Professor of Surgery and Pediatrics
Co-Director, Fetal Treatment Program
University of California, San Francisco
San Francisco, California

W. Allen Hogge, M.D.
Assistant Professor of Obstetrics and Gynecology and Pediatrics
University of Virginia
Charlottesville, Virginia
Director, Prenatal Diagnosis and Treatment Center
University of Virginia Hospital
Charlottesville, Virginia

Glenn Isaacson, M.D.
Adjunct Assistant Professor of Fetal Anatomy in Obstetrics and Gynecology
New York Hospital—Cornell Medical Center
New York, New York

x Contributors

Albert R. Jonsen, Ph.D.
Professor and Chairman
Department of Biomedical History and Ethics
School of Medicine
University of Washington, Seattle
Seattle, Washington

Charles S. Kleinman, M.D.
Professor of Pediatrics, Diagnostic Imaging, and Obstetrics and Gynecology
Yale University School of Medicine
Chief, Section of Pediatric Cardiology
Yale–New Haven Medical Center
New Haven, Connecticut

Frederick C. Koppitch III, M.S., C.L.S.p.(C.G.)
Research Assistant
Wayne State University School of Medicine
Supervisor
C.S. Mott Center Cytogenetic Laboratory
Detroit, Michigan

Russell K. Laros, Jr., M.D.
Professor and Vice Chairman
Department of Obstetrics, Gynecology and Reproductive Services
University of California, San Francisco School of Medicine
San Francisco, California

John W. Larsen, Jr., M.D.
Professor, Obstetrics, Gynecology and Genetics
Director, Wilson Genetics Center
George Washington University
Attending Physician
George Washington University Hospital
Washington DC

Chin-Chu Lin, M.D.
Professor, Department of Obstetrics and Gynecology
University of Chicago
Pritzker School of Medicine
Chicago, Illinois
Attending Physician
Chicago Lying-In Hospital
Chicago Illinois

Martha D. MacMillin, M.S.
Genetic Counselor
Wilson Genetics Center
George Washington University
Washington, D.C.

Donald R. Mattison, M.D.
Professor
Department of Obstetrics and Gynecology
University of Arkansas for Medical Sciences
Little Rock, Arkansas

S. Gene McNeeley, M.D.
Assistant Professor
Department of Obstetrics and Gynecology
University of Michigan Medical School
Ann Arbor, Michigan

E. Haavi Morreim, Ph.D.
Associate Professor
College of Medicine
University of Tennessee, Memphis
Memphis, Tennessee

Roy H. Petrie, M.D., Sc.D.
Professor of Obstetrics and Gynecology
Director
Division of Maternal-Fetal Medicine
School of Medicine
Washington University in St. Louis
Director of Obstetrics
Barnes Hospital
St. Louis, Missouri

Marilyn L. Poland, Ph.D., R.N.
Associate Professor
Department of Obstetrics and Gynecology
Wayne State University
Co-Director
Institute of Maternal/Child Health
Detroit, Michigan

Mary Helen Quigg, M.D.
Assistant Professor
Department of Obstetrics and Gynecology
Wayne State University School of Medicine
Detroit, Michigan

Philip Reilly, M.D., J.D.
Director of University Affiliate Program
Shriver Center for Mental Retardation, Inc.
Waltham, Massachusetts

David A. Richardson, M.D.
Assistant Professor
Wayne State University School of Medicine
Grace Hospital
Department of Obstetrics and Gynecology
Detroit, Michigan

John A. Robertson, J.D.
Baker and Botts Professor
School of Law
University of Texas at Austin
Austin, Texas

Alfred G. Robichaux, III, M.D.
Co-Director
Division of Maternal-Fetal Medicine
Ochsner Clinic
Clinical Assistant Professor
Louisiana State University Medical Center
Staff, Department of Obstetrics and Gynecology
Ochsner Foundation Hospital
New Orleans, Louisiana

Charles Rodeck, B.Sc., M.B.B.S., F.R.C.O.G.
Professor of Obstetrics and Gynecology
Royal Post Graduate Medical School
Institute of Obstetrics and Gynecology
Honorary Consultant
Queen Charlotte's and Chelsea Hospital
London, England

Wayne I. Roe, M.A.
President
Health Technology Associates
Washington, DC

Frederic M. Rosen, J.D.
Detroit, Michigan

Kenneth J. Ryan, M.D.
Professor and Chairman
Department of Obstetrics and Gynecology
    and Reproductive Biology
Harvard University Medical School
Chairman
Department of Obstetrics and Gynecology
Brigham and Women's Hospital
Boston, Massachusetts

Joseph D. Schulman, M.D.
Director
Genetics and IVF Institute
Attending Physician
Fairfax Hospital
Fairfax, Virginia
Professor of Human Genetics, Obstetrics
    and Gynecology, and Pediatrics
Medical College of Virginia
Richmond, Virginia

Thomas A. Shannon, Ph.D.
Professor of Religion and Social Ethics
Department of Humanities
Worcester Polytechnic Institute
Worcester, Massachusetts

Barbara W. Sholl, J.D.
Winnetka, Illinois

John S. Sholl, M.D., F.A.C.O.G.
Assistant Professor of Obstetrics and Gynecology
Northwestern University School of Medicine
Assistant Director of Obstetrics and Maternal-Fetal Medicine
Evanston Hospital
Evanston, Illinois

Ellen K. Silbergeld, Ph.D.
Director, Toxic Chemicals Program
Environmental Defense Fund
Washington, DC

Joe Leigh Simpson, M.D.
Professor and Chairman
Department of Obstetrics and Gynecology
University of Tennessee, Memphis
Memphis, Tennessee

Contributors

David C. Sobelsohn, J.D.
Formerly Visiting Associate Professor of Law
University of Detroit Law School
Detroit, Michigan
Member California, Illinois, and Michigan Bars

Robert J. Sokol, M.D.
Professor and Chairman
Wayne State University School of Medicine
Chief
Department of Obstetrics and Gynecology
Hutzel Hospital
Detroit, Michigan

James R. Sorenson, Ph.D.
Professor and Chair
Department of Health Behavior and Health Education
School of Public Health
University of North Carolina, Chapel Hill
Chapel Hill, North Carolina

Frank N. Syner, Ph.D.
Associate Professor
Department of Obstetrics and Gynecology
Wayne State University School of Medicine
Detroit, Michigan

Ilan E. Timor-Tritsch, M.D.
Professor
Department of Obstetrics and Gynecology
Columbia University College of Physicians and Surgeons
Director, Obstetric and Gynecologic Ultrasound, and Director, Obstetrics
Columbia-Presbyterian Hospital
New York, New York

LeRoy Walters, Ph.D.
Director, Center for Bioethics
Kennedy School of Ethics
Georgetown University
Associate Professor
Department of Philosophy
Georgetown University
Adjunct Professor
Department of Obstetrics and Gynecology
Georgetown University School of Medicine
Washington, D.C.

Robert A. Welch, M.D.
Assistant Professor, Department of Obstetrics and Gynecology
Wayne State University
Director, High Risk Pregnancy Unit
Hutzel Hospital, Detroit, Michigan

Dorothy C. Wertz, Ph.D.
Research Professor of Health Services
Boston University School of Public Health
Boston, Massachusetts

Acknowledgments

The editors are very grateful for the assistance of all the contributors and the J.B. Lippincott staff, and to Christine Palitti, Sue Rodriguez, and Shawn Grose for their help in preparing the manuscripts.

Foreword

The public is not always prepared to accept advances in science, particularly when application of these can be imagined to be either dangerous or not in the public interest. Public reaction to advances resulting from discoveries in molecular biology provides an excellent example of recent vintage. In the minds of many persons, the potential hazards exceeded the potential benefits of "tampering" with genes.

Advances in human reproductive physiology constitute another example of achievement for which the public was not prepared adequately. Over the past decade, in addition to in vitro fertilization, embryo transfer, and the plethora of applications of these technologies to solving problems resulting in infertility, there have been numerous technologic advances in methods applicable to diagnosis, treatment, and occasionally prevention of disorders that originate during gestation but result in postnatal morbidity of fetuses that survive. Indeed, rates of technologic development have outstripped considerations of the moral, ethical, legal, and social issues arising from introduction of these new methods into clinical practice. As a consequence, the suffering of potential beneficiaries is extended while these other issues are debated, inadequately considered ad hoc decisions complicate proper application of therapy, and public support for additional research is withheld.

Failure of science and the other disciplines to maintain the same cadence in relation to these problems arises in part from a lack of venues for exchanging information. Joint meetings of scientists, lawyers, and politicians are not customary. Moreover, the diverse skills and knowledge required to resolve conflicting issues among disciplines are rarely vested in the same persons, and finally, unfamiliarity with the language required to convey meaning to those not expert in science or law or sociology may complicate discussion.

Our lack of understanding leads to additional complications when rules, regulations, and even legal constraints are imposed not only on applications of techniques reflecting the "state of the art" but also on research designed to advance understanding, improve results, and extend applications. Additionally, an inadequately informed public sector complicates obtaining support for the research and its applications. Clearly, broadening our knowledge base and improving public understanding are desirable.

To these ends, Evans has succeeded in motivating recognized authorities on the scientific, legal, ethical, political, and sociologic issues related to human reproduction to contribute essays on current practice and prospects for future applications of therapies directed toward the fetus. For the most part, the essays may be regarded as free-standing, facilitating efficient use as references sources. For serious students of the issues, such a collection of essays provides sources of information to which they may return ad lib to familiarize themselves with perspectives of other disciplines on the problems posed. Furthermore, more intelligent interdisciplinary discussions should result from better understanding of the issues.

These essays are neither intended nor should they be regarded as the last word on the subject matter. Indeed, an entire section is devoted to new treatment modalities, not all of which are presently developed to the point of clinical application. Finally, perceptive persons will appreciate the need to repeat this exercise often lest our derelictions in addressing issues not presently recognized force us to withhold potentially useful therapies from the afflicted fetus and its parents, who are the ultimate beneficiaries of work in this field.

Griff T. Ross, M.D., Ph.D.[†]

[†] Our heartfelt thanks to Dr. Ross, whose recent demise makes his contribution even more meaningful.
— Editor

Contents

PART I
OVERVIEW OF CURRENT ISSUES

Chapter 1   Developing Issues in Reproduction — 3
SECTION 1:
SCIENTIFIC ISSUES — 3
  Mark I. Evans   Joseph D. Schulman
SECTION 2:
ETHICAL ISSUES — 4
  John C. Fletcher
SECTION 3:
LEGAL ANALYSIS — 8
  Alan O. Dixler
SECTION 4:
POLITICAL INVOLVEMENT IN HEALTH CARE — 10
  Ruth S. Hanft   Wendy J. Evans
SECTION 5:
SOCIOLOGIC ISSUES — 11
  James R. Sorenson
SECTION 6:
AN ANTHROPOLOGICAL PERSPECTIVE — 12
  Marilyn L. Poland

PART II
PRENATAL DIAGNOSIS AND SCREENING

Chapter 2 Prenatal Diagnosis of Chromosomal and
Mendelian Disorders ... 17
SECTION 1:
FIRST TRIMESTER PRENATAL DIAGNOSIS ... 17
 Mark I. Evans   Mary Helen Quigg   Frederick C. Koppitch III
 Joseph D. Schulman
SECTION 2:
SECOND AND THIRD TRIMESTER PRENATAL DIAGNOSIS ... 36
 John W. Larsen, Jr.   Martha D. MacMillin

Chapter 3 Prenatal Diagnosis of Congenital Malformations ... 44
SECTION 1:
ALPHA-FETOPROTEIN: MATERNAL SERUM AND AMNIOTIC FLUID
ANALYSIS ... 44
 Mark I. Evans   Robin L. Belsky Gold   Anne Greb
 Nancy Clementino   Frank N. Syner
SECTION 2:
ETHICAL ISSUES IN MATERNAL SERUM ALPHA-FETOPROTEIN
TESTING AND SCREENING: A REAPPRAISAL ... 54
 LeRoy Walters
SECTION 3:
ULTRASOUND DETECTION OF FETAL ANOMALIES ... 60
 Frank A. Chervenak   Glen Isaacson
SECTION 4:
TRANSVAGINAL ULTRASONOGRAPHY ... 71
 Arie Drugan   Ilan E. Timor-Tritsch

Chapter 4 Predictive Genetic Testing ... 84
 Kåre Berg

PART III
CLINICAL ISSUES

Chapter 5 Maternal Genetic Disease ... 94
SECTION 1:
TRANSMITTING GENETIC DISORDERS TO OFFSPRING OF MENTALLY
RETARDED INDIVIDUALS: PRINCIPLES UNDERLYING GENETIC
COUNSELING ... 94
 Joe Leigh Simpson
SECTION 2:
PREGNANCY IN PERSONS WHO ARE MENTALLY HANDICAPPED ... 101
 Thomas E. Elkins   S. Gene McNeeley

Chapter 6 Social and Environmental Risks of Pregnancy ... 114
SECTION 1:
CHEMICAL TERATOGENS ... 114
 Robert L. Anderson   Mitchell S. Golbus
SECTION 2:
ALCOHOL ... 140
 Ernest L. Abel   Robert J. Sokol

SECTION 3:
OCCUPATIONAL EXPOSURES AND FEMALE REPRODUCTION 149
Ellen K. Silbergeld   Donald R. Mattison   Joan E. Bertin

Chapter 7   Controversies Surrounding Antepartum Rh Immune Globulin Prophylaxis 172
James H. Beeson

PART IV
OBSTETRIC MANAGEMENT

Chapter 8   New Technology 183
SECTION 1:
EVOLUTION OF THE OXYTOCIN CHALLENGE TEST AS A DIAGNOSTIC TOOL 183
Gregory L. Glover   Alfred G. Robichaux
SECTION 2:
TECHNOLOGY ASSESSMENT AND REIMBURSEMENT: IMPLICATIONS FOR FETAL DIAGNOSIS AND THERAPY 187
Wayne I. Roe
SECTION 3:
LIABILITY AND EMERGING TECHNOLOGY 192
Frederic M. Rosen

Chapter 9   High Risk Situations: The Very Low Birth Weight Fetus 199
SECTION 1:
MEDICAL CONSIDERATIONS IN OBSTETRIC MANAGEMENT 199
Chin-Chu Lin
SECTION 2:
ETHICAL CONSIDERATIONS IN OBSTETRIC MANAGEMENT 233
E. Haavi Morreim
SECTION 3:
MULTIPLE GESTATION 242
Richard A. Bronsteen   Mark I. Evans
SECTION 4:
ETHICAL PROBLEMS IN MULTIPLE GESTATIONS: SELECTIVE TERMINATION 266
Mark I. Evans   John C. Fletcher   Charles Rodeck
SECTION 5:
BREECH PRESENTATION 276
Martin L. Gimovsky   Roy H. Petrie

Chapter 10   Keeping "Dead" Mothers Alive During Pregnancy 296
SECTION 1:
MATERNAL BRAIN DEATH DURING PREGNANCY 296
David R. Field   Russell Laros, Jr.
SECTION 2:
LEGAL ISSUES 307
Philip Reilly
SECTION 3:
ETHICAL ISSUES 311
Thomas A. Shannon

xx   Contents

Chapter 11   Delivery Methods   317
    SECTION 1:
    MIDFORCEPS DELIVERIES   317
        David A. Richardson   Mark I. Evans   Robert J. Sokol
    SECTION 2:
    CHANGES IN INDICATIONS AND INCIDENCE OF CESAREAN BIRTH   326
        Gregory L. Goyert   Robert A. Welch
    SECTION 3:
    LEGAL IMPLICATIONS OF DELIVERY OPTIONS   336
        Barbara W. Sholl   John S. Sholl

PART V
NEW TREATMENT MODALITIES

Chapter 12   In Vitro Fertilization   349
    SECTION 1:
    CLINICAL AND RESEARCH ASPECTS   349
        Joseph D. Schulman   María Bustillo
    SECTION 2:
    LEGAL ANALYSIS   356
        Alan O. Dixler
    SECTION 3:
    ETHICAL ISSUES IN CLINICAL AND RESEARCH APPLICATIONS   361
        John C. Fletcher

Chapter 13   **Surrogate Motherhood: Legal and Ethical Issues**   372
        Alexander Morgan Capron

Chapter 14   Immunologic Therapy   387
        James H. Beeson

Chapter 15   Fetal Therapy   395
    SECTION 1:
    SURGICAL MANAGEMENT OF FETAL MALFORMATIONS   395
        W. Allen Hogge   Mitchell S. Golbus
    SECTION 2:
    MEDICAL FETAL THERAPY   403
        Mark I. Evans   Joseph D. Schulman
    SECTION 3:
    DIAGNOSIS AND MANAGEMENT OF FETAL HEART DISEASE   412
        Joshua A. Copel   Charles S. Kleinman
    SECTION 4:
    GENE THERAPY   421
        W. French Anderson
    SECTION 5:
    LEGAL ISSUES IN FETAL THERAPY   431
        John A. Robertson
    SECTION 6:
    ETHICS IN EXPERIMENTAL FETAL THERAPY: IS THERE AN EARLY
    CONSENSUS?   438
        John C. Fletcher

PART VI
FATE OF FETUSES

Chapter 16 Federal Regulations for Fetal Research: A Case for Reform — 449
John C. Fletcher   Kenneth J. Ryan

Chapter 17 Primates and Anencephalics as Sources for Pediatric Organ Transplants: Medical, Legal, and Ethical Issues — 468
John C. Fletcher   John A. Robertson   Michael R. Harrison

Chapter 18 Allowing Babies to Die — 481
  SECTION 1:
  MEDICAL ISSUES — 481
    Anne B. Fletcher
  SECTION 2:
  LEGAL ISSUES — 488
    Leonard H. Glantz
  SECTION 3:
  ETHICAL ISSUES — 502
    Albert R. Johnsen

PART VII
NONMEDICAL ISSUES

Chapter 19 Government Involvement in the Doctor-Patient Relationship — 509
Ruth S. Hanft   Wendy J. Evans

Chapter 20 What About the Children? The Dilemma of Prematernal Liability — 520
Lynn D. Fleisher

Chapter 21 Government Funding of Abortions: The Constitutional Issues — 534
David C. Sobelsohn

Chapter 22 Sociologic Implications — 554
Dorothy C. Wertz   James R. Sorenson

Conclusion — 566
Duane F. Alexander

Index — 569

PART I
OVERVIEW OF CURRENT ISSUES

1

Developing Issues in Reproduction

SECTION 1: SCIENTIFIC ISSUES

Mark I. Evans and Joseph D. Schulman

Scientific progress occurs in many forums, from the juggernaut of mega-research centers to the creativity of the independent scientist. Despite cutbacks in federally funded programs which have shifted some of the focus from the former to the latter, the past decade has seen advancement in several areas, particularly reproductive technologies. Changes have occurred rapidly both in basic understanding of fundamental processes and in practical delivery of reproductive care.

The past ten years have brought a geometric increase in the scientific knowledge base about reproduction. In the mid-1970s, in vitro fertilization (IVF) was still a dream, ultrasound pictures were similar to watching a snowstorm, and mass prenatal screening tests such as alpha-fetoprotein (AFP) were available only in a few very select centers around the world. Certain technologies such as AFP screening and IVF have made the fundamental shift from theoretical and experimental to high-tech applied science. Prior to 1979, a presidential commission debated whether or not IVF was ethical. Now, there is almost a "corner store" mentality about the use of IVF in spite of papal teachings against interference in natural reproduction.

The "scientific" debate of the late eighties has focused on several therapeutic modalities including fetal therapy (surgical, medical, and genetic) and new applications of old techniques such as artificial insemination for surrogate motherhood. Fetal therapy has emerged as an intellectual challenge to complement increasing sophistication in prenatal diagnosis. The development of fetal therapy argues both *against* those who connect its use with abortion and *for* those who recognize prenatal diagnosis as a first step in diagnosis and treatment. The scientific groundwork for human therapy has been based on a series of animal models for surgical, pharmacologic, and now genetic therapies. Following animal work, advancement of the research requires courageous patients and physicians willing to attempt to solve problems with new solutions. For every new idea or treatment, someone has to be first.

Established methods of treatment have also undergone considerable changes, particularly in the area of obstetric care. The midforceps delivery and breech extraction are disappearing from the armamentarium of the obstetrician, having been pushed out not only by some scientific evidence, but more importantly by the threats of the legal system.

Similar co-opting of scientific protocol and development has been noted for maternal serum AFP (MSAFP) screening for neural tube defects and now also aneuploidy. The scientific database for MSAFP has expanded rapidly within the last few years. The serendipitous finding of the association between low MSAFP values and an increased risk of chromosomal abnormalities has created an opportunity to identify a high risk group of patients from among those who would normally never be offered prenatal diagnosis. Such possible identification of high risk patients becomes even more important in light of the fact that currently only about 12% of Down's syndrome fetuses are identified prenatally.

Another major change in the process of fetal assessment has been the ability to accomplish diagnoses earlier in pregnancy, both with the use of ever increasingly sophisticated ultrasound for structural studies and chorionic villus sampling for cytogenetic, biochemical, and molecular diagnosis. It is often possible to determine major problems even in the first trimester, thus allowing couples privacy in their reproductive decisions. Significant contributions have also been made in identifying risk factors for teratogenesis from compounds such as alcohol and environmental agents. Although much of the scare about alcohol and exposures to other drugs in small quantities may have been overstated, it is clear that with larger exposures such concerns are well founded.

Throughout this book, the editors and authors have tried to intertwine the "straight" scientific discussions with advice from experts on the ethical, legal, and political ramifications of the science. We believe that the intertwined approach allows for a well-rounded, honest assessment of hot topics in reproductive technology. In the ensuing overview sections, the authors will lay the groundwork for their respective methodologies and perspectives of their discipline. We suggest that the reader may gain a fuller perspective by reading these overviews before proceeding to a specific area.

SECTION 2: ETHICAL ISSUES
John C. Fletcher

ETHICS AND REPRODUCTIVE TECHNOLOGIES

What is the role of ethics in the development of fetal diagnosis and therapy? Ethics as a systematic human pursuit has two general purposes. Descriptive ethics involves the study of moral behavior, beliefs, and concepts in order to increase knowledge of moral experience. Normative ethics involves the commendation of guidance in the form of principles and rules to guide actions in the context of moral problems. Ethics should increase human knowledge as well as offer guidance in the proper use of freedom and the setting of proper limits to freedom.

Fetal research and experimental fetal therapy are controversial. In contemporary societies, it is difficult to resolve ethical controversies, because no single vision of the moral life can successfully unify the vast differences between the many moral traditions that co-exist in a pluralistic culture. Theologically based claims for ethical guidance exclude all individuals who cannot assent to theologic premises. Ethical arguments based on the power of human reason and the enlightenment that science supposedly confers have also not been able to prevail widely, even in highly developed technological societies.

In such a cultural context, how ought the tasks of normative ethics be pursued in regard to controversial fetal issues? My views are partly in sympathy with Englehardt's two-tier approach to ethics, similar in some respects to Hare's two-level analysis of moral reasoning.[1,3] At one level are the many, particularistic moral traditions that compete for dominance in everyday life. However, it is unrealistic to expect that any one view, or set of moral intuitions, about the moral life will successfully prevail. Because no particular moral tradition can provide sufficient guidance for an entire society on moral problems, one must seek a second, more critical, level for normative guidance. At a second level of "secular ethics" (or in this instance, secular bioethics), some common ground may be achieved by three commitments: (1) respect for persons and their communities, (2) evaluation of the prevailing moral approaches by a set of ethical principles whose general acceptance in a particular society will promote the best interests of all, and (3) the renunciation of the use of coercion and force in conflicts generated by moral problems.

Given this general perspective on ethics, the role of ethics in a systematic study of fetal diagnosis and therapy (or any other significant arena of sociomoral conflict) involves four interrelated steps.

Ethicists, like other investigators, must first accurately describe the major problems of moral choice in fetal diagnosis and therapy. Many examples of factual descriptions of ethical problems in fetal medicine and diagnosis are found in this volume. Second, the major contending ethical positions and approaches to ethical guidance for such problems must be described. If one approach to ethical problems is perceived as dominant in a society, prevailing in practice over other alternatives, such a dominant position must be shown actually to exist, based on studies of the evolution and prevalence of the approach. I see the general direction of ethical guidance for fetal diagnosis and therapy in this society evolving from the dominant approaches that currently exist in reproductive medicine and clinical genetics, as I will describe.

Third, if a dominant body of ethical guidance exists, the analysis should move to a test of the adequacy (for individuals, groups, and society) of this body of guidance. A selected set of ethical principles with wide respect across religious and cultural lines should be used to evaluate the inadequacies and contradictions of the dominant approach. The fourth step is to give indications, if any, for alteration of the dominant body of guidance in order to avoid wide divergence, harmful consequences, and lack of guidance on key problems.

The selection of basic ethical principles is obviously a crucial step in seeking common ground and in completing the third and fourth steps in the tasks of ethics. A cluster of basic ethical principles are widely applied in philosophic and theologic analysis of bioethical conflicts, which carry weight across cultural and religious lines:

1. Autonomy (respect for persons and their self-determination)
2. Non-maleficence (the non-infliction of harm on individuals or groups)
3. Beneficence (positive acts for benefits)
4. Justice (fairness and equality)

Different societies will order these principles differently, depending on the issue and other considerations in the society, such as stage of economic development, population, and level of health care.

A form of "rule-utilitarian" ethical theory has been sketched out above. This approach aims to harmonize the diverse goals and interests that arise in an evolving social life. It also encourages respect for the ordinary forms of moral and ethical guidance generated in society, but the higher aim is accountability, on a more impartial and general level, for the adequacy and effects of particular bodies of normative ethical guidance in everyday life.

ETHICAL GUIDANCE AND HUMAN REPRODUCTION

The general direction of ethical guidance for the use of new approaches to fetal diagnosis and therapy will evolve from older positions on sexuality and reproduction, as these positions are themselves affected by developments in technology and law. Ethics evolves from older to newer forms of guidance and from simpler to more complex forms. For example, existing ethical guidance for the use of older technologies, like prenatal diagnosis, also provides precedents to use with newer technologies, such as in vitro fertilization. However, the guidance that eventuates will be marked by the conflicts that accompanied the introduction of the new technology into society.

What are the prevailing ethical guidelines in sexuality and human reproduction? Since the 17th century, in Western nations and increasingly in other societies, these activities have been defined as voluntaristic social practices that ought to be governed largely by the claims of freedom and fairness, related to the ethical principles of autonomy and justice. Freedom is defined both negatively and positively. On the one hand it is freedom from external restriction, harm, and the disabling of voluntaristic activity. On the other hand, freedom is self-realization and the satisfaction of basic needs. Fairness is defined as impartial and equal treatment of those who participate in voluntaristic activities and as the obligation to live up to certain standards expected of all who participate in the activity.

Early modern societies saw the decline of kinship as the main organizing force of the society. The state assumed many of the social and economic functions that extended family members had once borne. The affection and companionship that bound the conjugal pair became more important, and the conjugal family became increasingly the seat of moral authority in family matters, rather than extrinsic religious authorities. The spread of concepts of individual choice and egalitarianism as espoused by Locke and others resulted in an 18th century ideal of marriage chosen for love and companionship rather than the traditional patriarchally arranged marriage.

Further, the institutions of marriage and family have been increasingly defined within a so-called private sphere of social existence, perceived as apart from immediate control of economic and political institutions. Within this private sphere it is believed that individual choice and autonomy can be protected and exercised. The relationship between the concept of privacy, as used by the Supreme Court in decisions related to contraception and abortion, and the historical development of a concept of a private sphere is extremely significant. The idea of a private sphere can also be understood as a product of secularization in that, with the reduction of influence of official religious guidance of individual choices, there needed to be an equivalent social definition of limits to political, social, and ecclesiastical interference with individual pursuit of happiness.

From these developments, an ethos has developed that protects the freedom of parents and physicians to apply knowledge gained from research and technology in order to avoid or achieve reproduction. At the same time it treats with fairness those who would not themselves, on moral grounds, use such freedom. On the practical level, this approach has been enacted by allowing knowledge and technology to be disseminated through a public filter of individual choice. Persons who want to practice contraception may do so; those who do not are not extrinsically punished. Persons who are at risk for genetic disease are counseled but are not prohibited from reproduction. Abortion decisions are overwhelmingly left as the choice of the woman. Mentally retarded persons are given sex education and equipped with contraception in some instances. It is increasingly considered morally blameworthy to sterilize another person involuntarily.

Does a dominant body of ethical guidance prevail for the moral problems associated with prenatal diagnosis? This question has been studied in the United States and 17 other nations.[2] The approach to problems of moral choice in prenatal diagnosis has three major features which enjoy strong consensus in practice:

1. Protection of parental and patient choices, including abortion
2. Full disclosure of findings of prenatal diagnosis
3. Voluntary programs of prenatal diagnosis

There is much more divergence on controversial indications for prenatal diagnosis, for example, maternal anxiety and sex selection unrelated to a sex-linked disease.

These practices provide another source of precedents upon which to develop approaches for problems presented by newer technologies. Some problems, however, are so novel as to fall totally outside the penumbra of such approaches. For example, should human embryos be created for the sake of research? An official commission in the United Kingdom held (by a 9-to-4 majority) that the scientific and medical benefits justified a limited and controlled possibility of such embryo research.[7] This same group voted to make commercial approaches to surrogate motherhood illegal and to discourage the practice, even as it gains a foothold in the United States.

COUNTERTRENDS IN FETAL ETHICS

Will the future see steady continuity of the prevailing approach of the past? Two countertrends to this general direction are worth noting.

Cases of court-ordered cesarean section[5] represent a new willingness to use force as well as a trend toward medical and legal activism and aggression in the interest of protecting the late-term fetus. Commentators like Robertson have suggested that if these court-ordered actions are correct, then "the state may have a far-reaching power to intrude on the mother's body and freedom of action for the benefit of the unborn child."[6] He extrapolates to scenarios of refused proven fetal therapy and coercion of the mother, if enough sociomoral support for such interventions exists. These cesarean cases should be seen against a wider challenge to the unlimited right of abortion, especially in the middle-to-late stages of pregnancy.[4] Willingness to override parental autonomy to protect the fetus would be the most significant change in the prevailing moral approach to reproductive technologies.

A second countertrend is the increasing, albeit unfounded, expectation of parents of perfection in terms of the health of their children. The rate of legal action against obstetricians has greatly increased, reflecting in part the higher expectation of parents. Sorenson and Wertz in Chapter 21 describe the trend toward perfectionism as one of the most important attitudes in reproduction now and in the future. Unless this trend is curbed, the future might well see abuses of genetic technology applied to reproduction for eugenic reasons, widespread use of sex selection, and routine abortion of fetuses with treatable disorders or carriers of deleterious genes. Any of these practices would violate the requirements of justice and fairness as applied to contemporary fetal diagnosis and therapy.

REFERENCES

1. Englehardt H Jr: The Foundations of Bioethics, pp 49–56. New York, Oxford University Press, 1986
2. Fletcher JC, Wertz DC, Sorenson JR, Berg K: Ethics and human genetics: A cross-cultural study in 17 nations. In: Vogel F, Sperling K (eds): Human Genetics, pp 655–672. Heidelberg, Springer-Verlag, 1987
3. Hare RM: Moral Thinking, pp 25–43. Oxford, Clarendon Press, 1981
4. Hilgers TW, Horan DJ, Mall D: New Perspectives on Human Abortion. Frederick, MD, University Publications of America, 1981
5. Kolder VB, Gallagher J, Parsons MT: Court-ordered obstetrical interventions. N Engl J Med 316:1192–1197, 1987

6. Robertson JA: Legal issues in fetal therapy. Semin Perinatol 9:140, 1985
7. United Kingdom Department of Health and Social Security: Report of the Committee of Inquiry into Human Infertility and Embryology, pp 58–69. Chairman, Mary Warnock. London, Her Majesty's Stationary Office, 1984

SECTION 3: LEGAL ANALYSIS

Alan O. Dixler

Despite all the interactions of medicine and the law, few physicians and scientists appreciate the very significant differences between a scientific and legal analysis of any given situation. Most medical professionals have little knowledge of the American legal system or understand the process of legal research and why, of necessity, legal adaptation will almost always come after scientific ones and cannot usually anticipate changes in technology.

American law is derived from the laws of England and from the methodology of English law. First, there is the so-called common law, essentially, judge-made law. With limited exceptions, there is an inherent power in judges to make rules of law in instances where there are none. Additionally, legislatures pass statutes, which are an additional source of legal rules. Finally, administrative agencies often have the power to issue regulations which are legally binding.

THE AMERICAN LEGAL SYSTEM

The United States is a federal republic and, as such, there are complete legal systems in each constituent state as well as that of the federal government, enacted by Congress. There are numerous federal administrative agencies, such as the Securities and Exchange Commission and the Federal Trade Commission, which are empowered to issue regulations that are legally binding. Additionally, there is a federal court system within which disputes are resolved, in the various district courts and in other courts of specialized jurisdiction. (One famous federal district court is the Federal District Court for the Southern District of New York, which is located in Manhattan.) Appeals from the district courts go to the various circuit Courts of Appeal, often based upon the geographic location of the district court in which the trial was held. For example, the Second Circuit includes New York, Connecticut, and Vermont; thus, an appeal from the Southern District of New York would go to the Second Circuit Court of Appeals, which is also located in Manhattan. The court of final appeal in the federal system is the United States Supreme Court in Washington, D.C.

Each state has a similar legal framework. The state legislature passes statutes. Each state also has administrative bodies which are empowered to issue binding regulations. Each state has a system of courts. There are trial courts (corresponding to the district courts on the federal side), and often intermediate appellate courts (corresponding to the Circuit Courts of Appeal on the federal side), and there is a state court of final appeal, often called the State Supreme Court (corresponding to the United States Supreme Court on the federal side). The State of New York is unusual in the way it has named its courts. In the New York system, the Supreme Court is a trial court. Intermediate appeals are taken to the Appellate Division of the Supreme Court, and the court of final appeal is the New York Court of Appeals.

Local legislative bodies such as city counsels also exist. Legislation issued on a municipal level is often referred to as ordinances. Municipalities are not an independent source of law, but rather, their authority is delegated to them by the state legislatures.

Questions of state law are usually litigated in state courts. State issues include such matters as corporation law, domestic relations law, property law, and tort law. In order to litigate in a federal court there must be a question of federal law at issue, or there must be a case in which a party from one state is suing a party from another. Federal issues include such matters as federal antitrust law, federal securities law, and federal income tax law. Both systems, state and federal, have a body of criminal law. Criminal cases are actions by the government to enforce a right to keep the peace. If Mr. A. were to punch Mr. B. in the nose, a crime and a tort would have been committed. The government (state or federal) would bring a criminal action against Mr. A. for the wrong that Mr. A. did to the public. Civil cases are actions by private parties to seek relief from wrongs done to them. Mr. B. could sue Mr. A. for money damages for the civil wrong that Mr. A. did to Mr. B. Civil wrongs other than breach of contract are called torts. In punching Mr. B. in the nose, Mr. A. committed the tort of battery.

Thus, having said that the American legal system is a composite of state and federal courts and legislatures, and that generally law is divided into criminal and civil actions, a word about legal methodology is in order.

LEGAL METHODOLOGY

There is a tendency for professional people who are well trained in a particular field to approach all of life's problems using the methods of analysis that are helpful to them in their professional lives. This should be guarded against. Legal issues must not be approached as if they were medical problems. A lawyer does not hear a fact pattern from a client and then prescribe a course of conduct generally viewed as correct. There is no *Washington Manual* for lawyers. Each matter is to some degree unique. Often, and far more frequently than a layman would suspect, there are no clear answers but only competing arguments which ultimately will be decided by a court when the proper case arises. Further, the law is far from static, and even the pace of change can vary. The law can at times be quite plastic, and the quality of advocacy can dramatically affect the content of a judicial decision. Thus, in advising a client, a lawyer frequently must use subjective judgment, and must, to some extent, "see over the horizon" to evaluate not only the existing legal authority, but also to identify issues which may cause legal pitfalls in the future.

It is in this frame of mind that the portions of this work dealing with legal issues should be read. Where the law is well settled, this state of affairs will be noted. However, there is never any assurance that a time-honored legal rule will not be re-thought if the rule no longer yields sensible results. Where the writers express their views on topics which have not been resolved, there can be no assurance that the expressed views will be followed by the court, administrative body, or legislature which, at some future time, must deal with the issue in an official capacity. It should also be noted that the law tends to be reactive rather than proactive. Accordingly, there may be no satisfactory legal solutions to problems posed by new technology at present. Legislatures usually do not enact statutes until a clear public need for the legislation is perceived. Administrative bodies generally do not issue regulations until a difficulty has surfaced which the administrators need to address. Case law is not made until there is an actual controversy which the parties are unable to settle among themselves.

Consequently, the medicolegal morass often encumbered in cases involving new philosophies and practices of medical therapies—surrogate motherhood, fetal treatment and rights, for example—can usually not be prevented a priori. Legislatures can establish codes of conduct for yet-to-be-performed acts, but the performers may often find themselves still in the middle of litigation aimed at further defining or modifying such conduct. Many of the ensuing legal chapters thus blend a combination of settled legal principles and case law with speculations on the outcome of issues yet to be fought.

SECTION 4: POLITICAL INVOLVEMENT IN HEALTH CARE

Ruth S. Hanft and Wendy J. Evans

Political involvement in health care and physician practice appears in many forms. Some political intervention is actually sponsored by physicians themselves who set standards for medicine and other health professions and effect supply or education programs. These standards are then reinforced through law or funding decisions. For example, the medical profession sets requirements imposed by programs such as Medicare that certain services must be provided by specified types of providers. Other forms of government intervention are inherent in resource allocation decisions for biomedical research funding or resource constraints such as reimbursement decisions. Political intervention also occurs through direct action of state or federal governments ranging from prohibiting certain procedures such as euthanasia or abortion to requiring prior approval for the use of certain drugs and devices, capital, and equipment. There are also numerous direct and indirect incentives that affect physician-patient interactions such as structure of health insurance benefits, tax policy on the deductibility of health insurance premiums, and fee schedules in public and private insurance programs.

The role of government in health care in a political and economic context is premised on the concept that some health care is a public good, not merely a private or consumer good. The effects of health care or lack of health care carry implications above and beyond individual benefit. For example, immunization policies directly affect the individual and also have a collective impact on epidemic control. Besides being an indivisible public good, health care plays a role in reducing premature death and disability. Prevention of premature death and disability affects the productivity of the nation and the costs to individuals and families and to social programs such as pension, disability, and workmen's compensation benefits. Specific public action can be arrayed against this basic philosophic construct. For example, licensure is designed to ensure that only persons of certain education and skill levels perform services which, if performed incorrectly, could result in harm to an individual and costs to society. The regulation of drugs and devices is based on the same harm avoidance concept.

Another rationale for government intervention defines the government as the purchaser of services. When the government underwrites the cost of care, it has the obligation to ensure a certain standard of care and to protect the public purse. Even the most extreme proponents of market economics, political libertarianism, and autonomy of the professions all concede that there is a legitimate government role in health care. At issue is the degree and precise mechanism of intervention. Chapter 19 will further discuss both government's direct intervention and its indirect influence through the use or withholding of economic resources. The areas of political-medical confrontation include the following:

Law and the courts
   Abortion
   Malpractice and liability
Protection of the population—Safety, efficacy, immunization
Supply control
   Credentialing, licensure, and accreditation of professionals: self-regulation enforced through law
   Certificate of need
Allocation of research resources
   The federal role in research funding
   Resource allocation and interest group politics
   Moratorium on certain research
   Informed consent and the researcher
Direct intervention in physician/patient relationships

Baby Doe and hot lines
Parent versus government authority
Squeal rules
Reporting of communicable diseases
Indirect intervention through insurance programs
  Structure of insurance programs
  Second surgical options
  Diagnostic Related Groups (DRGs) and fees
  Generic drugs
  Medicaid durational limits
  Investigational and experimental procedures

Moral and religious concepts affect the political dialog surrounding health care in such issues as patient autonomy (informed consent and free choice) and the sanctity of life (abortion and the withholding therapy). Often moral or religious concepts come into conflict in such areas as patient autonomy versus paternalism/physician autonomy, distributive justice versus individual choices of patients and providers, society's right to know versus privacy. It is in the political arena that a number of these issues are resolved and evolve over time.

SECTION 5: SOCIOLOGIC ISSUES

James R. Sorenson

A steady stream of biomedical developments over the past two decades has provided new reproductive options for many. These developments have covered a broad spectrum of reproductive issues, permitting increased control of the timing and spacing of pregnancies, earlier identification of fetuses with abnormalities, specification of maternal behaviors that are health risks to the fetus, and developments enabling previously infertile couples to become parents such as in vitro fertilization, embryo transfer, and surrogate motherhood. Further, there is the promise of more developments affecting other aspects of reproduction.

Not all segments of society have been interested in, nor stand to benefit equally from, such developments. For instance, effective control of the number and spacing of pregnancies has been adopted on a massive basis by some societal groups, profoundly affecting their fertility rates, while other groups have not favored fertility regulations. Of more limited impact have been the various advances surrounding the detection of abnormalities in utero, and of even more limited impact are developments involving in vitro technologies, embryo transfer, and surrogate motherhood.

It is important to emphasize, in reviewing the sometimes startling developments in biomedical science, that they define what is technologically feasible. How society, or more significantly, how individuals respond to these possibilities is determined by many things. At the risk of oversimplification, what people do is a function of what is technically possible, as well as what is culturally, socially, legally, and economically acceptable.

With the exception of the development of effective birth control methods, we do not have much understanding of how individuals might respond to new reproductive technologies. What we do have is some understanding of the cultural and social context surrounding pregnancy, reproduction, and child rearing in this society and in Western culture generally. Trends in social attitudes of reproduction and its control, as well as cultural values regarding parenting and children, are helpful in anticipating how individuals and society may respond to some of the new developments in reproduction.

Chapter 21 examines the effects on current developments in reproduction by such long-term trends as smaller families, a decline in infant mortality, an increasing reliance on scientific child rearing, changes in gender roles, and increasing medical assistance in reproduction. The authors identify a number of short-term trends, such as parenthood by choice, delayed childbearing, the feminist movement, and changes in the definition and composition of the nuclear family. Admittedly there is considerable speculation in this type of social forecasting. However, it is important to attempt to have some understanding of what the possibilities are so we may develop more enlightened and informed social policies concerning these new reproductive technologies.

New biomedical developments are not merely buffeted by existing social and cultural trends, of course, but such developments can, in time, change societal practices and even cultural values. Clearly, the availability of effective and efficient birth control technologies has changed not only societal practices, but cultural benefits and values regarding birth control. It is also possible that developments such as increased knowledge of maternal behavioral risk factors for abnormal birth outcomes, as well as the availability of prenatal diagnosis, will change societal practices and cultural beliefs regarding parental responsibility. How both the medical profession and the public will respond to reproductive technological development will depend on an understanding of the societal and cultural contexts in which such developments occur.

SECTION 6: AN ANTHROPOLOGICAL PERSPECTIVE
Marilyn L. Poland

Childbearing, while viewed by all societies as an important and necessary role of women, is also seen as a time of great uncertainty. A pregnancy may end poorly or the mother may die in childbirth. For this reason, all societies provide special protection for pregnant women in some form—amulets, prayers, pills, ceremonies, and prescribed behaviors.[1] While the underlying concern for the safety of the mother may be universal, the manner in which the mother, her attendants, and the larger society behave in relation to her pregnancy varies considerably.

Maternal conduct during pregnancy and the rules of conduct of those around her reflect how pregnancy is defined and managed. For example, societies that believe that spirits inhabit a woman's body to produce a baby if the gods will it, may have little use for biologic explanations and interventions and would therefore be less likely to hold the mother responsible for her fetus. Societies that believe the mother's behavior has direct biologic bearing on the fetus may dictate appropriate maternal behavior, such as receiving prenatal care, and may scorn those who do not participate.

Our society has based its understanding of pregnancy on scientific, biologic principles. Western biomedicine has increasingly colonized pregnancy, replacing the roles of midwife, spirits, and the family as monitors and protectors of pregnant women. As science has provided us with new and powerful instruments to produce conception, view the fetus, assess fetal chromosomes, and manage fetal conditions, the social roles of women and beliefs about the purpose and utility of technology have changed, thus altering our views of pregnancy and our perceptions of appropriate pregnancy-related behavior.

In this anthropological perspective on pregnancy and reproductive technology, two questions which characterize major social effects of technology are addressed: How has biotechnology altered the relationship between mother and fetus? How will cross-cultural differences in beliefs and values related to technologically directed reproduction be handled as technology becomes accepted (required) medical practice?

CHANGING SOCIAL ROLES OF WOMEN

Changes in social roles of women and in pregnancy technology are interrelated, each affecting the other. These interrelationships have biologic and social implications for present and future generations.

Social roles for women vary in our society, but in general, women are being defined less by childbearing and rearing functions and more by their work outside the home.[12] Women are marrying and bearing children later and limiting childbearing in order to obtain education and training necessary to establish themselves in the workplace.[7] But these social changes have a biologic effect. Delays in childbearing and exposure to chemical, physical, and psychological stress at work are associated with an increase in infertility, pregnancy complications, and birth defects.[2,4] But biotechnology has also had a dramatic effect on social roles of women. Many women feel that reliance on technology has given them more control over their reproduction, making it possible for them to plan their pregnancies around their other social roles in addition to increasing their likelihood of producing healthy children.

There is also evidence that while technology permits more freedom of choice in reproduction, it is exerting a new kind of social control. As sonograms and other prenatal tests permit us to view the fetus directly, and assess and correct medical conditions, the fetus assumes the status of patient with potential rights to diagnosis and treatment. Since the cooperation of the mother is necessary to assess and treat the fetus, maternal behavior becomes critical to the health of the fetus and is more assessable to public scrutiny.

In the past, women were urged to seek prenatal care in order to receive advice and reassurance and to monitor the course of pregnancy. Today, prenatal care involves more aggressive medical management. Maternal behaviors such as smoking and alcohol and drug abuse have clearer links to fetal health, and education and counseling programs are offered to reduce these unhealthy practices.[8] Technology has also altered expected maternal responsibility toward the fetus to include her participation in testing and treatments that may, for the first time, place her in some jeopardy. These include cesarean sections for fetal indications, and fetal surgery which involves operating on the mother to reach the fetus. Fetal surgery is presently seen as experimental and requires written, informed maternal consent. However, cesarean sections are seen as accepted medical practice, and mothers who have refused this surgery on themselves for the sake of the fetus have been overruled by the courts.[3,9] This alters the maternal role from one who carries the pregnancy and voluntarily uses technology, to one of whom it is required. This raises questions about control over other maternal behaviors, such as drinking alcohol or having prenatal testing, which may in the future involve legal controls. It would seem that the same technology that gave women control over reproduction has also removed some control.

HEALTH BELIEFS AND TECHNOLOGY

In all cultures, treatment stems from beliefs about what causes illness or an abnormal condition.[13] Biology, spirits, natural causes, and just bad luck are all explanations for illness which reflect the basic beliefs of a cultural system. Often, two explanations co-exist, as in this country when patients use folk medicine and biomedical treatments together to achieve a cure.

This variation in health beliefs also extends to explanations about pregnancy complications, the birth process, and causes of fetal/newborn abnormalities. For example, pregnancy is a time when women are subjected to cultural expectations about diet. These may include limited salt intake, increasing protein, routine use of vitamins, and appropriate weight gain. But these dietary practices are all open to cultural interpretation. Health professionals, for example, may base their recommended maternal weight gain of about 25 pounds over pregnancy on statistical correlations with ideal infant weight, but some of their patients believe in limiting weight gain to produce a smaller baby and an easier, safer birth.[6]

The use of prenatal technology is also open to cultural interpretation. Women have refused fetal transfusion and cesarean sections because of religious beliefs that prohibit the use of blood products.[5,11] Early registration for prenatal care, the basis for prenatal genetic testing, is seen as unnecessary by some poor women who reject the notion of preventive care. As one 36-year-old mother of four who received no prenatal care said, "As long as you feel okay, the baby moves, and you take your vitamins, you don't have to see the doctor. Poor people can't afford to see the doctor when nothing is wrong."[10] These beliefs are counter to prenatal medical risk profiles and would support later access to prenatal care by these women.

Differences in culturally derived beliefs about the purpose and value of reproductive technology can result in conflicts between health professionals and mothers over what constitutes an appropriate maternal role. The manner in which these conflicts are addressed will reflect underlying social values involving personal freedom of choice and the strength of our belief in the use of biomedical technology to define and solve health problems.

REFERENCES

1. Bates B, Turner AN: Imagery and symbolism in the birth practices of traditional cultures. Birth 12:29–35, 1985
2. Bayer R: Women, work and reproductive hazards. Hastings Center Report, Oct: 14–18, 1982
3. Bowes W, Selgestad B: Fetal vs. maternal rights: Medical and legal perspectives. Obstet Gynecol 58:209–214, 1981
4. Cecos B, Schwartz D, Mayaux MJ: Female fecundity as a function of age. N Engl J Med 306:404–406, 1982
5. Chernack B: Recovery for prenatal injuries: The right of a child against its mother. Suffolk University Law Rev 10:582–609, 1976
6. Fathaner GH: Food habits—An anthropologist's view. J Am Dietetic Assoc 37:335–338, 1960
7. Feldman SD: Impediment or stimulant? Marital status and graduate education. In Huber J (ed): Changing Women in Changing Society, pp 220–232. Chicago, University of Chicago Press, 1973
8. Hobel C, Hyvarinen M, Okada D, Oh H: Prenatal and intrapartum high risk screening: Predictions of the high-risk neonate. Am J Obstet Gynecol 117:1–9, 1973
9. Jefferson v Griffin Spalding Co. Hospital Authority, 247 Ga. 86, 274, SE 2nd, 457 (1981)
10. Poland M: Ethical issues surrounding access to prenatal care. Paper presented at American Anthropological Assoc, Washington, DC, 1985
11. Raleigh Fitkin-Paul Morgan Memorial Hospital v Anderson, 201 A. 2nd 537, 538 (NJ, 1964)
12. Ridley JC: The effects of population change on the roles and status of women. In Safilios-Rothchild C (ed): Toward a Sociology of Women, pp 382–386. Lexington, MA: Xerox Coll Publishing Co, 1972
13. Snow LE, Johnson SM: Modern day menstrual folklore: Some clinical implications. JAMA 237:2736–2739, 1977

PART II
PRENATAL DIAGNOSIS AND SCREENING

2

Prenatal Diagnosis of Chromosomal and Mendelian Disorders

SECTION 1: FIRST TRIMESTER PRENATAL DIAGNOSIS

*Mark I. Evans,
Mary Helen Quigg,
Frederick C. Koppitch III, and
Joseph D. Schulman*

Prenatal diagnosis has undergone a major revolution in the last five years, in particular with the introduction of first trimester diagnosis.

Mid-trimester amniocentesis has been the standard and mainstay of prenatal diagnosis dating back to the initial expansion of services following the 1973 Supreme Court decision of Roe v. Wade.[8,24,36,42] However, traditional genetic amniocentesis results usually have not allowed final diagnosis of a possibly severely affected fetus until nearly 20 weeks gestation. By that time, quickening has occurred with its associated emotional bonding to the fetus. The couple has usually made the transition from "being pregnant" to "going to have a baby." In this situation, the termination of an otherwise wanted pregnancy is frequently traumatic. In some cases, the grieving may be as great as with the loss of a liveborn child.

The development of chorionic villus sampling (CVS) has given at-risk couples a new, and perhaps better, alternative. CVS is usually performed between 9 and 12 weeks of gestation. The diagnosis of both cytogenetic and biochemical disorders can be made far earlier in pregnancy with this technique, thus allowing couples privacy in their information gathering and decision-making processes. If an abnormality is detected by CVS and if the couple elects termination, it can be performed by the safer and less psychologically traumatic first trimester methods.

A second important factor in the availability of first trimester diagnosis is the inherent controversy surrounding abortion. As the debate over abortion continues to flame, and with advances in neonatal survival, there will be increasing pressure to restrict or outlaw

17

second trimester terminations. As a result, prenatal diagnosis of cytogenetic, mendelian, and congenital malformations will likely be forced earlier and earlier in pregnancy.[5] We believe that ultimately there will be an uneasy truce on abortion, which will leave the first trimester a "demilitarized zone."

RISK FACTORS

Chromosomal Disorders

By far the most common reason for using prenatal diagnostic techniques is advanced maternal age. When such services first became available in the early 1970s, resources were severely limited. Amniocentesis was usually offered only to women in the highest risk categories such as those over age 40. With the increasing availability of services, the "magic" cut-off time fell to age 38. At present, the generally accepted age is 35. It must be recognized, however, that today there are more Down syndrome babies born to women under age 35 than there are to those over 35. With the present system, less than 15% of all Down syndrome fetuses are detected prenatally. Such statistics reflect the higher number of women in lower age brackets having children (Table 2-1). It must be recognized that while fear of trisomy 21 is the main reason that most patients present for prenatal diagnosis, trisomy 21 comprises only approximately half of the abnormal, prenatal chromosomal diagnoses.

Trisomy 21 is not the only chromosomal abnormality which is age-dependent. Trisomies 13 and 18, 47,XXX, and 47,XXY karyotypes also show increased incidence with maternal age.[34] The incidence of chromosomal abnormalities detected by mid-trimester amniocentesis (approximately 2%) is four times higher than that usually seen at term. The discrepancy is reflective of the normal spontaneous abortion rate in fetuses after 16 to 18 weeks. This loss rate has been reported as high as 2% to 3% of cytogenetically normal fetuses and is even higher in abnormal fetuses.

There is some controversy over the recurrence risk for a cytogenetic abnormality in parents with normal karyotypes. At younger ages, a recurrence risk of about 1% seems realistic, which is comparable to that normally quoted to a 38-year-old. At older ages, the risk may be only slightly higher than normal age-related risks. Therefore, all women with a previous abnormality, regardless of their age, should be offered the opportunity to undergo a genetic diagnostic procedure.

When the indication for prenatal diagnosis is a previous abnormality from a balanced reciprocal or Robertsonian translocation in one of the parents, the risk to subsequent offspring is higher than 1%. In Robertsonian translocations the risk varies depending on the specific chromosomes involved as well as whether it is the mother or the father who is the carrier.[33] While the theoretical risk of such an unbalanced translocation is 50%, actuarial data suggest that the risk usually approaches the 1% to 15% range[52] (Figure 2-1).

If either of the parents is aneuploid, antenatal cytogenetic studies are always indicated because the risk of offspring may be as high as 30%.[47] In instances in which the mother is a mosaic such as 45,X/46,XX, although there is insufficient data to quote accurate risks, there would appear to be a higher risk than normal age-related risks.

New evidence has suggested that the "fragile-X" syndrome may be responsible for a large proportion of previously idiopathic male mental retardation.[19] A recent editorial in Lancet has suggested "fragile-X" testing for all retarded males.[40] If all mentally retarded

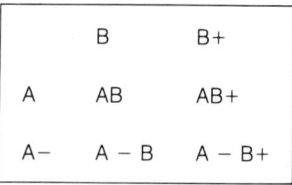

FIGURE 2-1. Of the four possibilities one (AB) is normal; one (AB+) would have excess material; one (A−B) would have missing material; and one (A−B+) would be a balanced carrier, the same as the parent.

Table 2-1. Risk of Having a Liveborn Child With Down's Syndrome or Other Chromosome Abnormality

Maternal Age	Risk of Down's Syndrome	Total Risk for All Chromosome Abnormalities
20	1/1667	1/526
21	1/1667	1/526
22	1/1429	1/500
23	1/1429	1/500
24	1/1250	1/476
25	1/1250	1/476
26	1/1176	1/476
27	1/1111	1/455
28	1/1053	1/435
29	1/1000	1/417
30	1/952	1/385
31	1/909	1/385
32	1/769	1/322
33	1/602	1/286
34	1/485	1/238
35	1/378	1/192
36	1/289	1/156
37	1/224	1/127
38	1/173	1/102
39	1/136	1/83
40	1/106	1/66
41	1/82	1/53
42	1/63	1/42
43	1/49	1/33
44	1/38	1/26
45	1/38	1/21
46	1/23	1/16
47	1/18	1/13
48	1/14	1/10
49	1/11	1/8

males were screened for "fragile-X" syndrome, it is possible that the etiology for thousands of cases of mental retardation would be identified. It is postulated that fragile-X syndrome is the second most common cause of mental retardation following Down syndrome.[30] However, the cost as well as the shear volume of work would seem to prohibit such mass screening.

Diagnoses of conditions featuring chromosome instability can be based on amniotic fluid cells and have been made in pregnancies at risk (Table 2-2). Fragile-X syndrome can be diagnosed clinically because of macroorchidism. Cytogenetically, when amniotic fluid cells are cultured in folate-deficient media, the fragile sites on the X chromosome can be identified. Unfortunately, the results are often equivocal. Detection of the carrier female is even less certain. DNA linkage analysis is now being used for diagnosis in this disorder.[29,37]

Exposure to chemotherapeutic agents or therapeutic radiation in the treatment of neoplasia has been suggested as an indication for prenatal diagnosis. The data on cytogenetic abnormalities in women exposed to nonmedical radiation have not shown any significant increase in aneuploid rates in the children, but there are many questions as to abortion rates and overall fertility.[3,47] Inadvertent diagnostic radiation exposure is not an indication for cytogenetic prenatal testing.

Mendelian Disorders

It is widely accepted that the risk of producing a fetus with a cytogenetic disorder varies with maternal age. Thus, many couples at increased risk can be identified independent of previous reproductive history. However, the diagnoses of most inborn errors of metabolism have no obvious screening mechanism and cannot be routinely applied to patients except those who are known to be at significant risk. As such, the prenatal diagnosis of mendelian disorders is usually sought for in a couple who already have an affected child.

Approaches to prenatal diagnosis of mendelian disorders can be made in one of several ways. With a metabolic enzymatic block such as 21 hydroxylase deficiency congenital adrenal hyperplasia, elevated levels of 17 hydroxyprogesterone in cell-free amniotic fluid can be measured.[54] In most conditions, however, the diagnosis can only be made following a culture of amniotic fluid cells. For example, in Hurler syndrome the measurement of alpha-iduronidase, or in Tay Sachs disease hexosaminidase A in cultured amniotic fluid cells can be diagnostic.[25,32] Since many of these conditions are very rare, there are often only a few laboratories in the world equipped to perform these sensitive assays. Attempts at prenatal diagnoses of these conditions need to be coordinated with the appropriate laboratories well in advance. It is beyond the scope of this chapter to discuss all diagnoses which are technically possible. A complete list of references would be staggering, and thus only a short representative list has been cited.[6,17,20,28,31,51,55] Many disorders commonly diagnosed or potentially diagnosable by analysis of amniotic fluid, amniotic fluid cells, or chorionic villi are listed in Table 2-3, and the list is constantly being expanded. Prior to informing a family there is no antenatal test available, the physician should contact the appropriate authorities for the current state of the art.

CLINICAL PROCEDURES

Chorionic Villus Sampling

Diagnoses of cytogenetic and many biochemical abnormalities can be accomplished by genetic amniocentesis performed in the mid-trimester of pregnancy. However, the late date at which amniocenteses are most often performed, plus the time necessary to complete

Table 2-2. Disorders of Chromosome Stability

Disease	Inheritance	Diagnostic Test
Ataxia telangiectasia	AR	Sister chromatic exchange
Bloom syndrome	AR	DEB-induced chromosome breaks and rearrangements
Fanconi anemia	AR	
Fragile "X" syndrome	XLR	Fragile sites in folate-deficient media
Xeroderma pigmentosum	AR	DNA "repair" synthesis after UVL exposure

(AR, autosomal recessive; XLR, X-linked recessive; DEB, diepoxybutane; UVL, ultra violet light)

Table 2-3. Prenatal Diagnosis of Genetic Disorders

I. DISORDERS OF CARBOHYDRATE METABOLISM
   1. Galactokinase deficiency (AR) — Galactokinase (D)
   2. Galactosemia (AR) — Assay:
      1) Galactokinase (D)
      2) Galactose-1-P uridyl transferase (D)
   3. Glucose-6-phosphate dehydrogenase deficiency (XLR) — Glucose-6-phosphate dehydrogenase (D)
   4. Glycerol kinase deficiency (XLR) — DNA analysis (M)
   5. Glycogen storage disease
      A. Type I Von Gierke's disease (AR) — Assay: Glucose-6 phosphatase (D)
      B. Type II Pompe's disease (AR) — Assay: acid alpha-1 glucosidase (D)
      C. Type III Cori's or Forbes disease (AR) — Assay: Amylo-1,6 glucosidase (D)
      D. Type IV Anderson's disease (AR) — Assay: Amylo-1,4:16-transglucosidase (D)
      E. Type VIII Liver phosphorylase deficiency (XLR) — Assay: phosphorylase kinase (D)
   6. Pyruvate carboxylase deficiency (AR) — Assay: pyruvate carboxylase (D)
   7. Pyruvate decarboxylase deficiency (AR) — Assay: pyruvate decarboxylase (D)
   8. Pyruvate dehydrogenase complex deficiency (AR) — Assay: pyruvate dehydrogenase (D)

II. INBORN ERRORS OF AMINO ACID METABOLISM
   1. Albinism, ocular (XLR) — DNA linkage (M)
   2. Gamma-aminobutyric acid aminotransferase deficiency (AR) — Assay: 4-aminobutyric acid aminotransferase (D)
   3. Argininemia (Arginase deficiency) (AR) — Assay: Arginase in erythrocytes (D)
   4. Argininosuccinic aciduria (Anginosuccinate lyase deficiency) (AR) — Assay: argininosuccinate lyase (D)
   5. Citrullinemia (Argininosuccinate synthetase deficiency) (AR) — Assay: Argininosucinate synthetase (D)
   6. Carbamylphosphate synthetase deficiency (AR) —
      1) DNA linkage (M)
      2) Assay: Carbamylphosphate synthetase
   7. Cystathioninuria (AR) — Assay: Cystathionase (D)
   8. Gamma-glutamyl synthetase deficiency (AR) — Assay: Gamma-glutamyl synthetase (D)
   9. Gamma-glutamyl transpeptidase deficiency (AR) — Assay: Gamma-glutamyl transpeptidase (D)
   10. Glutaric aciduria (AR) — Assay:
      1) Dicarboxylic acids (D)
      2) Glutaryl-CoA carboxylase (D)
   11. Glutathine synthetase (AR) — Assay: Glutathine synthetase (D)
   12. Glycinemia, ketoic, type I (Propionic acidemia I) (AR) — Assay: Propinyl-coa carboxylase (D)
   13. Histidinemia (AR) — Assay: Histidase (D)
   14. Homocystinuria (AR) — Assay: Cystathionine synthedase (D)
   15. 4-hydroxybutyric acidemia (AR) — Assay: Succinic semi-aldehyde dehydrogenase (D)

(Continued)

(AR, autosomal recessive; AD, autosomal dominant; XLR, X-linked recessive; D, diminished; E, elevated; H, histology; M, molecular; K, karyotype)

Table 2-3. Prenatal Diagnosis of Genetic Disorders (*Continued*)

16.	3-hydroxy-3-methyl glutaryl CoA lyase deficiency (AR)	Assay: 3-hydroxy-3-methyl glutaryl CoA lyase (D)
17.	Hyperlysinemia, persistent form (AR)	Lysine-keto glutarate reductase (D)
18.	Hyperphenylalanemia	
	A. Type I (Classic phenylketonuria) (AR)	DNA linkage analysis (M)
	B. Type IV (dihydropteridine reductase deficiency) (AR)	Assay: 1) Dihydropteridine reductase (D) 2) GTP cyclohydrolase (D)
	C. Type V (dihydrobiopterin synthetase deficiency) (AR)	Assay: 1) Neopterin (E) 2) Biopterin (D)
	D. Type VIII (tyrosinemia) hereditary (AR)	Assay: 1) fumarylactoactase (D) 2) Succinylactase (D)
19.	Hypervalinemia (AR?)	Assay: Valine transaminase (D)
20.	Isovalinic acidemia (AR)	Assay: 1) Isovalerylglycine (D) 2) Isovaleryl-CoA Carboxylase (D)
21.	3-ketothiolase deficiency (AR)	Assay: 3-ketothiolase (D)
22.	Maple syrup urine disease (AR)	Assay: Branch chain 2-ketoacid decarboxylase (D)
23.	3-methylcrotinyl glycinuria (AR)	Assay: 3-methylcrotinyl-CoA carboxylase (D)
24.	Methylmalonic acidemia (AR)	Assay: methylmalonic CoA mutase (D)
25.	Methylene tetrahydrofolate reductase deficiency (AR)	Assay: methyltetrahydrofolate reductase (D)
26.	Methyltetrahydrofolate methyl transferase deficiency (AR)	Assay: methyltetrahydrofolate methyltransferase (D)
27.	Multiple carboxylase deficiency (AR?)	Assay: 1) Amniotic fluid methyl citrate (D) 2) Acyl CoA carboxylase (D)
28.	Non-ketotic hyperglycinemia (AR)	Assay: Amniotic fluid glycine level and glycine/serine ratio (E)
29.	Ornithine transcarbamylase deficiency (XLR)	DNA linkage (M)
30.	Ornithine-alpha-ketoacid transaminase deficiency (AR)	Assay: Ornithine alpha-ketoacid transaminase (D)
31.	5-oxoprolinuria (AR)	Assay: Glutathione synthetase (D)
32.	Prolidase deficiency (Hyperimidodipeptiduria) (AR)	Assay: Prolidase (D)
33.	Propinic Acidemia (Ketolic hyperglycinemia) (AR)	Assay: Propionyl CoA carboxylase (D)
34.	Saccharopinuria (AR?)	Assay: 1) Lysine-ketoglutarate reductase (D) 2) Saccharopin dehydrogenase (D)

(*Continued*)

(AR, autosomal recessive; AD, autosomal dominant; XLR, X-linked recessive; D, diminished; E, elevated; H, histology; M, molecular; K, karyotype)

Table 2-3. Prenatal Diagnosis of Genetic Disorders (*Continued*)

35. Transcobalamin 2 deficiency (AR)	Assay: B_{12} incorporation (D)
36. Vitamin B_{12} metabolic defect (AR)	Assay: Vitamin B_{12} coenzyme (D)

III. DISORDERS OF LIPID METABOLISM
1. Abetalipoproteinemia (AR) — Assay: Apo-beta-lipoprotein (D)
2. Adrenoleukodystrophy (XLR) — DNA linkage (M)
3. Apolipoprotein C-II deficiency (AR) — DNA analysis (M)
4. Atherosclerosis, premature (AR) — DNA linkage of Apolipoprotein A-1 site (M)
5. Familial high-density lipoprotein deficiency (Tangier disease) (AR) — Assay:
   1) Apolipoprotein A-1
   2) DNA linkage of Apolipoprotein A-1 (M)
6. Familial hypercholesterolemia (AD) — Assay:
   1) Low-density lipoprotein cholesterol receptors (D)
   2) DNA linkage (M)
7. Familial lipoid adrenal hyperplasia (AR) — DNA linkage (M)
8. Phytanic acid storage (Refsum's disease) (AR) — Assay: Phytanic acid Alpha-hydroxylase (D)

IV. DISORDERS OF LYSOSOMAL STORAGE
1. Acid lipase deficiency (AR) — Assay: Acid lipase (D)
   A) Wolman's disease
   B) Cholesteryl ester storage disease
2. Acid phosphatase deficiency (AR) — Assay: Acid phosphatase (D)
3. Aspartylglycosaminuria (AR) — Assay: Beta-aspartylglucosaminidase (D)
4. Ceramidase deficiency (AR) Farber's lipogranulomatosis — Assay: Ceramidase (D)
5. Fabry's disease (XLR) — Assay: Ceramidetrihexoside galactosidase (D)
6. Fucosidosis (AR) — Assay: Alpha-L-fucosidase (D)
7. Galactosylceramide lipidosis (Krabbe's disease) (AR) — Assay: Galactosyl (D) ceramide Beta-galactosidase
8. Lactosyl ceramidosis (AR) — Assay: Lactosyl ceramidase (D)
9. Gangliosidoses
   A. GMI gangliosidoses, generalized (beta-galactosidase deficiency) (AR) — Assay:
      1) Beta-galactosidase (D)
      2) Galactosyl oligosuccharides (E)
   B. GM2 gangliosidosis, adult onset (AR) — Assay: Beta-hexosaminidase A isoenzymes (D)
   C. Sandhoff disease (infantile gangliosidosis GM2) (AR) — Assay: N-acetylglucosaminyl
      1) Oligosuccharides (E)
      2) Hexosaminidase A & B (D)
   D. Tay-Sachs disease (AR) — Assay: Hexosaminidase A & B (D)
10. Gaucher's disease (AR) — DNA analysis (M)
11. Mannosidosis (beta-mannosidosis) (AR) — Assay: Alpha-mannosidase (D) (beta-mannosidase) (D)

(*Continued*)

(AR, autosomal recessive; AD, autosomal dominant; XLR, X-linked recessive; D, diminished; E, elevated; H, histology; M, molecular; K, karyotype)

Table 2-3. Prenatal Diagnosis of Genetic Disorders (*Continued*)

12.	Medium-chain acyl CoE-A dehydrogenase deficiency (AR)	Assay: Octanoate oxidation (D)
13.	Metachromatic leukodystrophy (MLD) (AR)	Assay: Arylsulphatase A (D) Arylsulphatase A
14.	Mucolipidoses	
	A. Type I (AR)	Alpha-neuraminidase (D)
	B. Type II (AR) I-cell disease	Assay: Beta-galactosidase (D) EM: Increased inclusion bodies (H)
	C. Type III (AR) Bermann disease	1) Assay: N-acetyl glucosaminyl phosphotransferase (D) 2) EM: Increased inclusion bodies (H)
	D. Type IV (AR)	EM: Increased inclusion bodies (H) Assay: Ganglioside neuraminidase (D)
15.	Mucopolysaccharidoses	
	A. Type I (AR) Hurler syndrome Scheie syndrome	Assay: Alpha-L-iduronidase (D)
	B. Type II (XLR) Hunter syndrome	1) DNA analysis (M) 2) Assay: Alpha-L-iduronic acid-2-sulfatase (D)
	C. Type III (AR) Sanfilippo syndrome (AR)	
	i. Sanfillipo A disease (AR)	1) DNA analysis (M) 2) Assay: Heparin sulfatase (D)
	ii. Sanfilippo B disease (AR)	Assay: Alpha-N-acetylglucosaminidase activity (D)
	iii. Sanfilippo C disease (AR)	Assay: Acetyl CoA: alpha-glucosaminide N-acetyl transferase (D)
	D. Type IV Morquio syndrome (AR)	Assay: N-acetyl-1 Galactosamine 6-sulphate sulphatase (D)
	E. Type VI Maroteaux-Larriy syndrome (AR)	Assay: Arylsulfatase-B (D)
	F. Type VII (AR) Sly syndrome	Assay: Beta-glucuronidase (D)
16.	Multiple sulfatase deficiency (AR)	Assay: Multiple sulfatase (D)
17.	Niemann-Pick disease (AR)	Assay: Sphingomyelinase activity (D)
18.	Sialic acid storage disease, infantile (AR)	Assay: Sialic acid (E)
19.	Sialidosis (AR)	Assay: Glycoprotein neuraminidase (D)
V.	DISORDERS OF STEROID METABOLISM	
1.	Adrenogenital syndrome (AR)	Assay: Steroid hydroxylase (D)
2.	Congenital adrenal hyperplasia (21-hydroxylase deficiency) (AR)	DNA analysis (M)

(*Continued*)

(AR, autosomal recessive; AD, autosomal dominant; XLR, X-linked recessive; D, diminished; E, elevated; H, histology; M, molecular; K, karyotype)

Table 2-3. **Prenatal Diagnosis of Genetic Disorders** (*Continued*)

	3. Congenital adrenal hyperplasia (11-beta-hydroxylase deficiency) (AR)	Assay: 11-deoxycortisol and tetralydrocortisol
	4. Placental sulfatase deficiency (XLR)	Assay: Steroid sulfatase (D)
VI.	DISORDERS OF PURINE AND PYRIMIDINE METABOLISM	
	1. Adenosine deaminase deficiency (severe combined immunodeficiency disease) (AR)	1) DNA analysis (M) 2) Assay: Adenosine deaminase (D)
	2. Lesch-Nyhan syndrome (XLR)	DNA analysis (M)
	3. Nucleoside phosphorylase deficiency with immunodeficiency (AD)	Assay: Nucleoside phosphosylase (D)
	4. Ortic aciduria (AR)	Assay: Orotidylic pyrophosphorylase and decarboxylase (D)
	5. Purine nucleoside phosphorylase deficiency (AR)	Assay: Purine nucleoside phosphorylase (D)
VII.	DISORDERS OF METAL METABOLISM	
	1. Menkes' disease (XLR)	DNA analysis (M)
	2. Wilson's disease (AR)	DNA analysis (M)
VIII.	DISORDERS OF PORPHYRIN AND HEME METABOLISM	
	1. Acatalesemia (AR)	Assay: Catalase (D)
	2. Porphyrias Congenital erythropoietic porphyria (AR)	Assay: Uro-porphyrinogen III Co synthetase (D)
	3. Acute intermittent porphyria (AD)	Assay: Uro-porphyrinogen I synthetase (D)
	4. Hereditary coproporphyria (AD)	Assay: Coproporphyrinogin oxidase (D)
	5. Varigate porphyria (AD)	Assay: Proto-porphyrinogin oxidase (D)
	6. Porphyria, hepato-erythropoietic (AR)	DNA analysis (M)
IX.	DISORDERS OF CONNECTIVE TISSUE, MUSCLE AND BONE	
	1. Achondroplasia (AD)	DNA analysis (M)
	2. Amyloidotic polyneuropathy (AD)	DNA analysis (M)
	3. Alpha 1-antitrypsin deficiency (AR)	DNA analysis (M)
	4. Becker muscular dystrophy (XLR)	DNA analysis (M)
	5. Duchenne muscular dystrophy (XLR)	DNA analysis (M)
	6. Ehlers-Danlos syndrome (AD, AR, XLR)	DNA analysis (M) of alpha-1 (I) collagen
	7. Congenital hypophosphatasia (AR)	U/S and assay of alkaline phosphatase (D)
	8. Marfan syndrome (AD)	DNA analysis (M) of alpha-2 (I) collagen
	9. Myotonic dystrophy (AD)	DNA analysis (M)
	10. Osteogenesis imperfecta Congenita lethalis (AR)	DNA analysis (M) U/S
	11. Osteogenesis imperfecta Type IV, I (AD)	DNA analysis (M)
X.	DISORDERS OF BLOOD AND BLOOD-FORMING TISSUE Coagulation Defects	
	1. Antithrombin III (AD)	DNA linkage (M)
	2. Classic hemophilia Hemophilia A (XLR)	DNA linkage (M)

(*Continued*)

(AR, autosomal recessive; AD, autosomal dominant; XLR, X-linked recessive; D, diminished; E, elevated; H, histology; M, molecular; K, karyotype)

Table 2-3. Prenatal Diagnosis of Genetic Disorders (*Continued*)

	3. Christmas factor deficiency Hemophilia B (XLR) Factor IX deficiency	DNA linkage (M)
	4. Factor X deficiency (XLR)	DNA linkage (M)
	5. Factor XIIIA (AR)	DNA linkage (M)
	6. Von Willebrand's disease (AD)	1) Factor VIII procoagulant (D) 2) DNA linkage (M)
	Hemoglobin and Blood-Forming Tissue	
	7. Fancani's anemia (AR)	Rate of chromosome breakage (K)
	8. Glucose phosphate isomerose deficiency (AR)	Assay: glucose phosphate isomerase (D)
	9. Hereditary methemoglobinemia (congenital enzymopenic methemoglobinemia) (AR)	Assay: NADH-cytochrome b 5 reductase (D)
	10. Hereditary persistence of fetal hemoglobin (AD)	DNA analysis (M)
	11. Rhesus antigen (AR)	Immunofluoresces (H)
	12. Sickle cell anemia (AR)	DNA analysis (M)
	13. Alpha-thalassemia (AR)	DNA analysis (M)
	14. Beta-thalassemia (AR)	DNA analysis (M)
	15. Triose phosphate isomerase deficiency (AR)	Assay: Triose phosphate isomerase (D)
XI.	DISORDERS OF TRANSPORT	
	1. Cystic fibrosis (AR)	DNA analysis (M)
	2. Cystinosis (AR)	Assay: Accumulation of cystine (E)
XII.	DISORDERS OF THE IMMUNE AND OTHER MECHANISMS OF DEFENSE	
	1. Agammaglobulinemia (XLR)	DNA analysis (M)
	2. Chediak-Higashi syndrome (AR)	Intracellular inclusions (H)
	3. Chronic granulomatous disease (XLR)	DNA analysis (M)
XIII.	MISCELLANEOUS DISORDERS	
	1. Cat eye syndrome (AD)	DNA analysis (M)
	2. Charcot-Marie-tooth disease (AD)	DNA analysis (M)
	3. Choroideremia (XLR)	DNA analysis (M)
	4. Cleft palate and ankyloglossia (XLR)	DNA analysis (M)
	5. Fragile X (XLR)	DNA analysis (M)
	6. Growth hormone deficiency—type A (AR)	DNA analysis (M)
	7. Huntington's disease (AD)	DNA analysis (M)
	8. Polycystic kidney disease, autosomal dominant form (adult polycystic kidney disease) (AD)	DNA analysis (M)
	9. Retinoblastoma (AD)	DNA linkage (M)
	10. Retinitis pigmentosa (XLR)	DNA analysis (M)
	11. Sulfite oxidase deficiency (Sulfocyteinuria) (AR)	Assay: sulfite oxidase (D)

(*Continued*)

(AR, autosomal recessive; AD, autosomal dominant; XLR, X-linked recessive; D, diminished; E, elevated; H, histology; M, molecular; K, karyotype)

Table 2-3. **Prenatal Diagnosis of Genetic Disorders** (*Continued*)

	12. Tourette syndrome (AD)	DNA analysis (M)
	13. Zellweger syndrome (AR)	Assay: Acyl CoA: Dihydroxyacetase phosphate acyltransferase (D)
XIV.	CHROMOSOME DELETION SYNDROMES	
	1. 5 q syndrome	Chromosome 5 (K)
	2. Beckwith-Wiedmann syndrome	Chromosome 11* (K)
	3. Cri du chat syndrome	Chromosome 5* (K)
	4. Becker muscular dystrophy	Chromosome X* (K)
	5. Duchenne muscular dystrophy	Chromosome X* (K)
	6. Glycerol kinase deficiency	Chromosome X* (K)
	7. Norrie disease	Chromosome X* (K)
	8. Prader-Willi syndrome	Chromosome 15* (K)
	9. Retinoblastoma	Chromosome 13* (K)
	10. Wilms' tumor	Chromosome 11* (K)
	11. Wolfe-Hirschhorn syndrome	Chromosome 4* (K)

* Association noted in some families

(AR, autosomal recessive; AD, autosomal dominant; XLR, X-linked recessive; D, diminished; E, elevated; H, histology; M, molecular; K, karyotype)

laboratory results, sets the diagnosis of serious genetic disorders most commonly at about 20 weeks gestation. By this time, the patient is very visibly pregnant, quickening has occurred, and significant emotional bonding to the fetus has occurred, making a second trimester termination psychologically traumatic.[15]

The newer technique of CVS is usually performed between 9 to 12 weeks from the last menstrual period and offers many potential advantages.[18,43] Principally, diagnoses can be made much earlier in pregnancy. Early diagnosis allows for results to be available before quickening and its ensuing emotional bonding, and allows the couple privacy in their decisions. Termination of pregnancy, when chosen by the parents, can be performed by the first-trimester suction method, which is considered safer and can be less emotionally traumatic, and can be performed as an outpatient. Experience with CVS diagnoses is expanding rapidly.

Although CVS has tremendous theoretical advantages over amniocentesis, the risks of the procedure are probably greater. A major problem in determining risks, both for amniocentesis and CVS, is differentiating between background spontaneous abortion rates and procedure complications. For amniocentesis at 17 weeks, the accepted background spontaneous abortion rate is about 2% to 3%. Various authorities feel that the procedural loss rate may be 0.2% to 0.5% over and above the background rate of 3%.[1,16,27,49] For CVS, estimates of background spontaneous abortion rates at 8 to 10 weeks have been widely varied. Procedural risks cannot be derived from overall spontaneous first-trimester loss rates, but must be based on data obtained following a normal ultrasound at 8 to 10 weeks. Recent data suggest that a 3% to 4% spontaneous loss figure may be appropriate and that true rates vary significantly with maternal ages.[45] Until such data are confirmed, only educated guesses can be used for CVS-related losses. Over 55,000 procedures have been recorded in the CVS registry[23] and suggest a 0.5% to 2% risk in most centers. Because of the relatively high background loss rate, it will take tens of thousands of cases to obtain definitive statistics. Regardless of the exact figures, CVS procedural loss rates are slightly higher than for amniocentesis in most experienced hands.

The National Institute of Child Health and Human Development (NICHD) has sponsored a randomized trial of CVS and amniocentesis. Patient acceptance of randomization in the United States has been very poor, but their attitude is understandable, given the strong built-in bias of couples who present for CVS because they want information as early as possible. In other countries, it is more acceptable for physicians to control and limit patient access to technology. Ultimately, in most Western countries it must be the patient who decides whether a higher risk with earlier results is preferable to a lower risk and results later in pregnancy.

In our experience, patients presenting for possible CVS (as opposed to amniocentesis) are older, better educated, have higher incomes, and fewer children.[14] The use of new technologies has traditionally been initially monopolized by higher socioeconomic groups, but in the coming years we will

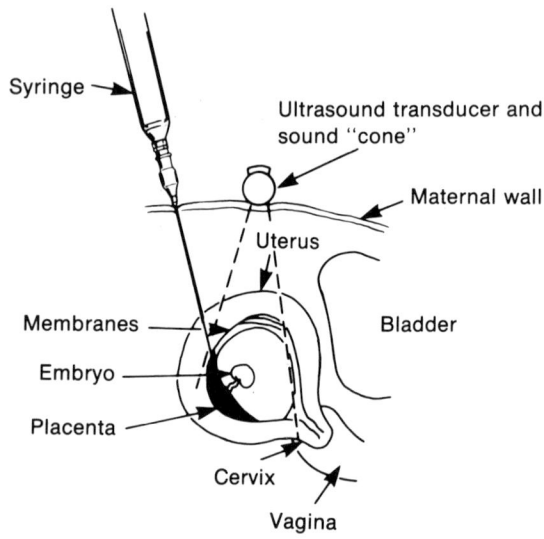

FIGURE 2-3. Transabdominal CVS using double-needle technique. An 18-gauge needle is passed through the skin and into myometrium. A longer 20-gauge needle can then be passed down the shaft of the 18-gauge needle into the placenta. Suction is created with a syringe, and villi aspirated. The 20-gauge needle can be reinserted multiple times without discomfort to the patient.

doubtless see an expansion to a larger population base.

Technology for obtaining chorionic villi has advanced over the past few years. Most centers currently use ultrasound-guided transcervical suction-aspiration techniques (Figure 2-2). There is also a growing trend to use a transabdominal route with either a single- or double-needle technique (Figure 2-3). Theoretical advantages of the transabdominal route include a possibly lower risk of infection as well as easier access to fundal placentas. In our experience, transabdominal sample size has been lower than from the transcervical route. In our program we have used, with success, the transabdominal route on high fundal placentas at 9 weeks or more. One important consideration in some centers has also been the ability to do transabdominal CVS with easily available spinal needles, which has exempted the procedure from the

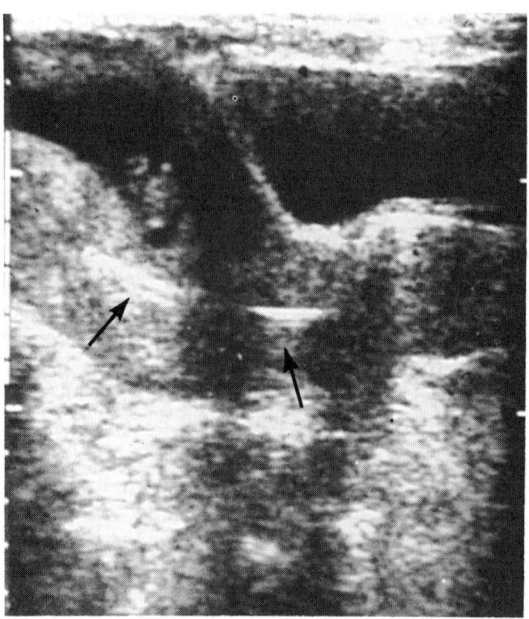

FIGURE 2-2. Ultrasound shows catheter (arrow) passing through cervix and about to enter placenta. Fetus can be seen within gestational sac.

Federal Drug Administration's "investigational device" authorization, as required for transcervical catheters.

Early Genetic Amniocentesis

We have also found performing genetic amniocentesis at 11 to 13 weeks to be a viable option (Figure 2-4). We have used early amniocentesis in circumstances when CVS was felt to be either too late, too risky such as with active herpes lesion, or because of an obstructed cervical canal.

Early amniocentesis can be considered an option in those pregnancies in which the placenta is inaccessible to either transcervical or transabdominal sampling, or in those that are beyond 11 weeks gestational age. Early amniocentesis fluid culture takes longer than fluid from older gestations, but the earlier time of amniocentesis more than compensates for the longer laboratory preparation time. Data from our center suggest that while there are limited circumstances under which very early amniocentesis might be appropriate, it is probably a safe and reasonable alternative.[13] Data on amniotic fluid alpha-fetoprotein are still being accumulated at early gestational ages, but in all probability will be satisfactory for neural tube defect diagnosis. Acetylcholinesterase often gives a weak positive band in early gestation, which can be differentiated from the broad band seen with open neural tube defects.

FIRST TRIMESTER LABORATORY DIAGNOSIS

Cytogenetic Data

There are two general approaches to obtaining cytogenetic information from CVS, direct and cultured preparations. In the direct preparation method, uncultured villi are prepared for direct use in cytogenetic studies. Many minor modifications of this basic technique have been published by several groups.[17] The major advantage of the direct technique as compared to using amniotic fluid cells is that even with a small villus sample, there are many more actively dividing trophoblast cells which can be karyotyped almost immediately. Results can be available within 24 to 48 hours of the procedure. In most large programs, however, due to the large volume of specimens, it may take up to a week or more to process the slides.

Until recently a major drawback associated with the direct technique was inferior quality of cytogenetic preparations. For this reason, laboratories would culture portions of the villus material and then karyotype the harvested fibroblastlike cells. Culturing the chorionic villus cells has produced better quality preparations and confirms the direct techniques. In our hands, direct processing has routinely yielded metaphases in the 300 to 350-band range. We use cultures with extremely small samples, to verify questionable direct results, and as a back-up to direct preps. An extremely small incidence of dis-

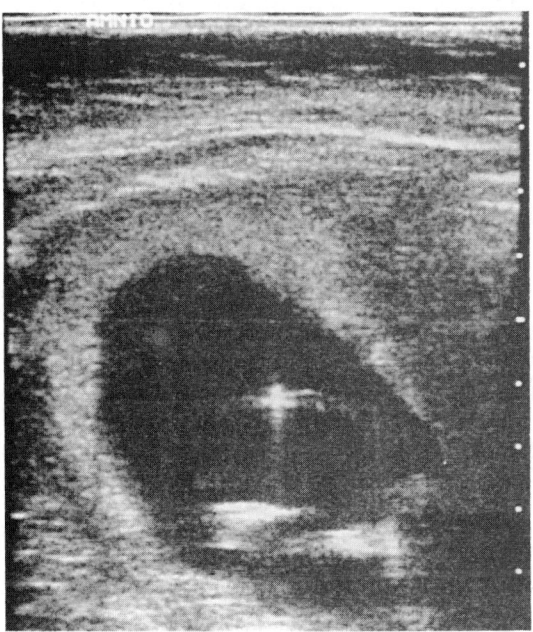

FIGURE 2-4. Ultrasound showing tip of 22-gauge amniocentesis needle in sac at 12 weeks. With sophisticated ultrasound, it is increasingly possible to aspirate fluid from extremely small pockets.

crepancies between fetal and direct prep karyotypes has been seen. In over 55,000 cases reported to the CVS registry,[23] there are a few known instances of a normal direct preparation with an abnormal long-term culture and amniocentesis.[41] Mosaicism in direct preparation will be seen about 1% of the time. Experience has taught that most of the time, such a pattern is not reflective of the true fetal karyotype. In this situation, culture is mandatory and in most, but not all, cases, long-term culture will show a normal result.

Biochemical Data

Many mendelian disorders previously diagnosable only by analysis of cultured amniotic fluid cells can now be diagnosed by either cultured or uncultured CVS specimens. The list of diseases for which diagnoses are now available is expanding geometrically as normal baseline levels are documented for many enzymes in chorionic villi or cells cultured from villi. But before attempting prenatal diagnosis, several theoretical questions need to be asked in establishing these normal biochemical levels. First, assuming that enzyme activity is demonstrable at all, the next question is whether there is a minimum gestational age before enzymatic activity would be expected in normal specimens. If so, then analysis of an at-risk specimen prior to a given gestational age would not be expected to be diagnostic.

In our experience, a gestational age barrier has not been the case for many enzymes tested; in general, CVS specimens have approximated fibroblast values.[12] Unfortunately, this is not always the situation. Differences between normal values for uncultured and cultured villi could create difficulties in using CVS for prenatal diagnosis of some biochemical disorders. However, a systematic approach of exploring normal values has been developed for many specific disease conditions.[2]

Molecular Diagnoses

The development of molecular biologic techniques has opened the door for a tremendous addition to the armamentarium of prenatal diagnosis. The biochemical diagnoses of mendelian disorders require the expression of gene products in cell culture. In many instances villi or amniotic fluid cells do not express the enzyme in question. Consequently, in these disorders an invasive technique such as a fetal liver biopsy, fetal skin biopsy, or fetal blood sampling has been required to obtain the tissue in which the enzyme is produced.[9,53] DNA from all cells contains all the information necessary to produce every gene product; direct DNA analysis will yield the same results regardless of the sample source. A major advantage of such studies is that by analysis of DNA itself, the problem of tissue specificity of gene expression is eliminated. For example, the diagnosis of sickle cell anemia previously required fetoscopic blood sampling, which carries a 3% to 5% risk of fetal loss. Because of the risk, fetoscopy has had very limited application.[10,35] Recently ultrasonically guided cordocentesis has become available for fetal blood sampling[7] (see Chapter 2, Section 2). Although safer than fetoscopy because of the smaller needle, cordocentesis still carries greater risks to the pregnancy than either CVS or genetic amniocentesis and usually cannot be performed until at least 18 or 19 weeks. However, molecular analysis of DNA obtained from uncultured amniotic fluid cells or chorionic villi allows for a much safer and earlier diagnosis of sickle cell anemia. The principles of molecular diagnosis open the entire spectrum of human disease to antenatal diagnosis.

There are three primarily related techniques by which molecular diagnoses have been accomplished. These are DNA hybridization, restriction endonuclease analysis, and linkage analysis. All of these strategies require an understanding of molecular events. They can be used when the approximate location of the disease gene is known, even when the gene product itself is not known. What is required is the localization of the gene to a region on a given chromosome.

A fourth technique, the polymerase chain reaction (PCR) has recently been developed. PCR will open the way to preimplantation diagnoses as it provides the possibility of achieving a diagnosis from even one cell.

DNA Hybridization

When the DNA sequence for the disease in question is known, radioactive complementary DNA (cDNA) can be made. In deletion diseases, the cDNA will not be able to bind appropriately to the subject's DNA, and diminished radioactivity will be found on autoradiography. For example, in alpha-thalassemia an alpha-globin probe is available and can be used for in utero diagnosis.[26] There are normally four copies of the alpha-thalassemia gene. A cDNA alpha-globin probe is used with DNA from amniotic fluid cells or chorionic villi. If all four copies of the globin gene are present, then a reaction of appropriate intensity is noted on autoradiography. If some or all of the copies of the globin are missing, a progressive decrease in the intensity of the reaction will be noted. In homozygous alpha-thalassemia, no reaction would be seen.[26]

Restriction Endonuclease Analysis

Restriction endonucleases are enzymes derived from bacteria which cleave double-stranded DNA at specific and consistent recognition sites. The resultant fragments are segregated electrophoretically into identifiable fragment lengths. When the restriction endonuclease cleaves at a gene known to cause a specific disease, the restriction fragments can be exposed to hybridized cDNA for identification and diagnosis by autoradiography. If the recognition site is not the gene itself, but rather located near the "disease" gene, then a diagnosis can be inferred under certain circumstances. In this situation, the confidence of such a diagnosis is inversely proportional to the distance between the gene of interest and the recognition site. This type of diagnosis is also contingent upon the analysis of DNA from multiple family members, as will be discussed with linkage analysis.

The classic example of restriction endonuclease analysis for prenatal diagnosis is sickle cell anemia. Ingram[21,22] demonstrated that the only difference between normal hemoglobin and sickle cell hemoglobin is a single amino acid substitution in the beta chain. In sickle cell hemoglobin, valine replaces glutamic acid in the sixth position from the N-terminal of the beta chain. This seemingly minor change results in an altered electrical charge and accounts for all of the clinical manifestations found in sickle cell anemia.

With the clear identification of the mutation, it is possible to make an accurate prenatal diagnosis in all at-risk pregnancies. Restriction endonuclease Mst 11's recognition site appears in the normal beta-globin chain at amino acids 5, 6, and 7. In sickle cell anemia, the substitution eliminates the recognition site. Subsequently the fragment lengths are different between normal beta-globin (1.1 kilobase) and sickle cell beta-globin (1.3 kilobase). By using radio-labeled probes and restriction endonucleases, autoradiography differentiates among normal hemoglobin, sickle cell hemoglobin, and sickle cell trait hemoglobin.[4]

Linkage Analysis

Whereas the antenatal diagnosis of sickle cell anemia relies on direct DNA analysis at the mutation site, the exact location of the "disease" gene is not known for the majority of disorders. In these cases, indirect methods must be used. Linkage analysis examines restriction fragment length polymorphisms (RFLPs) in the fetus and family members. Even though the exact gene location is unknown, if a small region of a chromosome is known to carry the gene, linkage analysis may be used. Conversely, the association (segregation) of a disease with a given polymorphism whose location is known can be used to learn the location of a gene. Such techniques, used in large families with multiple Huntington's disease patients, allow the localization of that gene to chromosome 4q.[17] Thus, the approach is backwards to that for sickle cell disease, in that the gene's location is known before the pathogenesis.

As with specific restriction endonuclease analysis, the DNA is cleaved with the formation of consistent fragment lengths. The closer the cleavage site is to the suspected gene location, the more reliable the information. The important factor in linkage analysis is not the specific gene, but rather the fragment lengths generated. Measurements of the RFLPs from the fetus, in association with those from an affected sibling, nonaffected sibling, parents, grandparents, and so on, infer gene carrier versus noncarrier status. The reliability of the test is based on the proximity of the gene to the cleavage site. The closer the two are associated, the greater the probability a diagnosis can be accurately made.

A classic example of linkage analysis is myotonic dystrophy (MD), an autosomal dominant condition, which until very recently could not be diagnosed directly prenatally. The gene for MD is known to be on chromosome 19 in close proximity to both the secretor locus and the Lutheran blood group locus. With this information, an indirect diagnosis is possible. To make an antenatal diagnosis, the family of the at-risk fetus must be "informative"; that is, the family must have (1) an affected member or the banked DNA from an affected member available for analysis, and (2) a heterozygous secretor locus or Lutheran blood group locus showing the expression of two alleles. The MD gene can either be on the same chromosome in the chromosome 19 pair as the known trait (coupling), or on the opposite chromosome of the pair (repulsion). If these conditions are present, the family is informative and prenatal diagnosis is possible.

The confidence of the diagnosis is inversely proportional to the distance between the MD gene and the reference gene, in this case, either the secretor locus or Lutheran blood group locus. The closer the genes, the greater the probability that the fetus will inherit the genes together because the chances of crossing over in meiosis is reduced. It is also possible, particularly with X-linked disorders, to offer diagnosis even if the affected individual is not available. If other normal males are present, then the missing puzzle piece, the abnormal X, can be deduced.

As more markers are identified, gene mapping studies will be better able to define the location of specific genes. This will enable researchers to diagnose disease states and carrier states with greater reliability. The number of disorders open to antenatal diagnosis expands daily, and the reliability of the diagnoses increases as more probes are used by numerous groups to "walk the gene" and eventually identify it.

At present, there are clear indications that if a gene product can be isolated, it will be possible to identify linked RFLPs of antenatally diagnostic value. The initial observation that RFLPs can be used for antenatal diagnosis was made by Kan, Golbus, and Dozy[26] and was a fundamental landmark in antenatal diagnosis.

A major ethical dilemma has occurred with the availability of DNA diagnosis. The situation that has received the most publicity is that of Huntington's disease. DNA analysis not only permits prenatal diagnosis of this devastating disease, but it also identifies the presymptomatic patient. The ethical storm centers on whether presymptomatic testing should be encouraged or even allowed, as well as who should be told test results. Though diagnosis in this disease has been technically possible for several years, the technology is only now beginning to be used clinically. Many of the medical, ethical, and legal issues in this disease remain unresolved.

POLYMERASE CHAIN REACTION

The polymerase chain reaction (PCR) is a technology for *in vitro* amplification of selective DNA sequences so that a larger amount than the original sample of pure DNA is available for analysis. The PCR technique is capable of producing selective enrichment of a specific DNA sequence by a factor of 10^6, enabling analysis to be performed on as little as 1 ng of DNA. (The amount of genomic DNA present in only 150 diploid cells).[44]

The procedure involves two oligonucleotide primers that flank the DNA segment to be amplified, and then repeated cycles of denaturation, oligonucleotide primer annealing to their complimentary sequences, and primer extension by DNA polymerase. Since the extension products are also complimentary and are able to bind primers, each successive cycle essentially doubles the amount of DNA synthesized in the previous cycle. Repeated cycles result in an exponential increase in copies of the region flanked by the primers.[45,46] Using a heat stable DNA polymerase (isolated from *Thermus aquaticus*) that is relatively unaffected by the denaturation process enables the use of a temperature system near the temperature optimum of the polymerase-catalyzed enzyme, which allows significant shortening and automation of the procedure.[45] A further improvement of the method involves attachment of a phase promoter onto at least one of the PCR primers.[50] The segments amplified by PCR are transcribed, thus further increasing the signal and providing an abundance of single stranded DNA, which increases the sensitivity and reduces the time required to sequence an allele. The success rate of genomic amplification with transcript sequencing may also be higher because the transcription reaction may compensate for suboptimal PCR and because the single-stranded template generated has a higher probability of being successfully sequenced than a linear, double stranded template.[50] The automation and heat stabilization of the process shortens to 3–4 hours an *in vitro* reaction that might otherwise take days or weeks of growth and purification.[45]

The clinical and research implications of PCR processes are enormous, as they provide quick and accurate analysis of very small amounts of DNA. Prenatal diagnosis of sickle cell anemia by these methods has already been accomplished in a rapid and sensitive process taking less than 8 hours.[11] Identification of viral specific DNA strands from HIV-1 in seropositive culture-positive patients has also been accomplished. The method of DNA amplification made it possible to obtain results within 3 days, whereas virus isolation takes 3–4 weeks.[38]

The speed and quantity of data obtainable by direct genomic sequencing will allow us to approach the date when the complete human genome will be mapped pure DNA strands, and identification of single base mutation will allow the use of small amounts of DNA in identification of the affected individual or the carrier state. With these techniques, diagnoses at the preimplantation stage should eventually be possible and will set the stage for early gene therapy.

Legal Issues

It is well established that failure to offer prenatal diagnostic services to women in appropriate at-risk categories constitutes medical malpractice.[39] There is significant precedence for the tort liability of physicians who have not appraised patients of the availability of such services. It is reasonable to anticipate that over the course of the next several years that liability may be extended beyond gross negligence from failure to discuss common indications such as advanced maternal age. There could be standards to require discussion of more esoteric issues, such as failing to take an adequate family history which might reveal susceptibility to certain metabolic disorders, or failure to screen patients in at-risk categories. Similarly, there will undoubtedly be litigation following complications to pregnancies for which unsure practices were performed on patients not clearly in high-risk groups but who "insisted" upon them. The impact of malpractice litigation has been felt particularly hard in both the obstetric and neonatal communities. There is no reason to believe that this trend will be reversed.

Legal issues to be debated in the next several years include the management of pregnancy when the fetus is discovered to have a genetic abnormality too late for parents who would have chosen to terminate the pregnancy to do so, or when they do not wish extraordinary measures to be taken.[27] There is general agreement that with a fetus who is very severely affected with a lethal condition such as anencephaly, labor can be induced even beyond the 20 to 24 week legal limit in most jurisdictions. Similarly, there is good precedence (legal and ethical) that the fetus with a minor malformation should be treated as though normal, notwithstanding the legal right to terminate any pregnancy before the gestational age limit. There is much controversy in the middle ground, however, with regard to reliably predictable severe handicaps, such as a large meningomyelocele, microcephaly, or trisomy 13 or 18. It is reasonable to expect that such cases will be at the forefront of medical and legal attention and precedence, and that each physician caring for such a patient will realize that his conduct in the particular case may result in medicolegal action and publicity, to be compared against the existing standards of given communities.

Ethical Issues

The purpose of prenatal diagnosis is to inform parents accurately and to present them with all appropriate options. Under no circumstances is the purpose of prenatal diagnosis to force or encourage the abortion of any fetus. All decisions regarding termination or continuation of pregnancy are to be made only by the parents after they have been given as thorough and complete counseling as possible.

One of the principal ethical complaints about prenatal diagnosis is that it is a "search and destroy" mission. With the advent of limited fetal therapeutic options, such as the correction of bladder obstruction or prevention of external genital masculinization in 21-hydroxylase deficiency (congenital adrenal hyperplasia), termination is not always the only option. Nevertheless, it is apparent that the ethics of abortion and the ethics of the fetus as patient are bound to collide. The point in gestation when it is reasonable to consider a fetus a potential viable being has been creeping earlier and earlier in gestation. It is reasonable to expect that the medical, legal, ethical, and public policy communities will be sensitive to such changes. Ultimately these communities will require earlier diagnosis before the mid-trimester fetus has rights which supersede those of the mother. The late 1980s and 1990s will clearly be an ethical battleground over which these issues will be fought on many fronts.

REFERENCES

1. Alexander DF: Workgroup paper: Risks of amniocentesis. In Gastel B, Haddow JE, Fletcher JC et al (eds): Maternal Serum Alpha-Fetoprotein: Issues in the Prenatal Screening and Diagnosis of Neural Tube Defects, p 20. Public Health Service, Government Printing Office, 1981
2. Ben Yoseph Y, Evans MI, Bottoms SF et al: Lysosomal enzyme activities in fresh and frozen chorionic villi and in cultured trophoblasts. Clin Chem Acta 161:307, 1986
3. Bloom AB: Induced chromosome aberrations in man. Adv Human Genet 3:99, 1972
4. Boehm C, Kazazian HH: Prenatal diagnosis of hemoglobinopathies by DNA analysis. CRC Crit Rev Oncol Hematol 4:155, 1985
5. Brock DJH: Early diagnosis of fetal defects, p 78. Edinburgh, Churchill Livingstone, 1982
6. Cooper DN, Schmidtke J: Diagnosis of genetic disease using recombinant DNA. Human Genet 73:1, 1986
7. Daffos F, Capello-Pavlovsky M, Forestier F: Fetal blood sampling during pregnancy with use of a needle guided by ultrasound: A study of 606 consecutive cases. Am J Obstet Gynecol 153:655, 1985
8. Doe v Bolton, 410 US 179, 1973
9. Elias S, Mazur M, Sabbagha R et al: Prenatal diagnosis of harlequin ichthyosis. Clin Genet 17:275, 1980
10. Elias S, Simpson JL: Fetoscopy. In Sciarra JJ (ed): Gynecology and Obstetrics, vol 5, chap 105, pp 1–6. Philadelphia, JB Lippincott, 1988.
11. Embury SH, Scharf SJ, Saiki RK et al: Rapid prenatal diagnosis of Sickle Cell Anemia by a new method of DNA analysis. N Engl J Med 316:656–661, 1987
12. Evans MI, Koladny E, Schulman JD et al: Lysosomal enzymes in chorionic villi, cultural amniocytes, and cultured skin fibroblasts. Clin Chem Acta 157:109, 1986

13. Evans MI, Koppitch FC, Nemitz B et al: Early genetic amniocentesis or chorionic villus sampling: Expanding the opportunities for early prenatal diagnosis. J Reprod Med 3:450, 1988
14. Evans MI, Moran P, Grevengood C et al: Opting for chorionic villus sampling: Correlation of increased genetic risk with accepting greater procedure risks. *Society for Gynecologic Investigation,* Atlanta, Georgia, May 18–21, 1987
15. Fletcher JC, Evans MI: Maternal bonding in early fetal ultrasound examinations. N Engl J Med 308:392, 1983
16. Golbus MS, Caughman WD, Epstein CJ et al: Prenatal diagnosis in 3000 amniocenteses. New Engl J Med 300;157, 1979
17. Gusella JF, Wexler NS, Conneally PM et al: A polymorphic DNA marker genetically linked to Huntington's disease. Nature 306:234, 1983
18. Gustavii B, Chester MA, Edvall H et al: First trimester diagnosis on chorionic villi obtained by direct direct vision technique. Hum Genet 65:373, 1984
19. Hagerman R, Smith ACM, Mariner R: Clinical features of the fragile X syndrome. In Hagerman RJ, McBogg PM (eds): The Fragile X Syndrome, p 17. Dilan, Co, Spectra, 1983
20. Harper K, Pembrey ME, Davies KE et al: A clinically useful DNA probe closely linked to hemophilia A. Lancet 2:6, 1984
21. Ingram VM: A specific chemical difference between the globins of normal human and sickle cell anemia haemoglobin. Nature 178:792–794, 1956
22. Ingram VM: The hemoglobins in genetics and evolution. New York, Columbia University Press, 1963
23. Jackson L: CVS Registry. Dept. of Medical Genetics, Jefferson Medical College, Thomas Jefferson University, no 20, March 1987
24. Jacobson CB, Barter RH: Intrauterine diagnosis and management of genetic defects. Am J Obstet Gynecol 99:795, 1967
25. Kaback M: Summary of Worldwide Tay Sachs Disease Screening and Detection. Los Angeles, University of California Press, 1981
26. Kan YW, Golbus MS, Dozy AM: Prenatal diagnosis of alpha-thalassemia. N Engl J Med 295:1165, 1976
27. Larsen JW Jr, Evans MI: Genetic causes. In Lin CC, Evans MI (eds): Intrauterine Growth Retardation, p 85. New York, McGraw-Hill, 1984
28. Lidsky AS, Guttler F, Woo SCL: Prenatal diagnosis of classic phenylketonuria by DNA analysis. Lancet 1:549, 1985
29. Mally JC, Dedlon AK et al: Linkage and genetic counseling for the fragile-X using probes 52A, F9, DX13, and ST14. Am J Med Gen 27:435–448, 1987
30. McGravan L, Maxwell F: Cytogenetic aspects of the fragile X syndrome. In Hagerman RJ, McBogg PM (eds): The Fragile X Syndrome. Dilan, CO, Spectra, 1983
31. McKusick VA: *Medelian Inheritance in Man,* 7th ed. Baltimore, Johns Hopkins University Press, 1986
32. McKusick VA, Neufeld EF: The mucopolysaccharide storage diseases. In Stanbury JB, Wyngaarden JB, Frederickson DS et al, (eds): The Metabolic Basis of Inherited Disease, p 751. New York, McGraw-Hill, 1983
33. Mikkelson M: Down's syndrome: Current stage of cytogenetic research. Hum Genet 12:1, 1971
34. Milunsky A (ed): Genetic Disorders and the Fetus. New York, Plenum Press, 1979
35. Modell B, Ward RHT: Antenatal diagnosis of the hemoglobinopathies. In Rocker I, Lawrence KM (eds): Fetoscopy, pp 87–145. Amsterdam, Biomedical Press, 1981
36. Nadler HL: Antenatal detection of hereditary disorders. Pediatrics 42:912, 1968
37. Oberle I, Mandel JL et al: Polymorphic DNA markers in prenatal diagnosis of fragile-X syndrome. Lancet 1:871, 1985
38. Ou CY, Kwok S, Mitchell SW et al: DNA—Amplification for direct detection of HIV-1 in DNA of peripheral blood mononuclear cells. Science 239:295–297, 1988
39. Phillips v United States, 566 F. Suppl I, 1981
40. Preventive screening for fragile-X syndrome. Lancet 2:1191–1192, 1986
41. Rosinsky BJ, Martin AO, Elias S et al: Accuracy of cytogenetic analysis of chorionic villus specimens is maximized by use of both direct preparation and culture. Am J Hum Gen 39:A264, 1986
42. Row v Wade, 410 US 113, 1973
43. Simoni G, Brambati B, Danesino C et al: Diagnostic application of first trimester trophoblast sampling in 100 pregnancies. Hum Genet 66:252, 1984
44. Saiki RK, Bugawan TL, Horn GT et al: Analysis of enzymatically amplified β globin and HLA-DQ DNA with allele-specific onconucleotide probes. Nature 324(13):163–166, 1986
45. Saiki RK, Gelfand DH, Stoffel S et al: Primer-directed enzymatic amplification of DNA with

a thermostable DNA polymerase. Science 239:487–491, 1988
46. Scharf SJ, Horn GT, Erlich HA: Direct cloning and sequence analysis of enzymatically amplified genomic sequence. Science 233:1076–1078, 1986
47. Simpson JL: Pregnancies in women with chromosomal abnormalities. In Schulman JD, Simpson JL (eds): Genetic Disorders and Pregnancy, pp 450–466. New York, Academic Press, 1982
48. Simpson JL: Fetal loss rate after normal ultrasound at eight weeks gestation: Implications for chorionic villus sampling. The diabetes in pregnancy project. Am J Hum Genet 36:1975, 1984
49. Simpson NE, Dallaire L, Miller JR et al: Prenatal diagnosis of genetic disease in Canada: Report of a collaborative study. Can Med Assoc J 115:739, 1976
50. Stoflet ES, Koeberl DD, Sarkar G, Sommer SS: Genomic amplification with transcript sequencing. Science 239:419–494, 1988
51. Tsui LC, Buchwald M, Barker D et al: Cystic fibrosis locus defined by a genetically linked polymorphic DNA marker. Science 230:1054, 1985
52. Verp MS: Antenatal diagnosis of chromosomal abnormalities. In Sciarra JJ: Gynecology and Obstetrics, vol 5, chap 102, pp 1–8. Philadelphia, JB Lippincott, 1988
53. Walser M: Urea cycle disorders and other hereditary hyperammonemic syndromes. In Stanbury JB, Wyndaarden JB, Frederickson DS et al (eds): The Metabolic Basis of Inherited Disease. New York, McGraw-Hill, 1983
54. Warsof SL, Larsen JW, Kent SG et al: Prenatal diagnosis of congenital adrenal hyperplasia. Obstet Gynecol 55:751, 1980
55. White R, Woodward S, Leppert M et al: A closely linked marker for cystic fibrosis. Nature 318:382, 1985
56. Wong C, Dowling CE, Saiki RK et al: Characterization of beta Thalassemia mutations using direct genomic sequencing of amplified single copy DNA. Nature 330:384–386, 1987

SECTION 2: SECOND AND THIRD TRIMESTER PRENATAL DIAGNOSIS

John W. Larsen, Jr., and Martha D. MacMillin

During the 1970s the prenatal diagnosis of chromosomal and mendelian disorders during the second trimester progressed from novelty to part of routine obstetric practice. Amniocentesis has proved to be an extremely safe method for obtaining the amniotic fluid cells necessary for analysis, and accurate laboratory testing of the cells has become standard. Fetoscopy and percutaneous umbilical cord puncture are additional techniques for second and third trimester diagnosis and therapy. This section will explore dilemmas and decisions with reference to the safety and accuracy of these techniques.

DIAGNOSTIC TECHNIQUES

Amniocentesis

Prior to its general use as a technique for prenatal genetic diagnosis, amniocentesis was developed as a diagnostic tool for research and clinical management studies of infections, Rh-sensitized pregnancies, fetal distress (meconium staining), and fetal lung maturity. The early studies antedated the development of obstetric ultrasound, and were guided by manual palpation of the fetus or, occasionally, x-ray films. Possible risks to the fetus due to needle puncture were substantially outweighed by the high likelihood of disease being diagnosed, particularly in the instance of Rh-sensitized pregnancy in which an abnormal spectrophotometric analysis was expected more than 50% of the time.

With the development of sonography for obstetric diagnosis during the 1970s, sonar guidance became part of routine amniocentesis technique. The first form of sonar guidance was the B-mode technique in which a picture or series of pictures of placenta and fetus were used to measure the distance from skin to amniotic fluid and to identify a point on the maternal abdominal wall through which a needle could be passed without puncturing the placenta. The B-mode sonar examination was generally performed remote in time and place from the amniocentesis.

The use of sonar prior to performing amniocentesis enabled the physician to estimate gestational age, count the number of fetuses present, detect myomas, confirm fetal viability, confirm gross fetal morphology, and locate the placenta. However, the advantage of placental localization was diminished by the general practice of transferring the patient from the sonar suite to another site for amniocentesis. The optimal point for needle insertion could change as the patient moved about or, in particular, emptied her bladder following the distention desired for a full diagnostic sonar study.

As sonar technology evolved and the cumbersome B-mode equipment was replaced by more compact and useful real-time equipment, sonar guidance came to mean sonar scanning immediately prior to and possibly during needle insertion.[3] The exact technique used remains a matter of operator preference and selection, as long as the end results of safety and accuracy are achieved. The loss rate of normal pregnancies due to amniocentesis and the rate of failure to obtain amniotic fluid should both be less than 1%. These figures are based on large published studies[7,8,15,22,34] and our personal experience with more than 7000 amnioceneteses.

Fetoscopy and Ultrasound-Guided Needle Aspiration

A tremendous surge of enthusiasm surrounding the use of the fetoscope occurred in the mid-1970s when it was realized that many biochemical disorders, which could not be diagnosed by enzymatic determination of amniotic fluid cells, could be determined by fetal blood sampling or biopsy of fetal organs, such as skin or liver. For example, there are multiple molecular defects that can cause the clinical picture of beta-thalassemia. While the majority of beta-thalassemia types can be detected antenatally by the molecular techniques described in the previous chapter, at present, the diagnosis of several of them requires direct blood analysis.[12,23] To a greater extent than with amniocentesis, the morbidity of the fetoscopy and ultrasound needle aspiration procedure is directly related to the experience of the operator. Fetal mortality from both procedures has fallen dramatically from the 10% range to less than 3% to 5% or lower in the most experienced hands.[12]

Although the development of molecular techniques has reduced the number of applications for fetoscopy, it is anticipated that the fetoscope or ultrasound-guided needle biopsy will continue to be used in four principle areas: fetal blood transfusion for Rh disease, fetal skin or other organ biopsy when histologic diagnosis is necessary, specific organ tissue retrieval for enzymatic study of organ-specific conditions (prior to the isolation of a gene probe), and visualization of the fetus for other indications (*e.g.*, polydactyly in Ellis van Creveld syndrome).[11]

Ultrasound guided sampling of cord blood during the second and third trimesters may be useful,[18,25] particularly in cases when rapid analysis is desirable in order to permit timely decisions regarding therapy or pregnancy termination. A specimen of fetal blood may permit a karyotype within a few days when there is not time to wait for conventional culture of amniotic fluid cells. When fetal demise is anticipated, a cord blood specimen can be obtained prior to fetal tissue necrosis that would preclude laboratory analysis. Alternatively, a placental biopsy can also be obtained by the same techniques as transabdominal chorionic villus sampling. Using direct preparation methods, a karyotype can be available within 24–48 hours.

For fetal therapy, ultrasound-guided fetal cord puncture has been particularly useful for intravascular transfusion of the isoimmunized fetus.[4,13] In cases that are potentially salvageable, the possible high risks of the procedure need to be considered in comparison to the anticipated benefits.[2]

PROBLEMS RAISED BY PRENATAL DIAGNOSTIC TECHNIQUES

PROBLEM 1

Should the generally trained obstetrician perform amniocentesis for prenatal diagnosis or refer to a subspecialist?

Graduates of obstetrics and gynecology residency training programs are expected to be familiar with both sonography and amniocentesis. However, these physicians are neither expected nor required to be expert at these techniques. Because of variability in personal aptitude and experience, individual obstetricians will vary considerably in their skill in performing amniocentesis. This has created a situation which favors referral of prenatal diagnosis patients when a skilled consultant is easily available and when the interaction among the patient, primary physician, and consultant does not undermine the relationship between the patient and her primary physician.

This issue of technical skill is part of the general expertise issue that always confronts any new, generally trained obstetrician-gynecologist. How can the new graduate be expert enough at anything to compete with an established practitioner? The feature that tends to distinguish amniocentesis from other procedures commonly performed during pregnancy is the perception of risk to the fetus. Fetal death or injury is a distinct endpoint for procedure-related hazard. In discussing the risks and benefits of an elective procedure, both patient and physician recognize the need to maximize safety for the fetus, particularly because the overwhelming majority of pregnancies tested will be normal.

Consultants who specialize in amniocentesis are sometimes, but not necessarily, board-certified in maternal-fetal medicine or medical genetics. There are not enough maternal-fetal medicine or medical genetics physicians in the United States to perform all the amniocentesis procedures indicated for the population, if the test were requested each time its use were appropriate. Thus, the generally trained obstetrician-gynecologist in many areas of the United States must be expected to perform amniocentesis when indicated in order to meet the needs of the pregnant women under his or her care.

PROBLEM 2

Who should have amniocentesis for prenatal diagnosis?

No pregnant woman is required to have an amniocentesis. However, the generally accepted standard of care requires the obstetrician to offer amniocentesis (or a referral to a consultant) if there is a medical indication for the test and if the diagnosis of pregnancy has been made in a timely manner. Medical indications for amniocentesis for prenatal diagnosis include the following:

Maternal age of 35 years or greater at the expected date of confinement
Previously diagnosed chromosomal abnormality in either parent or a prior child
Couples known to be at risk for a mendelian disorder that can be diagnosed in the fetus
Previous neural tube defects (see Chapter 3, Section 1) or abnormal maternal serum alpha-fetoprotein

While there are areas of controversy and indecision related to each medical indication for amniocentesis, there is a broader question related to general use of the procedure that should be considered first. Many obstetricians have asked, If amniocentesis is extremely safe, why not offer the test to any pregnant woman who wants it? For many years the main reason for a negative answer has been the limited number of laboratory facilities available to process the specimens.

Over time more laboratories have become active in amniotic fluid cytogenetic testing, so that in some areas of the country amniocentesis can now be offered for prenatal diagnosis to any pregnant woman who wants the test and can afford it. Medical insurance policies with obstetric benefits will pay at least part of the cost of prenatal diagnosis if there is a medical indication. The great majority of medical insurance policies do not cover purely elective amniocenteses.

In this situation, in which personal economics are in part replacing medical indications, it is important for those performing amniocentesis for prenatal diagnosis to continue to monitor the availability of the procedure for those individuals who in fact have a medical indication for diagnosis. It would be morally unacceptable to deny service to patients with medical indications because of too many already scheduled patients with only a personal preference indication.

When considering age as an indication for prenatal cytogenetic diagnosis, paternal age is also given some note. Maternal age was the original indication based on accumulated data that showed an increasing frequency of children born with Down's syndrome in relation to maternal age.[19,20] Subsequent data have suggested paternal age may be an additional risk factor but one given less statistical weight than maternal age.[17] In clinical practice, paternal age of 55 or greater has been considered by some centers to be a sufficient reason to offer prenatal diagnosis.

If "previously diagnosed cytogenetic abnormality" is the indication for prenatal diagnosis, these subsets of risk are also included in order of greatest risk:

- Those cases in which either parent has an abnormality. If the mother is a carrier of a group D/G balanced robertsonian translocation, her empiric risk for having a cytogenetically abnormal fetus is 10% to 15%; if the father has the translocation, the yield of cytogenetic abnormalities in the offspring is approximately 2%.[22,23] Risk figures for reciprocal translocation carriers are similar for female and male carriers.[27] Specific risks are generally unknown due to little or no accumulated and reported experience; however, the overall frequency of abnormal offspring has been estimated to be about 13% to 14% in a reciprocal translocation carrier.[27]
- Those parents who are known or expected to be cytogenetically normal, and the woman has had a chromosomal trisomy in a prior pregnancy. In clinical practice these women are given a recurrence risk for a cytogenetically abnormal pregnancy of 1% to 2% irrespective of maternal age. For women under age 30 this represents a significantly increased risk, but not for older mothers.[22] Some women may have a predisposing tendency to nondisjunction other than that related to age and chance alone. Women in this category are expected to receive reassurance of a cytogenetically normal pregnancy in the vast majority of cases, and prenatal diagnosis is offered explicitly for that purpose.
- In the lowest risk group, individuals whose prior pregnancy was affected by Turner syndrome (45,X) or by clinical speculation rather than proof of a cytogenetic disorder. Turner syndrome is not associated with advanced maternal age, and recurrence risks are considered low but unknown.[31] These women can be offered prenatal diagnosis for reassurance, if a high degree of safety can be expected.

In considering prenatal diagnosis for mendelian disorders, concern arises because of the inability to make an exact diagnosis because the basic biochemical defect of a disorder is unknown. Historically, for those X-linked recessive disorders, such as Duchenne muscular dystrophy (DMD), for which specific DNA diagnosis of the disease was not available, it was customary to offer prenatal diagnosis for sex alone. Abortion could then be performed on male fetuses, knowing that 50% of the aborted males would be normal. Recent advances in linkage studies have made it possible to predict the presence of several X-linked disorders more accurately.

Prenatal diagnosis and carrier detection

for DMD has been reported by Bakker and colleagues[1] using DNA marker loci on the short arm of the X chromosome. In 75% of patients a highly reliable diagnosis could be made. Conclusive results about the DMD status of the fetus or carrier mother could not be determined in all cases because of several limitations inherent to linkage analysis with restriction fragment length polymorphisms (RFLPs). These limitations included recombination between the marker and DMD loci, lack of informativeness of markers, and inability to identify the DMD X chromosome when neither an affected male nor healthy male sibling were available for DNA analysis. Prenatal diagnosis for these families had to be dependent on diagnosis of sex alone, as in the past. These limitations point out the importance of obtaining and storing DNA from living members affected with a potentially diagnosable mendelian disorder who may die prior to another conception.

Cystic fibrosis (CF) is a common autosomal recessive disorder for which an in utero diagnostic technique has long been sought. Every biochemical attempt at prenatal diagnosis of homozygotes has been hampered by problems of sensitivity and specificity of laboratory tests used.[6,24,32] False-positive diagnoses can lead to abortion of normal fetuses while false negatives can lead to birth of an affected child. Analysis of amniotic fluid intestinal enzymes has a reported accuracy of 96.5% with a false-positive rate of 1.4% and false-negative rate of 2.2%.[24] Prenatal diagnosis using DNA linkage analysis has recently become possible using the RFLPs on chromosome 7 thought to be closely linked to the CF loci.[26] Yet, accuracy again is limited, since molecular analysis is dependent on linked DNA polymorphisms and not the actual cystic fibrosis gene. Midtrimester diagnosis of CF which employs both the DNA technology and the biochemical approach with microvillar enzymes may increase the accuracy of prenatal diagnosis.

Presymptomatic testing for late-onset, autosomal-dominant disorders, such as Huntington's chorea and adult-onset polycystic kidney disease, is becoming available with the use of linked genetic markers.[16,28] These advances will allow prenatal diagnosis for these disorders to become technically possible. The option of pregnancy termination can be considered if an at-risk individual desires to have children free of the disease. This situation is significantly different from genetic diseases lethal in childhood or adolescence such as Tay Sachs, CF, and DMD. Termination of a fetus determined to be a carrier of the Huntington's gene would mean the abortion of an individual with the potential for decades of normal productive life prior to the onset of the disease.[5] Despite the great emotional burden that is part of the decision to terminate potential life of the fetus because of disease in the parent, the freedom to choose to terminate a pregnancy was established by the Roe v. Wade Supreme Court decision. Some parents may consider the use of selective abortions as the peak of social responsibility in order that their offspring not repeat the transmission of Huntington's chorea.

The results of maternal serum alpha-fetoprotein (MSAFP) testing can lead to a medically indicated amniocentesis. High MSAFP may mean that a fetal neural tube defect is present. (Issues related to high MSAFP are discussed in Chapter 3, Section 1.) Many centers are also using very low MSAFP as an indication for amniocentesis to look for cytogenetic disorders. Retrospective studies have shown that babies with chromosomal trisomies identified at birth had lower MSAFP measurements than did controls.[9,10,21] It is not known at this time what the degree of predictive value will be for using low MSAFP to predict trisomy in the fetus. However, on an investigational basis, the level of MSAFP obtained at 14 to 16 weeks has been used to adjust the patient's specific statistical risk given in pre-amniocentesis counseling regarding possible fetal trisomy.

PROBLEM 3

Should amniocentesis be offered for elective sex selection?

In clinical practice, some patients request elective sex diagnosis of the fetus in order to fashion their family by choice rather than chance. Reasons given include the desire to balance the sex distribution in a small family, or to have a child of the opposite sex after a series of children all of the same sex. There is also a strong male preference in certain ethnic groups.

Set against the selection wishes of individual parents is the concept of the generally perceived greater good for society. It is thought to be undesirable for any society to be composed of a preponderance of males or females. It could be argued that widespread availability of sex selection might force government regulation of the process in order to maintain social balance. Also, as a part of the greater good is contemporary American society's view of elective abortion as sexual discrimination. Many are opposed to discrimination based on sex. Loss of the potential life of a human fetus based merely on sex can be construed as a more violent act of discrimination than any of the currently debated and litigated acts that involve adults.

PROBLEM 4

Should the prospect of abortion be linked to pre-amniocentesis counseling?

When amniocentesis for prenatal genetic diagnosis was first being introduced, some centers made the technique available only to patients who agreed in advance to have an abortion if the laboratory testing indicated that an abnormality was present. However, upon reflection, it is obvious that a pre-amniocentesis agreement to have an abortion cannot be binding on the pregnant woman weeks later. Furthermore, heavy emphasis on abortion during pre-amniocentesis counseling can serve to heighten the patient's emotional tension needlessly, since only a few patients in every 100 will need to actually confront the abortion option at a time weeks removed from the original counseling. At the George Washington University, abortion is mentioned as an option in the initial patient information and then explained in detail only when directly pertinent to an individual case.

In those cases in which the patient chooses to abort, the secondary dilemma is related to choice of abortion technique. Prostaglandin-urea intraamniotic instillation is a technique that is generally available and relatively safe for the woman. Hysterotomy or hysterectomy for abortion is no longer recommended owing to the significantly higher complication rate when compared to instillation methods. It has been reported that laminaria dilation of the cervix followed by suction evacuation of the uterus may be safer than instillation up to 16 weeks gestation.[14] A few particularly skilled physicians can perform dilation and evacuation abortions safely at more advanced gestations. When this method is available, many patients prefer it in order to avoid the slower instillation techniques that essentially are an induction of labor. Nonetheless, in order to maximize safety for the pregnant woman, it should be reemphasized that the dilation and evacuation abortion technique can cause major pelvic and intraabdominal injuries, particularly if attempted by an unsupervised novice.

Many times it is scientifically desirable to confirm a prenatal diagnosis by studying abortus tissue. When instillation techniques have been used for abortion, there is usually great difficulty in obtaining further information if living cells are required (e.g., for cytogenetic studies); however, instillation techniques are preferred if the scientific goal is to obtain an intact fetus for anatomic dissection. Detailed anatomic studies are highly useful in establishing the data base used in counseling the woman regarding newly discovered cytogenetic rearrangements.

PROBLEM 5

Should prenatal diagnosis be performed after the age of viability has been reached?

With maximal neonatal intensive care technique, an otherwise normal premature human neonate can survive if born from 24 to 26 weeks gestation. A strong factor in selecting the time for routine prenatal diagnosis of genetic disorders is a desire to have the diagnosis made and abortion, if selected, done prior to this time.

Nonetheless, there are circumstances under which third trimester and late second trimester amniocentesis or fetal cord blood sampling for prenatal diagnosis may be recommended. For example, the clinical findings of fetal growth retardation and polyhydramnios are suggestive of trisomy 18 in the fetus. Trisomy 18 is likely to cause severe fetal distress during labor and possibly stillbirth; there is 100% anticipated neonatal mortality. The goal of prenatal diagnosis in this clinical situation is to permit selection of the route of delivery and the plan for neonatal care.[29,30] Knowing that the fetus will not survive, the obstetrician and family might plan to avoid cesarean delivery despite the anticipated detection of fetal heart decelerations. Without knowledge of the diagnosis of trisomy 18, the obstetrician might have advised an intensive antepartum program of fetal testing and maternal bed rest, culminating in a futile cesarean section and leaving the woman with a large scar, a large bill, and no surviving baby for the effort.

A second situation in which late prenatal diagnosis might be considered is the patient for whom fetal therapy is contemplated. If possible, it is desirable to know the cytogenetic status of the fetus before attempting a radical or innovative therapeutic intervention. For instance, an intrauterine shunt for draining of an intracranial sonolucent area would not be done if the fetus were known to have trisomy 13.

As third trimester prenatal diagnosis becomes a more common procedure, it is inevitable that nonfatal disorders such as Turner syndrome (45,X), Klinefelter syndrome (47,XXY), and others will be diagnosed. These cases will present a challenge for counseling and obstetric management. In order to resolve conflicts between the rights of the pregnant woman and the rights of her potential offspring in this situation, legal heirs to Roe v. Wade and Baby Doe may be produced.

REFERENCES

1. Bakker E, Bonten EJ, DeLang LF et al: DNA probe analysis for carrier detection and prenatal diagnosis of Duchenne muscular dystrophy: A standard diagnostic procedure. J Med Genetics 23:573, 1986
2. Benacerraf BR, Barss VA, Saltzman DH et al: Acute fetal distress associated with percutaneous umbilical blood sampling. Am J Obstet Gynecol 156:1218, 1987
3. Benacerraf BR, Frigoletto FD: Amniocentesis under continuous ultrasound guidance: A series of 232 cases. Obstet Gynecol 62:760, 1983
4. Berkowitz RL, Chitkara U, Goldberg JD et al: Intravascular transfusion in utero: The percutaneous approach. Am J Obstet Gynecol 154:622, 1986
5. Bird SJ: Presymptomatic testing for Huntington's disease. JAMA 53:3286, 1985
6. Brock DJH, Bedgood BD, Barron L et al: Prospective prenatal diagnosis of cystic fibrosis. Lancet 1:1175, 1985
7. Crandall BF, Howard J, Lebherz TB et al: Follow-up of 2000 second trimester amnioceteses. Obstet Gynecol 56:625, 1980
8. Cruikshank DP, Varner MW, Cruikshank JE et al: Midtrimester amniocentesis: An analysis of 923 cases with neonatal follow-up. Am J Obstet Gynecol 146:204, 1983
9. Cuckle HS, Wald NJ, Linderbaum RH et al: Maternal serum alpha-fetoprotein measurement: A screening test in Down syndrome. Lancet 1:26, 1984
10. Davis RO, Cosper P, Huddleston JF et al: Decreased levels of amniotic fluid alpha-fetoprotein associated with Down syndrome. Am J Obstet Gynecol 153:541, 1985
11. Elias S, Mazar M, Sabbagha R et al: Prenatal diagnosis of harlequin ichthyosis. Clin Gynecol 17:275, 1980
12. Elias S, Simpson JL et al: Fetoscopy. In Sciarra JJ (ed): Gynecology and Obstetrics, vol 5, pp 1–7. Hagerstown, MD, Harper & Row, 1987
13. Grannum PA, Copel JA, Plaxe SC et al: In utero exchange transfusion in severe erythroblastosis fetalis. N Engl J Med 314:1431, 1986
14. Grimes DA, Schulz K: Morbidity and mortality from second trimester abortions. J Repro Med 30:505, 1985
15. Golbus MS, Loughman WD, Epstein CJ et al: Prenatal genetic diagnosis in 3000 amnioceteses. N Engl J Med 300:157, 1979
16. Gusella JF, Wexler NS, Conneally PM et al: A

polymorphic DNA marker genetically linked to Huntington's disease. Nature 306:234, 1983
17. Hassold TJ, Jacobs PA: Trisomy in man. Ann Rev Genet 18:69, 1974
18. Hobbins JC, Grannum PA, Romero R et al: Percutaneous umbilical blood sampling. Am J Obstet Gynecol 152:1, 1985
19. Hook EB: Rates of chromosome abnormalities at different maternal ages. Obstet Gynecol 58:282, 1981
20. Hook EB, Chambers GM: Estimated rates of Down syndrome in live births by one year maternal age intervals for mothers aged 20–49 in a New York State study. Implications of the risk figures for genetic counseling and cost-benefit analysis by prenatal diagnosis programs. Birth Defects 13(3A):124, 1977
21. Merkatz IR, Nitowsky HM, Macri JM et al: An association between low maternal serum alpha-fetoprotein and fetal chromosome abnormalities. Am J Obstet Gynecol 148:886, 1985
22. Milunsky, A (ed): Genetic Disorders and the Fetus: Diagnosis Prevention, and Treatment, 2nd ed. New York, Plenum Press, 1986
23. Modell B, Ward RHT: Antenatal diagnosis of the hemoglobinopathies. In Rocker I, Lawrence KM (eds): Fetoscopy, pp 87–145. Amsterdam, Elsevier-North Holland, 1981
24. Mulivor RA, Cook D, Muller F et al: Analysis of fetal intestinal enzymes in amniotic fluid for the prenatal diagnosis of cystic fibrosis. Am J Med Genet 40:131, 1987
25. Nicolaides KH, Scothill PW, Rodeck CH et al: Ultrasound-guided sampling of umbilical cord and placenta blood to assess fetal well-being. Lancet 1:1065, 1986
26. Nugent CE, Gravius T, Green P et al: Prenatal diagnosis of cystic fibrosis by chorionic villus sampling using 12 polymorphic DNA markers. Obstet Gynecol 71:213, 1988
27. Petrosky DL, Borgaonkar DS: Segregation analysis in reciprocal translocation carriers. Am J Med Genet 19:137, 1984
28. Reeders ST, Brewing MH, Davies KH et al: A highly polymorphic DNA marker linked to adult polycystic kidney disease on chromosomes 16. Nature 317:542, 1985
29. Rochelson BL, Trunca C, Monheit AG et al: The use of a rapid in situ technique for third-trimester diagnosis of trisomy 18. Am J Obstet Gynecol 155:835, 1986
30. Schneider AS, Mennuti MT, Zackai EH: High cesarean section rate in trisomy 18 births: A potential indication for late prenatal diagnosis. Am J Obstet Gynecol 140:367, 1981
31. Smith DW: Recognizable Patterns of Human Malformations, 3rd ed. New York, WB Saunders, 1982
32. Szabo M, Teichmann F, Szeifert GT et al: Prenatal diagnosis of cystic fibrosis by trehalase enzyme assay in amniotic fluid. Clin Genet 28:16, 1985
33. Therman E: Human Chromosome: Structure Behavior, Effects, 2nd ed. New York, Springer-Verlag, 1986
34. Working paper on amniocentesis: An assessment of the hazards of amniocentesis. Br J Obstet Gynecol (Suppl 2) 85:1, 1978

3

Prenatal Diagnosis of Congenital Malformations

SECTION 1: ALPHA-FETOPROTEIN: MATERNAL SERUM AND AMNIOTIC FLUID ANALYSIS

Mark I. Evans, Robin L. Belsky, Anne Greb, Nancy Clementino, and Frank N. Syner

It has been over 15 years since Brock and Sutcliffe first described the application of amniotic fluid alpha-fetoprotein (AFP) for the diagnosis of neural tube defects (NTDs).[6] In the ensuing years, the measurement of AFP has evolved from a technique for the diagnosis of recurrent NTD in a very limited group of patients to a mass screening test for the entire prenatal population. While readily accepted in the United Kingdom and much of Europe by the mid- to late 1970s, political and emotional conflicts have retarded use of this valuable diagnostic screening technique in the United States.

It was only in 1983 when the U.S. Food and Drug Administration (FDA) finally permitted the release of test kits for maternal serum alpha-fetoprotein (MSAFP) measurements that the test became widespread. It was also in 1983 that the discovery of the association of low serum values with an increased risk of aneuploidy added an entirely new dimension to the application of AFP.[12,30] In this chapter we shall discuss the historical perspective of AFP screening and its more recent application to the detection of chromosome abnormalities.

DETECTION OF NEURAL TUBE DEFECTS

Incidence and Recurrence

The spectrum of NTDs, including anencephaly and spina bifida, comprises one of the most serious, common group of malformations observed in newborn infants. The overall incidence of NTDs is approximately 1 in 600 to 1 in 1000 in the United States, which is higher than the incidence of Down syndrome, a genetic disorder for which there is routine prenatal screening for patients considered at risk. The incidence of NTDs varies markedly, depending upon both the ethnic group, the geographic location, and socioeconomic status of the pregnant female.[23] The world's highest observed incidence rates are seen in Northern Ireland, where it is approximately 8 per 1000 births. For couples of Irish descent who have migrated to the United States, (best studied in New England), their risk is approximately halved. Japanese in Japan have one of the lowest rates of incidence of NTDs in the world. However, for individuals of Japanese ancestry in Hawaii (who therefore experience at least a partial western diet), the incidence of the disorder is doubled. In the United States, the highest incidence of NTDs is seen among the white, Appalachian population.[23] For any given locale there are marked racial differences between black and white patients.

NTDs follow a multifactorial pattern of inheritance. The risk of recurrence is correlated marginally with overall population rates, and no preconceptual markers are available to predict recurrence with great confidence. In the United States, the risk of recurrence of the defect following one affected child is said to be approximately 3%; in the United Kingdom, it is 5%.[23] Following the birth of two affected children within a family, the risk of a third is said to be about 10% to 20%. However, about 97% of all affected fetuses come from pregnancies not previously suspected to be at risk.[7]

Comparison of the prenatal diagnosis of cytogenetic (chromosomal) abnormalities and NTD reveals several major differences. Until recently the diagnosis of cytogenetic abnormalities was most often sought for patients without a positive family history, but who were defined as a group known to be at increased risk (i.e., due to advanced maternal age). For the prenatal diagnosis of NTD, patients who have had a previously affected child are defined to be at increased risk for recurrence. However, the vast majority of NTD births occur to couples not previously suspected to be at risk. Thus, inherent in a program to detect NTD is the necessity for mass-scale screening of nearly all pregnancies, rather than merely a small subset of the population that is known to be particularly at risk.

Amniotic Fluid AFP Analysis

An oncofetal analog of albumin, AFP is the principle protein in fetal plasma in early gestation.[27] AFP has many structural similarities to albumin but is antigenically distinct. AFP is synthesized by the fetal yolk sac and by the developing fetal liver. After 14 weeks gestation, fetal plasma levels decline as the fetal liver matures and synthesizes albumin. Fetal plasma AFP diffuses into the fetal urine and is excreted into the amniotic fluid. Part of the amniotic fluid AFP passes by diffusion into the maternal circulation via the amnion, while the remainder is swallowed and digested by the fetus.

The concentration of AFP in fetal plasma peaks at 12 to 14 weeks gestation (Figure 3-1), after which levels fall rapidly.[14,27] The levels in amniotic fluid parallel those in fetal plasma (Figure 3-2 and Table 3-1), but at about 1/200 the fetal plasma concentration. In contrast, MSAFP concentrations increase geometrically until 30 weeks gestation and then decline (Figure 3-3). Following birth, AFP levels in the mother and newborn fall rapidly, and by 6 months postpartum are at levels less than 10 mg/ml.

In 1972, the application of amniotic fluid AFP analysis to the detection of NTD was made by Brock and Sutcliffe.[6] They observed that fetuses with a communicating NTD such as anencephaly or meningomyelocele, had elevated levels of AFP in their amniotic fluid. Usually these elevations would be four to five standard deviations above the normal gestational age–adjusted median. However, given the large gradation of AFP levels between fetal serum and amniotic fluid, a very slight

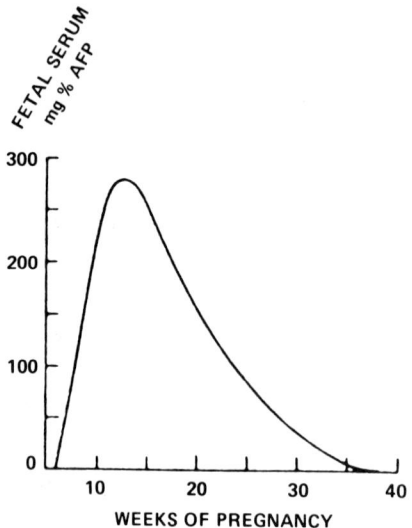

FIGURE 3-1. Fetal serum concentrations of alpha-fetoprotein showing peak concentrations at about 12 to 14 weeks.

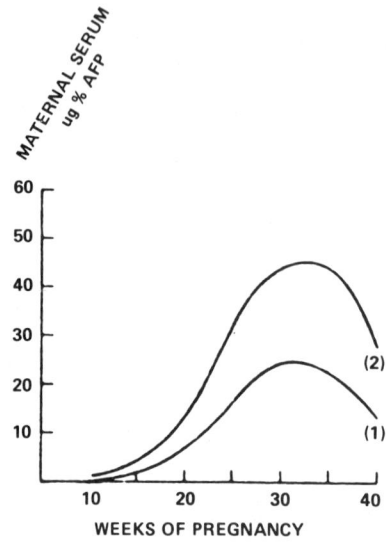

FIGURE 3-3. Maternal serum AFP levels rise into the third trimesters and then fall. (Median = 1, 95th percentile = 2)

fetal bleed could profusely affect the measurement of amniotic fluid AFP levels. Thus, a bloody amniocentesis could generate considerable confusion with regard to a diagnosis.

Fortunately, recent advances in methodology have increased the reliability of the diagnosis. In 1979, a relatively specific neural protein, acetylcholinesterase (ACHE) was discovered.[2,34] ACHE is found in the amniotic fluid when a NTD or abdominal wall defect is present. The addition of ACHE testing to the prenatal diagnosis of NTD has made the incidence of false-positive testing extremely small. Approximately 1 in 300 patients or fewer having an amniocentesis for AFP plus

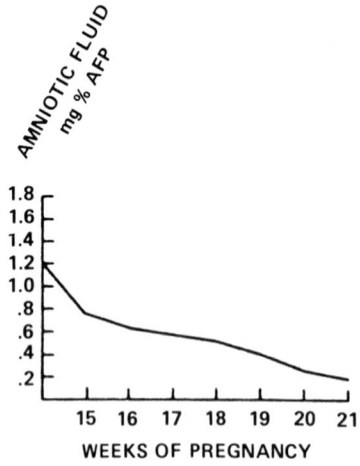

FIGURE 3-2. Amniotic fluid AFP levels fall with increasing gestational age.

Table 3-1. Maternal Serum and Amniotic Fluid Alpha-Fetoprotein Values

Weeks	Maternal Serum Median (ng/ml)	Amniotic Fluid Median (ng/ml)
15	24.1	16.8
16	30.1	13.4
17	33.4	11.2
18	41.5	9.09
19	48.0	8.13
20	55.5	6.62

(Wayne State University, Detroit, Michigan)

ACHE analysis (or about 1 in 20,000 from a serum screening program) will have a false-positive result.[2,9,10] ACHE has traditionally been interpreted as positive or negative. However, recently we have observed inconclusive results that represent a true but faint band. The implications of this finding depend upon gestational age. In early pregnancy (<15 weeks) approximately 10% of all ACHE will be inconclusive. Of this 10%, 15% will have a significant fetal abnormality. In later pregnancy only 3% will be inconclusive, but of these, 50% will have a significant malformation.

Some groups have proposed that ACHE analysis could replace AFP analysis.[35] However, most groups believe that AFP analysis should remain the primary test, with ACHE used concomitantly in cases of either an elevated AFP or a suspected anomaly.

Elevated levels of amniotic fluid AFP have also been found in conjunction with several other serious disorders such as omphalocele/gastroschisis, fetal death, and Turner syndrome[9,10]:

Congenital skin defects
Conjoined twins
Duodenal atresia
Exstrophy of cloaca
Tetralogy of Fallot
Fetal teratoma
Gastroschisis
Haemangioma of umbilical cord
Hydrocephalus
Meckel syndrome
Nuchal bleb
Oesophageal atresia
Osteogenesis imperfecta
Pilonidal sinus
Rh-isoimmunization
Turner syndrome

ACHE in amniotic fluid is elevated with some of these disorders. In most, a transudation of fetal blood or serum into the amniotic fluid can be hypothesized as a cause of the elevation.

Another identified high-risk group has been those patients who have an elevated amniotic fluid AFP, but a negative ACHE. The diagnosis of defects such as congenital nephrosis and omphalocele may arise in this group.[4] These can usually be identified through ultrasound examination. However, recent data have suggested that, for a large proportion of these patients with elevated AFP and negative ACHE, no fetal pathology will be observed.[37] However, another large segment of this population will suffer intrauterine demises with no known etiology.

Maternal Serum AFP Analysis

Despite the documented ability of amniotic fluid levels of AFP to predict serious NTD, it is clearly impossible to suggest that all women undergo amniocentesis for this diagnosis. Various collaborative studies have assessed the risk of amniocentesis over the past decade and have suggested an increased risk of abortion of 0.2% to 1% over background spontaneous abortion rates (about 2%–3% at 16 to 17 weeks).[19,31] Most authorities now believe that with the use of real-time ultrasound-guided needle entry, the risks in experienced hands are closer to the lower end of the spectrum.[26] While amniocentesis is a very safe procedure in experienced hands, the risk of the procedure is still greater than the overall incidence of the disease, and the cost to the medical system if all pregnant women required this procedure would be staggering.

Given that 97% of all NTD occur to couples not previously considered at risk, and since amniocentesis cannot be routinely performed on all patients, it follows that a screening test that could easily test all pregnancies would be very beneficial in identifying high-risk pregnancies. While amniotic fluid AFP measurements are necessary for the diagnosis of NTDs, a screening test which could limit the number of patients requiring invasive testing would have important public health and economic impact by increasing the detection and reducing the incidence of NTD.

In 1973, Brock, Bolton, and Monagham demonstrated that fetal AFP passes through the placenta and can be measured in the mother's serum.[5] As the pregnancy progresses, even in the second trimester, MSAFP levels increase[29] (see Table 3-1). A fetus with an open NTD will usually cause higher than normal amounts of AFP in maternal serum. Therefore, measurements of MSAFP can be used to identify the population of high-risk patients who require further testing, such as ultrasound and amniocentesis.

Threshold Values

Much debate and scientific study have surrounded the issue of establishing AFP threshold values for required further testing. Unlike amniotic fluid in which there is usually a wide differentiation between normal and abnormal values, MSAFP values are in three overlapping distributions of normal, open spina bifida, and anencephaly curves (Figure 3-4). It is well appreciated that the lower the threshold for proceeding to further testing, the higher the detection of affected fetuses, and the lower the sensitivity of the screening (i.e., many more false-positives). Thus, moving the threshold to the right (i.e., higher) will increase the proportion of abnormal fetuses detected among those chosen for invasive testing. Still, there will be many abnormal fetuses in the population who do not exceed the threshold and who will be missed. Moving the threshold to the left (i.e., lower) will increase the absolute number of abnormal fetuses detected, but will also increase the number of normal fetuses subjected to invasive and expensive tests to assess their status.

After several years of testing in multiple centers throughout the world, but particularly in the United Kingdom, a fairly standard testing protocol for the management of high MSAFPs was devised[36] (Figure 3-5). Because of variation between centers, it remains critical that each screening center have its own values. Since the curves do not always follow a statistically accepted normal distribution, nonparametric statistics were employed. An upper threshold point of 2.5 multiples of the median (MOM) gestational age of the individual population has been commonly used by most centers as the cut-off point for further testing. The 2.5 MOM cut-off is an arbitrary compromise to achieve a high yield of anomalies with exceptionally few false-positives.

Using these guidelines, of 1000 hypothetical women, approximately 5% will have an elevated MSAFP on the first test. The protocol requires that this blood testing be repeated in all cases of elevated values. Approximately 3% of the original population will have an elevated MSAFP twice. These patients are then referred for an immediate ultrasound to confirm gestational age and to search for the presence of another factor that might explain the elevated results. Exceptions can be warranted for going on immediately to ultrasound and possible amniocentesis following extremely high values (e.g., 5 MOM or more) or when gestational age approaches the cut-off point for offering termination in the particular jurisdiction.

Since MSAFP analysis is dependent upon accurate dating of the pregnancy, a more advanced gestational age than originally thought may explain a seeming elevation. In many centers with ready access to ultrasound, this second serum test may be performed after ultrasonic validation of

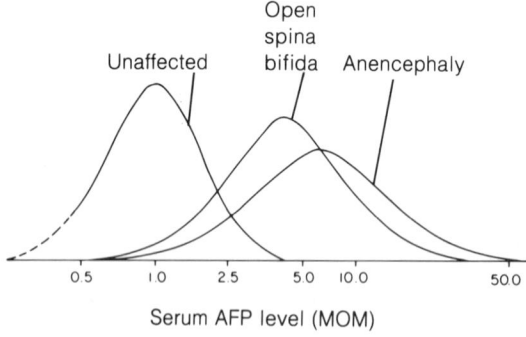

FIGURE 3-4. Overlapping distributions of maternal serum AFP values in normal, open spina bifida, and anencephalic pregnancies. (MOM, multiples of median)

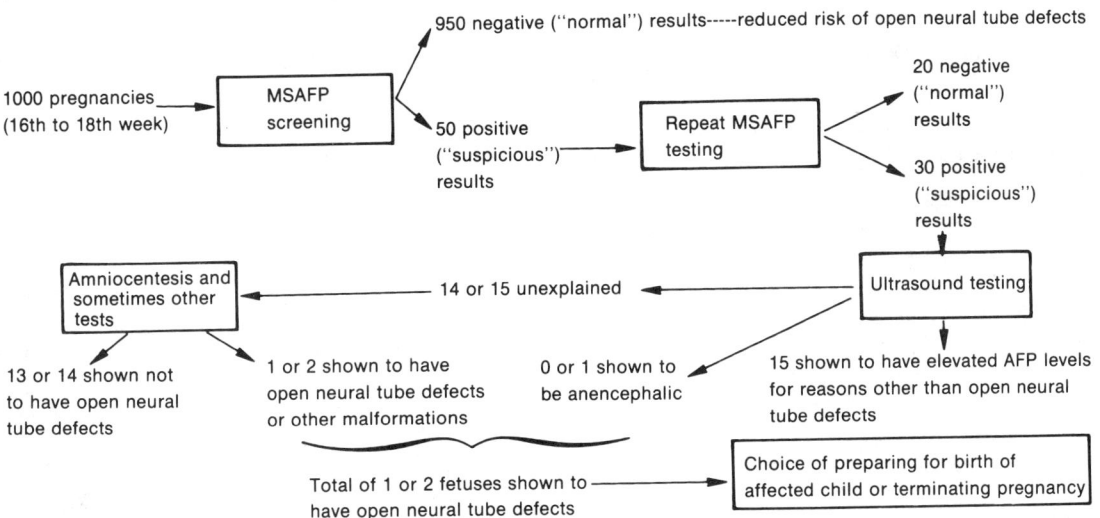

FIGURE 3-5. Flow chart shows course of 1000 hypothetical patients evaluated for neural tube defects (prior to advent of "low" for chromosomal anomalies). Of 1000 patients, 15 will have an indication for amniocentesis. The numbers of the chart are those expected if at each stage all women remaining in the high-risk category choose to undergo further testing.

dates. The presence of twins or other anomalies can also cause elevated MSAFP values. Levels are also known to be increased in fetal demise, multiple gestation, abdominal wall defects, and impending miscarriage.[29]

If, following two elevated MSAFPs and an ultrasound, no obvious reason for the elevations is found, a genetic amniocentesis is then recommended. Depending upon the exact patient population studied (i.e., the incidence of NTDs in the population) anywhere between 5% to 10% of such amniocenteses will be positive, suggesting a NTD or other significant anomaly such as ventral wall defect.

About 90% to 95% of amniocentesis specimens will have levels of AFP within the normal range for gestational age, and the cause of the elevated MSAFP will not be understood. Data from several sources have suggested that such patients may be at higher than background risk for having either preterm delivery or intrauterine growth retardation.[20] It is possible that the elevated MSAFP represents early placental dysfunction and could potentially be used as a marker for high-risk pregnancies.

Factors Affecting MSAFP Values

Several determinants are now known to affect serum levels. Probably the most important is maternal weight.[24] There is an inverse relationship between maternal weight and MSAFP, which is not surprising since a given amount of AFP is produced by the fetal liver. When distributed over a bigger mother, the resulting fetal concentration will be less. In our population prior to weight correlation, we observed tremendous variation in the percentage of cases considered outside the normal range at both high and low extremes of maternal weight. With correction, the discrepancies disappeared. Likewise, we have seen significant variation in median values between the two populations our program serves through two different laboratories. Despite the blind screening of samples showing only 2% to 4% variation in individual results, median values vary about 10% between a predominantly black, low-income population in Detroit, and a suburban, mostly white, middle-class population, which has led us to use different curves for black and white patients[3,17] (Table 3-2).

Table 3-2. Variation in Median MSAFP Values by Race

	\multicolumn{6}{c}{Weeks in Gestation}
	15	16	17	18	19	20
White or Other	26.1	29.3	32.3	38.0	43.1	44.4
Black	25.8	30.8	33.2	45.1	48.1	56.7

Blacks have MSAFP values as much as 20% higher at certain gestational ages. Failure to account for this variation could result in an excess of white patients with "low" values and blacks with "high" values.[17] Diabetic patients show decreased levels of MSAFP, for which adjustments need to be made.[31,36] Twins show approximately twice singleton values and also require adjustment.

DETECTION OF CHROMOSOME ANOMALIES

Within the past few years an entirely new application of MSAFP has emerged. Speculation about the meaning of low MSAFPs has been noted for years with the general consensus that it merely was an indication of too early gestation, nonpregnancy, or possibly trophoblastic disease.[7,13,14,25] In 1984, Merkatz and co-workers suggested that in the absence of any other indication, a low MSAFP may be correlated with a higher than expected incidence of chromosomal aneuploidy.[30] Other groups, including ours, have since confirmed these findings.

As MSAFP screening has become commonplace, many small laboratories with limited databases have entered the business creating concerns for quality control. We have found in the Detroit metropolitan area 15 laboratories whose medians vary by as much as 50% and whose use of correction factors varies widely.[18] Physicians utilizing MSAFP screening should be cognizant of these issues because they will impact the sensitivity and specificity of screening and ultimately could become entangled in the legal process.

As with the elevated MSAFP values, however, the threshold below which further testing is recommended is quite controversial. It has taken several studies for a concensus about the reliability of this screening to even begin to emerge. Initially, a low threshhold of 0.25 MOM was proposed which would define about 1% of the population. We felt such a low threshold defines too limited a population. Several groups, including ours, then tried 0.4 or 0.5 MOM with a 5% to 10% yield of "low" values. Empirically, since the a priori risk of aneuploidy is maternal age–dependent and the effort is designed to achieve a given even risk, then the MOM threshold should vary with maternal age. Hershey, Crandall, and Perdue were the first to publish an extrapolation of the prospect of MSAFP and maternal age risk.[22] We have slightly modified their slope and included data from Wald, and now use a weight-adjusted MOM with differing lower thresholds by maternal age (Table 3-3).

Considerable debate exists as to the efficiency of low level testing. Published data re-

Table 3-3. Adjusted Lower Thresholds Approximating Risk of a 35-Year-Old

Maternal Age	MOM
19–24	0.40
25–26	0.45
27–29	0.50
30	0.60
31	0.65
32	0.70
33	0.75
34	0.80
35	1.00

port a mean MOM for Down's syndrome of 0.72 and have suggested that 20% of aneuploidy might be detectable.[14] Others have speculated a somewhat higher pick-up rate.[34] Extrapolation of existing data is subject to many variables including the specific assay system and cut-off points. Debate will continue for several years before a best cut-off point or equation can be achieved.

The protocol to manage low MSAFP values is slightly altered from that following an elevated MSAFP value. The current prevailing opinion is that no repeat blood test is done and that the patient should proceed to ultrasound examination (for validation of the pregnancy dating), genetic counseling, and possible amniocentesis (to detect chromosomal abnormalities).[21] Depending upon the specific protocol used, approximately 3% to 8% of women screened through AFP analysis will have a low value, thus establishing a new application for the old protocol[17,33] (Figure 3-6). After ultrasound, approximately 70% of this group will have no obvious explanation for the low value; the low value must be believed and counseling and amniocentesis offered.

In our program we have seen an aneuploidy detection ratio of about 1%, mostly for women age 30 or younger, which is roughly comparable to other published results. This is consistent with our results for 35-year-olds and is slightly below the 2.2% seen overall in our advanced maternal age population.

The potential benefits of mass screening for chromosomal abnormalities are obvious.

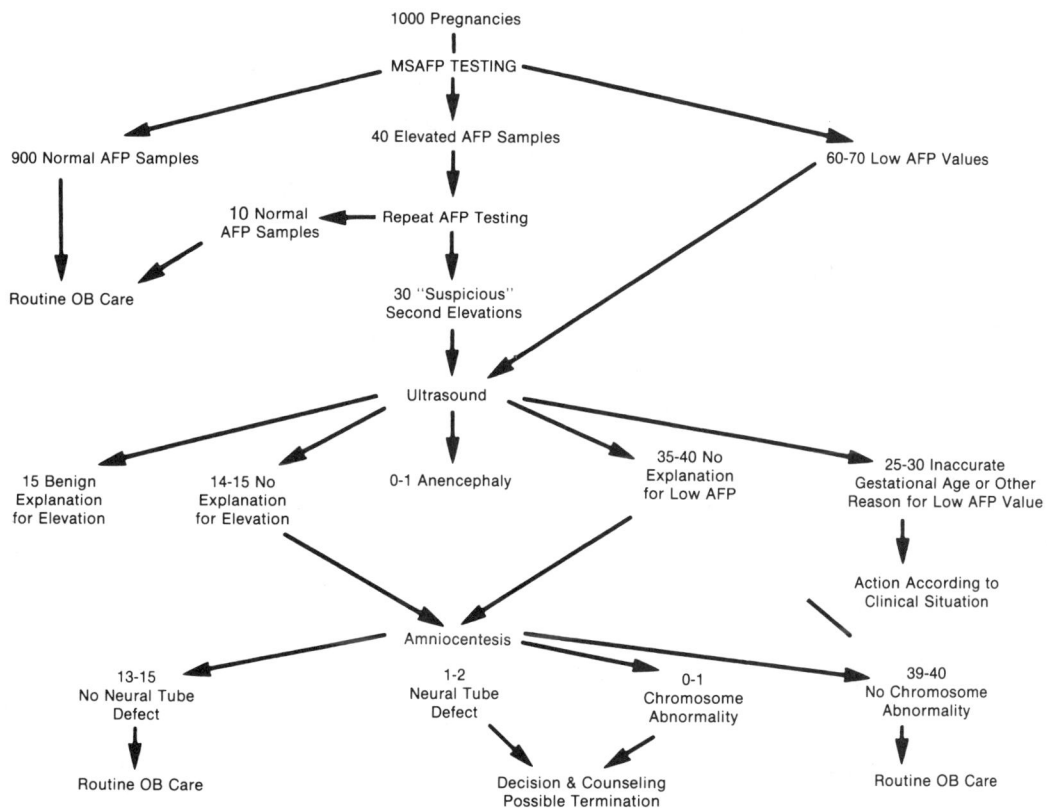

FIGURE 3-6. New MSAFP protocol including low MSAFP arm.

Currently, only about 12% of Down's syndrome fetuses are detected prenatally. Low MSAFPs allow women under age 35 who would not ordinarily be offered prenatal testing to be separated into a high-risk group who can be offered testing. It still remains to be seen whether this screening will be economical on a cost-benefit basis. While data on NTDs are convincing on this point, however, the costs of karyotyping far exceeds those of AFP and ACHE assays. Yet, since current data show detection rates comparable to the advanced maternal age population, we believe the economics as well as public health and parents' wishes will support testing. Our own experience suggests that low MSAFP values will detect enough chromosomal abnormalities to make this testing very beneficial.

THE FUTURE

MSAFP screening gained rapid acceptance in the United Kingdom and became an integral part of their obstetric care programs by the mid-seventies. The introduction of such screening, along with better ultrasound devices has profoundly reduced the incidence of NTDs in the United Kingdom, and the system appears to be cost beneficial.[11] In the United States, intense debate has continued for several more years, encompassing not only scientific but political, legal, and theological issues. Despite petitions by several pharmaceutical firms to the FDA as early as 1977, it was only in 1983 that the FDA agreed to allow test kits for MSAFP to become generally available. What statistics have been available on United States data have until now generally been generated by a relatively small number of large centers; however, such data have mimicked the results seen in the United Kingdom. Massive data from California's mandatory offering of MSAFP have confirmed all expectations.

The arguments against MSAFP screening have centered on the reliability of test procedures, access to follow-up testing, and the inevitable abortion arguments.[8,28] While it remains to be proven that mass utilization of the screening technique will have results equal to those seen in the United Kingdom, there is really very little reason to suspect that such will not be the case.

A final argument is the medicolegal risk. The American College of Obstetricians and Gynecologists warned its membership in May 1985 that failure to screen for NTDs, at the least, would likely be a probable cause for malpractice litigation if a child were born with an identifiable defect.[1] Such lawsuits have begun to emerge, and they will be undoubtedly more numerous in the future.

Delivery of MSAFP services has been subject to many pitfalls. With the emerging explosion of demand for MSAFP testing, many small laboratories have jumped into the business without establishing thorough protocols and reformed patterns. In the Detroit metropolitan area we have investigated variations in normal MSAFP values and handling of results from several laboratories. Even in the same area, there is as much as 50% variation in so-called normal values, and most small laboratories do not use any adjustments such as maternal weight, age, or race for computation risks. Such inconsistencies and lack of attention to detail may ultimately give MSAFP screenings an undeserved bad name.

On many occasions, we have had to deal with extremely distraught patients who have been given misleading and inaccurate information. Unfortunately, it is often impossible for any university program to coordinate a large, expert outreach program. We have addressed this issue by forming a collaborative program with a large, reputable commercial laboratory to mold a comprehensive approach of a commercial operation with the tertiary center capabilities of a keynote genetic center.[17] We speculate that similar collaboration efforts will become more common in the future as the need grows for "tertiary center technology" to be disseminated on a wider population basis.

REFERENCES

1. American College of Obstetricians and Gynecologists, Department of Professional Liability: Professional Liability Implications of AFP Tests, May, 1985
2. Amniotic fluid acetylcholinesterase electrophoresis as a secondary test in the diagnosis of anencephaly and open spina bifida in early pregnancy. Report of a collaborative study. Lancet 2:321, 1981
3. Baumgarten A: Racial difference and biological significance of maternal serum alpha-fetoprotein. Lancet 2:573, 1986
4. Brock DJH: The Early Diagnosis of Fetal Defects. Edinburgh, Churchill Livingstone, 1982
5. Brock DJH, Bolton AE, Monagham JM: Prenatal diagnosis of anencephaly through maternal serum alpha-fetoprotein measurements. Lancet 2:923, 1973
6. Brock DJH, Sutcliffe: Alpha-fetoprotein in antenatal diagnosis of anencephaly and spina bifida. Lancet 2:197, 1972
7. Collaborative study of Down syndrome using maternal serum alpha-fetoprotein and maternal age. Lancet 2:1460, 1986
8. Council on Scientific Affairs: Maternal serum alpha-fetoprotein monitoring. JAMA 247:1478, 1982
9. Crandall BF, Matsumoto M: Routine amniotic fluid alpha-fetoprotein in 34,000 pregnancies. Am J Obstet Gynecol 149:744, 1984
10. Crandall BF, Matsumoto M: Routine amniotic fluid alpha-fetoprotein assay: Experience with 40,000 pregnancies. Am J Med Genetics 24:143, 1986
11. Cuckle H, Wald N: The impact of screening for open neural tube defects in England and Wales. Prenatal Diagnosis 7:91, 1987
12. Cuckle HS, Wald NJ, Lindenbaum RH: Maternal serum alpha-fetoprotein measurement: A screening test for Down syndrome. Lancet 1:926, 1984
13. Davenport DM, Macri JN: The clinical significance of low maternal serum alpha-fetoprotein. Am J Obstet Gynecol 146:657, 1983
14. Doran TA, Cadesky K, Wong PY et al: Maternal serum alpha-fetoprotein and fetal autosomal trisomies. Am J Obstet Gynecol 154:277, 1986
15. Drusan A, Syder FN, Greb A, Evans MI: Amniotic fluid alphafetoprotein and acetylcholinesterase in early genetic amniocentesis. Obstet Gynecol 72:35, 1988
16. Drusan A, Syder FN, Belsky R et al: Amniotic fluid acetylcholinesterase: Implications of an inconclusive result. Am J Obstet Gynecol (in press)
17. Evans MI, Belsky RL, Clementino NA et al: Establishment of a collaborative university-commercial MSAFP screening program. A model for tertiary center outreach. Am J Obstet Gynecol 161:1441, 1987
18. Evans MI, Belsky RL, Greb AE et al: Wide variation in maternal serum alpha-fetoprotein reports in one metropolitan area. Concerns for the quality of prenatal testing. Obstet Gynecol (in press)
19. Golbus MS, Loughman WD, Epstein CJ et al: Prenatal genetic diagnosis in 3000 amniocenteses. N Engl J Med 300:157, 1979
20. Haddow JE, Palomaki GE, Knight GJ: Can low birth weight after elevated maternal serum alpha-fetoprotein be explained by maternal weight. Obstet Gynecol 70:26, 1987
21. Haddow JE, Palomaki GE, Wald N et al: Maternal serum alpha-fetoprotein screening for Down syndrome and repeat testing. Lancet 2:1460, 1986
22. Hershey DW, Crandall BF, Perdue S: Combining maternal age and serum alpha-fetoprotein to predict the risk of Down syndrome. Obstet Gynecol 68:177, 1986
23. Holmes LB: The health problem: Neural tube defects. In Gastel B, Haddow JE, Fletcher JC et al: Maternal Serum Alpha-Fetoprotein: Issues in the Prenatal Screening and Diagnosis of Neural Tube Defects, pp 1–4. US Government Printing Office, 1981
24. Johnson AM, Lingley L: Corrected formula for maternal serum adjustments. Lancet 2:812, 1984
25. Kjessler B, Hemmingson A, Nilsson BA et al: Early diagnosis of trophoblastic disease and fetal maldevelopment by determination of alpha-fetoprotein, human chorionic gonadotropin and amniography. Acta Obstet Gynecol Scand (Suppl)69:83, 1977
26. Larsen JW Jr, MacMillin MD: Prenatal diagnosis of chromosomal and mendelian disorders in the second and third trimester. In Evans MI, Fletcher JL, Dixler AO, Schulman JD (eds): Fetal Diagnosis and Therapy: Science, Ethics, and the Law. Philadelphia, JB Lippincott, 1989
27. Macri JN: Amniotic fluid alpha-fetoprotein evaluation. In Gastel B, Haddow JE, Fletcher JC et al: Maternal Serum Alpha-Fetoprotein:

28. Macri JN, Kasturi RV, Krawtz DA et al: Maternal serum alpha-fetoprotein screening: II. Pitfalls in low volume decentralized laboratory performance. Am J Obstet Gynecol 156:533, 1987
29. Main DM, Mennitu MT: Neural tube defects: Issues in prenatal diagnosis and counseling. Obstet Gynecol 67:1, 1986
30. Merkatz IR, Nitowsky HM, Macri JN et al: An association between low maternal serum alpha-fetoprotein and fetal chromosome abnormalities. Am J Obstet Gynecol 148:886, 1984
31. Milunsky A (ed): Genetic Disorders of the Fetus: Diagnosis, Prevention, and Treatment, 2nd ed. New York, Plenum Press, 1986
32. Milunksy A, Alpert E, Kitzmiller JL et al: Prenatal diagnosis of neural tube defects. VIII. The importance of serum alpha-fetoprotein screening in diabetic pregnant women. Am J Obstet Gynecol 142:1030, 1982
33. Simpson JL, Baum LD, Marder R et al: Maternal serum alpha-fetoprotein screening: Low and high values for detection of genetic abnormalities. Am J Obstet Gynecol 155:593, 1986
34. Smith AD, Wald, NJ, Cuckle HS et al: Amniotic fluid acetylcholinesterase as a possible diagnostic test for neural tube defects in early pregnancy. Lancet 1:685, 1979
35. Toftager-Larsen K, Wandrup J, Norgaard-Pederson B: Amniotic fluid analysis in prenatal diagnosis of neural tube defects: A comparison between six biochemical tests supplementary to the measurements of amniotic fluid alpha-fetoprotein. Clin Genet 26:406, 1984
36. United Kingdom collaborative study on alpha-fetoprotein in relation to neural tube defects: Maternal serum alpha-fetoprotein measurements in antenatal screening for aneuploidy and spina bifida in early pregnancy. Lancet 1:323, 1977
37. Wald NJ: Alpha-fetoprotein. International Symposium in Prenatal Diagnosis and Fetal Treatment, Kings College, London, November 1986

SECTION 2: ETHICAL ISSUES IN MATERNAL SERUM ALPHA-FETOPROTEIN TESTING AND SCREENING: A REAPPRAISAL

LeRoy Walters

Seven years ago I undertook an analysis of ethical issues in maternal serum alphafetoprotein (MSAFP) screening. At that time I discussed four issues:

1. What is the moral status of a fetus or newborn afflicted with a neural tube defect (NTD)?
2. What are the major potential benefits and risks of MSAFP screening?
3. What resource allocation questions are raised by MSAFP screening programs?
4. What issues of freedom and coercion do MSAFP screening programs raise?

These issues bear a striking resemblance to four much-debated topics in contemporary moral philosophy: personhood, beneficence, justice, and autonomy.

At the time of the original analysis, the United Kingdom Collaborative Study constituted, by a considerable margin, the largest body of MSAFP screening experience in the world. Two or three small regional screening programs were operational in the United States, and other pilot programs or studies were being planned. No commercial kits for MSAFP testing were available in the U.S. And the professional societies most likely to be directly involved with MSAFP testing—the American College of Obstetricians and Gynecologists, the American Academy of Pediatrics, and the American Society of Human Genetics—vigorously opposed government approval and release of commercial test kits in the absence of adequate mechanisms to ensure appropriate counseling and quality control.

In the intervening seven years much has

changed medically, ethically, and legally. It is difficult to identify the twelve most important events or trends with respect to MSAFP testing or screening during this period, even if one confines one's attention primarily to the situation in the United Kingdom and the United States. However, the following are among the most important events and trends from 1980 to 1987:

1. The apparent incidence of NTDs in the U.K. and the U.S. gradually declined.
2. The U.K. Collaborative Study continued, with gradually increasing acceptance rates among British pregnant women.
3. The number of private, regional programs offering MSAFP testing in the United States continued to grow, as did the annual number of pregnancies screened in such programs.
4. A qualitative assessment of a pilot MSAFP screening program in one Maryland county was undertaken by a team of researchers at Johns Hopkins University (April 1980–June 1982).
5. A randomized prospective study of whether primary prevention of NTDs could be achieved through preconceptional and prenatal vitamin supplementation was undertaken and debated in the U.K.
6. The Food and Drug Administration released commercial test kits for MSAFP screening (June 1983).
7. The use of MSAFP measurement as a screening test for Down's syndrome was proposed and increasingly employed.
8. A vigorous public debate about appropriate treatment for handicapped newborn infants, including infants afflicted with NTDs, occurred in the U.K. and the U.S.
9. The Department of Professional Liability of the American College of Obstetricians and Gynecologists recommended that member obstetricians offer MSAFP testing to all of their pregnant patients (May 1985).
10. It became clear that the lives of most, if not virtually all, infants born with NTDs (except anencephaly) could be prolonged to childhood and adulthood, given vigorous perinatal intervention.
11. The State of California established the first publicly funded, statewide program offering MSAFP testing to every pregnant woman resident in the state (April 1986).
12. A debate on the possible use of organs from anencephalic fetuses and infants for transplantation purposes was initiated.

With these intervening developments in view, I propose to return to the four questions raised in 1980. The questions will be modified slightly to include both MSAFP testing as a transaction based on discussion in the clinical relationship and MSAFP screening as a formally organized program offered to all pregnant women in a particular state or region. The line between testing and screening is obviously not clear in every case. Voluntary screening programs always include the offer of testing, but the offer of testing need not be part of a formally organized screening program.

I. What is the Moral Status of a Fetus or Newborn Afflicted with an NTD?

To speak of the moral status of an entity is to use a shorthand expression for a longer question, namely, Do we have moral obligations to this entity and, if so, why? This question could be called pre-ethical, or even metaphysical, for it identifies the moral universe in which moral rights, obligations, and virtues can be meaningfully discussed.

Since 1980 the moral status of anencephalics and newborns has been the object of renewed ethical interest and analysis. Two contexts have been considered, that of selective abortion after prenatal diagnosis and of organ transplantation. In the abortion context, Chervenak and associates argued that the selective abortion of an anencephalic fetus, even in the third trimester, is morally justifiable if freely chosen by a pregnant woman and if the diagnosis of anencephaly is reliably made. According to the authors, it is not possible to harm a being that has no cognitive function and no potential for developing cognitive capacities.[3]

A more recent essay by John Fletcher and associates considers the circumstances in which organs may legitimately be retrieved from anencephalic fetuses or newborns. The authors conclude that, just as the clinical management of other clearly dying but not yet brainstem-dead patients can, at a certain point, be reoriented toward the preservation of organs for the sake of potential recipients, so the treatment of not yet dead anencephalics could involve, for example, hydration and cooling to preserve organ function. If this method does not suffice for the preservation of organs, Fletcher and associates seem willing to consider classifying anencephalics as a special category of being to which the usual total brain death (including brainstem-dead) standard does not apply.[8]

This latter suggestion has considerable merit if one can formulate it in a way that does not, without further discussion, justify retrieving organs from living fetuses and newborns with normal developmental potential and from living patients that once had normal cognitive function but are now in a persistent vegetative state. A special standard for the determination of death could be limited to anencephaly (and perhaps a few similar, exceedingly rare conditions affecting the neocortex) if it stipulated that the fetus or infant in question must fulfill four criteria:

1. It currently has no neocortical function.
2. It never has had any neocortical function.
3. It has no potential for developing neocortical function even if given optimal life-sustaining treatment.
4. It would not have had the potential for neocortical function even if its development had continued.*

---

* This fourth criterion is required to exclude fetuses that have the potential for neocortical development and function but are aborted spontaneously or through induction.

In short, there is at least a trend in recent ethical discussions toward accepting the abortion of anencephalic fetuses even in the third trimester and toward justifying the treatment of dying anencephalic fetuses as potential sources of donor organs. Consideration is also being given to revising the definition of death in humans to include anencephalics that have a temporarily functioning brain stem.

The ethical debate about appropriate treatment for fetuses and infants with other open NTD† or Down's syndrome has been intense since 1980. Prenatally, a procedural solution has continued to be practiced in the U.S., the U.K., and most other developed countries. If a previable fetus is discovered to have an open NTD or Down's syndrome, the pregnant woman has the legal right to choose to terminate the pregnancy and thereby not to allow the fetus to develop to full term. For the period between viability and birth there has been little ethical or legal argument in favor of pregnancy termination, or early induced delivery, of fetuses with open NTD or Down's syndrome. In fact, the criteria developed by Chervenak and colleagues would clearly not justify the third-trimester abortion of fetuses with these conditions.

Postnatally, there is little support in the ethical literature for the direct, active induction of death in infants with open NTD or Down's syndrome. However, the ethical and legal discussion of appropriate management for newborns with open NTD or Down's syndrome continues. Adults are generally considered to have strong moral and legal obligations toward newborns afflicted with these handicapping conditions. Still, there continue to be disagreements about whether certain types of treatment—respiratory support and artificial means of nutrition and hydration—may legitimately be withheld or withdrawn from such newborns in special circumstances. These circumstances may include grave burdens to the child, to the family, and to the larger society. Most commentators, in-

---

† In the remainder of this essay, anencephaly and open NTD are treated as mutually exclusive categories.

cluding a recent presidential commission on bioethics, takes the position that the best interests of the infant—or, negatively expressed, grave burden to the infant—should be the primary consideration in decision-making about handicapped newborns.[15,18]

II. What are the Major Potential Benefits and Risks of MSAFP Testing and Screening?

A potential benefit of MSAFP testing on which both pro-choice and pro-life advocates can agree is that it can provide pregnant women and expectant couples with early information about a fetal health problem. Even if the couple is conscientiously opposed to selective abortion, this early knowledge can assist them in their preparation for the birth of a handicapped or dying child and can assist their health provider in counseling them about the management of pregnancy and delivery.

Beyond the agreement on the value of early knowledge, however, judgments about the potential benefits and risks of MSAFP testing and screening radically diverge. For proponents of the pro-life position, the selective abortion of a mid-trimester fetus afflicted with an open NTD or Down's syndrome constitutes a serious harm to the fetus. For proponents of the pro-choice position, selective abortion allows a couple to avert the birth of a handicapped infant and the subsequent problems that the rearing of such an infant may entail.

These radically divergent calculations of risk and benefit are based on differing assessments of the moral status of the mid-trimester fetus (see I above). There are no prospects for an early resolution of this metaphysical and moral dispute in the U.S., the U.K., and numerous other countries. However, public opinion polls in the U.S. have consistently revealed stronger public support for selective abortion of handicapped fetuses (79%–86%) than for abortion on request (39%–55%).[13]

Even if one accepts the moral legitimacy of selective mid-trimester abortion, there remain two major risk-benefit questions:

- What level of incidence of NTDs justifies initiating a general program of MSAFP testing or screening?
- Where should the cut-off level for positive results be set?

The answer to the first question has apparently changed in the United States within the past 7 years. In 1980 there was vigorous debate about the value of general MSAFP testing or screening programs in which the incidence of anencephaly and open NTDs is less than 1 in 1000. In 1987, for a variety of reasons including malpractice concerns and consumer initiatives, MSAFP testing or screening will be offered to most pregnant women in the U.S. and to all pregnant women in selected regions, such as California.

The setting of a cut-off point for any diagnostic test is based on a value judgment about the relative harm caused by false-positives and false-negatives. In MSAFP screening programs results reported between 1980 and 1987, the fraction of cases in which false-positive results led to the abortion of unaffected fetuses has been exceedingly low, in the range of 1 in 5000 to 1 in 10,000 women screened and 1 in 40 to 75 elevated amniotic fluid AFP levels. False-negative rates (including results from follow-up ultrasound diagnosis and amniotic fluid analysis) for anencephaly and open NTDs have been zero in three recent series of 34,000, 21,442, and 6344 pregnancies.[4,9,12] More refined algorithms that take into account the gestational age of the fetus and the weight and race of the pregnant woman are currently being evaluated.[1] In short, when supplemented with appropriate confirmatory tests, MSAFP testing and screening produce low-error rates. These rates may be further reduced by refinements in technique.

Quality control concerns remain in two spheres, however. First, questions have been raised about the accuracy of one of the commercial test kits released for use in MSAFP testing in the United States.[10] Second, if most obstetricians begin to offer testing to all of their pregnant patients and a substantial number of patients accept the offer, the serum samples are likely to be tested in a variety of diagnostic laboratories—at least if no established regional or statewide program exists. In the absence of well defined regional standards for performing and interpreting the assay, quality control may be difficult to achieve.

The State of California has instituted an exemplary quality control effort in its statewide program. The state has contracted with six private laboratories, to which it provides reagents for the assay. Quality control assessments are performed daily in each laboratory and reported on-line to the State Department of Health.[5]

III. What Resource Allocation Questions Are Raised by MSAFP Testing and Screening?

The central resource allocation question regarding MSAFP testing and screening is this: Who should have access to MSAFP testing, and at what cost? One approach to answering this question is through a cost-benefit calculus that takes into account the total cost of a testing or screening program and the total savings achieved through averting the birth and development to adulthood of a group of fetuses afflicted with open NTDs.

A second approach to the access question avoids some of the theoretical and practical difficulties of cost-benefit analyses. This approach raises the question, Does society have a moral obligation to provide an adequate level of health care to every one of its members? A recent presidential commission on bioethics argues (in my view convincingly) that society does have such a moral obligation.[17]

If the answer is affirmative, the crucial intermediate-level question becomes, Is MSAFP testing an essential component of an adequate level of prenatal care in the late 1980s in the U.S.? There is no easy answer to this question, especially given the contextual character of the notion of adequacy. However, the desire of a majority or perhaps even a substantial minority, of pregnant women to have the test, if it is available at reasonable cost, would constitute prima facie evidence that the test should be considered part of an adequate level of prenatal care. There is empirical evidence on this question from both the United Kingdom and the United States. In the U.K., where testing is covered by the National Health Service, the fraction of pregnant women accepting testing is over 80% at one center, the University College Hospital in London.[9] Preliminary data from the State of California suggest that just over 40% of pregnant women are willing to pay the $40 fee that covers all necessary diagnostic procedures.[5] In Maine's private regional program, 55% to 60% of all pregnancies are screened for elevated MSAFP; however, some pregnant women in the screened group may not be informed that their sera are being tested for MSAFP.[11]

The access question for most pregnant women in the U.S. is complicated by two types of financial uncertainties. The first is how far they will need to go in the testing process, for example, through real-time ultrasound or amniocentesis. The second uncertainty concerns the fraction of testing costs that will be covered by the pregnant woman's health insurance. For the foreseeable future, it seems likely that only pregnant women who can pay the costs of MSAFP testing, either directly or indirectly through private health insurance, will have access to this service, in the absence of public programs. Pregnant women who are poor or uninsured will not have access.

With its statewide MSAFP screening program the State of California has, de facto, designated MSAFP testing as part of an adequate level of prenatal care. The $40 fee for participation in the program more than covers the $8 to $10 cost of the initial serum screen. However, this modest fee is far exceeded by the approximate $1000 in costs that will be incurred by any pregnant woman who requires the entire series of NTD-related tests. Many women who are not able to afford the $40 participation fee in California are covered by the state's Medicaid program, Medi-Cal[14]; however, there may be other indigent women who do not qualify for Medi-

Cal and who find the $40 fee an insurmountable financial barrier.

IV. What Issues of Freedom and Coercion Do MSAFP Testing or Screening Programs Raise?

In my 1980 essay, I noted that Joseph Fletcher seemed to advocate mandatory screening programs for the prevention of birth defects: "mutual coercion mutually agreed upon."[7] However, no commentators on the specific question of MSAFP testing or screening have advocated that this set of diagnostic procedures be compulsory.

The majority position that has emerged in the United States for prenatal diagnostic services is that such services should be offered to every pregnant woman or expectant couple but not forced upon any woman or couple. (This offer may, of course, not provide a genuine option to some women or couples because of the resource allocation questions discussed above.) Until now, no mandatory prenatal screening programs have been instituted in the United States. This policy stands in sharp contrast to neonatal screening, for which mandatory programs exist in 46 states.[2]

Two interesting problems related to freedom and coercion remain, however. The first is whether pregnant women should receive their initial serum screen as part of routine obstetric care without being informed of the test and without giving their explicit consent. Since many pregnant women have well-informed and deeply held views on the ethical aspects of prenatal diagnosis, all pregnant women should, in my view, be informed of the proposed test and provided the option of accepting or declining it. This position is in accord with that adopted in the presidential commission report.[16]

A second question concerns the mode and effectiveness of various measures for informing pregnant women or expectant couples of their options. Two recent approaches to this issue deserve mention. A team of researchers at Johns Hopkins University School of Hygiene and Public Health developed a brochure, pitched at a tenth-grade reading level, to explain the various steps involved in MSAFP testing. Second, the State of California has developed a combination brochure and consent form, available in several languages and written at a sixth-grade level, for pregnant women who are being offered the serum screen.

The Johns Hopkins group conducted an empirical study designed to measure how much of the information contained in its simple-language consent form was retained by pregnant women at various intervals after they had received the brochure. The Hopkins investigators found that pregnant women performed significantly better on a multiple-choice recognition test than on an unprompted, free response test. However, 24% of women interviewed within a week of having consented to testing and having their blood drawn answered at least 25% of the multiple-choice items incorrectly.[5] This study suggests the need for interactive counseling, as well as understandable written information, if pregnant women and expectant couples are to be informed properly about MSAFP testing and about the implications of their decisions concerning such testing.

REFERENCES

1. Adams MJ, Windham GC, James LM et al: Clinical interpretation of maternal serum alpha-fetoprotein concentrations. Am J Obstet Gynecol 148:241–254, 1984
2. Andrews LB: State laws and regulations governing newborn screening. American Bar Foundation, Chicago, 1985
3. Chervenak FA, Farley MA, Walters L et al: When is termination of pregnancy during the third trimester morally justifiable? New Engl J Med 310:501–504, 1984
4. Crandall BF, Matsumoto M: Routine amniotic fluid alpha-fetoprotein measurement in 34,000 pregnancies. Am J Obstet Gynecol 149:744–747, 1984
5. Cunningham GC, Chief, Genetic Disease Branch, California Department of Health Services, July 11, 1986. Personal communication.
6. Faden RR, Chwalow AJ, Orel-Crosby E et al: What participants understand about a mater-

nal serum alpha-fetoprotein screening program. Am J Publ Health 75:1381–1384, 1985
7. Fletcher, JC: Humanhood: Essays in Biomedical Ethics. Buffalo: Prometheus Books, 1979, p 111
8. Fletcher JC, Robertson JA, Harrison MR: Primates and anencephalics as sources for pediatric organ transplants. Fetal Therapy 1:150–164, 1986
9. Hooper JG, Lucas M, Richards BA et al: Is maternal alpha-fetoprotein screening still of value in a low-risk area for neural tube defects? Prenatal Diagnosis 4:29–33, 1984
10. Knight GJ, Palomaki GE, Haddow JE: Letter: Maternal serum alpha-fetoprotein: A problem with a test kit. New Engl J Med 314:516, 1986
11. Kloza EM, Coordinator, AFP Prenatal Screening, Foundation for Blood Research, Scarborough, Maine, July 11, 1986. Personal communication.
12. Milunsky A, Alpert E: Results and benefits of a maternal serum alpha-fetoprotein screening program. JAMA 252:1438–1442, 1984
13. Sackett V: Split verdict: What Americans think about abortion. Policy Review 32:18–19, 1985
14. Steinbrook R. In California, voluntary mass prenatal screening. Hastings Center Rep 16 (October):5–7, 1986
15. US President's Commission for the Study of Ethical Problems in Medicine and Biomedical and Behavioral Research (1983). Deciding to forego life-sustaining treatment. Washington, DC, US Government Printing Office, 1983
16. US President's Commission for the Study of Ethical Problems in Medicine and Biomedical and Behavioral Research (1983). Screening and counseling for genetic conditions. Washington, DC, US Government Printing Office, 1983
17. US President's Commission for the Study of Ethical Problems in Medicine and Biomedical and Behavioral Research (1983). Securing access to health care. Washington, DC, US Government Printing Office, 1983
18. Weir RF: Selective nontreatment of handicapped newborns. New York, Oxford University Press, 1984

SECTION 3: ULTRASOUND DETECTION OF FETAL ANOMALIES

Frank A. Chervenak and Glenn Isaacson

Ultrasound, as no other diagnostic technique, has permitted detailed examination of the developing human baby to be performed commonly and safely. At the present time, no ill effect from diagnostic ultrasound has been documented reproducibly, but long-term studies are ongoing.[25,29,33]

Real-time ultrasound, which generates a continuous motion picturelike image of the moving fetus, is more easily used than static techniques and is of sufficient resolution to make many diagnoses. Structures as small as the lens of the eye and the semicircular canals of the ear can be visualized. Male and female genitalia can be reliably differentiated.[3] With this capacity, the vast majority of severe structural anomalies of the fetus can be diagnosed by ultrasound.

Examination for fetal anomalies is best performed between 16 and 20 weeks gestation when fetal structure are large enough to be studied, and subsequent examinations can be performed, if necessary, prior to fetal viability.

DIAGNOSTIC METHODS

There are six general ways in which the diagnosis of a fetal malformation can be made by ultrasound. These include absence of a normally present structure, presence of an additional structure distorting normal contour, dilatation behind an obstruction, herniation through a structural defect, abnormal fetal biometry, and absent or abnormal fetal motion. We will discuss each of these diagnostic categories and representative anomalies.

Absence of a Normally Present Structure

One class of fetal defects is characterized by the absence of a structure normally detectable by ultrasound. A dramatic example is fetal anencephaly: the absence of calvaria and much of the underlying brain. The ultrasound image of anencephaly is so clear that as early as 1972 a pregnancy was terminated on the basis of an ultrasound diagnosis.[4] The echogenic bones of the skull are absent (Figure 3-7) and the well-defined cerebral structures normally seen are replaced by a heterogeneous mass of cystic tissue called the area cerebrovasculosa. Over 100 cases of anencephaly have been reported with no false-positive diagnoses.[10]

Alobar holoprosencephaly describes the absence of certain midline cerebral structures as a result of incomplete cleavage of the primitive forebrain. The ultrasonic "midline echo" of the fetal head, normally generated by acoustic interfaces in the area of the interhemispheric fissure, is absent in this entity (Figure 3-8).[12] The same embryologic defect that causes incomplete cleavage of the forebrain in holoprosencephaly may produce hypotelorism, nasal anomalies, and facial clefts (Figure 3-9). The detection of both cranial and facial aberrations strengthens the diagnosis of holoprosencephaly.

The kidneys are normally seen as bilateral, ovoid, paraspinal masses with echo-spared renal pelves (Figure 3-10A). When they are not detectable, the diagnosis of renal agenesis is suspected. The presence of severe oligohydramnios and the inability to visualize the bladder support the diagnosis. There have been multiple reports of successful antenatal diagnoses of renal agenesis. However, false-positive and false-negative diagnoses continue to be made.[30] Problems with adequate visualization in the presence of oligohydramnios and simulation of the sonographic appearance of kidneys by ovoid-shaped adrenal glands lead to some of the confusion (Figure 3-10B).

Cleft lip and palate have been detected sonographically by meticulous examination of the fetal maxillary region in several anatomic planes (Figure 3-11).[18] Such diagnoses, however, have been sporadic and no good data are available concerning diagnostic accuracy.

Clearly the ability to detect the absence of a normal structure with certainty is dependent on consistent visualization of the normal structure.

Presence of an Additional Structure Distorting Normal Contour

The fetal surface contours are well visualized by ultrasound, owing to an acoustic interface between amniotic fluid and fetus. Masses that distort these familiar contours can thus be identified with ultrasound.

Fetal teratomas are the most common neoplasms of newborns. They are derived from pleuripotent cells and are composed of a

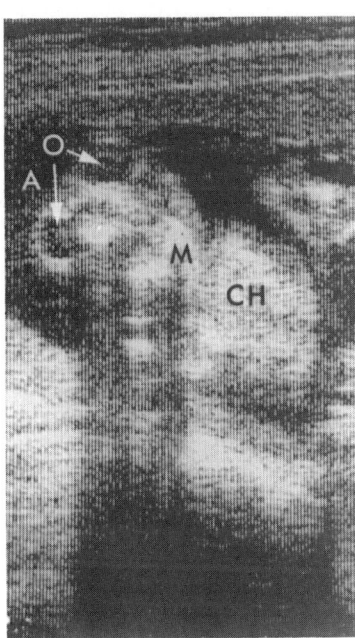

FIGURE 3-7. Sonogram of anencephalic fetus. (A, absent cranium; O, orbits; M, mandible; CH, chest) (Chervenak FA et al: When is the termination of pregnancy during the third trimester morally justifiable? N Engl J Med 310:501–504, 1984)

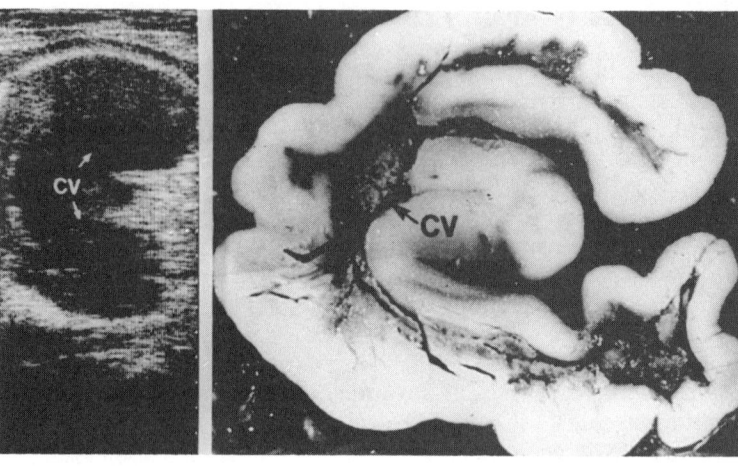

FIGURE 3-8. (A) Transverse sonogram through fetal skull demonstrates common ventricle (CV) and absence of midline structures. (B) Transverse section of fetal brain at autopsy demonstrates a collapsed CV, failure of cerebral hemispheres to separate, and absence of corpus callosum. (Chervenak FA et al: The obstetrical significance of holoprosencephaly. Obstet Gynecol 63:115–121, 1984)

diversity of tissues foreign to the anatomic site in which they arise. They may be seen as distortions in the fetal contour, often in the sacrococcygeal area (Figure 3-12) or, if elsewhere, usually along the fetal midline. Their characteristic internal sonographic appearance with irregular cystic and solid areas and occasional calcifications helps to identify these lesions.[15]

Fetal cystic hygromas are fluid-filled protrusions usually about the fetal neck, which arise from abnormal development of the lymphatic system.[11] They are generally echospared with scattered septations and often a

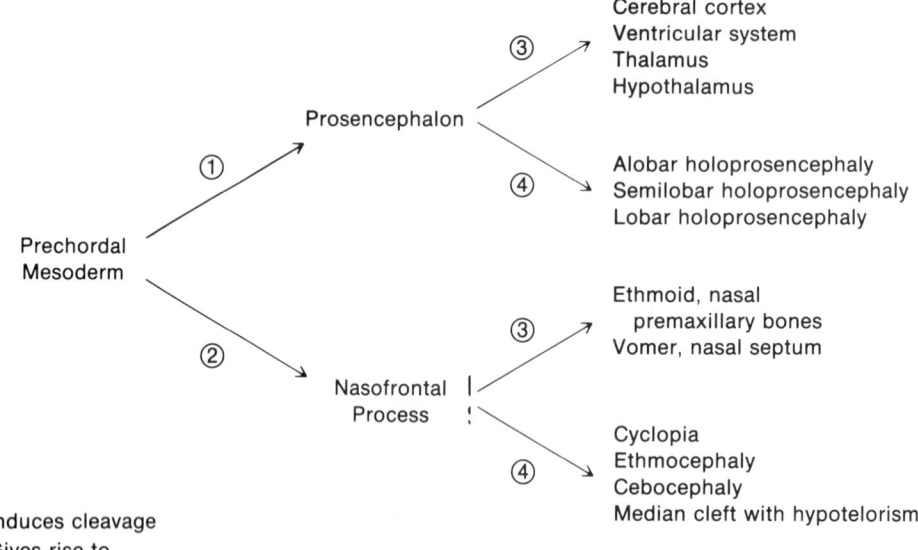

FIGURE 3-9. Embryology of holoprosencephaly and midline facial defects. (Chervenak FA et al: The obstetrical significance of holoprosencephaly. Obstet Gynecol 63:115–121, 1984)

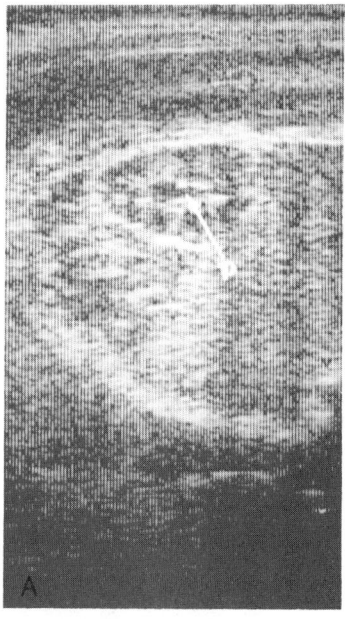
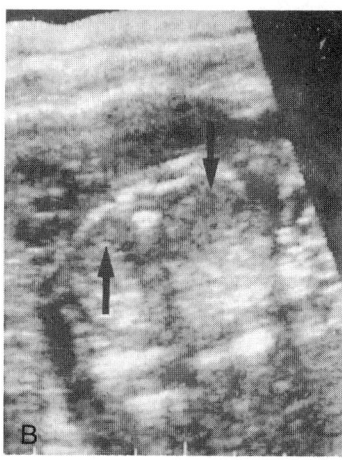

FIGURE 3-10. (A) Sonogram shows a normal kidney (P, renal pelvis). (B) Renal agenesis with severe oligohydramnios (arrows point to adrenal glands, not kidneys).

midline septum arising from the nuchal ligament[14] (Figure 3-13A). The generalized lymphatic disorder which produces these hygromas commonly leads to hydrops fetalis and intrauterine death (Figure 3-13B).[11]

Hydrops fetalis or fetal anasarca may be identified by the distortion of the normal fetal surface by skin edema.[23] Ascites and pleural and pericardial effusions may also be identified (Figure 3-14).

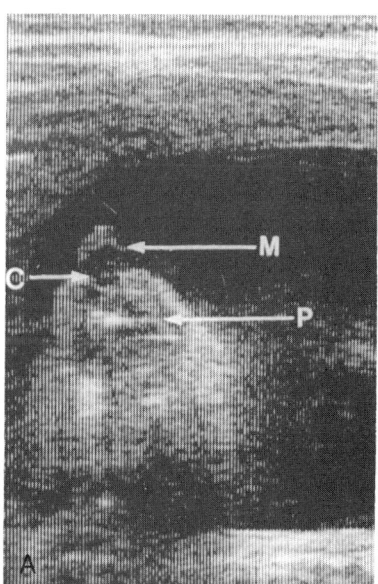
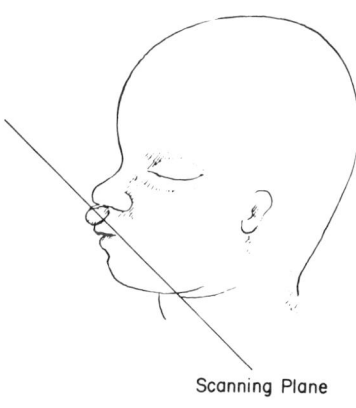

FIGURE 3-11. (A) Oblique scan through lower part of fetal face shows intact palate, cleft lip, and a mass protruding from lip (C, cleft; M, mass, P, palate). (B) Demonstration of scanning plane. (Chervenak FA et al: Antenatal diagnosis of median cleft face syndrome: Sonographic demonstration of cleft lip and hypertelorism. Am J Obstet Gynecol 149:94–97, 1984)

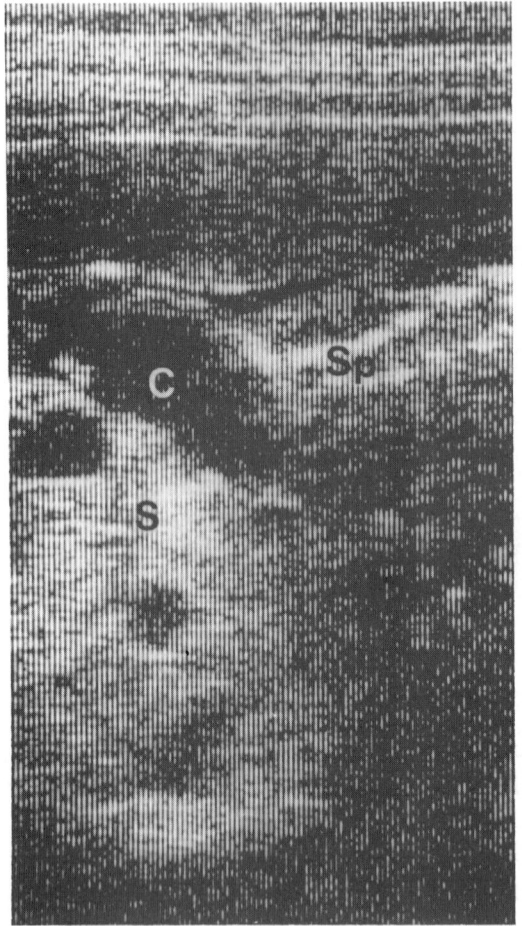

FIGURE 3-12. Antenatal sonogram reveals a predominantly solid mass (S) with irregular cystic areas (C) protruding from sacrococcygeal area, extrinsic to fetal spine (SP). (Chervenak FA et al: The diagnosis and management of fetal teratomas. Obstet Gynecol 66(5):666–671, 1986)

Dilatation Behind an Obstruction

Dilatation may be caused by obstruction to the normal flow of a variety of body fluids including cerebrospinal fluid, urine, or swallowed amniotic fluid. In this class of anomalies, the structural defect itself is rarely seen. Rather, what is observed is the distention of normal tissues behind that defect.

Hydrocephalus is characterized by a relative enlargement of the cerebroventricular system and often the fetal head by cerebrospinal fluid under pressure. It is most reliably diagnosed by comparing the width of the body of the lateral ventricle to the width of the fetal head. The location of the obstruction may be guessed by observing which portions of the ventricular system are enlarged. There is a frequent association of fetal hydrocephalus with other anomalies, especially spina bifida[5–8] (Figure 3-15).

Fetal small bowel obstruction may cause dilatation proximal to the area of obstruction. Duodenal atresia has been observed to produce its characteristic "double bubble" sign consisting of enlarged duodenum and stomach with narrowings at the pylorus and duodenum[24] (Figure 3-16).

Obstructions to urinary flow with proximal dilatation have been detected at the ureteropelvic and ureterovesicular junctions. Dilatation resulting from these two types of blockages is commonly unilateral. By contrast, bilateral ureteral dilatation is more common when the obstruction is at a posterior urethral valve and the bladder is enlarged (Figure 3-17).[22,32]

Herniations Through Structural Defects

A common theme in embryologic development is the formation of compartments containing vital structures by folding and midline fusion.[2] Incomplete fusion in a variety of locations can lead to defects and herniations of contained structures.

The neural tube and overlying mesoderm begin their closure in the region of the fourth somite, with fusion extending both rostrally and caudally during the fourth week of fetal life.[2] Incomplete closure at the rostral end produces cephaloceles, which are herniations of meninges and frequently of brain substance through a defect in the cranium[13] (Figures 3-18). Failed fusion at the caudal end produces spina bifida with protruding meningoceles and meningomyeloceles[9] (Figure 3-19). Sonographic diagnosis of each of these anomalies is dependent upon the demonstration of a defect in the normal structure

Prenatal Diagnosis of Congenital Malformations   65

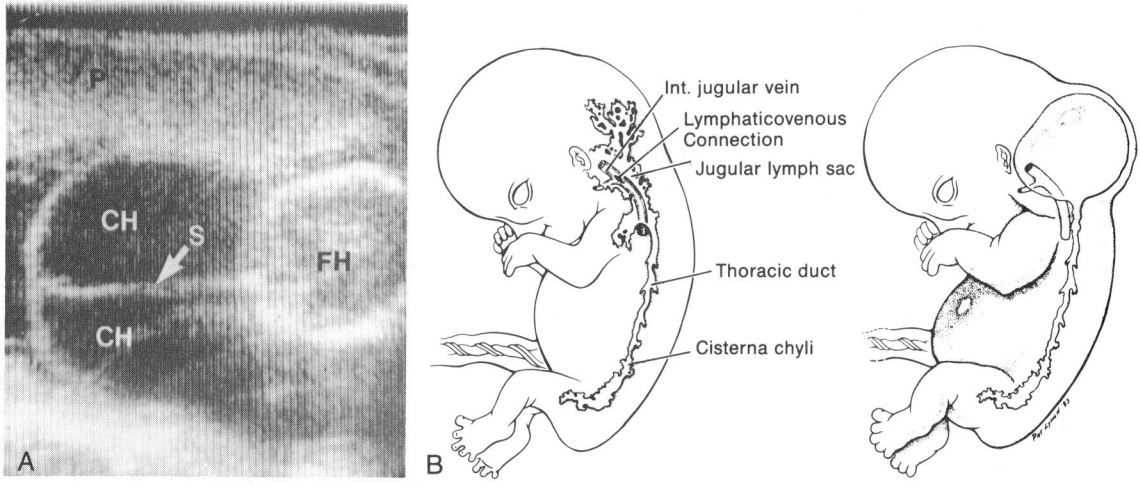

FIGURE 3-13. (*A*) Transverse sonogram demonstrating cystic hygroma with a midline septum (CH, cystic hygroma; S, septum; FH, fetal head; P, placenta). (*B*) Lymphatic system in normal fetus (left) with a patent connection between the jugular lymph sac and the internal jugular vein; on the right, a cystic hygroma and hydrops from a failed lymphaticovenous connection. (Chervenak FA et al: Fetal cystic hygroma. Cause and natural history. N Engl J Med 309:822–825, 1984)

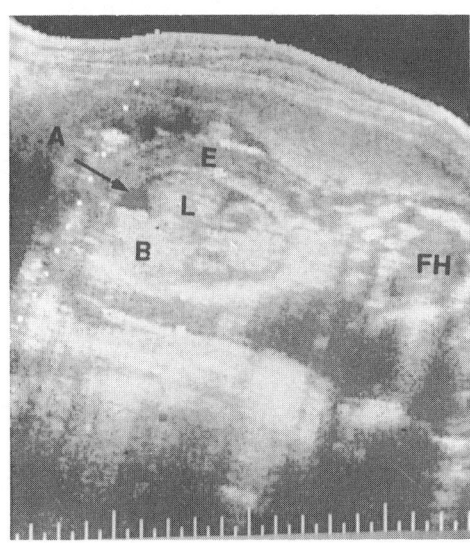

FIGURE 3-14. Longitudinal sonogram of hydropic fetus. (A, ascites; E, skin edema; L, liver; B, bowel; FH, fetal head)

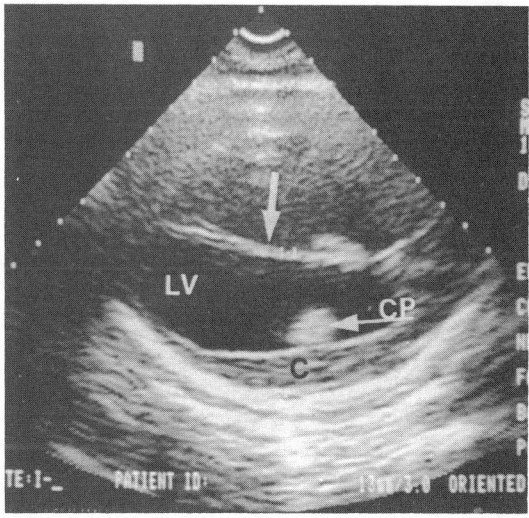

FIGURE 3-15. Transverse sonogram of fetal head demonstrates classic sonographic picture of fetal hydrocephalus. (LV, dilated lateral ventricle; CP, choroid plexus; arrow, midline echo; C, compressed cerebral cortex)

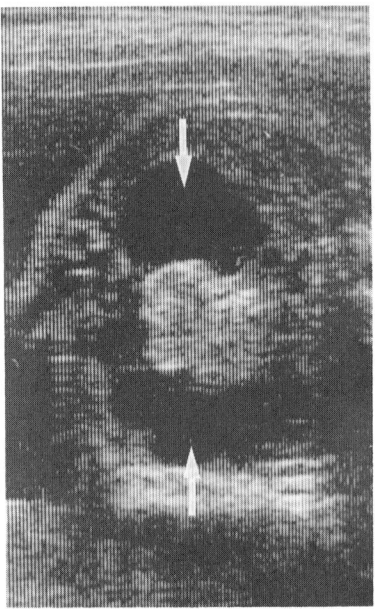

FIGURE 3-16. Sonogram reveals classic appearance of duodenal atresia; arrows point to the two echo-spared areas generating the "double bubble appearance."

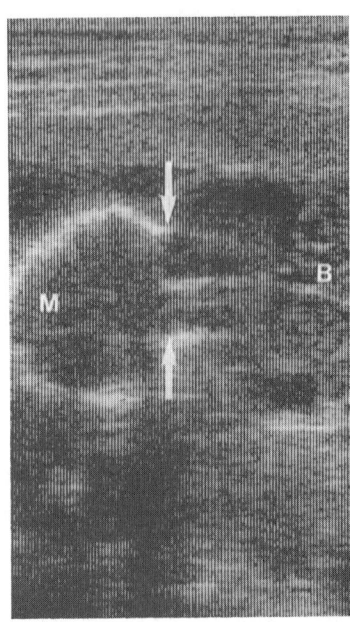

FIGURE 3-18. Oblique sonogram shows a large occipital encephalocele, arrows outline the defect in the skull (M, microcephalic skull; B, extruded brain tissue). (Chervenak FA et al: Diagnosis and management of fetal cephalocele. Obstet Gynecol 64:86–91, 1984)

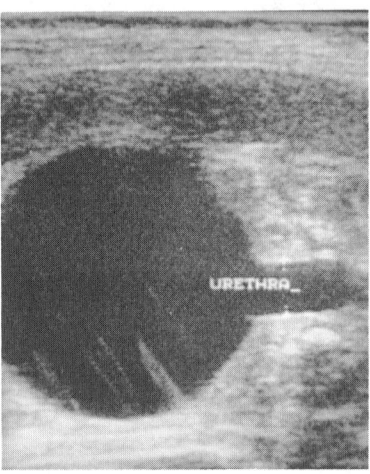

FIGURE 3-17. Sonogram is of a dilated urethra and bladder secondary to obstructed posterior urethral valves.

of the cranium or spine and of a protruding sac often containing tissue.

Omphaloceles result from failure of the intestines to retract from their temporary location in the umbilical cord and subsequent herniation of other abdominal contents.[2] Sonographically they are seen as the protrusion of abdominal contents, which may include both hollow and solid viscera, within a peritoneal sac[28] (Figure 3-20). Insertion of the umbilical cord into the sac helps to differentiate an omphalocele from gastroschisis, which may be eccentric in location and lack a peritoneal sac.

The diaphragm forms from four separate sources which fuse to separate the pleural and peritoneal cavities.[2] When a diaphragmatic hernia is present, abdominal contents may be visualized within the chest on transverse sonographic scanning (Figure 3-21), while a disruption of the diaphragm may be seen in the sagittal plane.[27]

Prenatal Diagnosis of Congenital Malformations 67

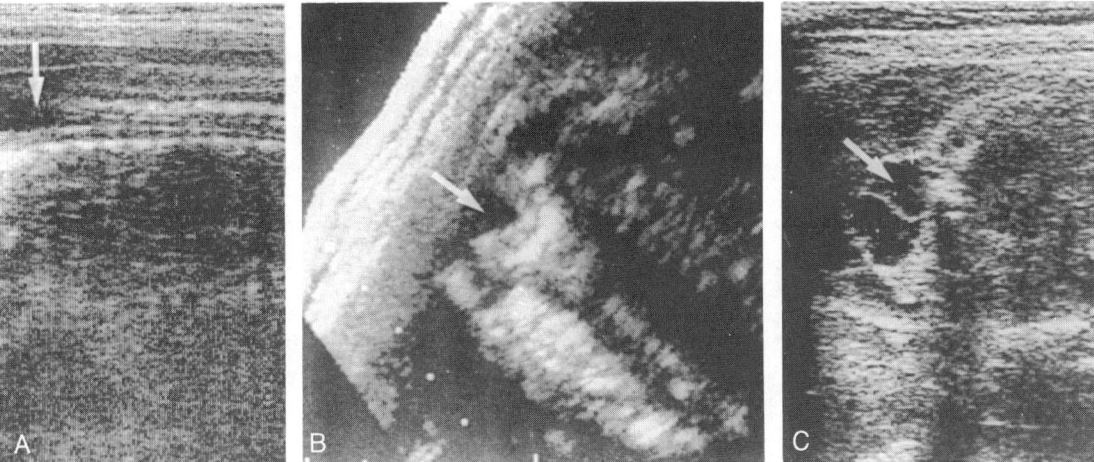

FIGURE 3-19. (A) Longitudinal sonogram of spina bifida (arrow). (B) Transverse sonogram of fetal spine with arrow pointing to spina bifida. (C) Transverse sonogram with arrow pointing to protruding meningomyelocele. (Chervenak FA et al: The diagnosis of fetal hydrocephalus. Am J Obstet Gynecol 147:703–716, 1983)

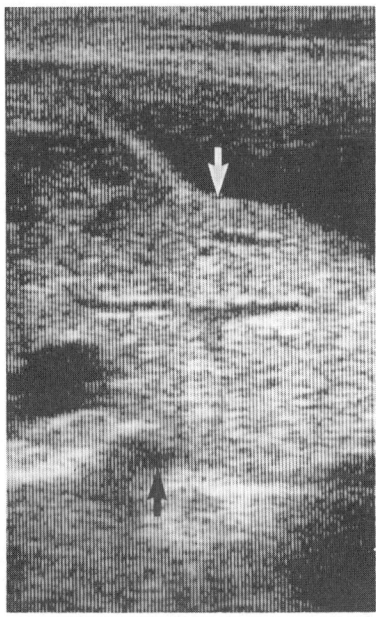

FIGURE 3-20. Sonogram of an omphalocele. Arrows point to a break in the abdominal wall.

Abnormal Fetal Biometry

Several fetal anomalies are best diagnosed not by observing alterations in shape or consistency, but by determining abnormalities in size. The science of fetal biometry has generated many nomograms defining norms for parts of the fetal anatomy at various gestational ages.

Fetal microcephaly is usually the result of an underdeveloped brain. Although commonly associated with cerebral structural malformations, microcephaly may be produced by a brain that is normal in configuration, but merely small. The accurate diagnosis of microcephaly has proved challenging, since compressive forces within the uterus may normally distort the shape of the fetal head. The best correlation between microcephaly diagnosed in utero and neonatal microcephaly is made when multiple parameters are measured and suggest a small head.[16]

A variety of skeletal dysplasias may affect the growth of long bones. Measurement may suggest a particular skeletal dysplasia, depending upon which bones are foreshortened. The shape of these long bones, their density, the presence of fractures, or the ab-

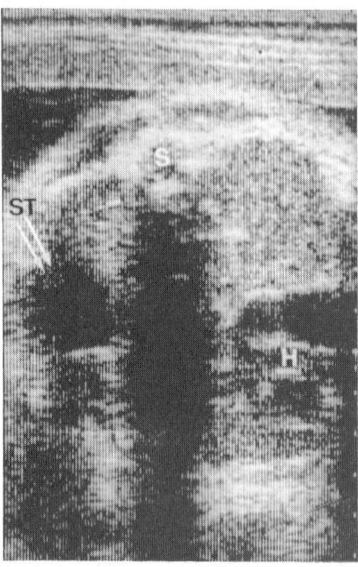

FIGURE 3-21. Transverse sonogram at the level of the fetal heart. The presence of abdominal contents, noticeably the stomach (ST), within the chest cavity suggests the diagnosis of diaphragmatic hernia. (S, spine; H, heart)

sence of specific bone may aid in differentiating the various boney abnormalities.

When interorbital distances are inconsistent with gestational age, hypotelorism or hypertelorism may be suggested (Figures 3-22 and 3-23). Abnormal distance between the orbits may serve as a clue to several malformation syndromes (e.g., alobar holoprosencephaly,[12] median cleft face syndrome[18]).

The internal architecture of the kidneys may be difficult to assess in the presence of oligohydramnios. The diagnosis of polycystic kidneys is thus aided by renal measurement. Polycystic kidneys are usually enlarged and thus display an abnormally increased kidney circumference—abdominal circumference ratio.[31]

Absent or Abnormal Fetal Motion

Abnormalities in fetal motion may suggest a malformation which cannot itself be seen. Although the fetus can normally assume contorted positions in utero, the persistence of such an unusual posture over time may suggest an orthopaedic or neurologic anomaly

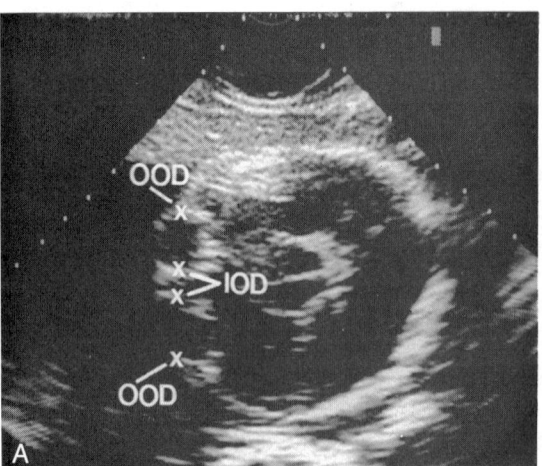
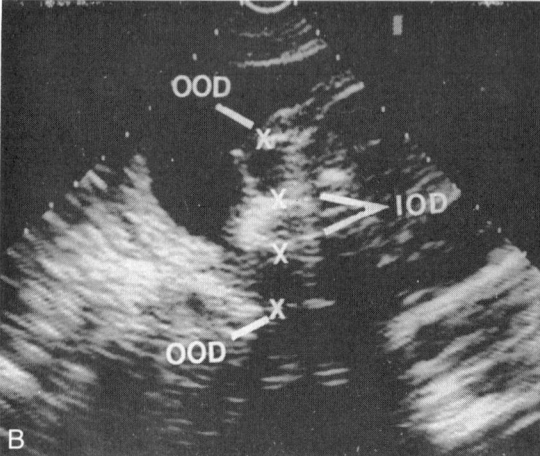

FIGURE 3-22. Transverse scans through orbits at 28 weeks of gestation are of (A) hypotelorism and (B) a normal fetus (OOD, outer orbital distance; IOD, inner orbital distance). Chervenak FA et al: The obstetrical significance of fetal holoprosencephaly. 63:115–121, 1984)

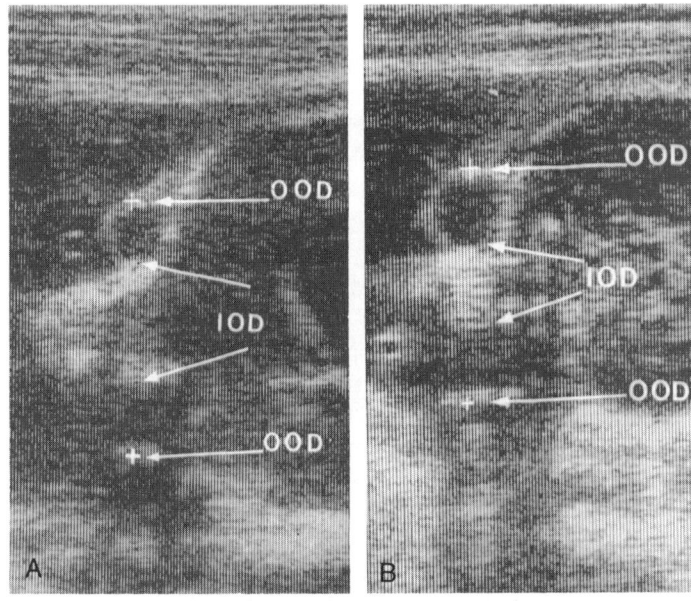

FIGURE 3-23. Transverse scans through orbits at 31 weeks gestation reveal (A) hypertelorism and (B) a normal fetus (OOD, outer orbital distance; IOD, interorbital distance). (Chervenak FA et al: Antenatal diagnosis of median cleft face syndrome: Sonographic demonstration of cleft lip and hypertelorism. Am J Obstet Gynecol 149:94–97, 1984)

such as clubfoot[17] (Figure 3-24) or arthrogryposis.[20]

The fetal heart is a most conspicuously dynamic part of the fetus. Although real-time ultrasound is of some value in diagnosing fetal cardiac anomalies, M-mode echocardiography better allows visualization and measurement of cardiac valvular motion,

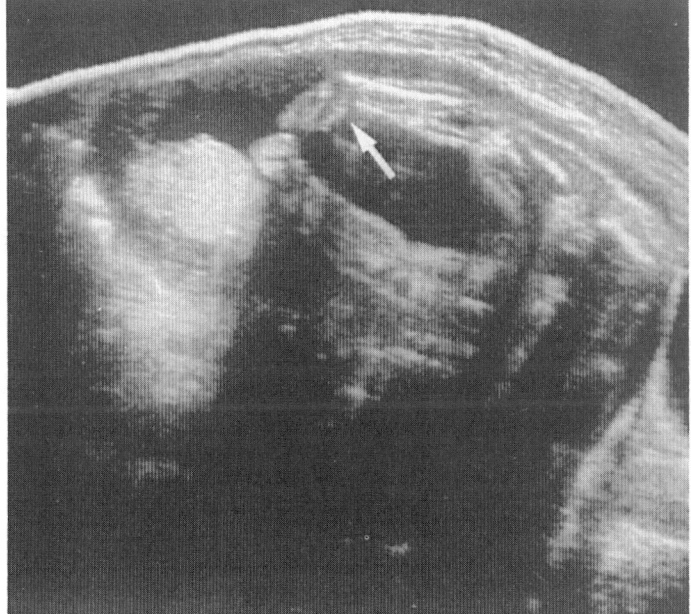

FIGURE 3-24. Longitudinal sonogram demonstrates lower legs with markedly inverted upper foot (arrow). Neonate was affected with clubfoot. (Chervenak FA et al: Antenatal sonographic diagnosis of clubfoot. J Ultrasound Med 4:49–50, 1985)

chamber size, and cardiac rhythm. The combination of these two modalities has permitted the diagnosis of a variety of major structural defects such as hypoplastic left heart syndrome and of dysrythmias including complete heart block.[1,19]

MANAGEMENT

Once an anomaly has been detected by ultrasound, a thorough search for associated anomalies as well as consideration of karyotype determination and serial ultrasound studies is warranted. This assessment of prognostic factors for an individual fetus aids the physician and parents to decide knowledgeably among various management options for the pregnancy. Elective abortion of a seriously malformed fetus, in utero therapy, alteration of timing or mode of delivery, or a decision not to intervene are among these options.[21,26] Transfer to a tertiary care center may be planned when the need for specialized medical or surgical care is anticipated.

REFERENCES

1. Allan LD, Crawford DC, Anderson RH, Tynan MJ: Echocardiographic and anatomical correlation in fetal congenital heart disease. Br Heart J 52:542–548, 1984
2. Arey LB: Developmental Anatomy. Philadelphia, WB Saunders, 1974
3. Birnholz JC: Determination of fetal sex. N Engl J Med 309:942–944, 1983
4. Campbell S, Johnstone FD, Hold EM, May P: Anencephaly: Early ultrasonic diagnosis and active management. Lancet 2:1226–1227, 1972
5. Chervenak FA, Berkowitz RL, Romero R et al: The diagnosis of fetal hydrocephalus. Am J Obstet Gynecol 147:703–716, 1983
6. Chervenak FA, Berkowitz RL, Tortora M et al: The diagnosis of ventriculomegaly prior to fetal viability. Obstet Gynecol 64:652–656, 1984
7. Chervenak FA, Berkowitz RL, Tortora M, Hobbins JC: The management of fetal hydrocephalus. Am J Obstet Gynecol 151:933–942, 1985
8. Chervenak FA, Duncan C, Ment LR et al: The outcome of fetal ventriculomegaly. Lancet 2:179–182, 1984
9. Chervenak FA, Duncan C, Ment LR et al: The perinatal management of meningomyelocele. Obstet Gynecol 63:376–380, 1984
10. Chervenak FA, Farley MA, Walters L et al: When is the termination of pregnancy during the third trimester morally justifiable? N Engl J Med 310:501–504, 1984
11. Chervenak FA, Isaacson G, Blakemore KJ et al: Fetal cystic hygroma. Cause and natural history. N Engl J Med 309:822–825, 1984
12. Chervenak FA, Isaacson G, Mahoney MJ et al: The obstetrical significance of holoprosencephaly. Obstet Gynecol 63:15–121, 1984
13. Chervenak FA, Isaacson G, Mahoney MJ et al: The diagnosis and management of fetal cephalocele. Obstet Gynecol 64:86–91, 1984
14. Chervenak FA, Isaacson G, Tortora M: A sonographic study of fetal cystic hygromas. J Clin Ultrasound 5:311–315, 1984
15. Chervenak FA, Isaacson G, Touloukian R et al: The diagnosis and management of fetal teratomas. Obstet Gynecol 66(5):666–671, 1986
16. Chervenak FA, Jeanty P, Cantraine F et al: The diagnosis of fetal microcephaly. Am J Obstet Gynecol 1449:512–517, 1984
17. Chervenak FA, Tortora M, Hobbins JC: Antenatal sonographic diagnosis of clubfoot. J Ultrasound Med 4:49–50, 1985
18. Chervenak FA, Tortora M, Mayden K et al: Antenatal diagnosis of median cleft face syndrome: Sonographic demonstration of cleft lip and hypertelorism. Am J Obstet Gynecol 149:94–97, 1984
19. Gertgesell HP Jr (ed): Symposium on Fetal Echocardiography. J Clin Ultrasound 13:227–273, 1985
20. Goldberg JD, Chervenak FA, Lipman RA et al: Antenatal sonographic diagnosis of arthrogryposis multiplex congenita. Prenat Diagn (In press)
21. Harrison MR, Golbus MS, Filly RA: The Unborn Patient. Prenatal Diagnosis and Treatment. Orlando, FL, Grune & Stratton, 1984
22. Hobbins JC, Romero R, Grannum P et al: Antenatal diagnosis of renal anomalies with ultrasound. I. Obstructive uropathy. Am J Obstet Gynecol 148:868–876, 1984
23. Holzgreve W, Curry CJR, Golbus MS: Investigation of nonimmune hydrops fetalis. Am J Obstet Gynecol 150:805–812, 1984
24. Lees RF, Alford BA, Brenbridge NAG et al: Sonographic appearance of duodenal atresia

in utero. Am J Roentgenol 131:701–705, 1978
25. Kremkau FW: Safety and long-term effects of ultrasound: What to tell your patients. Clin Obstet Gynecol 27:269–275, 1984
26. Manning FA, Lange IR, Morrison I, Harman C: Treatment of the fetus in utero: Evolving concepts. Clin Obstet Gynecol 27:378–390, 1984
27. Marwood RP, Dawson OW: Antenatal diagnosis of diaphragmatic hernias. Br J Obstet Gynecol 88:71–75, 1981
28. Nakayama DK, Harrison MR, Gross BH et al: Management of the fetus with an abdominal wall defect. J Ped Surg 19:408–413, 1984
29. National Institute of Child Health and Human Development: The Use of Diagnostic Ultrasound Imaging in Pregnancy. NIH Consensus Development Conference Process. Washington, DC, U.S. Government Printing Office, 1984
30. Romero R, Cullen M, Grannum P et al: Antenatal diagnosis of renal anomalies with ultrasound. III. Bilateral renal agenesis. Am J Obstet Gynecol 151:38–43, 1985
31. Romero R, Cullen M, Jeanty P et al: The diagnosis of congenital renal anomalies with ultrasound. II. Infantile polycystic kidney disease. Am J Obstet Gynecol 150:259–262, 1984
32. Sanders R, Graham D: Twelve cases of hydronephrosis in utero diagnosed by ultrasonography. J Ultrasound Med 1:341–348, 1982
33. Stark CR, Orleans M, Haverkamp AD, Murphy J: Short- and long-term risks after exposure to diagnostic ultrasound in utero. Obstet Gynecol 63:194–200, 1984

SECTION 4: TRANSVAGINAL ULTRASONOGRAPHY

Arie Drugan and Ilan E. Timor-Tritsch

Diagnostic ultrasound imaging of the female pelvic organs has been performed with increasing frequency over the last two decades. Although constantly evolving technology has improved resolution, very high resolution scanning of the female pelvis is still difficult to achieve transabdominally. This is because the distance from the abdominal wall to the pelvic organs is relatively long and precludes the use of high frequency transducers.

Although a 5-mHz transducer may be adequate for scanning the pelvis in a normal-size woman through the full bladder, a 3.5-mHz or 2.75-mHz transducer may be needed to obtain sufficient depth in a heavier woman. A lower frequency transducer gains focal depth at the price of axial and lateral resolution and, thus, fine details of the organ scanned are sacrificed. An intravaginal probe is positioned closer to the pelvic organs scanned, with most of the relevant anatomy being about 9 mm from the vaginal fornices as opposed to approximately 14 mm transabdominally through a full bladder. Thus, transvaginal higher frequency transducers (6.5–7 mHz) can be used with improved resolution due to minimal tissue attenuation.

Although there have been no clinical trials to ascertain patient compliance and subjective experience with transvaginal ultrasound to date, our experience and that of other authors[36,42] indicate that transvaginal ultrasound is superior to transabdominal ultrasound in several respects. Most obviously, transvaginal ultrasound does not require a full patient bladder. In addition to decreasing patient discomfort, this also means that patient procedures can be scheduled closer together, thus increasing the efficient use of the operator's time as well as reducing patient waiting time. Also, the earlier diagnosis of many anomalies decreases the psychological trauma to the patient. The advantages of transvaginal-ultrasound-guided oocyte monitoring and retrieval are discussed later.

We have used the Elscint ESI ED 65TV vaginal probe, attached to the ESI 1000 mechanical sector scanner at Rambam Medical Center in Israel. The scanner is a 6.5-mHz mechanical sector probe in a cylindrical case of 25.4-mm width. The rounded 10.5-mm spherical acoustic window houses a 10-mm transducer crystal. The performance characteristics of the probe include a variable frame

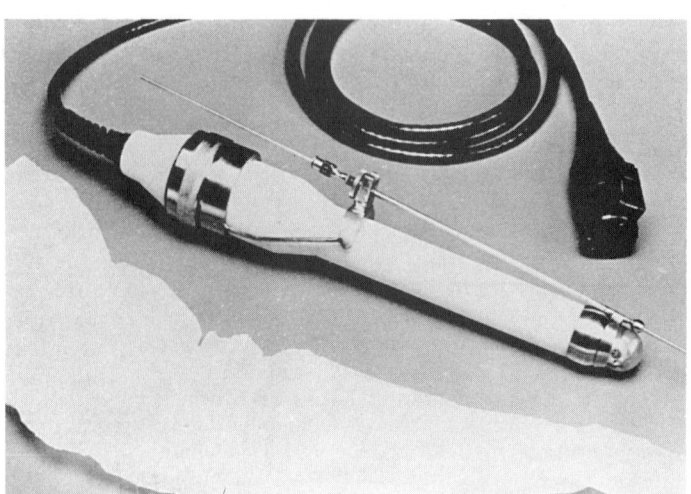

FIGURE 3-25. The transvaginal transducer fitted with needle guide, needle and sterile drape.

rate of 10 to 70 frames per second, a scan angle extendable to 105 degrees, an axis resolution of 0.45 mm, and a lateral resolution of 1.3 mm at the focal point. The focal zone is 20 mm to 70 mm and it is acoustically focused at 40-mm depth. The probe can be fitted with a needle guide for biopsy or oocytes pick-up, as shown in Figure 3-25.

TRANSVAGINAL SONOGRAPHY IN EARLY PREGNANCY

The human blastocyst implants into the congested and thick endometrial stroma 7 to 8 days postovulation. The trophoblast is thicker on the deep aspect of the implanted blastocyst, secondary to better nutrition, and forms the future placenta. The amniotic cavity forms from the inner cell mass of the blastocyst. At about 2 weeks postconception, the germinative layer, located between the amniotic cavity and the yolk sac, progressively differentiates to form the fetus. A simple circulatory system with a pulsating fetal heart is established in the fetus about 21 days postconception.[21] A pulsating fetal heart can be detected by transvaginal sonography about 4 weeks from conception (6 weeks gestational age from the last menstrual period [LMP]) in the 3-mm to 4-mm embryo, that is, within a week of its development.

Using the transvaginal probe, the gestational sac can be first detected about 15 to 18 days postovulation. At this stage, the gestational sac measures 4 mm to 5 mm in diameter, and the serum Beta HCG is between 400 to 800 mIU/l. These data represent a considerable refinement over Kadar's[25] pioneer data, which defined a "discriminatory zone" of 6500 mIU/ml serum for ultrasound detection of a gestational sac, usually at the end of the sixth week of gestation from LMP. More recently, Nyberg[31] showed that the gestational sac could be consistently demonstrated when serum Beta HCG levels are above 1800 mIU/ml.

An important characteristic of the early gestational sac is the double contour, which differentiates it from other intrauterine collections, such as intrauterine bleeding or the decidual reaction called "pseudogestational sac" described in ectopic pregnancy.[1,41] The demonstration of a "true" gestational sac—double-contoured and with peculiar laminar structures appearing at one pole (caused by maternal blood flow to the implantation site)—will effectively rule out the diagnosis of ectopic pregnancy, as the incidence of combined intra- and extrauterine pregnancies is very low (in the range of 1 in 20,000–30,000). This data can be obtained by transvaginal ultrasound (Figure 3-26) with great confidence about 7 to 10 days earlier than by transabdominal ultrasound.

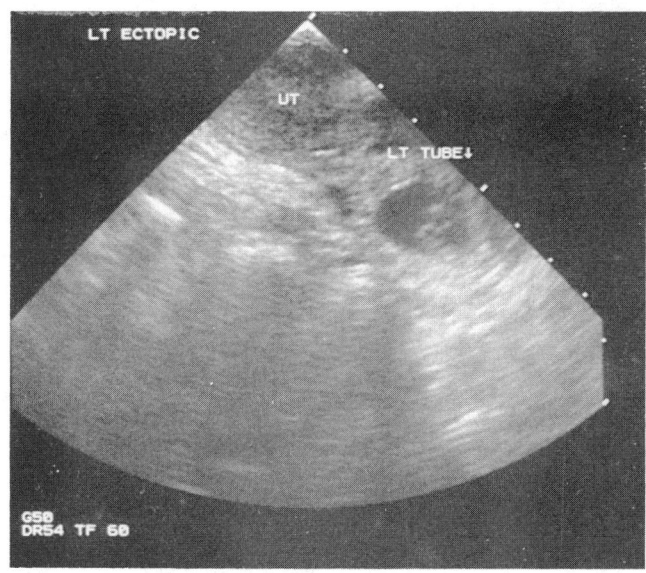

FIGURE 3-26. Ectopic pregnancy. Note empty uterus and viable pregnancy with fetal heart beats in left tube at 7 weeks gestation.

Abnormalities of the gestational sac may be the first sign of an abnormal pregnancy destined to abort, although generally other signs such as vaginal bleeding precede and are the indicators for the ultrasonographic study. Nyberg[32] recently described the morphology of the abnormal gestational sac. The gestational sac is considered abnormal if the following are true:

It is larger than 24 mm without an embryo.
It has a distorted shape.
There is a lack of the typical gestational double contour and the sac is greater than 10 mm in size.
The sac is in very low position within the lower uterine segment.
It has a thin choriodecidual reaction which measures 2 mm or less and no yolk sac is present.

The yolk sac becomes evident at about 5 weeks gestation. At this age it fills about one-third of the gestational sac and measures about 4 mm in diameter. A nonexistent yolk sac (usually diagnosed in conjunction with an anembryonic gestation), a smaller-than-4-mm yolk sac, or an irregularly shaped or fragmented yolk sac is a sign of abnormal gestation. The importance of the yolk sac in organogenetic congenital anomalies was appreciated only recently.[30,33] If the yolk sac is seen but no fetal pole is evident, or if a small-for-date and free-floating yolk sac is appreciated by real-time sonography, the diagnosis of missed abortion can be made[24] (Figure 3-27).

The fetal pole can be seen on transvaginal ultrasound by the end of the fifth week of gestation. The gestational sac is demonstrated as a 15-mm cystic structure with the 2-mm to 3-mm echogenic embryo adjacent to a cystic yolk sac. At the beginning of the sixth week, fetal heart beats should be demonstrable. Failure to see fetal heart beats 6.5 weeks from LMP, with accurate dating, indicates impending abortion.[39]

After 7 weeks gestation, measurements of the gestational sac are less informative and the measurement of crown-rump length (CRL) achieves more meaning. The high resolution obtained with transvaginal sonography provides precise CRL measurements on the fetal pole, with the membranes appearing clearly on the eighth week. The embryo can be seen moving actively in the amniotic cavity.

In the ninth week, the distinct parts of

74 Fetal Diagnosis and Therapy

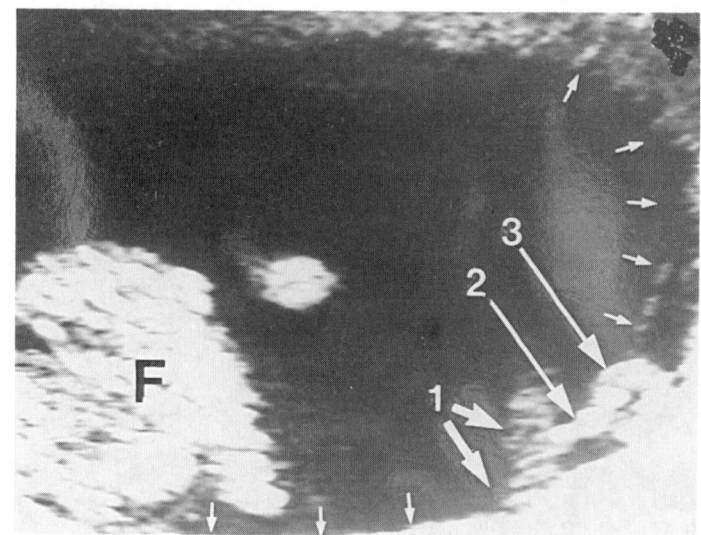

FIGURE 3-27. At 8 weeks, gross section of fetal body (F), chord (1), yolk stalk (2), and yolk sac (3) reveals that the amniotic membrane is separate from the uterine cavity (small arrows). The yolk sac is an extraamniotic structure.

the embryo—head, trunk, and limbs—appear and can be measured on transvaginal sonography. The head, which is already bigger than the yolk sac, appears to be filled with fluid (Figure 3-28). Close to the end of the ninth week, the choroid plexus is sometimes observed. At this stage the placenta appears clearer and its relationship to the uterine cavity is more obvious. Vaginosonographic-guided chorionic villus sampling (CVS) at 10 weeks gestation has been described.[16]

The ventricular system with its highly echogenic choroid plexus is easily seen at the

FIGURE 3-28. At 9 weeks, a distinct fetal head (larger than the abdomen) and limb buds are observed.

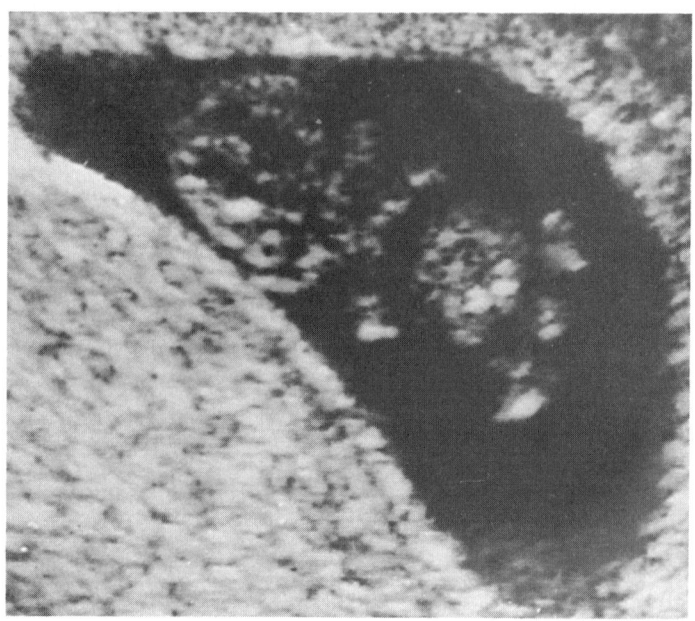

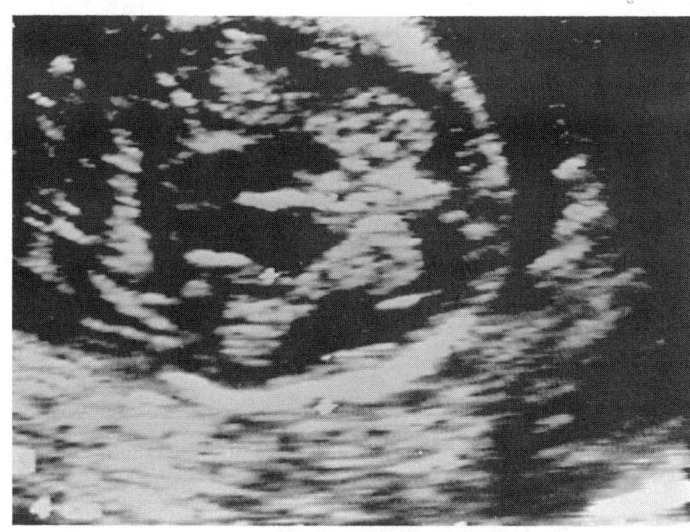

FIGURE 3-29. Fetal head at 12 to 13 weeks gestation. Note ventricular development and prominent choroid plexus.

end of the first trimester, at gestational age of 11 to 13 weeks (Figure 3-29). At about 12 weeks gestation, thalamus, brain stem, third ventricle, and cerebellum, as well as the base of the skull can be identified and measured. A normal view of the posterior cranial fossa will rule out an Arnold Chiari malformation or Dandy-Walker syndrome. Recent sonographic evaluation of cerebellar growth by Goldstein and co-workers[18] demonstrated a linear relationship with gestational age during the second trimester. Although able to identify the cerebellum at 12 weeks, actual data in their study is between 15 to 39 weeks gestational age.

The face and lips can be observed by transvaginal sonography at 12 to 13 weeks. A normal chin contour will, in effect, rule out the Pierre Robin syndrome (mandibular hypoplasia, with or without cleft palate). This syndrome may be part of a variety of skeletal and muscular syndromes, some with mendelian inheritance (e.g., congenital myotonic dystrophy). Cleft lip and palate, a midline fusion disorder, can be isolated or part of a more complete syndrome, and may be seen as part of chromosomal abnormalities such as trisomies 13 or 18, part of syndromes with mendelian inheritance like chondrodysplasia punctata (Conrad's syndrome) or diastrophic dwarphism (both autosomal recessive disorders), as part of non-mendelian-diseases together with congenital heart disease, or as a result of maternal teratogens during pregnancy (e.g., hydantoin or warfarin). Hypertelorism (increased interorbital distance) is seen as part of a few chromosomal abnormalities, the most common being trisomy 21.

The lens is observed in the fetal eye starting from the 12th to 13th week. Eye movements can be appreciated and the interorbital distance measured. Congenital cataract has an incidence of 1 in 250 live births, most commonly caused by an environmental (e.g., rubella infection) or other primary disorder (e.g., galactosemia or hypoparathyroidism or a syndromal association like Conrad's disease). Most genetic forms without a metabolic cause follow autosomal-dominant inheritance, with risks for siblings in an isolated case of about 10%.[23] Lens dislocation is a feature of Marfan syndrome (in conjunction with arachnodactily and pectus excavatus and aortic complications) or homocystinuria, but can be also an isolated event.

Fetal limbs and digits are observed using transvaginal ultrasound from the tenth week on, but measurement of the different bones and appreciation of specific limb movement is best performed during the 12th or 13th

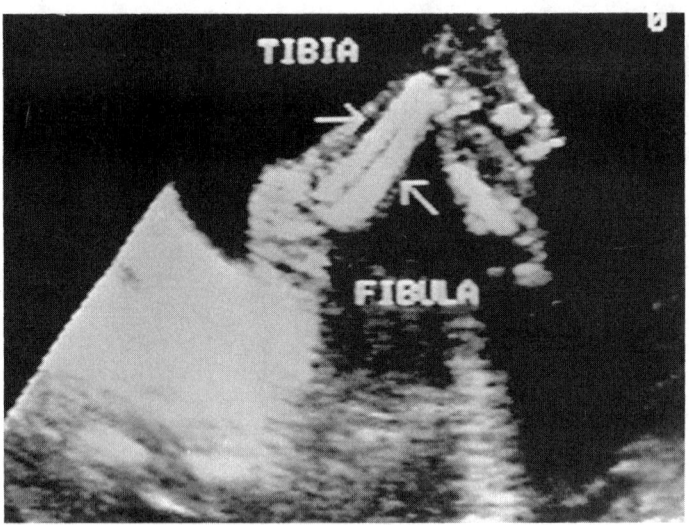

FIGURE 3-30. Tibia, fibula, and foot at 14 weeks gestation. (Reproduced courtesy of Dr. M. Bronstein, Rambam Medical Center, Haifa, Israel)

week of gestation (Figure 3-30). Fetal limb defects can be unilateral or bilateral. Most unilateral defects are of nongenetic origin, for example, damage caused by amniotic bands or by teratogens (the notorious effects of thalidomide or effects associated with injection of sex hormones like synthetic progestins or oral contraceptives during pregnancy).[22] Most bilateral limb lesions are genetic in origin and follow the rules of mendelian inheritance, for example, bone dysplasias which affect all bones, or syndromes affecting mainly the upper limbs like Fanconi's pancytopenia or thrombocytopenia-absent radius (TAR) syndrome, both with autosomal recessive inheritance. Fetal fingers or toes can be seen and counted (Figure 3-31) and their movement assessed in an attempt to rule out syndactyly or polydactyly. Syndactyly can be unilateral such as part of Poland syndrome

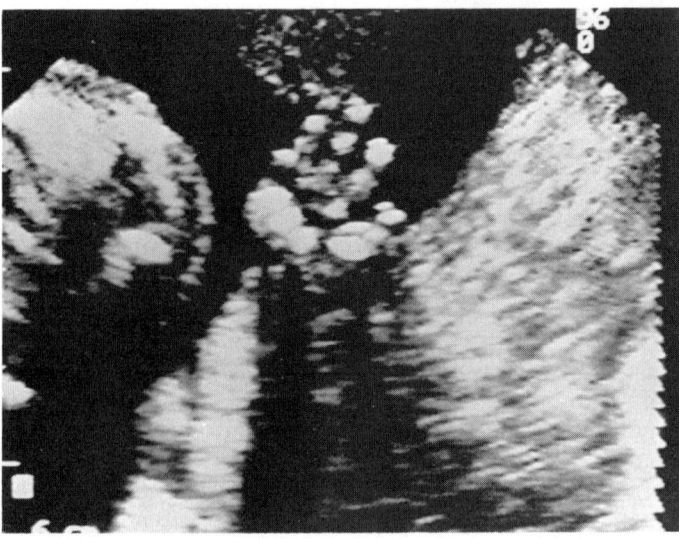

FIGURE 3-31. Palm and fingers at 16 weeks gestation. Note distinct interphalangeal joints. (Reproduced courtesy of Dr. M. Bronstein, Rambam Medical Center, Haifa, Israel)

(unilateral syndactyly with pectoral muscle aplasia), which is nongenetic and possibly related to abortifacients.[7] Bilateral isolated syndactyly of the hands or feet has several forms, all autosomal dominant. Important syndromes include orofacial digital syndrome, a dominant X-linked syndrome, lethal in males. Polydactyly in its isolated form is a relatively common condition inherited as an autosomal dominant trait with incomplete penetrance. More complex disorders with polydactyly include trisomy 13, Ellis-van Creveld syndrome (an autosomal recessive and frequently lethal bone dysplasia), and the autosomal-recessive Bardet-Bredle syndrome (with retinitis pigmentosa, hypogonadism, and mental retardation).

Using transvaginal ultrasound, fetal thoracic measurements may be obtained as early as 12 weeks, as compared with the most recently used nomograms which start at 16 weeks gestational age.[5] Thoracic dimensions are measured at the level of the four-chamber view of the heart. A low thoracic circumference–abdominal circumference ratio is found in pulmonary hypoplasia and in some of the lethal bone dysplasias such as thanatophoric dwarfism (in which most cases are de novo mutations). A normal four-chamber view of the fetal heart can rule out a fetal heart anomaly with a high degree of confidence. Congenital heart disease occurs in about 1% of live births, and is generally of unknown etiology or of polygenetic inheritance. The risk of congenital heart disease increases with advanced maternal age, by about 2% for women age 40 or more. Environmental causes (e.g., rubella), mendelian disorders (e.g., Marfan or Ellis-van Creveld syndromes) and non-mendelian syndromes (vertebral, anal, cardiac, thoracic, esophageal, renal, and limb [VACTERL] anomalies) are associated with congenital heart disease. Measuring heart circumference at the level of the four-chamber view and comparing it with thoracic circumference can facilitate the diagnosis of fetal heart failure in cases of nonimmune hydrops or cardiomyopathy.

A scan of the fetal abdomen at 13 weeks reveals the umbilical vein and stomach, and more commonly, the kidneys and fetal bladder. Polycystic kidneys and bladder obstruction are easily diagnosed. Abdominal wall defects can be detected by 12 weeks gestational age, as the return of the intestine into the peritoneal cavity and its rotation and fixation to the posterior abdominal wall should be completed at 10 to 11 weeks. Schmidt and colleagues demonstrated the sonographic visualization of a physiologic anterior abdominal wall hernia in the first trimester, which is caused by the relative rapid growth of the midgut starting at 6 weeks. This normal herniation of the midgut disappears by the tenth to 11th week as the intestine slides rapidly into the peritoneal cavity. Failure of midgut folding may cause abdominal wall defects such as omphalocele (incidence 1 in 5000 live births) or gastroschisis (incidence of 1 in 10,000–12,000). These lesions may be associated with anomalies of other organ systems (chromosomal 30%, genitourinary 40%, cardiovascular 16%–20%, and central nervous system 4%).[35] Disorders such as abdominal wall defects, bladder exstrophy, or the "prune belly" syndrome (abdominal muscle deficiency, megaureters, megacystis, undescended testes) are all amenable to prenatal diagnosis by maternal serum alpha-fetoprotein screening.

Fetal sex can be easily determined by transvaginal ultrasound at 13 weeks gestational age. This is of particular importance in the diagnosis of X-linked hereditary disorders, especially if prenatal diagnosis by chorionic villus sampling (CVS) or amniocentesis of the specific disease involved is not feasible.

These anomalies form an incomplete list of disorders which can be diagnosed by ultrasound. While almost all can be diagnosed by transabdominal sonography, they can be diagnosed more easily (due to better resolution) and earlier (1–3 weeks) by transvaginal sonography. Earlier diagnosis facilitated by transvaginal ultrasound should shorten the period of ambiguity and psychological trauma to the patient in the event of a decision to terminate an affected pregnancy. However, as a full description and nomograms of fetal dimensions at this early age are not yet available, and as most of ultrasonographic diagnoses of syndrome associations were not yet described by transvaginal sonography, care should be exercised in the near future regarding operative decisions until more data are available.

The distance between the transducer's top and the "target" organ lengthens concomitant with fetal growth, and the scanning becomes progressively more difficult in the late second and third trimesters. This problem can be partially solved by external manipulation of the fetal part to be examined toward the transducer.

ULTRASONOGRAPHIC EVALUATION OF THE CERVIX IN PREGNANCY

The first ultrasonographic description of a dilated cervix in pregnancy was published by Sarti in 1979.[34] Data published since then have emphasized the importance of a full patient's bladder[3] for measurement of cervical length, as well as demonstration of membrane herniation into the cervical canal and bulging with an hour-glass appearance into the vagina.[15,29] Using transabdominal ultrasonography, Michaels and associates showed that the development of cervical incompetence is a dynamic rather than a constant process. Quite often, changes occur at the level of the internal os, and are inaccessible by routine examination. Sonographic changes may thus be the earliest indication of incipient cervical failure. However, once they have occurred, the time elapsing to clinical prolapse of membranes is unpredictable.[29] Brown and co-workers[4] compared the evaluation of the cervix and lower uterine segment by the transabdominal and transvaginal routes. They found that the abdominal technique adequately depicted the correct status of the cervix and lower uterine segment in 76% of cases, compared to 83% using the transvaginal approach. Although this difference was not statistically significant, these results suggest that the transvaginal technique may be superior in obtaining an adequate evaluation of the lower uterine segment and cervix, and may have an advantage over a fully distended bladder for evaluation.

Placental localization and relation of placental site to cervix may also be evaluated by transvaginal sonography. Because the optimal point of examining the cervix and lower uterine segment is about 2.5 cm away from the external os, slight vaginal bleeding or suspected placenta previa should not preclude its careful use, even in the late second or third trimester.

TRANSVAGINAL SONOGRAPHY IN INFERTILITY

Involuntary infertility affects 15% to 20% of couples with serious economic and psychologic sequelae. About 40% to 50% of infertile couples suffer from ovulation disorders, and about 15% of infertile women suffer from mechanical infertility. A substantial proportion of the latter group will need in vitro fertilization and embryo transfer (IVF/ET). About 5% to 10% of the female population will need induction of ovulation.

Ovulation Induction

Until recently, ovulation induction was monitored by clinical and hormonal parameters. Ultrasonographic monitoring of ovulation induction is based on the pioneer work of Hackeloer,[20] who correlated follicular size by ultrasound with 17-beta-estradiol (E_2) measurements.

Using the 6.5-mHz vaginal probe, follicles are distinct starting at a diameter of 3 mm, but reaching clinical significance at about 10 mm.[12] This happens approximately 6 days before ovulation; later on in the natural ovarian cycle, only one follicle dominates. Hackeloer showed that the rate of growth of the dominant follicle is constant and averages 2 mm/day in the 5 days before ovulation. The diameter of the dominant follicle just prior to ovulation ranges between 18 mm and 24 mm, with an average of 20 mm to 22 mm.[19] Because the amount of estrogen produced by a single follicle increases as the follicle matures, and because 95% of the circulating E_2 level derives from the dominant follicle,[2] Hackeloer and associates found a linear correlation between follicular diameter and E_2 serum level in the natural cycle.[20]

In ovulatory cycles induced with clomiphene citrate (CC) or human menopausal gonadotropins (HMG), generally more than one dominant follicle develops. In these cases, although E_2 serum levels and follicular diameters seem to increase linearly, the correlation between the two is significantly lower than in the natural cycle.[8] In induced cycles, total follicular volume shows the highest correlation with serum E_2, since the rate of growth of the individual follicle and the leading follicle can change during the cycle.[40] Using ultrasonic follicular monitoring, we can withhold HCG administration when E_2 serum level is preovulatory but derived from multiple small follicles, thereby avoiding premature atresia of these follicles.

Follicular measurements are performed placing the patient in a lithotomy position with an empty bladder. Useful landmarks are the uterus, which appears while scanning in the transverse plane as an ovoid structure with enhanced echogenicity in its middle (endometrial response), and the iliac vessels which appear on the lateral side of the screen (near the pelvic wall) as prolonged anechoic structures, with pulsation and flow observed clearly. The ovaries are usually located medial to the iliac vessels, but their location may change, secondary to previous surgery or pelvic inflammatory disease (PID) adhesions.

Follicular volume (V) is calculated using the following formula for an ovoid:

$$V = \pi/6 \times A \times B \times C$$

where A, B and C are the largest diameters obtained measured on three planes.

When only two planes are available, the formula should be:

$$V = \pi/6 \times A \times B \times B$$

where A is the largest diameter measured and B is the smallest.

For most purposes, follicular volume is not calculated and the mean diameter of the leading follicles is used instead for assessment of ovarian response and decision for further treatment (Figure 3-32).

The changes in the endometrium in response to rising hormonal levels were sonographically observed and described by Smith.[37] Both reflectivity (the comparison of the gray scale texture of the endometrium to

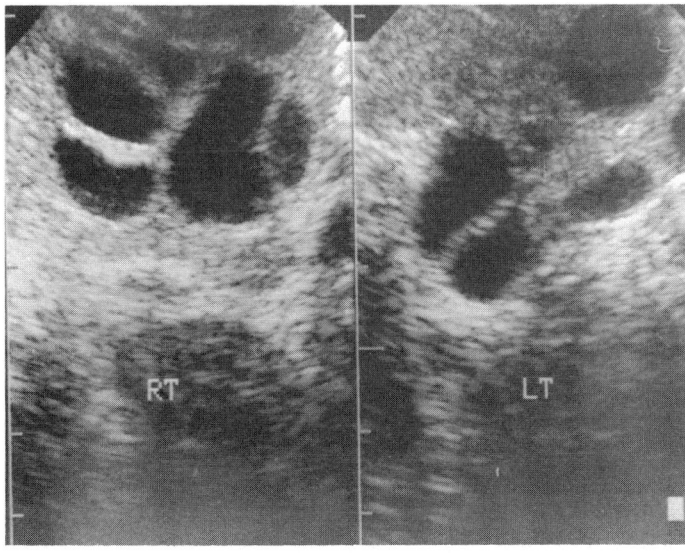

FIGURE 3-32. Preovulatory ovarian follicles just prior to oocyte pick-up. Note distinct follicular borders.

that of the myometrium) and thickness of the endometrium are enhanced by rising estrogen levels. The thickness of the endometrium is measured on both sides of the midline, through the central longitudinal axis of the uterus. Four patterns of endometrial response were described by Smith:

Grade D: An almost anechoic endometrium in the presence of a prominent midline echo. This endometrial pattern is characteristic of the early follicular phase with low estrogen levels. Thickness of the endometrium is less than 5 mm.

Grade C: Characterized by a solid area of reduced reflectivity and appearing darker than the surrounding endometrium. Endometrial thickness in this stage is about 5 mm, in response to rising estrogen levels.

Grade B: The endometrium is comparable in reflectivity with the surrounding myometrium and is indistinguishable in its gray scale appearance. The initial appearance of an endometrial halo is noted.

Grade A: The endometrium appears brighter than the myometrium, with an approximate thickness of about 10 mm, characteristic of ovulation.

In Smith's study, endometrial grades A and B were associated with higher estradiol levels, more mature oocytes at pick-up, and a higher fertilization and pregnancy rate. Due to the higher resolution of the transvaginal probe, these changes can be measured with greater precision, providing more accurate data for clinical decisions.

Ovulatory events were ultrasonographically observed by DeCrespigny.[9] Responding to levels of follicle-stimulating hormone (FSH) and luteinizing hormone (LH) and specifically the LH surge, the cumulus mass undergoes mucification and expands. This mucoid consistency enables visualization of the cumulus in about 60% to 65% of preovulatory follicles, 12 to 24 hours before ovulation. No change in size or appearance of the follicle is observed until after release of antral fluid and follicular collapse has occurred. Follicular rupture may be very rapid or take up to 35 minutes. During the ensuing hours the corpus hemorrhagia develops (the follicle area fills with echogenic shadows) and the expelled follicular fluid collects in the Douglas' Pouch. This ultrasonographic picture and the blurring of the follicular borders are accepted as signs of ovulation. However, especially in induced cycles with hyperovulation, an amount of fluid (up to 50 ml) may be observed in the cul-de-sac before actual ovulation occurs. This collection of fluid is caused by transudation from the dominant follicles, perhaps in response to high estrogen levels.[8]

Oocyte Retrieval for in vitro Fertilization and Embryo Transfer

The use of laparoscopy for retrieval of oocytes was introduced by Edwards and Steptoe in 1980,[38] and has become the standard procedure for IVF/ET. In 1981, Lenz[28] described the technique of ultrasonic-guided transvesical oocyte retrieval. With improved equipment and increased technical expertise, ultrasound-guided follicular aspiration has become as good as or superior to laparoscopic retrieval of oocytes.[13]

Disadvantages of this method are that transversing the bladder is psychologically stressful to the patient and penetration of the unanesthetized posterior bladder wall is painful. Urine contamination of the follicular fluid may occur, and transient hematuria has been reported (4 out of 30 cases by Lenz).[27] Moreover, the transvesical approach is not feasible if the ovaries are located deep in the Douglas' Pouch, posterior to the uterus.

In 1983, Gleicher[17] announced a single case of transvaginal oocyte retrieval. Dellenbach and co-workers later published their transvaginal oocyte retrieval technique and results using transabdominal ultrasonic guidance.[10,11] The procedure requires two operators, one controlling the transducer on the abdomen and the second performing the aspiration of the follicles transvaginally. This technique yields relatively low results (2.2 oocytes/patient)[11] and can be dangerous, with two reported cases of iliac vein lacerations.[6]

These complications were probably due to the lack of alignment between the abdominal transducer and the needle tip, as well as the free hand-operated vaginal needle. In 1986, Kemeter and Feichtinger described their experience with transvaginal oocyte retrieval using a vaginal sector scan probe combined with an automatic puncture device.[26] They reported a 98.3% transvaginal oocyte recovery with a mean 4.5 oocytes/patient and 21.3% clinical pregnancies/oocyte pick-up. These results in 61 patients are better than the results obtained in 371 patients with transabdominal ultrasonic-guided oocyte retrieval in their institution.[14]

Transvaginal oocyte retrieval has been practiced at Rambam Medical Center since December 1985. The 6.5-mHz vaginal probe is fitted with a needle guide for this procedure, whose line is parallel to the axis and 1.5 cm lateral to the axis line. The Elscint ESI 1000 sector scanner, a viewing angle of 105 degrees, and a rate of 14 images/second are employed. Patients undergo induced hyperovulation with combinations of cc/HMG/HCG or FSH/HMG/HCG, and are monitored by serum E_2 levels and transvaginal ultrasound scanning of the ovaries. The day before and the morning of follicular aspiration, povidone iodine vaginal suppositories are inserted in order to obtain sterile vaginal mucosa. Systemic antibiotics are not used routinely. Follicular aspiration is performed with the patient in the lithotomy position with an empty bladder. After diagnostic scanning to rule out ovulation, the vagina is thoroughly cleaned with povidone iodine solution and rinsed with sterile normal saline. The patient is draped and sterile covers are used for the sector scanner and the transducer. A dose of 50 to 150 mg pethidine hydrochloride (Demerol) and 10 to 15 mg diazepam (Valium) are injected intravenously, depending on the patient's weight and sensitivity, to achieve sedation. This dose is generally enough to keep the patient hypoanesthetized, relaxed, and awake, or in a superficial sleep.

The draped transducer fitted with a needle guide is introduced deep into the vagina and the largest diameter of the target follicle is aligned with the biopsy line. The follicle is entered with a 25-cm, 1.4-mm internal diameter, stainless steel serrated needle (manufactured by Izmel Ltd., Israel) and the follicular contents are aspirated under a suction pressure of 100 mm Hg into sterile culture flasks. If the oocyte cumulus complex is not discovered in the first sample, the follicle is flushed with culture medium and can be seen to enlarge. The injected flushing fluid contains micro air bubbles and appears turbulent on the screen. A new needle is used every time the needle tip passes the vaginal mucosa. After all follicles have been entered and aspirated, the pelvic organs are scanned to rule out active bleeding from puncture sites.

With this technique, 219 procedures of oocyte pick-up were performed in our hospital. Since December 1985, vaginal harvesting has yielded an average of 5.2 oocytes/patient, and a 12.8% clinical pregnancy rate per oocyte pick-up. These results are comparable to laparoscopic oocyte pick-up during the same period. Over a period, as the operators gained more experience with the vaginal procedure, there was a clear shift of methods to transvaginal harvesting. Laparoscopy is now done only in cases that need observation of the pelvic organs or in cases of unexplained infertility scheduled for gamete intrafallopian transfer.[12]

CONCLUSIONS

Transvaginal ultrasonography, using a higher frequency transducer and directing the tip of the transducer nearer to the organs scanned, produces a high-resolution, clear view of the pelvic organs.

In early pregnancy, developmental events can be seen using a vaginal probe approximately a week earlier than can be seen transabdominally. A quicker and more accurate appraisal of early pregnancy pathology (imminent abortion, ectopic pregnancy, fetal anomalies) can be achieved using transvaginal sonography. In cases requiring intervention, (e.g., conservative surgery for ectopic pregnancy) this can be done earlier, minimizing physical and emotional damage to the patient.

For follicular aspiration for IVF/ET, the transvaginal approach has several outstanding advantages:

Higher resolution images of the ovaries and surrounding organs are produced.
With a shorter distance between the transducer and the ovary, the distance transversed by the needle is shorter too, decreasing the probability of bowel or blood vessel injury.
The bladder is not penetrated.
The procedure is quite painless, well tolerated by most patients, and does not require local or general anesthesia, thus minimizing the risk to the patient.
As the recovery is quick, it is done as an outpatient procedure, minimizing the cost of the procedure.

For research purposes, the transvaginal approach could be used for early pregnancy developmental events, for flowmetry in early abortion and intrauterine growth retardation studies, and early detection of fetal anomalies. Early detection of multiple implantation after multiple embryo replacement should enable a choice of fetal reduction by the transvaginal or transvesical way. More experience is to be achieved with the transvaginal guidance for chorionic villus sampling.

REFERENCES

1. Abramovici H, Auslander R, Lewin A: Gestational-pseudogestational sac—A new ultrasonic criteria for differential diagnosis. Am J Obstet Gynecol 145:377–379, 1983
2. Baird DT, Fraser IS: Blood production and ovarian secretion rates of estradiol and estrone in women throughout the menstrual cycle. J Clin Endocrinol 38:1009–1015, 1974
3. Bowie JD, Andreotti RF, Rosenberg ER: Sonographic appearance of the uterine cervix in pregnancy—The vertical cervix. Am J Radiol 140:737–740, 1983
4. Brown JE, Thieme AG, Shah MD et al: Transabdominal and transvaginal endosonography: Evaluation of the cervix and lower uterine segment in pregnancy. Am J Obstet Gynecol 155:721–726, 1986
5. Chitkara U, Rosenberg J, Chervenak AF et al: Prenatal sonographic assessment of the fetal thorax—Normal values. Am J Obstet Gynecol 156:1069–1074, 1987
6. Cohen F, Debache C, Pez FP et al: Transvaginal sonographically controlled ovarian puncture for oocyte retrieval for in vitro fertilization. J In Vitro Fertil Embryo Transfer 3(5):309–313, 1986
7. David TJ: Nature and etiology of the Poland anomaly. N Engl J Med 287:487–489, 1972
8. DeCherney AH, Laufer N: The monitoring of ovulation induction using ultrasound and estrogens. Clin Obstet Gynecol 27:993–1002, 1984
9. DeCrespigny L, O'Herlihy C, Robinson HP: Ultrasonic observation of the mechanism of human ovulation. Am J Obstet Gynecol 139:616–640, 1981
10. Dellenbach P, Nisand I, Moreau L et al: Transvaginal sonographically controlled ovarian follicle puncture for egg retrieval. Lancet 1:1462–1472, 1984
11. Dellenbach P, Nisand I, Moreau L et al: Transvaginal sonographically controlled follicle puncture for oocyte retrieval. Fertil Steril 44:656–661, 1985
12. Drugan A, Blumenfeld Z, Erlik J et al: The use of transvaginal sonography in infertility. In Timor-Tritsch IE, Rottem S (eds): Transvaginal Sonography, pp 109–123. New York, Elsevier, 1987
13. Feichtinger W, Kemeter P: Laparoscopic or ultrasonically guided follicle aspiration for in vitro fertilization. J In Vitro Fertil Embryo Transfer 1:244–246, 1984
14. Feichtinger W, Kemeter P: Ultrasound guided of human ovarian follicles for in vitro fertilization. In Saunders RC, Hall M (eds): Ultrasound Annual, pp 25–37. New York, Raven Press, 1986
15. Fried A: Bulging amnion in premature labor: Spectrum of sonographic findings. Am J Radiol 136:181–185, 1981
16. Ghirardini G, Popp WL, Camurri L, Stoeckenius M: Vaginosonographic guided chorionic villi needle biopsy. Europ J Obstet Gynecol Reprod Biol 23:315–319, 1986
17. Gleicher N, Friberg J, Fullan N et al: Egg retrieval for in vitro fertilization by sonographically controlled vaginal culdocentesis. Lancet 2:508–509, 1983
18. Goldstein I, Reece AE, Pilu G et al: Cerebellar

measurements with ultrasonography in the evaluation of fetal growth and development. Am J Obstet Gynecol 156:1065–1069, 1987
19. Hackeloer BJ: Ultrasound scanning of the ovarian cycle. J In Vitro Fertil Embryo Transfer 1(4):217–220, 1984
20. Hackeloer BJ, Fleming R, Robinson HP: Correlation of ultrasonic and endocrinologic assessment of human follicular development. Am J Obstet Gynecol 135:122–128, 1979
21. Hamilton WJ, Boyd JD, Mossiman HW: The implantation of the blastocyst and the development of the fetal membranes, placenta and decidua. In: Human Embryology, pp 49–76. Cambridge, W Heffer & Sons, 1945.
22. Hill JA, Pickens AG, McDonough PG, Cunningham JJ: Ultrasound diagnosis of multiple anomalies associated with prenatal oral contraceptives. Med Ultrasound 6:116–118, 1982
23. Harper PS: The Eye in Practical Genetic Counseling. Bristol, England, J Wright & Sons, 1984
24. Hurwitz RS: Yolk sac sign—Sonographic appearance of the fetal yolk sac in missed abortion. J Ultrasound Med 5:435–438, 1986
25. Kadar N, Devore G, Rowen R: Discriminatory HCG zone: Its use in sonographic evaluation for ectopic pregnancy. Obstet Gynecol 58:156–161, 1981
26. Kemeter P, Feichtinger W: Transvaginal oocyte retrieval using a transvaginal sector scan probe combined with an automated puncture device. Human Reprod 1:21–26, 1986
27. Lenz S, Lauritsen JG: Ultrasonically guided percutaneous aspiration of human follicles under local anesthesia: A new method of collecting oocytes for in vitro fertilization. Fertil Steril 38:673–677, 1982
28. Lenz S, Lauritzen JG, Kjellow M: Collection of human oocytes for in vitro fertilization by ultrasonically guided follicular puncture. Lancet 1:1163–1169, 1981
29. Michaels WH, Montgomery C, Karo J et al: Ultrasound differentiation of the competent from the incompetent cervix—Prevention of preterm labor. Am J Obstet Gynecol 154:537–546, 1986
30. Naftolin F, Diamond MP, Pinter E et al: A hypothesis concerning the general basis of organogenetic congenital anomalies. Am J Obstet Gynecol 157:1–4, 1987
31. Nyberg DA, Filly RA, Mahoney BS et al: Early gestation—Correlation of HCG levels and sonographic identification. AJR 144:951–954, 1985
32. Nyberg DA, Laing FC, Filly RA: Threatened abortion—Sonographic distinction of normal and abnormal gestational scars. Radiology 158:397–400, 1986
33. Pinter E, Reece AE, Leranth CZ et al: Yolk sac failure in embryopathy due to hyperglycemia. Ultrastructural analysis of yolk sac differentiation associated with embryopathy in rat conceptuses under hyperglycemic conditions. Teratology 33:73–84, 1986
34. Sarti DA, Sample WF, Hobel CF, Starsek KY: Ultrasonic visualization of a dilated cervix during pregnancy. Radiology 130:417, 1979
35. Schmidt W, Yarkoni S, Crelin ES, Hobbins JC: Sonographic visualization of physiologic anterior abdominal wall hernia in the first trimester. Obstet Gynecol 69:911, 1987
36. Schwimer SR, Lebovic Y: Transvaginal pelvic ultrasonography: Accuracy in follicle and cyst size determination. J Ultrasound Med 4:61–63, 1985
37. Smith B, Porter R, Ahuja K, Craft I: Ultrasonic assessment of endometrial changes in stimulated cycles in an in vitro fertilization and embryo transfer program. J In Vitro Fertil Embryo Transfer 1(4):233–238, 1984
38. Steptoe PC, Edwards RG: Laparoscopic recovery of preovulatory human oocytes after priming the ovaries with gonadotropins. Lancet 1:683–687, 1970
39. Timor-Tritsch IE, Rottem S, Blumenfeld Z: Pathology of the early intrauterine pregnancy. In Timor-Tritsch IE, Rottem S (eds): Transvaginal Sonography, pp 109–123. New York, Elsevier, 1987
40. Vargyas JM, Marrs RP, Kletzki DA, Mishell DR: Correlation of ovarian follicular size and serum estradiol levels in ovulatory patients following Clomiphene Citrate for IVF/ET. Am J Obstet Gynecol 144:569–573, 1982
41. Weiner C: The pseudogestational sac in ectopic pregnancy. Am J Obstet Gynecol 139:959–961, 1981
42. Yee B, Barnes RB, Vargyas JM, Marrs RP: Correlation of transabdominal and transvaginal ultrasound measurements of follicle size and number with laparoscopic findings for in vitro fertilization. Fertil Steril 47:828–832, 1987

4

Predictive Genetic Testing

Kåre Berg

All the analyses described in this section could reasonably be referred to as predictive tests, since they predict the health of a child to be born several months after the tests have been conducted. However, the analyses hitherto described detect actual disease or malformation in the fetus, and they are therefore better referred to as diagnostic tests.

For the present purpose, the term *predictive tests* will be used for analyses that have predictive value with respect to future disease risk in persons or fetuses that do not have an illness at the time of testing, or in offspring of the individuals analyzed. The term *screening* will be limited to mass analyses of populations or population groups that are being conducted without previous knowledge of a specific disease risk in any given individual. With these definitions, the vast majority of tests conducted on fetuses today are diagnostic rather than predictive, and for the purpose of the present discussion it is therefore necessary to also consider predictive testing conducted after birth.

TECHNOLOGIES FOR PREDICTIVE GENETIC TESTING

Predictive genetic testing can be conducted by scoring for any genetic trait that has been shown to invariably or very frequently occur in a given disease or that is known to exhibit population association of some strength with a given disease.

Deficiency of the serum protein, alpha-1 antitrypsin, is caused by a mutant gene at one single locus. It has been known for several years that persons with this inherited anomaly are at increased risk to develop obstructive pulmonary disease. This disease can be greatly incapacitating and it is therefore important to try to prevent it if at all possible. Exposure to cigarette smoke or other air pol-

---

This chapter was written while the author was a Scholar in Residence, Fogarty International Center, National Institutes of Health, Bethesda.

lutants significantly increases the risk to develop obstructive pulmonary disease in people with this genetic trait. This example of interaction between genetic and environmental factors clearly points to the importance of considering genes *and* environment in the etiology of diseases, rather than considering genes *or* environment. Alpha-1 antitrypsin deficiency is an example of a disorder in which predictive testing could be used in a beneficial way, to urge individuals to cease cigarette smoking and avoid air pollution to prevent or delay the development of the disease to which they are genetically predisposed.[1-3]

It is important to realize that alpha-1 antitrypsin deficiency in many instances is compatible with normal or nearly normal life, although some bearers of this trait are born with liver disease. Nevertheless, the characteristics of this genetically determined condition is such that mass screening of fetuses is not called for. On the other hand, prenatal diagnosis could be an option to couples who have had a child with this disorder and severe liver disease.

Predictive tests are not limited to single, qualitative phenomena such as alpha-1 antitrypsin deficiency. Thus quantitative parameters that are influenced by several genes as well as environmental factors (such as total cholesterol level) could contribute to disease risk (e.g., for early-onset coronary heart disease). Existing methodologies and knowledge already make it possible to test for several simply inherited genetic traits and to measure many quantitative parameters that have predictive value with respect to atherosclerosis.[4,6]

In recent years, the combined use of specific DNA probes and restriction enzymes that split DNA at specific base sequences has made it possible to study the genetic material itself, in health and disease. It is already possible to examine a high number of human genes, and normal genetic variation in the DNA itself has been uncovered at many human gene loci or in areas flanking known genes. This includes loci for several physiologically or clinically relevant proteins such as apolipoproteins. Claims have already been made concerning the association between DNA variation and atherosclerotic or other diseases, that if confirmed could be used in predictive testing.[11,12]

Regardless of the ultimate fate of disease associations that have been reported up to now, it can safely be predicted that the new DNA technology will greatly increase the possibilities of conducting predictive tests over the next few years. There can be little doubt that the capacity to detect genes for simply inherited disorders prior to disease manifestations, as well as genes contributing to the risk for multifactorial diseases, will be greatly improved. The former category of disease will be relatively rare, and detection of the gene in question will often imply that the disease is unavoidable, whereas the latter category comprises several frequent diseases and the predictive tests will only uncover an increased (or decreased) risk compared to the population at large. From the point of view of predictive testing, these two categories of disorders are so different that they need to be treated separately.

PREDICTIVE TESTS FOR SIMPLY INHERITED DISORDERS

Although the great majority of simply inherited, serious diseases manifest themselves shortly after birth or in early infancy, some very serious monogenic disorders do not manifest themselves until adult life. When such diseases are dominantly inherited, it implies that a son or daughter of an affected person has a 50% risk of having inherited the gene and therefore of becoming ill in adult life. Huntington's disease, a disorder with severe central nervous system manifestations and dementia, is a particularly relevant example of such a disease, although autosomal dominant hypercholesterolemia is much more frequent.[8,10] Huntington's disease will most frequently last for many years, create a number of clinical and social problems, and be a very severe burden to the whole family. Familial hypercholesterolemia, although carrying a significantly increased risk of myocardial infarction, sudden death, or angina pectoris at a relatively young age, is compatible with normal life for a great proportion of the person's life span; several patients have a close to normal life span, and there is reasonable hope for therapeutic and preventive progress in this disorder.

Hypercholesterolemia

The characteristics of autosomal dominant hypercholesterolemia are such that screening for this disorder may be meaningful if safe, lifelong treatment that will normalize serum cholesterol can be developed. The disease would be detected in programs aimed at detecting coronary heart disease risks in general. Prenatal diagnosis of the disease is possible and may be wanted by some people who themselves have the disease or have seen its consequences in their family. Whereas prenatal diagnosis to detect familial hypercholesterolemia in its usual, heterozygous form may be ethically questionable, there can be little doubt about the justification of conducting prenatal diagnosis of the homozygous form (which can occur only if both parents have the disease in the heterozygous state). Homozygotes for familial hypercholesterolemia may contract myocardial infarction by age 2 and most of them die at a very early age, often in their teens. Unfortunately, safe lifelong treatment permitting normal life is unlikely to be developed for the homozygous form in the foreseeable future.

Mass fetal screening and selective abortion for familial hypercholesterolemia would be extremely costly and ethically doubtful because of the characteristics of the disease in its heterozygous form, and would only extremely rarely lead to the unsuspected detection of a fetus that has the disease in its very rare homozygous form.

Huntington's Disease

Whereas cloning of the gene causing familial hypercholesterolemia[13] has made it possible to detect the disease with certainty using DNA from various cell types including cultured fetal cells, the gene for Huntington's disease can at present be detected only in an indirect manner. DNA variation in an area close to the Huntington's disease locus can in many families make it possible to follow the segregation of the gene for the disease.[9] This approach, however, carries a significant degree of uncertainty because recombination can occur between the disease locus and the DNA region that serves as a tag for the gene, resulting in wrong predictions. With a disease such as Huntington's, very little uncertainty can be tolerated in a predictive test.

The main importance of the discovery of a DNA variation linked to the gene for Huntington's disease is the promise it holds for developing DNA probes for the Huntington's disease locus itself. There can be little doubt that gene-specific probes will be developed in the near future, and it is therefore timely to discuss the use of predictive tests for Huntington's disease, assuming that definite DNA tests will soon be developed.

There is no causal therapy and no effective preventive measure available for Huntington's disease, and it could be argued that it is better to abstain from predictive testing in this situation. The choice of a person at risk to not take a predictive test should be respected. The individual should have a right to refuse knowledge about his or her own health prospects if there is no therapy or prevention available and provided that this refusal does not hurt or seriously affect the lives of other people. However, it can be argued that a person with a 50% risk for Huntington's disease would be able to make more responsible choices and plans for his or her life if it were known for certain that he or she carried the gene. Such choices may include not to have children or, at the very least, to inform a prospective spouse about the test result and the risk to offspring. Importantly, a reliable predictive test would make it possible to definitely reassure half of the high-risk individuals that they did not carry the gene, information that would probably have consequences for family planning and other important decisions.

Those people whose test results show that they definitely carry the gene raise the most problematic and controversial issue in connection with predictive testing for Huntington's disease. There is a need to develop adequate counseling and support systems before extensive predictive testing for Huntington's disease is initiated. Most important, the medical profession must listen to the viewpoints of the at-risk persons and their organizations. It seems clear that a high number of people at risk for Huntington's disease do indeed want a predictive test conducted when it becomes available, and this wish should be respected. It must be remembered that by ignoring the knowledge of the genetic risk and by acting as if it were not there, the at-risk individual may indeed pass on very severe problems to other persons, such as a spouse who will be left with a hopelessly ill husband or wife, the offspring who will have to live with the knowledge of their risk, and the whole family who may face many years with difficult social and emotional problems. These consequences of ignoring a risk situation form a moral argument in favor of active genetic counseling and of making predictive tests available to families where Huntington's disease segregates. The disease is so rare that mass screening of the general population would be out of the question.

A definite DNA test for the Huntington's disease gene would be applicable also to cells from a fetus, so that predictive prenatal testing is a realistic option in the future. Thus, couples of whom one is at risk are capable of having children that do not have the disease gene; a pregnancy in which the fetus with the Huntington's disease gene could be terminated. The characteristics of the disease seem to fully justify the termination of pregnancy in such situations.

If the test were gene-specific, a positive result with fetal cells would necessarily mean that the at-risk parent (of the fetus) definitely possessed the Huntington's disease gene (even if that parent had not been tested). It is, however, possible to use DNA technology for prenatal diagnosis in a more indirect way that would not pass the burden or relief of definite knowledge on to the at-risk parent. DNA marker areas close to the Huntington's disease locus may be probed for this purpose, since they would serve as markers of the relevant area of chromosome 4.*

A fetus (like any other human being) has four grandparents: the two parents of a parent at risk and the two parents of the spouse. Since chromosomes occur in pairs, a given individual would possess only two of the four grandparental chromosome 4. If the DNA markers used were suitable to differentiate between all grandparental chromosomes, the test would consist in determining if a given fetus had a chromosome 4 from the grandparent with Huntington's disease. If not, there would be no risk of Huntington's disease in the future. If the fetus had one of the relevant chromosomes from the affected grandparent, the strategy would be to terminate the pregnancy, although one would not know if the chromosome in the fetus was indeed carrying the Huntington's disease gene or was the member of the chromosome pair that carried the normal allele. Consequently, the fetus would be genetically normal in half of the cases where the pregnancy would be terminated. Although this loss of healthy fetuses is undesirable, it would have to be weighed against the problems of informing the person at risk that he or she will develop Huntington's disease. One may argue that it is ethically questionable to create a family when there is a 50% risk that one of the parents will become severely ill while the children are still young, but the individual couple's right to an autonomous decision should be the overriding principle.[7]

It may be concluded that in the future both gene-specific technologies and technologies detecting a 50% risk in the fetus will become available options. This will make it pos-

---

* A DNA marker that is much closer to the locus for Huntington's chorea than previously used markers has recently been reported by Gilliam et al. (Gilliam TC, Bucan M, MacDonald ME et al: A DNA segment encoding two genes very tightly linked to Huntington's disease. Nature 238:950–952, 1987).

sible for couples of whom one is at risk for Huntington's disease to have children that do not have the gene for the disease. This type of analysis is likely to remain limited to known risk situations, since mass screening of fetuses for risk for diseases such as Huntington's disease can hardly be justified.

PREDICTIVE TESTS FOR FREQUENT DISORDERS

Several of the frequent major diseases have genetic as well as environmental factors to their etiology. The genetic component may primarily relate to a single, well-defined polymorphism, as is the case for HLA-associated diseases, or may comprise several genes each of which contribute to disease susceptibility. The genetic factors alone may not cause disease; it is primarily when unfavorable environmental or nutritional conditions interact with the products of susceptibility genes that disease develops. There is, for example, no doubt that myocardial infarction, occurring at a relatively young age, has strong genetic determinants.[4,6] Nevertheless, the frequency of this disease has varied significantly in this century, showing that even those with an inherited susceptibility can avoid disease if environmental circumstances are favorable. It becomes important, therefore, to identify individuals at risk in order to make it possible for them to make life-style changes in a healthier direction and to take full advantage of any other preventive measures.[4,6*]

Persons with susceptibility genes are not doomed to contract the disease in question. Importantly, a number of the genes that contribute to susceptibility to diseases such as atherosclerosis belong to normal genetic polymorphisms and their bearers may well have had advantages with regard to survival under totally different living conditions in the distant past.

Although several genes that contribute to coronary heart disease risk or to a risk-factor level are known, it may be predicted that over the next few years the new DNA technology will significantly improve identification of individuals at risk.[†] Although many genes may contribute to atherosclerosis susceptibility, in the future a limited number of highly predictive genetic tests may be selected for mass-screening purposes. Atherosclerosis is a heavy burden on society and individuals, and attempts to prevent the disease have been given high priority for several years. Unfortunately, the importance of genetic factors has been ignored in several extensive studies, and it is not yet possible to fully evaluate the relative importance of each single genetic risk factor, combinations of such factors, or combinations of such factors and environmental or nutritional factors. The already existing knowledge is, however, sufficient to envisage a system of voluntary screening of young adults for the purpose of reducing changeable risk factors in those who are highly at risk. Hopefully, the effects of preventive actions will improve when such measures are started at a young age, and those who know that they are at risk will necessarily have a stronger motivation to avail themselves of preventive measures than the population at large.

Predictive tests for fetuses with respect to genes predisposing to common diseases of adult or middle age, combined with selective

---

* The study of DNA polymorphisms at apolipoprotein loci has led to the detection by several workers of a definite association between a marker at the apolipoprotein B locus and lipid levels (Law A, Powell LM, Brunt H et al: Common DNA polymorphism within coding sequence of apolipoprotein B gene associated with altered lipid levels. Lancet i:1301–1303, 1986; Berg K: DNA polymorphism at the apolipoprotein B locus is associated with lipoprotein level. Clin Genet 30:515–520, 1986).

† Two claims of direct association between DNA variation at apolipoprotein loci and coronary heart disease have been reported (Ordovas JM, Schaefer EJ, Salem D et al: Apolipoprotein A-I gene polymorphism associated with premature coronary artery disease and familial hypoalphaproteinemia. New Engl J Med 314:671–677, 1986; Hegele RA, Huang L-S, Herbert PN et al: Apolipoprotein B-gene DNA polymorphisms associated with myocardial infarction. New Engl J Med 315:1509–1515, 1986). There is in both cases a need for confirmatory studies.

abortion, should not be contemplated, since the presence of susceptibility genes does not necessarily cause disease. Many of the susceptibility genes form part of man's normal genetic variation, and mass fetal screening with selective abortion would be absurd. In contrast, the best predictive tests for various disorders should be made available to young adults on a mass scale for purposes of disease prevention. Such tests should be voluntary and there must be strict rules concerning the test results in order to prevent such information from being used to the person's disadvantage.

PROTECTION OF PREDICTIVE TESTING DATA

Predictive genetic testing introduces a new element in medical, social, and professional relationships that is at best difficult to handle with existing experience and traditions. Established practices seem to be based on an assumption that, although there is in general a high degree of protection of data, certain consumers of health data have a legitimate right to know.

Traditionally, health information includes previous and present diseases and predictable complications to existing disorders; it is not concerned with future disease risks in people who are currently healthy. Thus, existing experience and traditions may not be adequate for managing predictive health information. A need exists to develop ways to handle results of predictive tests on healthy persons which are significantly different from present practices concerning information about actual illnesses.

Insurance companies, pension funds, employers, educational institutions, and the military may, at present, have a right to obtain information about a person's previous or present diseases. Although the use that they make of the data could be beneficial to the individual, their main motivation for asking for information may be to limit expenses or to exclude persons with a variety of diseases from certain professions, services, or pension or insurance programs. It is easy to see how certain disorders or slight anomalies would be incompatible with some professional careers (for example, color blindness and work requiring safe understanding of signal lights), but I question the ethics involved in disclosing personal data to health information consumers in the present system. Since life insurance rates or pension fund payments are generally calculated on the basis of total mortality and morbidity, there is no easy ethical justification for insurance companies asking for predictive health information that could exclude the person in question from an insurance program. It would seem that the increased profits for the insurance company come at too high a cost to the less fortunate.

Results of predictive tests on healthy persons should be strictly protected to secure extensive beneficial use of such tests. If people have reason to believe that predictive tests could be used to their disadvantage, they may be skeptical to being tested or may try to conceal the results. Access of health data consumers to predictive tests could have an unfortunate discriminatory effect on highly responsible individuals who have tests conducted in order to promote their health. Such disclosure would also introduce an unacceptable element of randomness, since chance events may decide which diseases can be predicted by tests available at any given time or in a given geographic area. Making disclosure of test results to health data consumers optional to the individual would not be a solution, since those who refuse disclosure or refuse to take a test could very well be subject to discrimination.[5]

Consumers of health data have functioned well so far without access to predictive tests. Increased profits or reduced costs can hardly serve as ethical justification for imposing hardship on a significant part of the population. In the matters of life insurance, health insurance, and pensions, the overriding principle should be that the community at large absorb the cost of the less fortunate. Although questions of safety may make it desirable to exclude persons with certain genes from certain professions, great caution should be exerted in allowing access to predictive testing results. Individual results of such tests are not an urgent need of the society.

A break with existing traditions for handling information concerning a person's previous or present diseases seems justified, since the person in question is healthy at the time of testing and therefore has a right to be treated as healthy; he or she may indeed stay healthy for many years. Furthermore, in the majority of diseases, the genes are part of the normal predisposing genetic variation in man, and most of the bearers of such normal genes will have a life span and a disease profile that resemble those of the population at large.

A practicable procedure to handle these problems and pave the way for extensive beneficial use of predictive genetic testing would be to make the results of such tests the exclusive property of the person in question, so that only he or she could decide to whom the information should be disclosed, presumably to medical and paramedical personnel who would advise the person on preventive measures and help carry them out.[5] It would have to be explicitly forbidden for any consumer of health information to ask about predictive tests or to make any transaction, admission, or appointment dependent on such tests. Finally, it should also be explicitly forbidden for third parties such as doctors or laboratories to disclose results of predictive tests to anybody but the tested person, or to indicate that such tests have been conducted. It is urgent that such rules be given the strength of law, and since developing new laws may take a long time, it is essential that preparatory discussions and work be started as soon as possible.

It could be argued that different rules should be established for information on genes that invariably cause serious disease. In this situation, disclosure could be made to prevent harm to third parties, but not to meet any wish from insurance companies, pension funds, educational institutions, or employers in general. The preferred principle even when it comes to the safety and well-being of other persons may be to make test results the property of the tested person.

Extensive use of predictive tests will necessitate the establishment of an elaborate system for informing the public and counseling the tested people about the test results. It will be a formidable task and counseling should probably be provided at several levels. If adequate counseling and education are provided, most people will probably make rational and responsible choices concerning career goals or change of career. Education and counseling combined with responsible choices by the individuals in question may go a long way to achieve what society could otherwise be tempted to try to achieve through obligatory predictive testing.

Weighing all of the above and other considerations, the preferable approach would seem to be to apply the same strict rules for data protection to all predictive genetic testing.

CONCLUDING REMARKS

Predictive genetic testing is to an extent already possible for certain common disorders as well as some rare monogenic diseases that manifest themselves in adult or middle age. Such testing holds great promise for attempts to control common diseases, and for reducing anxiety and promoting responsible decision-making in families with certain rare genetic diseases.

Existing experience and practices do not form a safe and acceptable basis for handling data concerning predictive tests on persons who are healthy at the time of testing and may remain so for many years. As a consequence, it is proposed that results of predictive genetic tests should be made the exclusive property of the tested individual who would be the only person with the right to pass on the information.[5] It is furthermore proposed that it should be explicitly forbidden for traditional consumers of health information to request predictive testing or even to inquire about tests that may have been conducted. In several countries, such protection of the individual would require new laws. It is strongly recommended that preparatory discussions and planning be started soon to secure extensive beneficial use of predictive genetic testing.[5]

Predictive testing of the fetus will in the foreseeable future most likely be done only for some of the most severe diseases of adult life such as Huntington's disease. There is no place for testing fetuses for genes predisposing to common disorders, and selective abortion based on results of such tests would be ethically questionable. Voluntary screening to prevent common diseases in middle age should take place in early adult life or, in some instances, even in childhood. Predictive tests for serious rare disorders such as Huntington's disease should in relevant cases be made available in early adult life so that test results can be taken into consideration in family and career planning.

REFERENCES

1. Berg K: Inherited variation in susceptibility and resistance to environmental agents. In Berg K (ed): Genetic Damage in Man Caused by Environmental Agents, pp 1–25. New York, Academic Press, 1979
2. Berg K: Occupational and industrial problems in population monitoring. In Bora KC, Douglas GR, Nestmann ER (eds): Chemical Mutagenesis, Human Population Monitoring and Genetic Risk Assessment, pp 63–74. Amsterdam, Elsevier Biomedical Press, 1982
3. Berg K: Ethical problems arising from research progress in medical genetics. In Berg K, Tranöy KE (eds): Research Ethics, pp 261–275. New York, Alan R Liss, 1983
4. Berg K: Genetics of coronary heart disease. In Steinberg AG, Bearn AG, Motulsky AG, Childs B (eds): Progress in Medical Genetics, vol V, pp 35–90. Philadelphia, WB Saunders, 1983
5. Berg K: Problems in monitoring population groups at high risk. Hereditas (June 19–22) 100:175–177, 1984
6. Berg K: Genetics of coronary heart disease and its risk factors. In Berg K (ed): Medical Genetics: Past, Present, Future, pp 351–374. New York, Alan R Liss, 1985
7. Fletcher JC, Berg K, Tranöy KE: Ethical aspects of medical genetics. A proposal for guidelines in genetic counseling, prenatal diagnosis and screening. Clin Genet 27:199–205, 1985
8. Goldstein JL, Brown MS: Familial hypercholesterolemia. In Stanbury JG, Wyngaarden JB, Fredrickson DS et al (eds): The Metabolic Basis of Inherited Disease, 5th ed, pp 672–712. New York, McGraw-Hill, 1983
9. Gusella JF, Wexler NS, Conneally PM et al: A polymorphic DNA marker genetically linked to Huntington's disease. Nature 306:234–238, 1983
10. Heiberg A, Berg K: The inheritance of hyperlipoproteinemia with xanthomatosis. A study in 132 kindreds. Clin Genet 9:203–233, 1976
11. Owerbach D, Billesbolle P, Schroll M et al: Possible association between DNA sequences flanking the insulin gene and atherosclerosis. Lancet 2:1291–1293, 1982
12. Rees A, Stocks J, Shoulders CC et al: DNA polymorphism adjacent to human apoprotein A-1 gene: Relation to hypertriglyceridemia. Lancet 1:444–446, 1983
13. Yamamoto T, Davis CG, Brown MS et al: The human LDL receptor: A cysteine-rich protein with multiple Alu sequences in its mRNA. Cell 39:27–38, 1984

PART III
CLINICAL ISSUES

5

Maternal Genetic Disease

SECTION 1: TRANSMITTING GENETIC DISORDERS TO OFFSPRING OF MENTALLY RETARDED INDIVIDUALS: PRINCIPLES UNDERLYING GENETIC COUNSELING

Joe Leigh Simpson

Pregnancy in mentally retarded individuals not only creates dilemmas concerning the circumstances of the conception and its consequences, but also raises questions concerning transmission of genetic disorders from parent to offspring. Although it is impractical here to review every genetic disorder in which a mentally retarded female may become pregnant or a mentally retarded male may sire a pregnancy, this section will review applicable principles governing transmission of chromosomal abnormalities or mutant genes.

CHROMOSOMAL ABNORMALITIES

Approximately 1 of every 150 individuals in the general population has a chromosomal disorder.[14] About half of such abnormalities are due to autosomal abnormalities; the other half are due to sex chromosomal abnormalities.[17]

Autosomal Trisomy

Empiric Observations

Autosomal disorders are associated with such profound mental retardation (IQ, 20–30) that reproduction almost never occurs.[28] In only a few types of nonmosaic autosomal trisomy do individuals survive sufficiently long for pregnancy to be possible. For example, individuals with trisomy 13 and trisomy 18 rarely survive past infancy, and none has become pregnant. In fact, females with these trisomies also show ovarian dysgenesis.[20,24] Other trisomies in which pregnancies could theoretically occur include trisomy 8, 9, and 22; however, in all three the incapacitated nature of affected individuals makes pregnancy socially unlikely, even if ovarian function is normal. Of course, gonadal mosaicism could also occur in phenotypically normal individuals whose germ cells contain a trisomic line. Indeed, parental germinal mosaicism is an often-assumed and sometimes proven[18] explanation for recurrent aneuploid offspring.[15]

The one trisomy that has been associated with reproduction is Down's syndrome (trisomy 21). Twenty-seven pregnant females with trisomy 21 were reviewed by Van de Velde-Staquet and co-workers in 1973.[32] Since then, other cases have been observed, including one of which I am aware. Pregnancy and labor by trisomy 21 females are not characterized by unusual clinical features, at least as reported by investigators who are not obstetricians. Nine of the 27 liveborn offspring tabulated by Van de Velde-Staquet's group[32] had trisomy 21; no other chromosomal abnormalities occurred. Although the occurrence of trisomic offspring was relatively frequent (33%), the number of offspring was still less than expected (50%) on the basis of theoretical predictions. Nonetheless, amniocentesis or chorionic villus sampling should be offered to all pregnant trisomy 21 females. A related observation is that chromosomally normal offspring of trisomy 21 mothers have been purported to show nonspecific malformations in greater than expected frequency.[25] However, additional data are necessary to exclude biases of ascertainment or reporting.

There are no confirmed reports of offspring sired by males having numerical autosomal abnormalities. In fact, sterility is believed characteristic of Down's syndrome males, probably as a result of meiotic breakdown.

Theoretical Considerations

The fewer than predicted trisomic offspring born to trisomy 21 mothers is a finding consistent with expectations based upon behavior in plant trisomies. To understand these basic observations, one must recall that the presence of three homologous chromosomes should lead to formation of a trivalent at the pachytene stage of meiosis I.[26,28] At any given point along the chromosome length, only two of the three chromosomes can pair; however, at another point, two different chromosomes can pair. Alternatively, one bivalent and one univalent can form; such a situation is more likely to occur if small chromosomes (e.g., chromosome 21) are involved. At anaphase I, two chromosomes (a bivalent) usually pass to one pole, whereas the remaining chromosome passes to the opposite pole. This results in equal numbers of $n + 1$ and n gametes.

Because similar phenomena surely apply in man, several principles derived from plant studies are worth summarizing. First, a univalent is subject to secondary cytologic abnormalities irrespective of its complementary product (i.e., bivalent in the above case). In fact, it is often the irregular behavior of the univalent that contributes to lower than expected (50%) proportions of $2n + 1$ progeny in plants. Second, females transmit the additional chromosome more often than do males. For example, the six trisomies of *Triticum durum* (Emmer wheat) are transmitted through females at an average frequency of 23%; through males the transmission frequency is only 2%.[30] Failure of transmission could be due to elimination of the additional chromosome during meiosis, or to reduced viability of $n + 1$ embryos. The different transmission rates in males and females further suggest that elimination during meiosis is the most salient mechanism in plants. Of special relevance to trisomy 21 in humans is that small chromosomes are most frequently eliminated in plants, presumably because their short length minimizes the opportunity for chiasmata formation. Third, trisomies for other chromosomes may also occur, presumably caused by either a generalized interference with disjunction or an induction of univalents in other chromosomes.

Sex Chromosomal Abnormalities

47,XXX females should theoretically produce equal numbers of 23,X and 24,XX secondary oocytes, which at fertilization could theoretically yield equal numbers of 46,XX; 46,XY; 47,XXX; and 47,XXY zygotes. However, most progeny of 47,XXX females are chromosomally normal. Although there is no unassailable explanation, one could surmise that the situation is analogous to that occurring in trisomy 21. The specific cytologic mechanism could involve either preferential segregation of the 24,XX product into the first polar body or decreased fertilizing ability of the 24,XX oocytes.

The above observations notwithstanding, 47,XXX and especially 46,XX/47,XXX women have indeed had chromosomally abnormal offspring, albeit at far less than theoretically expected frequencies. Barr and colleagues[3] recorded that 1 of 20 47,XXX women had a 47,XXY son; 3 of 8 46,XX/47,XXX women had 47,XXX or 46,XY/47,XXY sons; and 1 of 8 had a 46,XX/47,XXX daughter. At least one 47,XXX female has had a 47,XX,+21 child,[18] and another has had a 45,X child.[13] Several 46,XX/47,XXX women have had offspring with Klinefelter's syndrome,[2,16,29] and one 46,XX/47,XXX mother had a 48,XXYY son.[34] In addition, 45,X/46,XX/47,XXX mothers have borne offspring with sex chromosomal mosaicism[5,12] and with Down's syndrome.[1,16]

Although these reports raise the possibility that women with a 47,XXX cell line show increased liability for chromosomally abnormal offspring, caution is warranted. Biases of ascertainment and reporting clearly exist. For example, sometimes the maternal complement was detected only after birth of an abnormal proband.[6,26] Still, it seems prudent to offer antenatal chromosomal studies to pregnant 47,XXX and 46,XX/47,XXX women. Discussion with these women should include not only the possibility of 47,XXY and 47,XXX offspring, but also the possibility of other chromosomal abnormalities.

Structural Chromosomal Abnormalities

Deletions

Mental retardation may be associated with a variety of structural chromosomal abnormalities. Loss or duplication of significant portions of any autosome would be expected to produce profound mental retardation. For social reasons alone, reproduction would not ordinarily be expected. Indeed, I am aware of no examples of a deleted autosome being transmitted from a mentally retarded individual to her offspring. However, if pregnancy should occur in a retarded individual having an autosomal deletion, the theoretical likelihood that the aberration will be transmitted is 50%—either the deleted chromosome or the normal chromosome must be transmitted. If the deleted chromosome is transmitted, mental retardation would, of course, be anticipated.

Reproduction by individuals with large deletions is improbable, but the phenomenon could occur with small deletions or with deletions of sex chromosomes. In fact, many dominantly transmitted disorders are actually the result of minute deletions. Moreover, transmission of a deleted X chromosome has been observed,[7,21,27] albeit unassociated with retardation. Still, the general cytogenetic principle for autosomal trisomy should apply as well to transmission of chromosomal abnormalities. Fewer than the theoretically expected 50% offspring would be affected. Such counseling would be applicable if reproduction ever occurs in a female with an autosomal deletion.

Ring Chromosomes

Ring chromosomes originate by breaks in both the long and short arms. Distal acentric fragments are lost, and proximal long and short arm fusion occurs. Secondary rearrangements are common. The loss of genetic loci makes the clinical consequences similar to that for deletions.

Transmission of ring chromosomes is usually by females and not by males, who are often sterile due to meiotic breakdown. Although transmission has usually involved normal women, there are at least three examples of retarded women with ring chromosomes who transmitted the ring to offspring. Fujimaki and co-workers[10] observed a slightly retarded woman who transmitted ring 15 to her growth-retarded son. Palmer and associates[22] observed transmission from a retarded mother with ring 21 to her retarded offspring with ring 21. Bower and colleagues[4] studied a similar phenomena involving ring 14.

Translocations

The structural chromosomal abnormality about which questions of transmission by mentally retarded individuals will most often arise is that of translocation. Individuals with balanced translocations, either reciprocal or robertsonian, are known to produce unbalanced gametes as a result of normal meiotic segregation.[26,28] Of course, heterozygous (balanced) individuals are not ordinarily retarded; thus, their reproduction is not immediately relevant to this communication.

Individuals with unbalanced translocations show duplications or deficiencies that would ordinarily be expected to confer profound retardation; these individuals would not be expected to reproduce. However, they theoretically could become pregnant. If so, specific risk figures would need to be estimated on the basis of the particular translocation involved. It is worth noting, however, that both normal and abnormal products are possible, even if the mother or father is unbalanced. More than one type of chromosomal abnormality could occur in the offspring. Affected females would probably be more likely to reproduce than affected males, who would probably be sterile due to meiotic breakdown. If both sexes were fertile, transmission rates to offspring would probably be higher for mothers than fathers. Of course, prenatal cytogenetic studies could detect any chromosomal abnormalities present in the offspring.

MENDELIAN DISORDERS

Pregnancies can occur in women who are retarded as a result of a host of mendelian mutations. The list of potentially relevant disorders is far too long to consider in a single chapter. Again, however, it is appropriate to review the principles governing transmission of the mutant gene to offspring.

Autosomal Dominant Disorders

Pregnancy may occur in individuals having an autosomal dominant disorder characterized by mental retardation. The likelihood that the mutant gene would be transmitted to any given offspring, male or female, is 50%, in accordance with basic tenants of mendelian inheritance. The actual clinical outcome, however, might not be as dire.

There are several reasons for clinical outcome to differ from theoretical exceptions. First, autosomal dominant disorders are usually characterized by varied expressivity and even lack of penetrance. In fact, a woman who is retarded as a result of an autosomal dominant disorder might well have a milder form (minimal expression) of the disorder. Indeed, only individuals with minimal expression are capable of reproducing. Therefore, it need not follow that mental retardation in the pregnant mother will be transmitted to the offspring, even if the mutant gene is transmitted. (The gene in the offspring could be even more minimally expressed.) Thus, the likelihood is 50% that the mutant gene will be transmitted to any given offspring, but not necessarily 50% of those offspring will actually be retarded.

One clue toward deducing probable outcome is to search for intrafamilial variability. If multiple family members have been affected with a given disorder, the likelihood that a family member with the gene will be retarded can be estimated. The likelihood that the pregnancy in question can produce a mentally retarded offspring can thus be better estimated.

Autosomal Recessive Disorders

An individual having an autosomal recessive disorder conferring mental retardation would ordinarily be less likely to reproduce than individuals with autosomal dominant disorders; however, those who do become pregnant usually have genetically normal offspring. The reason is that it is unlikely for the partner to be heterozygous for the same mutant allele.

The exact probability of offspring being affected depends upon the frequency of the condition in the population. As an example, if the incidence of an autosomal recessive disease is 1 in 10,000, then the heterozygote frequency is 1 in 50 ($q^2 = 1/10,000$; $q = 1/100$; $2pq = 2/100$ or $1/50$). Now, the affected individual must transmit the mutant gene to all offspring; however, his or her partner has only 1 chance in 50 of being a carrier. Thus, the overall likelihood that any given offspring will be affected is $1 \times 1/50 \times 1/2 = 1/100$. If heterozygote detection tests exist, they obviously should be performed to exclude that possibility, particularly if prenatal diagnosis is available.

One circumstance in which an autosomal recessive disorder in a parent might be transmitted to offspring involves an incestuous mating. If a normal brother impregnated his mentally retarded female sibling, the likelihood that he would be heterozygous for the same mutant gene is 2/3. A heterozygous brother would have one chance in two of transmitting the mutant allele. Thus, the likelihood that their offspring would be affected would be $1 \times 2/3 \times 1/2 = 2/6 = 1/3$. Fortunately, such circumstances arise only rarely.

The Fragile X Syndrome

The X-linked recessive disorder most likely to raise queries concerning reproduction in the mentally retarded is the fragile-X syndrome, a common disorder whose incidence is approximately 1 in 2000 males.[31] The locus (or fragile site) involves region Xq27 (Figure 5-1).

There are many puzzling aspects of this condition. One would expect hemizygous males to be always retarded and heterozygous females to be phenotypically normal. Certainly this is often observed. However, females with the fragile X sometimes show mental retardation, and males with the fragile X may be normal. Moreover, both phenotypically normal and cytogenetically normal males may transmit the fragile X to descendents, who have then been retarded. That

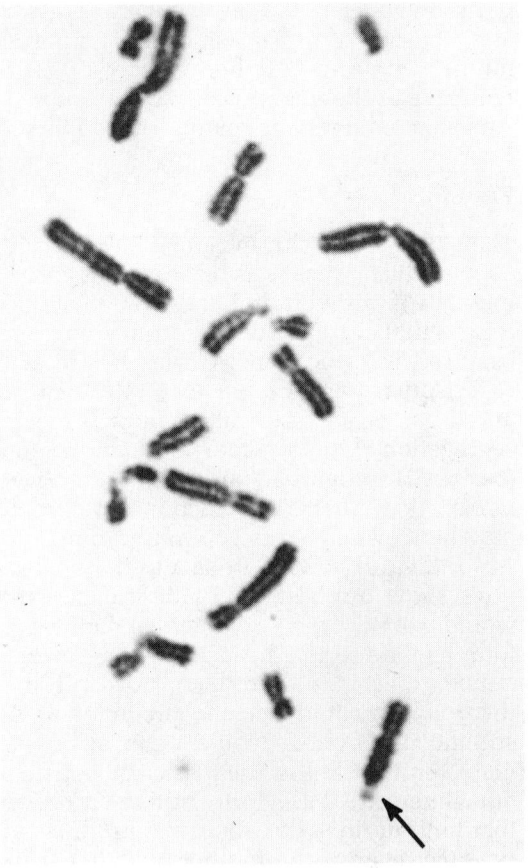

FIGURE 5-1. Metaphase shows fragile X chromosome. (Preparation by Dr. Avirachan Tharapel, University of Tennessee, Memphis)

there are few apparent sporadic cases further verifies that the fragile-X phenomena may show lack of penetration. The most popular hypothesis to explain the above findings is the existence of an autosomal "suppressor" factor (gene).[9,17] Other possibilities have also been voiced.[8,33]

Puzzling aspects of expression and penetrance notwithstanding, however, one would expect to observe retarded females with the fragile X who are capable of reproducing and transmitting the mutant X to male offspring. Sons inheriting the X would thus be hemizygous and probably be retarded. On average, one would expect 50% of male offspring to be affected, as well as more severely affected than the mother. Retarded fragile-X males could also reproduce, transmitting the mutant X to half of their daughters. These daughters would not ordinarily be expected to be affected. However, that possibility could not be excluded categorically.

Other X-Linked Recessive Disorders

Males having other X-linked recessive disorders characterized by mental retardation could also be fertile, yet there are no definite examples. Again, any fertile male would be predicted to transmit the mutant X to none of their sons and to all of their daughters. Those daughters who inherit the mutant X would be heterozygous but not affected.

POLYGENIC/MULTIFACTORIAL DISORDERS

Surely some individuals with mental retardation are affected on the basis of polygenic/multifactorial etiology. Some of their offspring will thus be retarded as a result of the same etiology. However, risks to offspring should be relatively low.

The difficult part is determining when this particular form of inheritance is applicable to an individual having mental retardation. One would expect polygenic/multifactorial inheritance to be a more likely explanation for mental retardation in individuals whose IQ is 50 to 70 because they represent the lower end of the normal Gaussian distribution. Retardation in such cases might involve as few as two genes.[28] (Similar reasoning applies as well to neural tube defects, facial clefts, and all disorders affecting only a single organ system.) An individual having a polygenic/multifactorial trait carries a recurrence risk of 1% to 5% for affected offspring. One would thus expect comparable recurrence risks in polygenic/multifactorial mental retardation. The degree of mental retardation in affected offspring would ordinarily be expected to be comparable, but not necessarily identical to that of the proband (parent).

Reliable empiric data are difficult to obtain because, in virtually all reported samples of individuals with "idiopathic" mental retardation, mendelian or cytogenetic disorders could have passed unrecognized. In an older study by Reed and Reed,[23] among offspring of a single mentally retarded parent, 11% were similarly affected (Table 5-1). Once a retarded parent had a retarded child, the risk for subsequent retarded offspring rose to 20%. If both parents were retarded, 40% of the offspring were affected. By contrast, two normal parents having a retarded child incur only 1% recurrence risk in any subsequent pregnancy.

Table 5-1. Empiric Risk Figures for "Idiopathic" Mental Retardation*

Parents	Previous Children	Risk of Retardation in Subsequent Pregnancy
Both normal	Normal (or none)	1%
Both normal	One retarded	6%
One retarded	Normal (or none)	11%
One retarded	One retarded	20%
Both retarded	Normal (or none)	40%
Both retarded	One retarded	42%

* These data were published by Reed and Reed[23] in 1965, prior to many modern advances that surely would have allowed some of these "idiopathic" cases to be recategorized into mendelian or cytogenetic etiologies.

A polygenic/multifactorial trait may not always cause mental retardation per se. However, complications arising secondary to the defect may produce retardation. For example, spina bifida can clearly be transmitted (2% likelihood) from parent to child. Hydrocephaly may or may not be associated, but if it is, mental retardation may result. Likewise, offspring may inherit a cardiac abnormality which might, through cyanosis and hypoxemia, secondarily lead to mental retardation.

A final comment is that recurrence risk figures specific for parent-to-child transmission may not be available for all polygenic/multifactorial disorders. However, the recurrence risks are the same for all first-degree relatives (parents, siblings, offspring). That is, one would offer the same recurrence risks for 1) offspring of one affected parent, and 2) offspring of two normal parents who have one affected child. The recurrence risk for polygenic/multifactorial traits in second-degree relatives (uncles, aunts, nephews, nieces, grandchildren) is considerably lower, usually 1% or less, but still higher than that of the general population.

REFERENCES

1. Armendares S, Buentello L, Sanches J, Oritz M: XO/XX/XXX mosaicism without Turner stigmata. Lancet 2:840, 1970
2. Baike AG: XXY son of a possible XX-XXX mother. Lancet 1:697, 1972
3. Barr ML, Sergovich FR, Carr DM, Shaver EL: The triplo-X female: An appraisal based on a study of 12 cases and a review of the literature. Can Med Assoc J 101:247, 1979
4. Bower RS, Buckton KE, Ratcliff SG, Syme J: Inheritance of a ring 14 chromosome. J Med Genet 18:209, 1981
5. de Toni E, Massimo L, Vanello MJ, Podesta F: La casistica di un anno di attivita del Centro di Studi cromosomici della clinica Pediatrica di Genova nel campo dell malformazioni aessuali. Minnerva Pediatr 17:583, 1965
6. Dewhurst J: Fertility in 47,XXX and 45,X patients. J Med Genet 15:132, 1978
7. de Fitch N, Saint VJ, Richer CL et al: Premature menopause due to a small deletion in the long arm of the X chromosome: A report of three cases and a review. Am J Obstet Gynecol 142:968, 1982
8. Friedman JM, Howard-Peebles PN: Inheritance of fragile X: An hypothesis. Am J Med Genet 23:701, 1986
9. Froster-Iskenius U, Schulze A, Schwinger E: Transmission of the marker X syndrome trait by unaffected males: Conclusions from studies of large families. Hum Genet 67:419, 1984
10. Fujimaki W, Baba K, Tatara K et al: Ring chromosome 15 in a mother and her children. Hum Genet 76:302, 1987
11. Geisler M, Svejcar J, Degenhart K: XXY son of an XX/XXX mother. Lancet 1:159, 1972
12. Giraud F: La fertile des femmes: 45,X/46,XX et 45,X/46,XX/47,XXX. Ann Genet 15:256, 1973
13. Guzman-Toledano R, Ayala A, Zarate A, Jimenez M: Triple X female and Turner's syndrome offspring. J Med Genet 13:516, 1976
14. Hook EB, Hamerton JL: The frequency of chromosome abnormalities detected in consecutive newborn studies—Differences between studies—Results by sex and by severity of phenotypic involvement. In Hook EB, Porter IH (eds): Population Cytogenetic Studies in Humans, p 63. New York, Academic Press, 1977
15. Hsu LYF, Hirschhorn K, Goldstein, A, Barcinski MA: Familial chromosomal mosaicism, genetic aspects. Ann Hum Genet 33:343, 1970
16. Hsu LYF, Palo-Garcia F, Grossman D et al: Fetal wastage and maternal mosaicism. Obstet Gynecol 40:98, 1972
17. Israel M: Autosomal suppressor gene for fragile-X: An hypothesis. Am J Med Genet 26:19, 1987
18. Kadonti T, Ohama K, Makino S: A case of 21-trisomic Down's syndrome from the triplo-X mother. Proc Jpn Acad 46:709, 1970
19. Kaffe S, Hsu LYF, Hirschhorn K: Trisomy 21 mosaicism in a woman with two children with trisomy 21 Down's syndrome. J Med Genet 11:378, 1974
20. Kennedy JF, Freeman MG, Benirschke K: Ovarian dysgenesis and chromosome abnormalities. Obstet Gynecol 50:13, 1977
21. Krauss CM, Turksay RN, Atkins L et al: Familial premature ovarian failure due to an interstitial deletion of long arm of the X chromosome. N Engl J Med 317:125, 1987
22. Palmer CG, Hodes ME, Reed T, Kujetin J: Four new cases of ring 21 and 22, including familial transmission of ring 21. J Med Genet 14:54, 1977
23. Reed RW, Reed SC: Mental retardation. A

Family Study. Philadelphia, WB Saunders, 1965
24. Russell P, Altschuler G: The ovarian dysgenesis of trisomy 19. Pathology 7:149, 1975
25. Scharra S, Stengel-Rutkowski S, Rodewald-Rudescu A et al: Reproduction in a female patient with Down's syndrome. Hum Genet 26:207, 1975
26. Simpson JL: Pregnancies in women with chromosomal abnormalities: In Schulman JD, Simpson JL (eds): Genetic Diseases in Pregnancy: Maternal Effects and Fetal Outcome. New York, Academic Press, 1981
27. Simpson JL: Genetic control of sexual development. Proceedings 12th World Congress on Fertility and Sterility, pp 165–173. Parthenon, Lancaster, 1987
28. Simpson JL, Golbus MS, Martin AO, Sarto EG: Genetics in Obstetrics and Gynecology. New York, Grune & Stratton, 1982
29. Tsuang ML, Miller JR, DeBault LE: Klinefelter's syndrome and maternal XX/XXX mosaicism. J Med Genet 12:114, 1975
30. Tsuneuski K: Transmission of monosomes and trisomes in Emmer wheat. Wheat Inf Serv 17–19:34, 1964
31. Turner G, Opitz JM, Brown WT et al: Conference report. Second International Workshop on the Fragile X and X-Linked Mental Retardation. Am J Med Genet 23:11, 1986
32. Van de Velde-Staquet MR, Breynaert R, Walbaum R et al: La descendance des meres trisomiques 21. J Genet Hum 21:187, 1973
33. Van Dyke DL, Weiss L: Maternal effect on intelligence in Fragile X males and female. Am J Med Genet 23:723, 1986
34. Ziska J, Balicek P, Nielsen J: XXYY son of a triple-X mother. Humangenetik 26:159, 1975

SECTION 2: PREGNANCY IN PERSONS WHO ARE MENTALLY HANDICAPPED

Thomas E. Elkins and S. Gene McNeeley

When pregnancy occurs in a person who is mentally handicapped a multitude of medical, psychosocial, ethical, and legal concerns become prominent considerations. Any management plan to be effective must therefore use a multi-disciplinary approach.

In reality, ongoing pregnancy is one of the least common reasons for clinic visits at the University of Michigan model clinic program for the reproductive health concerns of mentally handicapped persons (Table 5-2). This agrees with other studies that show a relatively low rate of pregnancy among women who are mentally handicapped, especially those who are moderately, severely, or profoundly mentally handicapped. However, it is the crisis of a pregnancy in a person who is mentally handicapped that emphasizes the many concerns surrounding reproductive health in this population.

The incidence of childbearing among persons who are developmentally disabled has been difficult to study. The number of persons who are mentally handicapped and who give birth to children appears relatively small when the entire population is considered (educable as well as noneducable mentally handicapped). In the University of Michigan program for persons with developmental disabilities, 10 of the first 250 patients seen had experienced a total of 20 pregnancies. All of these patients were mentally handicapped to a moderate or lesser degree. No statistics are available for those minimally impaired persons who routinely delivered children outside of this clinic program. In general, it is very uncommon for persons with severe or profound impairment to reproduce, but it becomes more common as the

Table 5-2. Reasons for Clinic Visits (175 Patients)

Medical Problem	No. of Patients
Pelvic exams	44
Menstrual problems (Bleeding or pain)	43
Premenstrual syndrome	39
Sex counseling (6 males)	25
Sterilization (2 males)	18
Vaginitis	13
Sexual abuse	6
Birth control pills	6
Menopause	4
Masturbation problems	4
Pregnancy	3

(From University of Michigan model clinic program)

level of mental retardation improves and as the opportunity for social interaction becomes more prominent.

Many people support the myth that mentally handicapped persons are unusually fertile and have prolific numbers of children if allowed to do so. Indeed, the occasional patient is seen who has had six children, and reared none of them. However, in those studies of persons with developmental disabilities who have become parents, the data indicate that most have average-size families. A study by Charles conducted in Nebraska in the early 1950s showed an average of 2.12 children per family in this population.[6] Scally reported a study of 342 married couples with developmental disabilities in Ireland in 1973, and found that the average number of children was 2.3 per family (slightly lower than the overall average for the region).[28] A study by Laxova and colleagues in Great Britain recently revealed a rate of 1.8 children born per woman in a sample of 53 women who had at least one child and had been institutionalized at some point.[20a] In a further review by Floor and co-workers, only 37% of 214 previously institutionalized persons had married, and only 32 children had been born to 54 couples.[13] In contrast to these low figures, three studies have shown a higher rate of childbearing among developmentally disabled persons than among the nonhandicapped population.[15,22,28] In general, these studies tended to document family sizes in lower socioeconomic areas. The overall summary of the data does not indicate a higher rate of childbearing by mentally handicapped persons than by others in their region.

With the recent trends of de-institutionalization, improved medical prognosis of handicapped persons, innovative educational programs for this population, and increased community living and socialization, higher pregnancy rates among the mentally handicapped may be anticipated. Management of these situations begins with an understanding of basic principles underlying health care for this particular population.

The founding policies of the University of Michigan clinic, adopted from prior policies of a similar clinic at the University of Tennessee, include the following ethical guidelines:

- Each patient is to be considered as a unique individual regardless of the level of mental retardation.
- Each person is to be considered as representing an entirety of needs who requires a variety of management approaches.
- Treatment should always consider the least harmful alternative in care or the least restrictive means of management.
- Even though societal and familial interests are important, the attempt is made, generally, to provide care that is in the patient's best interests.
- Decisions regarding care should reflect a knowledge of societal opinion, and thus a societally based advisory committee is involved in appropriate medical-ethical-legal decision-making.
- Because of the question of the capacity to provide informed consent in this population and the respect for the positive value of mentally handicapped persons, mandatory review is required before invasive or controversial care is provided.[10,12]

In reviewing the management of the

many problems of reproductive health for persons who are mentally handicapped we have focused discussion on the problems directly related to pregnancy, parenting, and the prevention or planning of future pregnancies in patients who are mentally handicapped. Many of the issues considered must be covered very briefly, but more in-depth coverage is available in several excellent texts.[7,14,21]

PROBLEMS DIRECTLY RELATED TO PREGNANCY

Medical Concerns of Prenatal Care

Patients who are mentally handicapped are only a portion of the larger population of "developmentally disabled persons" who have a variety of physically or mentally handicapping disabilities. The number and variety of physical/medical problems seen in a series of 45 consecutive patients who came to the clinic for reproductive health concerns in Tennessee are shown in Table 5-3.

Many mentally retarded patients have serious medical problems including congenital heart disease and seizure disorders. Early consultation with the cardiologist is mandatory and co-management during pregnancy may be helpful. Termination of pregnancy is reserved for traditional maternal indications. Pregnancy does not have a predictable affect on seizure disorders. Anticonvulsant therapy is frequently used in this population and a variety of complications in the infants may be attributed to such therapy.

The fetal phenytoin syndrome includes growth retardation, microcephaly, and craniofacial anomalies, and the risk for fetal anomalies increases with phenobarbital use. Deficiencies in vitamin K–dependent clotting factors may occur; laboring women should receive 1 g of vitamin K during labor in addition to treatment of the newborn. Carbamazepine (Tegretol) may be associated with decreased head size in the infant. Valproic acid used during pregnancy may be associated with neural tube defects, spina bifida, and skeletal malformations. Trimethadione is contraindicated during pregnancy.

A significant number of women who are mentally handicapped also have severe musculoskeletal deformities. Pregnancy in these patients raises great concern about immobility and the development of deep vein thrombosis. A high hepatitis carrier rate within institutions requires prenatal screening of this population. Finally, in a study by Salerno, underdeveloped pelvic organs were common in patients who were mentally handicapped, especially in those with Down's syndrome.[26] Because of this, and the high incidence of sexual abuse in this population that begins in early adolescence,[5] an increased rate of cephalopelvic disproportion may be anticipated in parturition.

In addition to the direct physical concerns that are prominent in pregnancy, there are social health concerns. Dietary habits of persons with mental retardation may be inadequate to support a pregnancy. Dietary consultation should be obtained and social services can arrange for supplemental food stuffs during pregnancy. Vitamin and iron supplements should be prescribed. Ultrasonography should be performed as needed to demonstrate appropriate fetal growth in this population at risk for intrauterine growth retardation.

Table 5-3. Associated Medical Problems in Clinic Patients

Medical Problem	No. of Patients
Hearing loss	6
Obesity	6
Visual loss	5
Down's syndrome and chromosomal disorders	5
Cardiac disease	3
Congenital rubella	2
Chondrodystrophy	2

(Elkins TE, Gafford S, Muram D: A model clinic approach to the reproductive health concerns of the mentally handicapped. Obstet Gynecol 68[2]:186, 1986. Reprinted with permission from The American College of Obstetricians and Gynecologists.)

Incidence of Mental Retardation in the Offspring

Numerous studies have documented a tendency for persons with mental retardation to give birth to children who have a higher IQ score than their own. Brandon showed that in a group of mothers with mental retardation, 91% of children had normal IQ scores, with an average IQ of 74.[4] Charles noted a similar finding in offspring with an average IQ of 95, even though the mothers had a mean IQ of 81.[6a] Other studies further substantiated these findings.[20b,29a]

However, all studies of offspring are not positive. Johnson showed that 65% of offspring of mothers with mental retardation also were retarded.[16] A second study by Mickelson showed that only 33% of children were normal when their mothers were known to be mentally retarded.[24a] An increased number of these children are known to need special education, with one British study showing an 11.6% incidence (17 times greater than normal), and another study showing a 22% incidence.[20b,29b] In a 1965 study of 7778 children by Reed and Reed, when both parents had an IQ of under 70, nearly 40% of the children were mentally retarded; when only one parent was mentally retarded, 15% of the children were mentally retarded; and when neither parent was mentally retarded, only 1% of the children were mentally retarded.[26]

Three-fourths of mentally handicapped persons originate from "cultural-familial" or "socially deprived" homes.[25] Numerous researchers have shown that an altered environment or extensive early social and educational support can improve mentally handicapping conditions recognized early in childhood. This underscores the need to arrange social agency support for pregnant, mentally handicapped patients prior to delivery for the benefit of both the mother and the newborn child.

Finally, concerns about the mental capabilities of offspring of mentally handicapped parents are especially prominent when a parent has a genetically transmissible disorder that causes mental retardation. The classic example of such a disorder is Down's syndrome. No male with Down's syndrome has been reported to have fathered a child. However, pregnancy in women with Down's syndrome does occur, although uncommonly. A review of 30 pregnancies to 26 women with Down's syndrome resulted in 10 children with Down's syndrome, 18 children without Down's syndrome, and 3 spontaneous abortions.[3] Of some concern is that 6 of the 17 offspring without Down's syndrome had other congenital anomalies, a much higher than usual number.

Difficulties Anticipated in Labor and Delivery

It is difficult for anyone to adapt to the uncertainty, the loss of control, the pain, and the anxiety of labor and delivery. For the person who is mentally handicapped, it may be an impossible task. However, there are mentally handicapped patients who can understand the contraction-relaxation process, the pushing efforts needed in the second stage, and the relaxation required to facilitate postpartum genital repair. Again, third trimester education about the process of labor and delivery must be accomplished with mildly and moderately handicapped patients to avoid an excessively high operative delivery rate. In Bovicelli's study of patients with Down's syndrome 7 of 21 reported births were by cesarean section, 2 were breech extractions, and 1 was a forceps delivery.[3b] Despite all educational efforts, an operative-controlled delivery may be the safest choice for some severely or profoundly handicapped patients who progress in pregnancy to term gestation.

Concerns about Pregnancy Termination

Often pregnancy represents a tragedy, rather than a joy, for the sexually abused and confused mentally handicapped person. Patients who are incest victims with life-threatening heart disease, or who are abuse victims so puzzled by their growing abdomens that they beat themselves unless constantly restrained make even the most conservative physicians sympathetic to pregnancy termination. However, legal constraints on such procedures vary widely, and many states have rigid rules preventing pregnancy terminations in any mentally handicapped person. Although the Supreme Court has allowed pregnancy termination in a particular situation, regional or state laws must be considered and legal counsel must be obtained.

At the University of Michigan a process similar to that used for sterilization requests is applied to any request for pregnancy termination. A societally based advisory committee aids in decision-making by reviewing an assessment of the patient's decisional capacity (which is usually honored when present) and determining the medical "best interests" for the pregnant patient when decisional capacity is absent.[11]

PARENTING FOR PERSONS WITH DEVELOPMENTAL DISABILITIES

Many myths and uncertainties exist concerning the parenting role of persons with developmental disabilities. Although many within society still object strongly to the idea of allowing these persons to become parents, the fact remains that many do function in a parenting role.

Given the lack of agreement as to what constitutes adequate child care in our society, the reliability of any data collected will also be questioned. In 1947, Mickelson followed 90 families in which one or both parents were mentally retarded, and found that 42% of the families were given satisfactory parenting ratings (with another 32% being questionable).[24] A "satisfactory parenting rating" implied that children were well fed, well clothed, attended school, and that no complaints from child protection agencies had been received. The unsatisfactory group had a high correlation with the presence of mental illness in this group of mothers, as well as mental retardation. Those with satisfactory ratings made more effective use of social agencies.

Educational Needs

Other studies have documented the need for supporting social agencies to prevent a proponderance of neglectful child rearing by mentally handicapped parents.[2,21] In a 1947 study by Mitchell, mothers who were mentally handicapped were portrayed as inadequate housekeepers and parents, although they showed love and concern for their children.[25] Furthermore, in only one-third of the cases, did social work intervention improve child care in her study. A British study showed that one-third of families in this population had one or more children removed from the home for child neglect,[29b] which also occurred in 39% of the families in Mickelson's study.[24b] In Scally's large study from Ireland, only 30% of families were satisfactorily raising their children in the home.[28] A general conclusion is that childbearing, although a distinct possibility for the mentally handicapped person, does not imply that adequate child rearing will occur. Extensive use of social support agencies and home support is required to ensure adequate parenting for effective child care in most instances.

With these facts in mind, those patients who enter the third trimester of pregnancy, are educable, and want to keep their child are offered parenting instruction. Social support agencies are contacted to organize assistance prior to childbirth.

A nursing education program at the University of Wisconsin-Milwaukee for prospective parents who are mentally handicapped includes these five topics: handling the small infant; child growth and development; food, recreation, and discipline; hazards, emergencies, and safety measures; and use of health care and community resources.[20b] In a recent instance at the University of Michigan, a call for assistance to the local county association for retarded citizens was answered by 16 different social agencies willing to provide support for a mother with mental retardation, and to provide follow-up prenatal education in the home. Many physicians are simply unaware of the help available to handicapped families in most major communities in the

United States, which underscores the need for patient–social service contact prior to childbirth whenever parenting is seen as an issue.

Developing a Policy During Pregnancy for Potential Parenting

As noted by Haavik and Menninger, one of the major problems encountered in ethical and legal discussions about reproduction among mentally handicapped persons is separating the rights and responsibilities of marriage from the rights, responsibilities, and duties of parenthood.[14] Although society has deemed many persons as unfit parents, including alcoholics and psychotics, only the retarded have been legally denied the right to procreate in some states. Part of the reason for this is the generally negative attitude toward the person who is mentally handicapped as a parent in our society. In several surveys of parents and care providers of persons who are mentally handicapped, only 4% to 12% of those surveyed believed that the mentally handicapped persons with whom they were associated would ever be capable of parenting.[1,9,29b] However, none of these studies looked only at higher functioning persons who are mentally handicapped, in which the results of similar studies might vary.

It is not uncommon for patients who are mentally handicapped to express a strong desire to become a parent. It is generally agreed that health care providers during the pregnancy are not the ones responsible for determining a person's capacity to parent. Neither is it helpful to maintain overly generalized negative or positive ideas about the parenting capacity of *all* persons who are mentally handicapped. Therefore, a program has been developed for managing pregnant patients in the third trimester under the following guidelines:

- Each person is viewed as a unique individual with distinct capacities and needs.
- Each person should be encouraged and assisted to achieve reasonable goals for parenting to the limit of his or her capabilities (physically, mentally, and spiritually).

Child neglect and child abuse are never acceptable alternatives in parenting. Steps necessary to avoid this possibility should be considered prior to childbirth, whenever possible.

With these basic principles as guidelines for management, every pregnant patient who is mentally handicapped is assigned to a clinic nurse and social worker for evaluation, observation, and educational programs. Initial interviews are used to assess a knowledge base about parenting and especially infant child care. An individualized education program about parenting responsibilities and child care is then developed for those who want to keep custody of their children. This is then expanded to include education about and use of supportive services, as indicated, to help in the home. Careful records are kept regarding patient reliability in taking prenatal medications and attending appointments, predelivery preparations made for the newborn (e.g., purchasing furniture and baby clothes), and the patient's ability to manage the newborn while in the hospital postpartum. All of these notations are helpful in legal custody discussions, should they arise.

POSTPARTUM COUNSELING REGARDING SEXUALITY, CONTRACEPTION, AND STERILIZATION

Sexuality Education and Counseling

Concerns about expressions of sexuality within the population of persons with mental retardation have long been discussed. The "normalization" emphasis of the 1970s brought worldwide attention to the issue. Kempton made a clear listing of a consensus of what normalization means to persons with mental retardation:

- The right to receive training in social-sexual behavior that will open more doors for

social contact with people in the community
- The right to all the knowledge about sexuality that can be comprehended
- The right to enjoy love and to be loved by the opposite sex, including sexual fulfillment
- The right for the opportunity to express sexual impulses in the same form that is socially acceptable for others
- The right to birth control services that are specialized to meet their needs
- The right to marry
- The right to have a voice in whether or not they should have children
- The right for supportive services which involve those rights as they are needed or feasible.[17]

Again, the crisis of pregnancy emphasizes the need for sex education for persons who are mentally handicapped. Craft and Craft stated

> The vast majority of retarded people will develop normal secondary sex characteristics and they need more help not less in understanding these changes and the accompanying emotions. They need knowledge which will give them some protection against exploitation. And lastly, it is unrealistic of society to demand responsible sexual behavior from people who have never been taught what constitutes responsibility and irresponsibility in sexual matters.[7]

Today, many resources, manuals, slide series, and curricula have been developed as aids for teaching sexuality to persons who are mentally handicapped.

At the University of Michigan, an initial evaluation of sexuality knowledge is made using a modification of the Edwards Assessment Scale (a program of positive and negative social-sexual behavior patterns shown with pictures). Counseling is then conducted on an individual basis when indicated, or within weekly group sessions, according to the needs of the patient.

Although a detailed description of counseling techniques is beyond the scope of this chapter, it must be mentioned that the emphasis in these programs is on the development of responsible sexual activity patterns and the avoidance of sexual abuse. The response to these sessions is usually very positive, when long-term reinforcement and follow-up is achieved. Kempton reviewed 31 courses involving 430 persons with mental retardation and reported that these sessions resulted in improvement in social behavior, increased self-respect, more openness, fewer feelings of guilt, and no increase in inappropriate behavior.[18]

The avoidance of sexual abuse is a major focus in sexuality education. Mentally handicapped persons are often passive and friendly, especially nonassertive and easily led. As noted by others, this makes them especially susceptible to sexual exploitation.[19] From interviews within our clinic setting, it appears that 10% to 30% of patients brought to the clinic have experienced some form of sexual abuse. With all of these considerations, it is apparent that any postpartum management should include socialization and sexuality training programs for the mentally handicapped and for their caretakers. The keys to any educational program for the mentally handicapped include patience, repetition, reinforcement, and follow-up.

Contraception and Sterilization

The prevention of future pregnancies is often a major concern after pregnancy has occurred and individual problems associated with pregnancy are recognized. Past studies indicated that persons with mental retardation did not use family planning services, even when special opportunities were offered.[8] This attitude of denial is still seen in many families and caretakers, but is rarely a problem post partum and is being seen much less in current programs generally.

Contraceptive technology has been helpful to many persons with mental retardation. However, certain methods are less applicable than others. Intrauterine devices may seem very convenient, but are often associated with increased menstrual bleeding and cramping in someone already having difficulty with menstrual hygiene. Furthermore, IUDs may increase pelvic infection rates and in many patients (especially those with Down's syndrome) may cause a decreased immune response to infection. Therefore, little use of IUDs has been made in the current clinic program.

Barrier methods, although excellent in theory, generally require more manual dexterity, willful self-control, and planning than many of these patients are capable of providing.

Low-dose oral contraceptives have been especially helpful in limiting the duration and amount of menses, controlling the psychosocial distress associated with irregular, anovulatory cycles, and providing contraception. However, some patients experience increased seizures or persistent irregular bleeding. Oral contraceptives are contraindicated for preexisting cardiovascular disease.

Depo Provera, a long-lasting injectable form of medroxyprogesterone acetate, has been useful in limiting menstrual problems, diminishing cyclic discomfort, and (secondarily) providing contraception. It remains somewhat controversial, however, and is not used as a first choice routinely.

Finally, sterilization is one of the most controversial areas of concern for persons with mental retardation, and the legal guidelines vary greatly in different regions. The American College of Obstetricians and Gynecologists has recently offered a statement concerning this issue, and it is affixed to this chapter as an appendix to provide a brief guideline to health care providers.

REFERENCES

1. Alcorn D: Parental views on sexual development and education of trainable mentally retarded. J Special Ed 8:126, 1974
2. Berry J, Shaprio A: Married mentally handicapped patients in the community. Proceedings of the Royal Society of Medicine 68(12):27, 1975
3. Bovicelli L, Orsini LF, Rizzo N et al: Reproduction down syndrome. Obstet Gynecol 59:13S(a), note 25(b) 1982
4. Brandon MWG: A survey of 200 women discharged from a mental deficiency hospital. J Mental Sci 106(442):355, 1960
5. Chamberlain A, Rauh J, Passer A et al: Issues in fertility control for mentally retarded female adolescents. I. Sexuality activity, sexual abuse, and contraception. Pediatrics 73(4):445, 1984
6. Charles D: Ability and accomplishments of persons earlier judged mentally deficient. Genet Psychol Monogr 47:3(a), note 1(b), 1953
7. Craft A, Craft M: Sex Education & Counseling for Mentally Handicapped People. Baltimore, University Park Press, 1983
8. David HP, Smith JD, Friedman E: Family planning services for persons handicapped by mental retardation. Am J Public Health 66(11):1053–1057, 1976
9. Deisher RW: Sexual behavior of retarded in institutions. In de la Cruz F, LaVeck GD (eds): Human Sexuality and the Mentally Retarded. New York, Brunner/Mazel, 1973
10. Elkins TE, Gafford S, Muram D: A model clinic approach to the reproductive health concerns of the mentally handicapped. Obstet Gynecol 68(2):185, 1986
11. Elkins TE, Heaton C, McNeeley SG, DeLancey JO: Use of an advisory committee to aid in sterilization decisions for the mentally handicapped. Presented at the Second Annual Adolescent and Pediatric Gynecology Society Meeting, Cleveland, Ohio, September 1987
12. Elkins TE, Strong C, Wolfe AR, Brown D: An ethics committee in a reproductive health clinic for mentally handicapped persons. Hastings Center Report, June 1986, pp 20–22
13. Floor L, Baxter D, Rosen M, Zisfein L: A survey of marriages among previously institutionalized retardates. Mental Retardation 13(2):33, 1975
14. Haavik SF, Menninger KA II: Sexuality, law, and the developmentally disabled person. In Legal and Clinical Aspects of Marriage, Parenthood, and Sterilization. Baltimore, Paul H Brookes, 1981
15. Heber R, Garber H: The Milwaukee project: A study of the use of family intervention to prevent cultural familial mental retardation. In Friedlander B, Sterritt G, Kirk G (eds): Exceptional Infant—Assessment and Intervention, vol 3. New York, Brunner/Mazel, 1975
16. Johnson B: Study of cases discharged from the

Laconia state school from July 1, 1924, to July 1, 1934. Am J Ment Defic 50:437, 1946

17. Kempton W: The mentally retarded person. In Gochros H, Gochros J (eds): The Sexually Oppressed. New York, Association Press, 1977
18. Kempton W: Sex education for the mentally handicapped. Sexuality Disability 1(2):137–146, 1978
19. Kempton W, Forman R: Guidelines for Training in sexuality and the Mentally Handicapped. Philadelphia, Planned Parenthood Association of Southeastern Pennsylvania, 1976
20. Laxova R, Gilderdale S, Ridler MAC: An aetiological study of fifty-three female patients from a subnormality hospital and of their offspring. J Ment Defic Res 17:193(a), note 3(b), 1973
21. Macklin R, Gaylin W: Mental Retardation and Sterilization: A Problem of Competency and Paternalism. New York, Plenum Press, 1981
22. Madsen MK: Parenting classes for the mentally retarded. Mental Retardation 12(4):195, 1979
23. Mattinson J: Marriage and Mental Handicap. Pittsburgh, University of Pittsburgh Press, 1971
24. Mickelson P: The feebleminded parent: A study of 90 family cases. Am J Ment Defic 51:644(a), note 5(b), 1947
25. Mitchel SB: Results in family casework with feeble-minded clients. Smith College Studies in Social Work 18(1):21, 1947
26. Reed EW, Reed SC: Mental Retardation: A Family Study. Philadelphia, WB Saunders, 1965
27. Salerno LJ, Park JK, Giannini MJ: Reproductive capacity of the mentally retarded. J Reprod Med 14(3):123, 1975
28. Scally BG: Marriage and mental handicap: Some observations in Northern Ireland. In de la Cruz F, LaVeck GD (eds): New York, Brunner/Mazel, 1973
29. Shaw C, Wright C: The married mental defective—A follow-up study. Lancet 1:273(a), note 6(b), 1960
30. Whitcraft CJ, Jones JP: A survey of attitudes about sterilization of retardates .Ment Retard 12(1) 30, 1974

Appendix

AMERICAN COLLEGE OF OBSTETRICIANS AND GYNECOLOGISTS ETHICS COMMITTEE STATEMENT: STERILIZATION OF WOMEN WHO ARE MENTALLY HANDICAPPED

The Committee on Ethics recognizes the need to preserve the principle of free and informed consent before performing a sterilization procedure. This statement is designed to provide background information and guidance to the Fellows of the American College of Obstetricians and Gynecologists when sterilization is being considered for mentally handicapped persons whose ability to provide informed consent is questionable or absent. Although sterilization for mentally handicapped males may be analogous in many ways, other issues exist that are best addressed by other professional groups. This statement therefore pertains only to issues involved in sterilization of females who are mentally handicapped. **Furthermore, the presence of a mental handicap alone does not, in itself, justify either sterilization or its denial.**

I. HISTORICAL BACKGROUND

In the United States, public policy regarding the sterilization of mentally handicapped persons has passed through three historical phases. The first was evident early in this century, when state laws encouraged compulsory sterilizaton of mentally handicapped persons, and judicial decisions gave approval to such actions based on eugenic principles and societal interests.[1]

The second phase was marked by growing social disapproval of mandatory sterilization. This became manifest in 1942, when the U.S. Supreme Court proclaimed reproduction to be a fundamental human right.[2] In many jurisdictions this decision initiated legislative and judicial actions that prohibited sterilization of persons with mental disabilities.[3] In 1979 federal regulations denied the use of federal funds for the sterilization of any mentally incompetent person.[4]

As the third phase of public policy now emerges, widely differing viewpoints are expressed in state laws, which permit sterilization in some cases, prohibit it in others, or most commonly, offer no legal guidance. In each of these phases serious abuses and injustices have been committed: either persons who were objectively capable of parenting but who were incorrectly considered incapacitated were deprived of their procreative rights, or persons for whom pregnancy was a serious burden or harm were denied opportunity for a full range of contraceptive options.

II. CLARIFICATION OF TERMS

For the sake of brevity, persons with mentally handicapping disabilities are described within this document as mentally handicapped persons. The term "mentally handicapped" may be similar in some ways to other phrases, such as "mentally retarded," "mentally impaired," "mentally disabled," or "mentally deficient" that are not used in this document because of their unclear connotations. None of these terms, however, including the one we have chosen to use, describes the person's ability to give informed consent.

It is important to distinguish between the terms "mental capacity" and "mental competency." Within this document, a person's "mental capacity" (to give informed consent) is a functional determination made by appropriate professionals after evaluation of a particular patient. A person's "mental competency" to give informed consent is a determination made by a court of law.

III. ETHICAL CONSIDERATIONS

It is important that obstetrician-gynecologists be aware of the ethical issues inherent in sterilization procedures involving mentally handicapped persons, and of the need to give each sterilization request careful, individual consideration. A systematic approach is necessary in the consideration of sterilization of mentally handicapped patients.

III.A. EVALUATION OF CAPACITY TO PROVIDE INFORMED CONSENT

Individuals who are mentally handicapped are not necessarily incapable of providing informed consent for sterilization or other medical procedures. A person's capacity to provide informed consent for any medical procedure is often difficult to determine. The determination of the capacity to provide informed consent involves the patient's understanding of reasonable alternatives, risks and benefits of the procedures, and the ability to express her personal choice. These elements of informed consent are the same for handicapped and non-handicapped persons. In mentally handicapped individuals, however, impairments of communication skills and mental abilities exist, and vary from person to person and in the same person over time. For this reason, certain precautions must be undertaken to ensure that informed consent is achieved. Ensuring that decisions to request sterilization are not coerced and not transient may require multiple interviews with the patient alone over an appropriate time period. Obtaining the assistance of professionals trained in communicating with mentally handicapped persons is essential in seeking to assess capacity. These professionals may include special educators, psychologists, attorneys familiar with disability law, and physicians accustomed to working with persons who are mentally handicapped. In most jurisdictions, court action is not usually required to proceed with a sterilization procedure, even when a patient is mentally handicapped, if there is agreement among these consultants that an individual is capable of consenting.

Practices to determine a patient's mental capacity to make decisions differ among various legal jurisdictions. If the capacity to provide informed consent remains uncertain despite the aforementioned assessment attempts, a court determination of mental competency may be required by law before a sterilization procedure is performed.

For sterilization, the consent of minors, or of parents on their behalf, may not be recognized in certain jurisdictions under any circumstances. Because state laws vary widely, physicians need to know the laws in their jurisdictions.

III.B. PHYSICIAN RESPONSE WHEN A PATIENT CANNOT GIVE INFORMED CONSENT

If a patient is mentally incapacitated or is adjudicated mentally incompetent, serious consideration should be given to a variety of issues before a sterilization procedure is performed. The initial premise should be that nonvoluntary sterilization is generally not ethically acceptable in our society because of the violation of privacy, bodily integrity, and reproductive rights that it may represent. In some unusual situations, however, sterilization may be considered a reasonable part of a mentally incapacitated or incompetent person's overall health care.

Four categories of concern should be considered in any decision to sterilize a mentally incapacitated or incompetent person: 1) identification of an appropriate decision-maker, 2) alternatives to sterilization, 3) best interests of the mentally incapacitated or incompetent person, and 4) current understanding of applicable laws.

III.B.1. DECISION-MAKERS

In most medical settings, parents, immediate family members, or legal guardians are given the power to provide proxy consent for medical treatment for mentally incompetent or incapacitated persons. The best interests of the patient are generally served by immediate family members who have maintained a close, long-term, positive relationship with the mentally incapacitated or incompetent person. Reliance upon proxy consent (by family or guardians) alone, however, increases the risk of sterilization abuse because a conflict of interest may exist. Some states do not even allow family members or guardians to authorize a sterilization procedure. Therefore, in cases involving proxy consent, the physician should evaluate whether the best interests of the patient will be served. Consultation with other professionals should be considered. These may include pediatricians, neurologists, psychiatrists, psychologists, social workers, attorneys, special educators, or clergy. Input from institutional ethics committees may be desirable, and court opinion may be required except in those states where specific guidelines have already been developed.

III.B.2. ALTERNATIVES TO STERILIZATION

In responding to requests for sterilization of patients who cannot consent because of mental incapacity or incompetence, due consideration should be given to alternative methods of management before any invasive procedure such as surgical sterilization is selected as the most appropriate alternative:

- Noninvasive modalities, such as socialization training, sexual abuse avoidance training, menstrual hygiene training, family counseling, and sexuality education should be considered in lieu of, or concomitant with, requests for sterilization.
- Although medical treatment is usually preferable to surgery, the risks associated with long-term medical contraception or hormonal treatment may be as great or greater than those of a single definitive surgical procedure.

III.B.3 BEST INTERESTS OF THE PATIENT

With all requests for sterilizaton of a mentally incapacitated or incompetent person the primary consideration is the best interests of the patient.

Certain facts should be ascertained in order to protect these interests:

- The mental incapacity or incompetency should be a permanent condition, and not one in which the functional capacity to choose or the capacity to be a parent would change.
- There should also be a reasonable likelihood that the patient is fertile and may experience sexual intercourse unless her social freedom is restricted.
- It should be determined whether pregnancy represents a serious, objective physical risk (e.g., severe heart disease) to the patient.
- Even if no health risks would be incurred through pregnancy, the burdens to the patient of childbearing, parenting, or menstrual hygiene problems should be considered. When the harms to the patient are less direct or less immediately apparent, more careful appraisal of benefits versus burdens is warranted to be certain of the best ethical choice.

There may be cases in which other factors override sole consideration of the best interests of the patient. This can occur either when there is difficulty in determining the patient's best interests or when other concerns are so serious as to merit consideration in themselves. Examples of such concerns may include the following:

- In some cases pregnancy would represent a significant risk that the infant would be born with a serious genetic or congenital problem.
- Pregnancy or preserving reproductive function may significantly increase the difficulty of caring for the patient; an infant would make further demands on the same caretaker or necessitate the shift of that responsibility to other individuals or institutions.

In some situations, particularly when requests for surgical sterilization are based on concerns about burdens to others, the apprehensions about these burdens may or may not be realistic, particularly in the case of the very young patient.

When factors such as these appear to override the best interests of the patient, additional review is indicated, such as by an institutional ethics committee.

Finally, if a surgical method is employed, the selection of the sterilization procedure should represent the most appropriate method of care that will achieve the intended benefits.

III.B.4. LEGAL CONSIDERATIONS

It is essential to recognize municipal, county, state and federal statutes, regulations, or legal decisions that control the practice of sterilization of mentally incapacitated or incompetent persons.

Used with the permission of the American College of Obstetricians and Gynecologists.

REFERENCES

1. *Buck v. Bell*, 274 U.S. 200 (1927)
2. *Skinner v. Oklahoma*, 316 U.S. 535 (1942)
3. *Relf v. Weinberger*, 372 F Supp. 1196 (D.D.C. 1974)
4. Making Health Care Decisions-President's Commission

6

Social and Environmental Risks of Pregnancy

SECTION 1: CHEMICAL TERATOGENS

Robert L. Anderson and Mitchell S. Golbus

Teratology is the study of abnormal development and congenital malformations. This includes the classification, frequency, causes, and mechanisms of anomalous embryonic and fetal development. Until recently it was believed that the mammalian fetus developed in the shielded environment of the maternal uterus and that, therefore, external factors were not a significant influence on development. This was consistent with the popular mendelian principles of inheritance, which had been rediscovered by Garrod.[60]

In the 1940s two different types of reports appeared which were to introduce the age of modern experimental teratology. First, Gregg[69] recognized the association between maternal rubella infection and abnormal fetal development. Second, Warkany and his associates[237,238] published a series of articles demonstrating the adverse effect of environmental factors on intrauterine mammalian development. Articles concerning the effects of experimental environmental manipulation on embryogenesis continued to accumulate over the ensuing 15 to 20 years, but the recognition of the significance of teratology to the practicing obstetrician occurred only after a drug-induced catastrophe. In 1961 Lenz[114] and McBride[128] simultaneously reported that an epidemic of limb-reduction malformations in newborns was due to maternal ingestion of the sedative thalidomide early in pregnancy. This finding had obstetric, legal, pharmaceutical, and governmental regulatory repercussions which are still ongoing. Today every physician should be exquisitely discriminating in his use of medication during pregnancy.

CONTRIBUTING FACTORS

A comprehensive review of experimental teratology is no longer possible due to the immense accumulation of reports, nor would it best serve the interests of the practicing physician. It is, however, worthwhile to comprehend the general principles involved in the mechanisms by which environmental agents lead to congenital defects.

The long-standing argument about nature (genetics) versus nurture (environment) has been resolved with the understanding that both play an intertwined role in development. Any potential teratogen exerts its influence on a background of over 20,000 genes which vary from individual to individual. For example, when considering multifactorially inherited anomalies which rely on both genetic and environmental factors, fraternal twins have significantly less concordance for any defect than identical twins. This is a reflection of the fraternal twins' dissimilar genetic constitution. This point is magnified when comparing effects in strains or species. For example, thalidomide in low doses causes its characteristic defects only in humans and higher primates; most other mammals are resistant.

Critical Periods

Data from the thalidomide experience made it evident that only women who had taken the drug between the 20th and 40th day after conception delivered infants with drug-induced malformations.[104] There are, then, *critical periods* in development, defined as times of greatest susceptibility of a specific developing organ to a specific teratogen. The most important variable is which particular tissues of the embryo are undergoing organogenesis at the time of insult. The same dose of thalidomide that causes ear malformations if taken 22 days after conception will cause amelia of the lower extremities if taken 28 days after conception.

Because various organs develop at different rates, the incidence of teratogenesis may differ for different organs. Neural tissue, which has a long period of development, is susceptible to environmental influences throughout almost all of gestation. In contrast, the palate, which begins to develop during the fifth week of gestation, is completely fused by 12 weeks; thus, a much shorter critical period exists. Most teratologic effects occur early in gestation because this is the period of most active organogenesis.

A second contributory factor to this timing is that drugs are metabolized by degradation, oxidation, reduction, and hydrolysis. These are all functions of liver microsomal enzymes, which first appear at approximately midgestation. The generalization that earlier developmental stages are more susceptible to environmental influences should be tempered by noting some exceptions. The pre-implantation stages of development tend to be resistant to malformation induction. In part this is because a smaller dose of teratogen is delivered to the embryo, which does not yet have a circulatory connection to the mother. Additionally, cleavage of this totipotential stage leads either to cell replacement with no noticeable effect or to embryo death.

Underlying Mechanisms

As the literature in experimental teratology accumulated it became apparent that different agents could produce identical defects. This led to the concept that underlying mechanisms or early events caused by environmental agents existed such that a common defect was the result of a common pathway initiated by a specific underlying mechanism. Just as there are a limited number of changes that can occur in developing cells, tissues, and organs that do not cause embryonic death, there are a limited number of pathways and, therefore, a certain commonality to the malformations produced. The following initial changes at the molecular level are recognized as basic teratologic mechanisms:

Mutation (gene or chromosome)
Mitotic interference
Altered RNA synthesis or function

Lack of precursors, substrates, or coenzymes for biosynthesis

Disruption of aerobic- or anerobic-metabolism that alters energy sources

Membrane alterations with abnormal membrane transfer or altered cell recognition

Osmolar imbalance

Specific enzyme inhibition.[241]

Each of these mechanisms is capable of producing imbalances in growth and differentiation. The final defect is preceded by a series of abnormal morphogenic events which in total represent the pathogenesis of the abnormal development. Modern teratology is devoted to the study and understanding of these abnormal morphologic events; this chapter also examines the mechanisms of determination and differentiation.

Abnormal development can be manifested in only a few ways. Organism death due to cell loss during early embryogenesis or due to a lethal biosynthetic mutation represents the most severe result. Malformations are the manifestation most often recognized in the newborn. Many recognized constellations of anomalies are due to secondary and tertiary adjustments to an original single defect. Damage during the fetal period after organogenesis is most likely to be manifested as growth retardation. In this respect, malnutrition with its lack of biosynthetic substrates and the resultant intrauterine growth retardation may be considered a teratologic event.

Functional disorders are the fourth type of manifestation and may be explained by nonlethal cellular depletion. These disturbances may be the most sensitive indicator of teratogenicity. Only by employing a variety of maturational and behavioral measurements at various times of life will we be able to recognize behavioral or latent effects of teratogens. It is unknown to what extent the fulfillment of human potential is limited by drug-induced functional aberrations.

Dosage

The total dose of an environmental agent that reaches the conceptus depends upon many variables: the amount of the agent administered and its form (solid, liquid, or gas) are among the most obvious. The result can range from having no effect to causing death.

Maternal detoxification processes are paramount in protecting the fetus, and it must be recognized that these genetically controlled capabilities will vary with the individual. The placenta has been greatly overrated as a fetal protector. It now appears that most unbound compounds in the maternal serum cross the placenta at a rate controlled by compound size, charge, lipid solubility, and its tendency to protein binding. Some compounds, such as amino acids, are preferentially transported against a gradient to the fetal side of the placenta. This can occasionally work to the detriment of the fetus, as with phenylpyruvic and phenyllactic acid, which accumulates in maternal phenylketonuria and whose transfer causes mental retardation in the nonphenylketonuric offspring.

It seems clear that in teratogenesis there is a demonstrable threshold below which no embryotoxic effect occurs. This is in contrast to mutagens and carcinogens, which appear to have a straight-line dose-response curve with no practical lower limit of response. This may be because mutagens and carcinogens reflect single cell alterations while teratogenesis requires alteration of a critical number of cells beyond the embryonic restoration capability.[243]

TERATOGENIC DRUGS

The scope of the problem of fetal teratogenesis is revealed by the list of 900 different drugs taken by pregnant women in the National Institutes of Health (NIH) Collaborative Perinatal Study.[82] Pregnant women take an average of almost four drugs excluding nutritional supplements during pregnancy with only 20% of pregnant women abstaining from drug usage.[52,123] Perhaps even more significant is that 40% of the women took medication during the first trimester, and that approximately one-half of the total drug consumption during pregnancy occurred during the period of organogenesis.[52,192]

Comparison of drug administration during pregnancy in 1960[163] and in 1981[20] is not very encouraging. The later study found that 45% of pregnant women took at least one prescribed medication in pregnancy, with many taking as many as three. Rayburn[175] found that 75% of patients took one drug exclusive of prenatal vitamins and iron. Nearly half of the drugs consumed were over-the-counter types rather than prescription medications.

Wilson[243] has tried to place the problem in perspective by pointing out that 65% to 70% of developmental defects are of unknown origin and only 2% to 3% are known to be due to drugs and environmental chemicals. This is somewhat less than reassuring in view of the overwhelming size of the unknown category. It is difficult to trace specific defects or constellations of defects to specific drugs because of many confounding factors. These include:

- The drug may be administered as therapy for an illness which itself causes the malformation.
- The fetal malformation may cause maternal symptoms which are treated with a specific drug.
- The drug may inhibit the abortion of an already malformed infant.
- The drug may commonly be employed in combination with a second drug which causes a malformation

A second problem is that the congenital malformation study group may include only structural malformations, all congenital defects, or all disorders with a possible prenatal etiology. As the structural malformation group is progressively diluted, the likelihood of assigning causality decreases.[102] Additionally, because most studies do not contain appropriate controls, the clinical teratology literature is a source of semi-useful data.

Any statement about human teratogenesis must, by definition, be incomplete. The obstetrician is therefore inevitably left in a quandary. Many drugs and environmental agents have not been studied adequately for their teratogenic potential. Only a few have been studied well enough to define their hazards or to pronounce them safe. Even if an agent is found to be teratogenic, there is a long lag time before reports appear in the literature and the evidence accumulates. This evidence may well be published in sources unfamiliar to the practicing obstetrician. The articles used to reference this chapter make the point. Only 21% of the articles were published in obstetric journals, whereas 31% were in general medical journals, 13% in teratology or genetic publications, 13% in specialty publications other than obstetrics or pediatrics, 9% in pediatric journals, and 13% in foreign publications.

With this caveat it is nevertheless possible to categorize many drugs as positively or possibly teratogenic and to indicate some drugs which under normal conditions of use involve little or no teratogenic risk. In addition we would suggest exposing the pregnant patient only to the most necessary therapeutic agents, and only then after considering the "fetal side" of the patient complex. Perhaps such a policy, widely applied, would influence the 65% to 70% of developmental defects of unknown origin.

Antineoplastic Agents

Antineoplastic agents kill cells. They work best against rapidly dividing cells, a characteristic not only of a neoplasm but also a fetus. Therefore, it is not surprising that these compounds are among the most potent teratogens known. Antineoplastic agents may be classified as alkylating agents, antimetabolites, or miscellaneous cytotoxic drugs. Hormones and antibiotics, which may be used as anti-tumor medications, will be discussed in their respective sections.

Alkylating Agents

Alkylating agents substitute in protein and nucleic acids and form cross-links with DNA, causing its inactivation. The most commonly used alkylating drugs are busulfan, chlorambucil, cyclophosphamide, nitrogen mustard, triethylenemelamine (TEM) and triethylenethiophosphoramide (thio-TEPA).

Currently, busulfan therapy for chronic granulocytic leukemia probably accounts for the greatest number of exposed fetuses. Thirty-five cases of busulfan use during pregnancy have been reported with 4 anomalous fetuses resulting. Diamond, Anderson, and McCreadie[40] described an infant with growth retardation, cleft palate, microphthalmus, cloudy corneas, hypoplastic ovaries, and poorly developed external genitalia. The mother had been irradiated and received 6-mercaptopurine in addition to busulfan during pregnancy. de Rezende and colleagues[38] reported an abortus with numerous unspecified malformations from a mother receiving only busulfan. Boros and Reynolds[18] described an infant with growth retardation, absence of the right kidney, hydronephrosis of the left kidney, and hepatic subcapsular calcifications born to a patient treated with busulfan and allopurinal. Pyloric stenosis has been described in one infant exposed only after the first trimester. Of the 12 infants exposed to busulfan in utero for whom a birth weight and gestational age was reported, 8 have manifested severe intrauterine growth retardation. A recurrent problem with numbers such as these is that the likelihood is greater for a positive rather than a negative case report to be published, and thus the number of affected neonates is probably inflated. Nevertheless, busulfan should be considered as a teratogen causing both malformations and intrauterine growth retardation.

Chlorambucil administration has been reported to result in two fetuses with unilateral renal and ureteral agenesis.[204,214] Cyclophosphamide has resulted in 6 malformed infants with extremity defects from first trimester exposures.[30,68,220,227] Nicholson[151] reviewed 11 pregnancies exposed to nitrogen mustard, which resulted in 7 normal infants, 1 induced abortion, and 3 spontaneous abortions. Since then 2 other infants with malformations who were exposed to nitrogen mustard as part of a multiple drug therapy have been reported.[59,132] At least 9 fetuses have been exposed in utero to TEM or thio-TEPA with no resulting anomalies.[152]

Antimetabolites

The antimetabolites are structural analogues of naturally occurring substances; they either cause a deficiency of, or replace, the corresponding compound. From a teratogenic point of view the most infamous antimetabolite is the folic acid antagonist aminopterin, which was used as an abortifacient in the 1950s.[65,223,224] Seventy percent of the pregnancies exposed to this agent aborted, and many of the abortuses demonstrated abnormalities. One-third of the remaining pregnancies resulted in malformed infants. The anomalous fetuses and newborns (one was also exposed to thalidomide) demonstrated striking bony maldevelopment with a globular head, abnormal triangular facies, small ears, and markedly retarded growth.

Another commonly used folic acid antagonist, methotrexate, also has been linked causally with infants born with multiple skeletal defects in eight first-trimester exposures.[141,170] Studies have shown that methotrexate may persist in human tissue for prolonged periods after termination of treatment, and no safe interval has yet to be established.[29,234] The recent enthusiasm for using methotrexate to treat psoriasis probably will lead to an increased number of fetal exposures.

Other Cytotoxic Drugs

Interestingly, significant numbers of pregnancies have been treated with purine antagonists without adverse effects. Of 62 infants exposed to 6-mercaptopurine, the only one with anomalies was also exposed to busulfan.[151] Another purine antagonist of great importance is azathioprine (Imuran), an immunosuppressant used in the ever-increasing number of women with renal transplants who are undertaking pregnancy. There have been over 125 reported conceptions in transplant recipients, with the only reported structural defect being one infant with pulmonic stenosis.[164] One infant whose father was taking azathioprine was born with a myelomeningocele and, secondarily, bilateral dislocated hips and bilateral talipes equinovarus.[221]

The number of anomalies reported do not differ from that expected in a control population. There have been, however, a number of newborns exposed to azathioprine in utero who were born with lymphopenia, adrenal insufficiency, growth retardation, and an increase in chromosome breakage.[154] More extensive surveillance of the development, immunocompetence, and chromosomal complement in neonates exposed to azathioprine is required before the apparent safety of this drug can be verified. Procarbazine, although frequently used in combination with other drugs, appears to be the common agent in four first-trimester exposures that resulted in malformed fetuses.[225]

Several infants have been exposed in utero to vinblastine and vincristine, and the only anomalies occurring in the newborn were felt to be related to the other agents used in combination. For each of these drugs, individually, very few pregnancies have occurred in treated women; however, the absence of reported defects should not be interpreted as evidence for a total lack of teratogenicity.

Catanzarite and Ferguson[27] reviewed the outcome of 47 pregnancies associated with acute leukemia and exposure to combination chemotherapy involving multiple drugs. Forty treated pregnancies resulted in 31 surviving infants, 5 abortions, 3 perinatal deaths, and 1 infant in grave condition. The 7 untreated patients had pregnancies resulting in 1 abortion, 2 perinatal deaths, and 4 living infants. In the 40 liveborn infants, there were 2 with neutropenia but no malformations. Intrauterine growth retardation was noted, with most exposed infants falling in the 10th to 25th percentile for gestational age. However, Catanzarite notes that this may be a result of the maternal disease rather than the chemotherapy received during the pregnancy.

Antimicrobial Agents

Antibiotics

The sulfonamides may be a hazard to the newborn because of their competition with bilirubin for albumin-binding sites; however, they present little danger as a teratogen. Although Nelson[150] reported that a higher proportion of mothers of infants with anomalies than of control mothers took sulfonamides during pregnancy, this was not verified by other studies.[161,178] The combination of trimethoprim and sulfamethoxazole has been advocated for therapy of urinary tract infections and is of some concern because both components have been found to be teratogenic to rats.[230] Williams and associates[241] reported that no abnormalities were observed in ten pregnancies exposed to this combination during the first trimester. Nevertheless, until more animal and human data are available, this combination therapy should be avoided during pregnancy unless there are no suitable alternatives.

Penicillin has been widely used during pregnancy for the last 20 years without any implication of teratogenicity, and may be considered a safe drug during pregnancy. However, there has been no systematic epidemiologic study of the prenatal effects of the new drugs chemically related to penicillin.

Chloramphenicol is another antibiotic that has been used widely during pregnancy with no demonstrable adverse fetal effects. It is, however, quite toxic to the newborn and causes the so-called *gray syndrome* of abdominal distention, cyanosis, and vascular collapse. Maternal chloramphenicol therapy in labor may result in a neonate with toxic blood levels; therefore, this antibiotic should be restricted in late pregnancy.

Erythromycin exposure during pregnancy has been associated with one infant with exencephaly and other defects.[118] However, examination of a published photograph indicates that the fetus had amniotic band syndrome, a known sporadic malformation complex; thus, the anomalies should not be attributed to the erythromycin exposure.

Metronidazole significantly increases chromosome aberrations in treated patients' lymphocytes.[142] Peterson and associates[166] studied 206 pregnancies exposed to metronidazole and found no increase in the overall prevalence of congenital anomalies, but did find four infants with malformations among the 55 exposed during the first trimester. Morgan[145] studied 880 patients diagnosed with *Trichomonas vaginalis* in pregnancy. The 597 who were symptomatic were treated, and the 283 asymptomatic patients were not treated. Of those treated, only 62 received metronidazole in the first trimester. No differences in growth retardation, prematurity, or malformations were noted in these two groups. The significance of these findings to the individual patient or to the fetus is unclear, but discretion suggests that in the first trimester of pregnancy this drug should be avoided if possible.

Tetracycline forms a chelated complex with calcium orthophosphate and becomes incorporated into bones and teeth if present during the period of calcification. This property is common to all tetracyclines. Deciduous teeth (but not permanent teeth) begin calcifying during the fifth month of fetal life and, if exposed to tetracycline, will appear yellow and fluoresce a bright yellow with an intensity directly proportional to the total tetracycline dosage.[235] After years of exposure to light, the yellow color of the teeth turns gray to brown. In addition to this cosmetic problem, teeth containing tetracycline are more susceptible to cavities and display enamel hypoplasia. Bones begin calcifying at two months of fetal life and also can incorporate tetracycline if exposed in utero; however, tetracycline-containing bones do not appear to be more liable to fracture.[228] The suspicion that tetracycline might be implicated in developmental anomalies of the extremities has been raised, but numerous studies of tetracycline administration at the critical time for limb development have not corroborated this concern.

Many antibiotics inhibit DNA or RNA synthesis making them potential antiviral and antineoplastic agents. Those which have been studied (actinomycin D, mitomycin C, adenine arabinoside, fluorodeoxyuridine, and idoxuridine) are all teratogenic in rodents. Stephens and colleagues[217] reported one first-trimester exposure to 5-fluorouracil (5-FU) that resulted in a fetus with multiple anomalies of the extremities as well as gastrointestinal and urinary tract malformations. However, there have been no other published reports associating 5-FU or other drugs in this group with human fetal malformations, but neither have there been any series of negative cases attesting to their safety.

Antituberculins

Streptomycin and dihydrostreptomycin have been used extensively as antituberculosis agents. The ototoxity known to occur in adults also can occur in the fetus; more than 30 cases of hearing deficit and eighth nerve damage have been reported in infants exposed to streptomycin derivatives in utero. The risk of fetal ototoxicity has ranged from 3%[174] to 11%.[58] Other aminoglycosides (e.g., neomycin, kanamycin, and gentamicin) are also potentially ototoxic. Nine of 391 infants exposed in utero to kanamycin had a hearing loss.[54] Aside from ototoxicity, however, the aminoglycoside antibiotics have shown no other teratologic effect.

The standard drugs used as antituberculosis agents have been isoniazid (INH) and para-aminosalicyclic acid (PAS). Studies of large cohorts of pregnant women treated for tuberculosis have revealed no increased incidence of anomalies in their offspring.[98,122] Potworowska and co-workers[169] reported that 7 of 23 infants of mothers treated with ethionamide had anomalies, with central nervous system (CNS) defects being the most common. Although this has not been verified in other studies,[13,250] it seems advisable to avoid this drug during pregnancy. The newer antituberculosis agents, rifampin and ethambutol, have been used in hundreds of pregnant women without evidence of any teratogenic effect.[98] The manufacturers of rifampin have collected data on 229 conceptions during which this drug was administered; 6 of

202 exposed infants had malformations.[215] No control data were reported, but this 3% malformation rate does not appear significantly higher than expected.

Antimalarials

Antimalarial agents have been suspected of being teratogenic, but no systemic or epidemiologic surveys are available. Maternal ingestion of quinine was reported to cause neonatal deafness over one hundred years ago.[180] Winckel[245] reviewed 17 cases of congenital anomalies of the ear or eye following in utero exposure to quinine, but in view of the widespread use of the drug he felt a causal relationship was tenuous. Large doses of quinine also have been used as an abortifacient. Tanimura[223] surveyed the literature and found 20 malformed infants who had been exposed in this manner; however, the total sample size was not stated.

Chloroquine has replaced quinine as an antimalarial drug, and is also employed in the therapy of systemic lupus erythematosus. The only report implying teratogenicity concerns a woman who, while taking chloroquine during pregnancy, had one spontaneous abortion and gave birth to three children with congenital defects (one with Wilms' tumor and hemihypertrophy; one with sensorineural deafness; and one with sensorineural deafness, and mental and physical delayed development. She had three normal children when not taking chloroquine during pregnancy.[80]

A third antimalarial agent, quinacrine hydrochloride, has been associated with a single newborn with renal agenesis, spina bifida, and megacolon.[234] Pyrimethamine is a folate antagonist used as an antimalarial and its use in pregnancy has been discouraged in the past. However, its use in large prophylactic programs and in high doses for treatment of toxoplasmosis has resulted in a large number of early pregnancy exposures without malformations or other problems being noted.[46] Folinic acid supplementation is recommended when pyrimethamine is prescribed in pregnancy. In the absence of sufficient systemic studies it is difficult to arrive at a final conclusion regarding the antimalarial compounds; thus, any pregnant woman taking these drugs should be apprised of this uncertainty.

Hormones and Anti-Hormones

Adrenal and Pituitary Steroids

Adrenal corticosteroids are potent palatal teratogens in rodents, and clinicians are therefore wary of these widely employed drugs. Literature surveys of 688 fetuses exposed in utero to corticosteroids or adrenocorticotropic hormone (ACTH) revealed 20 infants with congenital anomalies, a frequency no different from control data.[17,195] Although only 6 cases of acute adrenal insufficiency in the neonate have been reported, this is a risk to which the pediatrician should be alert. The risk of stillbirth or placental insufficiency with intrauterine growth retardation is difficult to evaluate, because no appropriate untreated control population exists. It is more likely that these latter complications are associated with the underlying maternal disease requiring corticosteroid therapy than with the drug itself.

Other than gonadotropins, the only pituitary hormone implicated as having a possible deleterious fetal effect is oxytocin. Mast and group[124] first suggested a relationship between the use of oxytocin and neonatal hyperbilirubinemia, and verification by others has followed.[28,37] Hyperbilirubinemia secondary to oxytocin is independent of gestation age, birth weight, or Apgar score, but whether it is caused by a redistribution of blood between fetus and placenta or by a mechanism involving red blood cell breakdown or hepatic enzyme maturation is unknown.

Androgens

Androgens, including 19-nortestosterone derivatives found in some birth control pills, can masculinize the female fetus. Labioscrotal fusion is seen if exposure occurs prior to the 12th week of gestation; clitoral and labia majora enlargement without labioscrotal fusion are seen when the exposure occurs only in the second and third trimesters. The incidence of fetal masculinization varies according to the drug and dosage. An 18% incidence of masculinization was noted for female infants exposed to norethindrone,[92] compared to only 1% of those exposed to medroxyprogesterone.[24] Male fetuses do not appear to be adversely affected, but may have genital development somewhat advanced for their gestational age. In animals the antiandrogen cyproterone acetate may induce feminization of the male fetus.[216]

Estrogens

The possibility of transplacental chemical carcinogenesis emerged in 1971 when Herbst and associates[85] reported eight cases of vaginal adenocarcinoma in young women, seven of whom had been exposed to stilbesterol in utero. Although over 200 cases of vaginal adenocarcinoma associated with prenatal stilbesterol exposure have been reported, probably 500,000 patients were at risk; thus, the chances of developing cancer during the first two to three decades of life is low. In addition, the carcinoma-in-situ prevalence rate among these patients is 1.4%.[126] A prevalence rate of 30% to 90% for vaginal adenosis has been reported, but its bearing on future development of cancer is unknown.[71,201] Male fetuses exposed to stilbesterol in utero have a 25% incidence of epididymal cysts, hypotrophic testes, and capsular induration of the testes, and a 32% incidence of pathologic spermatozoal analyses.[62]

The only other estrogenic compound implicated teratologically has been clomiphene citrate. There have been approximately a dozen case reports of malformed infants conceived after clomiphene stimulation, with half of these having a neural tube defect; no denominator is available for a critical evaluation of these reports. Two surveys totaling 321 similarly treated pregnancies contained only four infants with major malformations, certainly within expected limits.[73,77]

A question regarding the association of clomiphene and gonadotropins with meiotic nondisjunction has been raised by some soft data. Oakley and Flynt[159] reported twice the expected rate of trisomy 21 among offspring who were conceived following an induced ovulation. In addition, spontaneous abortions of pregnancies conceived the month of or month following ovulation induction by clomiphene or menotropins have a significantly higher incidence of aneuploidy.[19] Because the pregnancies which continued were not studied, it is impossible to know if more aneuploid pregnancies were conceived or if a higher proportion of those conceived were spontaneously aborted. Kurachi and colleagues[110] reviewed the outcome of 1034 pregnancies following clomiphene-induced ovulation. Spontaneous abortion and ectopic and molar pregnancies accounted for 99 losses (14.8%). In the 935 infants born, there were 21 with visible anomalies (2.3%), not significantly different from the incidence of 1.7% with malformations in over 30,000 infants conceived after spontaneous ovulation. The malformations noted in the clomiphene group were similer in type and frequency to those occurring in the spontaneous ovulation group. The data should be recognized as being only "mildly suggestive," and monitoring of pregnancies conceived following ovulation induction should resolve these questions over the next few years. Until the question of whether ovulation induction is related to meiotic nondisjunction rates is answered, women who conceive during such therapy may be apprised of the possibility of amniocentesis to verify the chromosomal normality of the fetus.

Progestational Agents

Progestogens or combinations of estrogens and progestogens (birth control pills) have been employed widely in early gestation, either as a withdrawal pregnancy test or to support a threatened abortion. In addition, women have continued to take birth control pills after conceiving, unaware of their pregnancy. The teratologic implications of this exposure to progestogens have been debated for the last 15 years. In 1967, Gal, Kirman, and Steen[55] reported that women who gave birth to infants with meningomyelocele or hydrocephalus were significantly more likely than control women to have had a withdrawal pregnancy test in the first trimester. However, at least two studies[113,228] have failed to confirm this association. In 1973, Levy and co-workers[116] reported six cases of transposition of the great vessels in offspring exposed to hormonal pregnancy tests during the first 6 weeks of pregnancy. Again, a similar retrospective study[148] failed to confirm this relationship.

The Jerusalem Perinatal study[78] of 11,468 infants and a prospective study[157] of 100 exposed pregnancies both found an increased incidence of cardiac anomalies in newborns with a history of progestogen exposure. The NIH Collaborative Perinatal Project report[82] in 50,282 pregnancies and a matched case control study[94] in 70 newborns with cardiac defects found relative risks of 2 to 6.5 for progestogen exposure. The VACTERL (vertebral, anal, cardiac, tracheoesophageal, renal, and limb anomalies) complex was felt related to oral contraceptive exposure by two reports[155] but the association could not be supported by at least two other authors.[36,82]

Four reports have noted an association between early fetal progestogen exposure and hypospadias in the male neonate.[2,78,83,120] Another large, prospective study of over 14,000 pregnancies found the relative risk for hypospadias after progestin exposure to be 1.75 (confidence limits 0.5–4.4).[126] Limb reduction defects secondary to oral contraceptive exposure in early pregnancy have been noted in three reports,[84,95,130] but the data from the NIH Collaborative Perinatal Study were inconclusive.[82] Studies of overall malformation rates following progestin exposure are inconclusive or negative.[67,78,160] In a 1985 review, Simpson summarized all available data on these various defects and progestin exposure and concluded that such exposures did not substantially increase the risk of anomalies above that expected in nonexposed pregnancies.[205]

The absolute increase in the risk of having an infant with a congenital anomaly appears to be small with progestogen exposure, and the influence of confounding factors and of specific hormone preparations is still not clear. Although inadvertent exposure of the fetus to progestogens will continue to occur, iatrogenic exposure appears unwarranted as there is no evidence that this is an effective therapy for threatened abortion[64]; there are simpler, quicker, and more accurate pregnancy tests.

Thyroid and Related Drugs

Thyroid hormones have been used as a reproductive panacea for many years, but they appear to cross the placenta very poorly if at all. In spite of widespread use, there have been only a few isolated case reports of children with congenital malformations after maternal thyroid ingestion. However, congenital goiter and hypothyroidism attributable to maternal intake of antithyroid drugs or iodine are well documented. The thiourea agents, which block the iodination of tyrosine and the coupling of diiodotyrosine, are widely used in the therapy of maternal hyperthyroidism. These drugs readily cross the placenta and may cause fetal hypothyroidism and a compensatory hypertrophic goiter. Neonatal goiter induced by thiourea derivatives tends to be small and does not usually cause respiratory obstruction. Cretinism is avoided by controlling the mother with a minimal maintenance dose, and signs of neonatal hypothyroidism disappear over a 2 to 6 week period. Breastfeeding is contraindicated if the mother continues on thiourea therapy.

Burrow and colleagues[23] compared children exposed to propylthiouracil in utero to unexposed siblings and found no significant difference in intelligence, height, or bone age. Only one particular drug, methimazole, has been associated with a specific ulcerlike midline scalp defect; five infants showed this defect following in utero exposure.[135,147]

Inorganic iodides also have been used to treat hyperthyroidism and are often used as a mucolytic agent in the treatment of asthma. Iodides readily cross the placenta, interfere with fetal thyroid production, and may cause massive thyroid enlargement. The huge goiter may prevent fetal swallowing leading to polyhydramnios, and has been responsible for a number of neonatal respiratory obstruction deaths. A high percentage of the survivors demonstrated varying degrees of cretinism.[25,247] The excessive use of iodides during pregnancy for either thyroid or respiratory disorders, and breastfeeding by women taking iodide-containing medications should be avoided.

Finally, because the fetal thyroid concentrates iodine after 10 weeks of pregnancy,[200] radioactive iodine ingested by the mother after this time will destroy fetal thyroid tissue. The use of I-131 during pregnancy, even for diagnostic purposes, is, therefore, contraindicated.

Insulin and Hypoglycemic Agents

Given the known increased incidence in congenital anomalies in the offspring of diabetic women, it is difficult to evaluate the teratogenicity of hypoglycemic agents. The patterns of malformation in babies of nondiabetic and diabetic mothers (except for caudal regression syndrome) are similar, and the increased incidence of anomalies in offspring of nontreated class-A diabetic women makes it improbable that insulin, per se, is teratogenic. The oral hypoglycemic agents, particularly sulfonylureas, have been criticized as potential teratogens. However, in spite of their marked teratogenicity in rodents, there is no evidence of an increased rate of anomalies in general nor of any specific anomaly in human neonates exposed in utero.

Socially Used Drugs

Alcohol

One of the most significant teratogenic risks to the fetus arises from the maternal use of alcohol. Alcoholism is the most common drug abuse problem in contemporary society, affecting 1% to 2% of women of childbearing age. In 1973 Jones and co-workers[100] reported eight unrelated children with a similar malformation pattern born to mothers with chronic alcoholism. The characteristic findings and the frequency of their occurrence in fetuses of alcoholic mothers noted in the NIH Collaborative Perinatal Project were as follows: an IQ of 79 or less (44%), intrauterine growth retardation (32%), ocular anomalies (25%), joint anomalies (25%), and cardiac murmurs (25%).[99] Additionally, these neonates may go through an alcohol withdrawal reaction.[167]

More moderate alcohol consumption during pregnancy may carry a significant risk.[220] Of 16 women who drank 2 ounces or more of alcohol daily, 19% delivered infants with evidence of the fetal alcohol syndrome (FAS). Of 54 women who consumed between 1 and 2 ounces of alcohol daily, 11% of the children had at least partial features of the fetal alcohol syndrome. Rosett and associates[183] evaluated over 450 women and studied neonatal outcome related to alcohol consumption. In the subgroup of heavy drinkers who abstained or reduced their intake in the last half of pregnancy, the incidences of low birth weight, short stature, and small head size were all reduced below that noted for moderate drinkers. However, the morphologic features of FAS occurred at the expected frequency. This suggests that these decreased growth parameters are either reversible or late developing, and strongly supports counseling the heavy drinker to abstain in later pregnancy to prevent some of the serious FAS sequelae. Twelve infants with FAS have been followed for up to 20 months and compared with normal controls. These affected infants exhibited delayed mental and motor development as well as physical abnormalities and growth retardation when compared to the controls.[66] Alcohol is discussed in detail in Section 2.

Tobacco

Maternal smoking is a well established cause of intrauterine growth retardation.[206] There is also evidence that smoking increases the risk of a stillbirth, particularly for the woman who is already at risk,[186] and increases the perinatal death rate.[133] The influence of maternal smoking on the incidence of congenital malformations is unclear; half of the studies report an increased incidence, whereas the other half claim a decreased incidence.

Maternal narcotic addiction can be directly related to such obstetrical complications as intrauterine growth retardation, premature labor, breech delivery, and toxemia. The neonate has a 65% to 75% chance of undergoing withdrawal, which has an associated 3% to 5% mortality rate. Several large series have demonstrated that there is no increased risk of congenital anomalies, per se.[176,250] Neonatal withdrawal also has been reported following excessive maternal propoxyphene use.

LSD and Marijuana

Lysergic acid (LSD) use during pregnancy has been the subject of a number of reviews. Long[119] studied 161 children born to parents who ingested LSD before conception, during the pregnancy, or both. He felt the only suspicious finding was in five infants with limb deficiency anomalies, which ostensibly could be explained in no way other than attributing them to the LSD usage. It must be recalled, however, that these patients often have a history of multiple drug ingestion and are generally at an increased reproductive risk. Jacobson and Berlin[93] studied 148 pregnancies of LSD users and found five more infants with limb bud anomalies and a 9.6% incidence of nervous system defects. In view of this last finding it might be appropriate to offer LSD users sonography or a maternal serum alpha-fetoprotein determination. This type of prospective data eventually will help establish the risk of a prenatally detectable neural tube defect. There has been much discussion of the effect of LSD on chromosomal breakage, but Dumars[45] karyotyped 41 infants whose parents were LSD users and found no increase in chromosomal breakage or rearrangements.

The teratogenicity of marijuana remains an unanswered question. There is no evidence of human teratogenicity, but likewise there is no assurance that marijuana exposure is safe for the fetus. Patients who have smoked marijuana during pregnancy may be reassured but should be asked to desist.

Psychotropic Drugs

Thalidomide

This class of drugs is of particular interest because it contains the classic teratogen, thalidomide. Thalidomide is a hypnotic agent that was widely used outside the United States as a tranquilizer and sedative. The experience with thalidomide has led to particular wariness regarding psychotropic agents as potential teratogens. The spectrum of thalidomide embryopathy includes reduction deformities of the limbs, ear anomalies, nasal abnormalities, defects of the middle lobe of the right lung, cardiac malformation, pyloric or duodenal stenosis, and gastrointestinal atresias. The observation that an affected girl showed müllerian aplasia suggests that gynecologists may become more involved with these patients.[89]

Tranquilizers

The antipsychotic agents, or major tranquilizers, include many phenothiazine derivatives, haloperidol, and lithium. Debate about the teratogenicity of the phenothiazine compounds has raged for almost two decades and still continues. Two large surveys serve to summarize the dilemma. A prospective French survey (INSERM) included 12,764 women, of which 315 took phenothiazines during the first trimester.[185] The malformation rate among the exposed infants was significantly higher than in the control group. Specifically, phenothiazines with a 2- or 3-carbon aliphatic side chain, rather than those with piperazine or piperidine side chains, appeared to be implicated as teratogens. However, the NIH Collaborative Perinatal Project data showed no increase in anomalies among phenothiazine-exposed neonates.[208] As to specific malformations, only cardiovascular defects showed a significantly increased standardized relative risk, and even this association is doubtful in the context of multiple comparisons. So long as such uncertainty about the safety of these drugs remains, they should be employed in pregnancy only after consultation between psychiatrist and obstetrician, and only when absolutely necessary.

Lithium carbonate has been widely employed for patients with manic-depressive psychosis. Because of concern about potential teratogenicity, a registry of lithium babies was established first in Scandinavia and later in California. To these two registries 183 infants have been reported; 20 had malformations, 15 involving the heart and great vessels. The most common defect is the rare Ebstein's anomaly, which has occurred in at least 5 infants.[240] A follow-up of the lithium-exposed children born without malformations showed no increased frequency of physical or mental problems.[194] At this time, the conclusion must be that lithium is a teratogen, and its use in pregnant women and in women likely to conceive should be avoided. Because lithium is present in breast milk it also may be advisable for mothers receiving lithium not to nurse their infants.

Haloperidol, a butyrophenone derivative, is used to treat schizophrenia and agitated psychoses. There have been two case reports of limb malformations in infants exposed to haloperidol early in the first trimester.[41,107] However, there were no malformations among 189 infants exposed in utero when their mothers took haloperidol as an antiemetic.[233] Until the safety of this drug in pregnancy is better established it should be employed only when no safer alternative is available.

The antianxiety agents or minor tranquilizers are among the most commonly used drugs by American women. Several prospective studies have examined the safety of meprobamate and chlordiazepoxide. The best study is also the most disturbing. Milkovich and van den Berg[136] observed severe anomalies in 12.1% of infants exposed to meprobamate, in 11.4% of infants exposed to chlordiazepoxide, and in 2.6% of infants born to mothers diagnosed as anxious but not treated. Drug exposure occurred in the first 43 days after the last menstrual period and the children were followed for five years. In sharp contrast, Hartz and colleagues[81] reported the NIH Collaborative Perinatal Project data and found no increased risk of anomalies from exposure to these two drugs. This project reported all malformations found in the first year of life and had a base rate almost three times as high as the previous study. Thus, if the main drug effect was either severe defects or defects more likely to be noticed after the first year of life, the different results of these studies would be understandable. One other smaller study recorded malformations noted in the first 6 weeks of life.[34] No adverse effects attributable to chlordiazepoxide were demonstrated, but meprobamate exposure in the first trimester was associated with a significant excess of malformations. The safety of meprobamate and chlordiazepoxide should be considered questionable, but no definitive answer is currently available.

Most studies on diazepam are retrospective case-control comparisons. Suspicions were first raised by a report from the Centers for Disease Control (CDC), which demonstrated that in infants exposed to diazepam during the first trimester there was a fourfold relative risk for cleft lip with or without cleft palate.[187] However, this association was found during a multiple association search and thus needs to be interpreted with caution, as noted by the authors. This report prompted review of the *Finnish Register of Congenital Malformations*, which confirmed a significant increase in cleft palate in neonates with first-trimester exposure to diazepam.[190] Further confirmation was furnished by a Norwegian study, which found a sixfold increase in oral clefts among newborns who had been exposed to diazepam during the first trimester.[1] Shiono and Mills[202] in a prospective review of the NICHD/Kaiser-Permanente data of over 33,000 pregnancies, identified 854 gravida who were exposed to diazepam in the first trimester of pregnancy. In this group, only one case of oral clefting was noted, while 31 such lesions were noted in the 32,000 nonexposed pregnancies. In addition, in a case-control review, Rosenberg and co-workers[182] compared over 600 infants with cleft lip, cleft palate, or both with 2498 controls. The relative risks for diazepam exposure were 1 for cleft lip with or without cleft palate, and 0.8 for cleft palate alone. These findings do not support any association between diazepam exposure and oral clefts. Pregnant women inadvertently exposed to diazepam should be told that any association is very weak, and it must be remembered that even a sixfold increase in oral cleft will produce less than a 1% incidence of affected infants.

Antidepressants

The spectre that tricyclic antidepressants might cause limb reduction defects was raised by McBride,[129] but no support for the teratogenicity of these compounds was found in later retrospective studies.[9,173]

The amphetamine CNS stimulants are also phenothiazine derivatives. A large retrospective study reported more congenital malformations among infants exposed in utero to amphetamines than to those not exposed,[153] and a case-control survey of newborns with cardiovascular anomalies revealed an association with prenatal amphetamine exposure.[158] The one large prospective study that speaks to the issue found neither an association with severe anomalies, per se, nor with cardiovascular defects; however, a suggestive association with oral clefts was observed.[137] Four cases of biliary atresia have been reported in newborns exposed to amphetamines in the second and third gestational months, and this is noteworthy because of the rarity of the lesion.[115] Thus, there may be some teratogenic risk of amphetamines and continued surveillance is warranted.

Anticonvulsants

Approximately 1 in 200 pregnant women is epileptic, and anticonvulsant therapy is usually continued throughout the pregnancy. The teratogenicity of antiepileptic drugs was first questioned in 1964 by Janz and Fuchs,[97] who retrospectively surveyed 246 epileptic women and found five malformed infants in the treated group and none among the untreated cases. Because only liveborns were studied and the numbers were small, they were unwilling to draw any conclusions. Over the next 8 years there were many positive case reports and a few series which suggested that cleft lip with or without cleft palate occurred more frequently among infants exposed to antiepileptic medications in utero.[48,131] There also were intermittent publications indicating these drugs were generally safe for human fetuses. Starting in late 1972, however, more data implicating this class of drugs as teratogens were reported without indicating which specific agents were implicated. Speidel and Meadow[213] found a threefold increase in the malformation rate among infants exposed in utero to antiepileptics compared to control infants, and similar ratios were reported by others.[14,121,139]

At this time Niswander and Wertelecki[153] claimed that one confounding factor was that untreated epileptic women were at increased risk of delivering a malformed infant. However, many other studies have found no difference in the malformation rate among control infants and infants of untreated epileptics.[4,48,108,121,144,212] Whether or not a woman actually experienced convulsions during the pregnancy does not influence the rate of either minor or major malformations among her offspring.[198] Our analysis of the literature indicates that exposure of the fetus to antiepileptics introduces a two- to fivefold increase in the risk of having an infant with anomalies, with specific increase in oral clefts and congenital heart defects.[4,87,96]

The concept of a specific syndrome caused by a specific anticonvulsant agent arose when digital hypoplasia and nail dysplasia were associated with diphenylhydantoin exposure.[10] A recognizable syndrome of intrauterine growth retardation, microcephaly, mental retardation, a ridged metopic suture, inner epicanthal folds, eyelid ptosis, a broad depressed nasal bridge, nail or distal phalangeal hypoplasia, and hernias was identified as the fetal hydantoin syndrome.[74-76] A prospective study of 35 infants and a review of 104 infants from the NIH Collaborative Perinatal Project, all of whom were exposed in utero to diphenylhydantoin, indicated that 11% of exposed newborns had sufficient features to be classified as having fetal hydantoin syndrome, and an additional 31% displayed some features compatible with the syndrome.[75] Buehler[22] has reported a decrease in epoxide hydralase activity in infants affected with the hydantoin syndrome in comparison to the enzyme level in their unaffected siblings. This assay may allow identification of fetuses at risk for effects of maternal hydantoin. Because of this data, we recommend that epileptic women consider changing from hydantoin to phenobarbital under the direction of a neurologist prior to their attempting conception or, if not previously seen, at their first prenatal visit.

Valproic acid, another anticonvulsant, was first reported by Robert and Guibaud[179] in 1982 to be associated with lumbosacral neural tube defects. Bjerkedal[15] also found this same association. In a review of 72 cases with such defects, 9 were born to epileptic mothers who were treated with valproic acid in pregnancy.[46] DiLiberti and group[42] has defined the fetal valproate syndrome as extended epicanthal folds, flat nasal bridge, small upturned nose, long upper lip with a shallow philtrum, a thin upper vermillion border, and down-turned angles of the mouth. Other reviews have failed to confirm this association.[26,125] However, it would seem advisable to avoid the use of valproic acid in pregnancy.

Trimethadione, used to treat petit mal epilepsy, also has been implicated as causing a specific malformation syndrome.[61,249] The fetal trimethadione syndrome includes growth and development delay, V-shaped eyebrows, epicanthal folds, low-set ears, palatal anomalies, and irregular teeth. Serious cardiovascular and visceral anomalies have occurred in some affected individuals. Eighty-seven percent of the 53 reported pregnancies with in utero exposure to trimethadione or paramethadione resulted in either fetal loss or in a child with the fetal trimethadione syndrome.[51]

Phenobarbital has been in use for more than 60 years, and from a teratologic point of view, appears to be the safest antiepileptic. The NIH Collaborative Perinatal Project[83] reviewed over 50,000 pregnancies and found 1415 with first-trimester exposure to phenobarbital without evidence of increased major or minor anomalies. There has been only one report raising a question of a phenobarbital-induced dysmorphic syndrome.[12] In view of this safety record we recommend a change to this medication when possible for epileptic patients considering pregnancy. Although barbiturates carry an addiction liability and could cause neonatal withdrawal symptoms, at the dosage levels usually required for epilepsy control, fetal addiction should be an extremely rare complication.

Anticoagulants

Warfarin derivatives are competitive inhibitors of vitamin K, causing decreased synthesis of clotting factors II, VII, IX, and X. It has been known for over 30 years that warfarin crosses the placenta and can produce fatal fetal hemorrhage.[232] Chronic anticoagulation in patients with deep thrombophlebitis or with prosthetic cardiac valves accounts for the greatest use of warfarin in pregnancy. As patients with valve replacements began attempting pregnancy in the 1960s, the number of fetuses exposed to warfarin increased. Several reports of malformed neonates were published in that decade,[43,101,171] but a well defined warfarin syndrome was not delineated until 1975.

In 1975–1976 approximately 20 cases of abnormal infants exposed to warfarin in utero were collected.[91,162] First-trimester exposure appears to result in nasal hypoplasia, chondrodysplasia punctata, and possibly retardation, whereas second- and third-trimester exposure results in retardation, optic atrophy, and microcephaly. Prospective estimates of the risk of embryopathy are not available, but estimates as high as 25% to 50% in the first trimester have been offered.[199]

Heparin is a large molecule that does not cross the placenta and, therefore, causes neither fetal hemorrhage nor malformations. A minor obstacle to using this agent for long-term anticoagulation during pregnancy is that the patient must be taught to self-administer the medication.[88,218] Nonetheless, in pregnancy, heparin is the anticoagulant of choice, and the use of warfarin derivatives is contraindicated.

Miscellaneous Drugs

Anesthetics

General anesthesia is employed for surgery for 15,000 to 30,000 pregnant women annually in the United States. Early retrospective studies found no association between anesthetics in pregnancy and congenital malformations.[203,209] A series of surveys have presented data suggesting a two- to fourfold increase in the rate of spontaneous abortion in women chronically exposed to inhalation anesthetics (i.e., anesthesiologists and operating room nurses), and some studies even have implicated that the wives of male anesthesiologists are at higher risk.[8,31,105] Problems with these studies are that they are not well controlled, that no specific agent is implicated, and that there is no information as to the nature of the aborted conceptuses. Some surveys observed an increased rate of congenital anomalies in neonates exposed in utero,[33,105] while others found no difference in malformation rates.[31]

The issue must be considered unresolved, awaiting a well constructed prospective study that includes pathologic and chromosomal examination of abortuses. Until such data become available, each woman working in the operating room will have to make a personal decision whether or not to stop working before undertaking a pregnancy. The issue may be moot because the last decade has seen the introduction of better instruments for delivering anesthesia which lower the exposure of personnel in the operating rooms. Thus far, no adverse effects on human embryos from local anesthetics have been reported.

Salicylates

Acetylsalicylic acid and other salicylates are ingested by over 80% of pregnant women some time during their pregnancy. Some case-control surveys of aspirin teratogenicity have found significantly increased risks of malformations in exposed fetuses,[52,103,177,191] whereas others have found no association between aspirin and anomalies.[35,207,230] These studies indicate that if aspirin has a teratogenic effect, the risk must be exceedingly low, and that there is no specific malformation syndrome implicated. Chronic consumption of large doses of aspirin does prolong the length of gestation and increase the perinatal mortality rate.[32,117] Aspirin interferes with platelet aggregation and factor XII synthesis, and the resultant bleeding predisposition in both mother[32,117] and newborn[16] is probably the cause of the increased perinatal mortality. Occasional consumption of lesser amounts of aspirin, as generally employed by American women, was not associated with any increased perinatal mortality.[197] Nevertheless, it appears prudent not to encourage aspirin usage for trivial reasons in the third trimester.

Antinausea and Antihistaminic Drugs

Antinausea medications have been widely used during the first trimester, meclizine and Bendectin being the two most commonly prescribed drugs. After the thalidomide publicity several small retrospective surveys implicated meclizine as a potential teratogen;[165,239] however, more extensive prospective studies found no association between meclizine and malformations.[137,210,248]

Similar large prospective studies have demonstrated the safety of the commonly used combination of dicyclomine, doxylamine, and pyridoxine (Bendectin) during pregnancy.[90,134,196,211] A prospective review of first-trimester exposures to many medications[7] revealed an increased occurrence of cleft lip, cleft palate, congenital heart disease, and undescended testes in 1580 infants exposed to Bendectin. However, the statistical significance of these findings is borderline, and casts doubt on any strong relationship between exposure to Bendectin and these defects. Nevertheless, the manufacturer removed Bendectin from the market because of the deluge of lawsuits alleging teratogenicity of the product.

Another drug in this class, diphenhydramine, is used for its antihistaminic and mild sedative actions. Although not extensively studied, one retrospective case-control investigation of children with oral clefts showed a significant association between cleft palate and first-trimester exposure to diphenhydramine.[189] However, the NIH Collaborative Perinatal Project reviewed over 50,000 pregnancies, with 595 first-trimester exposures to diphenhydramine and found no increase in either major or minor malformations.[83]

Diuretics

Many diuretics are teratogens to rodents, but none has been found harmful to human embryos. Thiazides given to the mother have been associated with bone marrow depression, causing extremely low platelet counts in the newborn.[181] However, this reaction occurred in only a small group of infants, and the magnitude of the risk is not well defined. None of the cardioactive drugs has been associated with congenital anomalies, but both hypoglycemia and bradycardia may occur in the newborn after propanolol administration to the mother.[63,72]

Antihypertensives

Antihypertensive agents do not appear to have human teratogenic actions, but they may still compromise the neonate in other ways. Reserpine taken by the mother during the 24 hours before delivery causes nasal discharge and congestion in 10% to 16% of the exposed newborns.[21,39] Hexamethonium compounds cross the placenta and cause a fetal ganglionic blockade leading to paralytic ileus.[146]

Vitamins

Excess or substandard intake of vitamins has been a classical tool of experimental teratologists, but appears to have limited significance in human gestation. Vitamin A is the most suspect, because two cases of urinary tract malformation were reported in infants exposed to excessive retinol in the first trimester.[11,168] Gal and associates[56] found higher maternal serum vitamin A levels in mothers of infants with CNS malformation than in control mothers. Two children malformed in association with hypovitaminosis A have been described; one had microcephaly and anophthalmia,[188] whereas the other had microphthalmia and coloboma.[111] Vitamin D also has drawn attention. Friedman[53] correlated high doses of vitamin D and infantile hypercalcemia with supravalvular aortic stenosis as part of a characteristic syndrome (Williams' syndrome). However, excessive maternal intake of vitamin D has not been consistently seen in either the mothers nor the infants with this lesion.[5,184]

Retinoic acid, a modified form of vitamin A, is a known teratogen in many animal strains. Following its introduction for the treatment of acne, a number of first-trimester exposures resulted in severe fetal malformations, including microcephaly, ear abnormalities, cardiac defects, and CNS lesions. The CDS registry lists 57 first-trimester exposures in continuing pregnancies resulting in 12 spontaneous abortions, and malformations in 21 of the 45 liveborn infants.[112] In an attempt to avoid the risk of teratogenicity, Harms and co-workers[79] attempted to use isotretinoin topically. However, in their controlled study, the topical form was not effective in the treatment of moderate acne. The oral use of this drug should be avoided, or contraception ensured, in females in the menstruating age group.

D-Penicillamine

D-penicillamine is employed as a chelating agent in therapy for Wilson disease and cystinuria. One neonate was born with generalized connective tissue defects, including lax skin, hyperflexible joints, vessel fragility, and impaired wound healing after the mother was treated throughout pregnancy with 2 g D-penicillamine daily for cystinuria.[143] Gal and Ravenel[57] summarized this and four similar cases. In addition, they noted 2 infants born with severe contractures but felt the defects could possibly be secondary to CNS lesions rather than the penicillamine taken by the mother. However, a review of 27 women treated with unknown quantities of D-penicillamine for rheumatoid arthritis or cystinuria reported only 1 infant with a small ventricular septal defect in 43 offspring.[70] Nineteen of these women were exposed only in the first trimester, whereas 8 took the drug throughout pregnancy. A review of 18 women with Wilson disease treated with D-penicillamine before and during 29 pregnancies resulted in no congenital anomalies in the offspring.[193]

The therapeutic maintenance dose of D-penicillamine for Wilson disease is usually 1 g daily, and this may be an argument for using the lowest possible maintenance dose during pregnancy. Alternatively, the excess maternal copper in this condition may absorb the penicillamine and thus protect the fetus.

Rubella Immunization

Rubella immunization has been contraindicated immediately prior to and during pregnancy from the time the vaccine was first made available. However, inadvertent exposures have occurred and the CDC has studied 630 such pregnancies that were carried to term.[171] There were no rubella-related defects in the group. Although immunization during pregnancy should continue to be avoided, this information is reassuring and helpful in counseling couples who have been exposed.

ENVIRONMENTAL AGENTS

Naphthalene is an example of an environmental chemical that can harm a specific group of fetuses at risk because of their genetic predisposition. The agent is representative of a large number of oxidizing agents that produce hemolytic anemias in individuals lacking normal erythrocyte glucose-6-phosphate dehydrogenase (G6PD) activity. Naphthalene and many of the other oxidizing agents cross the placenta and can cause hemolysis in a susceptible fetus.[6,252] In both reported cases, the mother had ingested mothballs during the third trimester.

Environmental agents need not be ingested by the mother to affect the fetus, as demonstrated by the chlorobiphenyls. An epidemic of skin eruptions in 1968 in Japan was caused by cooking oil that was contaminated with chlorobiphenyls. Nine pregnant women were affected, and each delivered an infant with dark brown–stained skin. Two infants were stillborn, and five showed intrauterine growth retardation.[140] In addition, various environmental agents related to specific employment situations such as laboratory solvents[219] and the chemicals involved in printing[49] have been implicated as teratogens.

Fetal toxicity from organic mercury has been known for years,[3] but has come to public attention only recently because of sporadic epidemics caused by the consumption of mercury-containing fish. Infants exposed in utero demonstrate a syndrome of CNS damage including cerebral palsy, chorea, ataxia, seizures, and mental retardation.[149] Because maternal exposure to methylmercury occurs primarily by fish consumption, it has been recommended that women of childbearing age should eat no more than 350 grams of fish per week.[106]

Agent Orange, a chemical defoliant used extensively in Southeast Asia in the 1960s, has been noted as a possible cause of birth defects in offspring of the exposed military fathers. Erickson's group[50] studied over 7000 infants born with severe defects in the Atlanta area between 1968 and 1980 and compared them with case controls, identifying those whose fathers were Vietnam veterans, and evaluating the possibility of their prior exposure to Agent Orange. The primary conclusion of this study was that men exposed to this herbicide were not at greater risk of fathering a child with serious defects. A similar study performed by the Australian health authorities [44] matched over 8500 cases with appropriate controls and found no increased risk of structural defects in offspring of Australian Vietnam veterans. In addition, review of Vietnamese hospital records fails to reveal an increased incidence of defects in pregnancies possibly exposed to this agent.[109] Although these three studies do not prove a lack of effect, they suggest that if a teratogenic effect exists with Agent Orange, it is a weak one, or acts in only a limited manner.

REFERENCES

1. Aarskog D: Association between maternal intake of diazepam and oral clefts. Lancet 2:921, 1975
2. Aarskog D: Maternal progestins as a possible cause of hypospadius. N Engl J Med 300:75, 1979
3. Alfonso J, De Alvarez R: Effects of mercury on human gestation. Am J Obstet Gynecol 80:145, 1960
4. Annegers JF, Elveback LR, Hauser WA, Kurland LT: Do anticonvulsants have a teratogenic effect? Arch Neurol 31:364, 1974
5. Antia AU, Wiltse HE, Rowe RD et al: Pathogenesis of the supravalvular aortic stenosis syndrome. J Pediatr 71:431, 1967
6. Anziulewicz JA, Dick HJ, Chiarulli EE: Transplacental naphthalene poisoning. Am J Obstet Gynecol 78:519, 1959
7. Aselton P, Jick H, Milunsky A, Hunter J, Stergachis A: First trimester drug use and congenital disorders. Obstet Gynecol 65:451, 1985
8. Askrog V, Harvold B: Teratogenic effects of inhalation anesthetics. Nord Med 83:498, 1970
9. Banister P, Dafoe C, Smith ESO, Miller J: Possible teratogenicity of tricyclic antidepressants. Lancet 1:838, 1972
10. Barr M Jr, Poznanski AK, Schmickel RD: Digital hypoplasia and anticonvulsants during gestation: A teratogenic syndrome? J Pediatr 84:254, 1974
11. Bernhardt IB, Dorsey DJ: Hypervitaminosis A and congenital renal anomalies in a human infant. Obstet Gynecol 43:750, 1974
12. Bethenod M, Frederich A: Les enfants des antiepileptiques. Pediatrie 30:227, 1975
13. Bignall JR: Study of possible teratogenic effects of ethionamide. Bull Int Union Tuberc 36:53, 1965
14. Bjerkedal T, Bahna SL: The course and outcome of pregnancy in women with epilepsy. Acta Obstet Gynecol Scand 52:245, 1973
15. Bjerkedal T, Czeizel A, Goujard J et al: Valproic acid and spina bifida. Lancet 2:1096, 1982
16. Bleyer WA, Breckenridge RT: Studies on the detection of adverse drug reactions in the newborn. II. The effect of prenatal aspirin on newborn hemostasis. JAMA 213:2049, 1970
17. Bongiovanni AM, McPadden AJ: Steroids during pregnancy and possible fetal consequences. Fertil Steril 11:181, 1960
18. Boros SJ, Reynolds JW: Intrauterine growth retardation following third-trimester exposure to busulfan. Am J Obstet Gynecol 129:111, 1977
19. Boue J, Boue A, Lazar P: Retrospective and prospective epidemiological studies of 1500 karyotyped spontaneous human abortions. Teratology 12:11, 1975
20. Bracken MB, Holford TR: Exposure to prescribed drugs in pregnancy and association with congenital malformations. Obstet Gynecol 58:336, 1981
21. Budnick IS, Leikin S, Hoeck LE: Effect in the newborn infant of reserpine administered antepartum. Am J Dis Child 90:286, 1955
22. Buehler BA: Epoxide hydralase activity and the "fetal hydantoin syndrome." Clin Res 33(1):129A, 1985
23. Burrow, GN, Bartsocas C, Klatskin EH, Grunt JA: Children exposed in utero to propylthiouracil. Am J Dis Child 116:161, 1968
24. Burstein R, Wasserman HC: The effect of provera on the fetus. Obstet Gynecol 23:931, 1964
25. Carswell F, Kerr MM, Hutchison JH: Congenital goitre and hypothyroidism produced by maternal infestion of iodides. Lancet 1:1241, 1970
26. Castilla E: Valproic acid and spina bifida. Lancet 2:683, 1983
27. Catanzarite VA, Ferguson JE: Acute leukemia and pregnancy: A review of management

and outcome, 1972–1982. Obstet Gynecol Surv 39:663, 1985
28. Chalmers I, Campbell H, Turnbull AC: Use of oxytocin and incidence of neonatal jaundice. Br Med J 2:116, 1975
29. Charache S, Condit PT, Humphreys SR: Studies on the folic acid vitamins. IV. The persistence of amethopterin in mammalian tissues. Cancer 13:236, 1960
30. Coates A: Cyclophosphamide in pregnancy. Aust NZ J Obstet Gynaecol 10:33, 1970
31. Cohen EN, Belville, JW, Brown BW: Anesthesia, pregnancy and miscarriage: A study of operating room nurses and anesthetists. Anesthesiology 35:343, 1971
32. Collins E, Turner G: Maternal effects of regular salicylate ingestion in pregnancy. Lancet 2:335, 1975
33. Corbett TH, Cornell RG, Endres JL, Lieding K: Birth defects among children of nurse-anesthetists. Anesthesiology 41:341, 1974
34. Crombie DL, Pinsent RJ, Fleming DM et al: Fetal effects of tranquilizers in pregnancy. N Engl J Med 293:198, 1975
35. Crombie DL, Pinsent RJFH, Slater BC et al: Teratogenic drugs—RCGP Survey. Br Med J 4:178, 1970
36. David TJ, O'Callaghan SE: Birth defects and oral hormone preparations. Lancet 1:1236, 1974
37. Davies DP, Gomersall R, Robertson R et al: Neonatal jaundice and maternal oxytocin infusion. Br Med J 3:476, 1973
38. deRezende J, Coslovsky S, deAguiar PB: Leucemia et gravidez. Rev Ginecol Obstet 117:46, 1965
39. Desmond MM, Rogers SF, Lindley JE, Moyer JE: Management of toxemia of pregnancy with reserpine. Obstet Gynecol 10:140, 1957
40. Diamond I, Anderson MM, McCreadie SR: Transplacental transmission of busulfan (Myleran) in a mother with leukemia. Pediatrics 25:85, 1960
41. Dieulangard P, Coignet J, Vidal JC: Sur un cas d'ectrophocomelie, peut-etra d'origine medicamenteuse. Bull Fed Soc Gynecol Obstet Fr 18:85, 1966
42. DiLiberti JH, Farndon FA, Dennis NR, Curry CJR: The fetal valproate syndrome. Am J Med Genet 19:473, 1984
43. Disaia PJ: Pregnancy and delivery of a patient with a Starr-Edwards mitral valve prosthesis. Obstet Gynecol 28:469, 1966
44. Donovan JW, MacLennan R, Adena M: Vietnam service and the risk of congenital anomalies: A case-control study. Med J Aust 140:394, 1984
45. Dumars KW Jr: Parental drug usage: Effect upon chromosomes of progeny. Pediatrics 47:1037, 1971
46. Editorial: Valproate and malformations. Lancet 2:1313, 1982
47. Editorial: Pyrimethamine combinations in pregnancy. Lancet 2:1005, 1983
48. Elshove J, Van Eck JHM: Aangeboren misvormingen, met name gespleten lip met of zonder gespleten verhemelte, bij kinderen van moeders met epilepsie. Ned J Geneesk 115:1371, 1971
49. Erickson JD, Cochran WM, Anderson CE: Birth defects and printing. Lancet 1:385, 1978
50. Erickson JD, Mulinare J, McClain PW et al: Vietnam veterans' risks for fathering babies with birth defects. JAMA 252:903, 1984
51. Feldman GL, Weaver DD, Lovrien EW: The fetal trimethadione syndrome. The American Society of Human Genetics 28th Annual Meeting, Program and Abstracts, p 41A. San Diego, CA, 1977
52. Forfar J, Nelson M: Epidemiology of drugs taken by pregnant women: Drugs that may affect the fetus adversely. Clin Pharmacol Ther 14:633, 1973
53. Friedman WF: Vitamin D and the supravalvular aortic stenosis syndrome. Adv Teratol 3:85, 1968
54. Fujimori H: Influence of kanamycin on hearing acuity in the neonate and suckling. Presenting at the 10th Anniversary of the Kanamycin Conference, Tokyo, 1967
55. Gal I, Kirman B, Steen J: Hormonal pregnancy tests and congenital malformations. Nature 216:83, 1967
56. Gal I, Sharman IM, Pryse-Davies J: Vitamin A in relation to human congenital malformations. Adv Teratol 5:143, 1972
57. Gal P, Ravenel SD: Contractures and hydrocephalus with penicillinamine and maternal hypotension. J Clin Dysm 2:9, 1984
58. Ganguin G, Rempt E: Streptomycinbehandlung in der Schwangerschaft und ihre Answirkung auf des Gehor des Kindes. Z Laryng Rhinol 49:496, 1970
59. Garrett MJ: Teratogenic effects of combination chemotherapy. Ann Intern Med 80:667, 1974
60. Garrod AE: Inborn errors of metabolism (Croonian lectures). Lancet 2:1, 73, 142, 214, 1908
61. German J, Kowal A, Ehlers KH: Trimetha-

dione and human teratogenesis. Teratology 3:349, 1970
62. Gill WB, Schumacher GFB, Bibbo M: Pathological semen and anatomical abnormalities of the genital tract in human male subjects exposed to diethylstilbestrol in utero. J Urol 117:477, 1977
63. Gladstone GC, Hordof A, Gersony WM: Propranolol administration during pregnancy: Effects on the fetus. J Pediatr 86:962, 1975
64. Glass RH, Golbus MS: Habitual abortion. Fertil Steril 29:257, 1978
65. Goetsch C: An evaluation of aminopterin as an abortifacient. Am J Obstet Gynecol 83:1474, 1962
66. Golden NL, Sokol RJ, Kuhnert BR, Bottoms S: Maternal alcohol use and infant development. Pediatrics 70:931, 1982
67. Goujard J, Rumeau-Rouquette C: First-trimester exposure to progestagen/oestrogen and congenital malformations. Lancet 1:482, 1977
68. Greenberg LH, Tanaka KR: Congenital anomalies probably induced by cyclophosphamide. JAMA 188:423, 1964
69. Gregg N: Congenital cataracts following German measles in the mother. Trans Ophthalmol Soc Aust 3:35, 1941
70. Gregory MC, Mansell MA: Pregnancy and cystinuria. Lancet 2:1158, 1983
71. Gunning JE: The DES story. Obstet Gynecol Surv 31:827, 1976
72. Habib A, McCarthy JS: Effects on the neonate of propranolol administered during pregnancy. J Pediatr 91:808, 1977
73. Hack M, Brish M, Serr DM et al: Outcome of pregnancy after induced ovulation. Follow-up of pregnancies and children born after clomiphene therapy. JAMA 220:1329, 1972
74. Hanson JW: Fetal hydantoin syndrome. Teratology 13:185, 1976
75. Hanson JW, Myrianthopoulos NC, Harvey MAS, Smith DW: Risks to the offspring of women treated with hydantoin anticonvulsants with emphasis on the fetal hydantoin syndrome. J Pediatr 89:662, 1976
76. Hanson JW, Smith DW: The fetal hydantoin syndrome. J Pediatr 87:285, 1975
77. Harlap S: Ovulation induction and congenital malformations. Lancet 2:961, 1976
78. Harlap S, Prywes R, Davies AM: Birth defects and oestrogens and progesterones in pregnancy. Lancet 1:682, 1975
79. Harms M, Philippe I, Ceyrac D, Saurat J-H: Isotretinoin ineffective topically. Lancet 1:398, 1985
80. Hart CW, Nauton RF: The ototoxicity of chloroquine phosphate. Arch Otolaryngol 80:407, 1964
81. Hartz SC, Heinonen OP, Shapiro S et al: Antenatal exposure to meprobamate and chlordiazepoxide in relation to malformations, mental development, and childhood mortality. N Engl J Med 292:726, 1975
82. Heinonen OP, Slone D, Monson RR et al: Cardiovascular birth defects and antenatal exposure to female sex hormones. N Engl J Med 296:67, 1977
83. Heinonen OP, Slone D, Shapiro S: Birth Defects and Drugs in Pregnancy. Littleton, MA, Publ Sciences Group, 1977
84. Hellstrom B, Lindsten J, Nilsson K: Prenatal sex-hormone exposure and congenital limb-reduction defects. Lancet 2:372, 1976
85. Herbst AL, Ulfelder H, Poskanzer DC: Adenocarcinoma of the vagina. Association of maternal stilbesterol therapy with tumor appearance in young women. N Engl J Med 284:878, 1971
86. Hill R: Drugs ingested by pregnant women. Clin Pharmacol Ther 14:654, 1973
87. Hill RM, Verniaud WM, Horning MG et al: Infants exposed in utero to antiepileptic drugs. Am J Dis Child 127:645, 1974
88. Hill WC, Pearson JW: Outpatient intravenous heparin therapy for antepartum iliofemoral thrombophlebitis. Obstet Gynecol 37:785, 1971
89. Hoffman W, Grospietsch G, Kuhn W: Thalidomide and female genital malformations. Lancet 2:794, 1976
90. Holmes LB: Teratogen update: Bendectin. Teratology 27:277, 1983
91. Holzgreve W, Carey JC, Hall BD: Warfarin-induced fetal abnormalities. Lancet 2:914, 1976
92. Jacobson BD: Hazards of norethindrone therapy during pregnancy. Am J Obstet Gynecol 84:962, 1962
93. Jacobson CB, Berlin CM: Possible reproductive detriment in LSD users. JAMA 222:1367, 1972
94. Janerich DT, Dugan JM, Standfast SJ, Strite L: Congenital heart disease and prenatal exposure to exogenous sex hormone. Br Med J 1:1058, 1977
95. Janerich DT, Piper JM, Glebatis DM: Oral contraceptives and congenital limb-reduction defects. N Engl J Med 291:697, 1974

96. Janz D: The teratogenic risk of antiepileptic drugs. Epilepsia 16:159, 1975
97. Janz D, Fuchs U: Are antiepileptic drugs harmful when given during pregnancy? Ger Med Mon 9:20, 1964
98. Jentgens H: Antituberculise chemotherapre und Schwagerschaftsabbusch. Prax Pneumol 27:479, 1973
99. Jones KL, Smith DW, Streissguth AP, Myrianthopolous NC: Outcome in offspring of chronic alcoholic women. Lancet 1:1076, 1974
100. Jones KL, Smith DW, Ulleland CN, Streissguth AP: Pattern of malformation in offspring of chronic alcoholic mothers. Lancet 1:1267, 1973
101. Kerber IJ, Warr, OS, Richardson C: Pregnancy in a patient with a prosthetic mitral valve. JAMA 203:157, 1968
102. Klemetti A: Definition of congenital malformations and detection of associations with maternal factors. Early Hum Dev 1:117, 1977
103. Klemetti A, Saxen L: The Finnish Register of Congenital Malformations. Helsinki, Health Services Research of the National Board of Health in Finland, 1970
104. Knapp K, Lenz W, Nowack E: Multiple congenital abnormalities. Lancet 2:725, 1962
105. Knill-Jones RP, Rodrigues LV, Moir DD, Spence AA: Anaesthetic practice and pregnancy. Lancet 1:1326, 1972
106. Koos BJ, Longo LD: Mercury toxicity in the pregnant woman, fetus and newborn infant. Am J Obstet Gynecol 126:390, 1976
107. Kopelman AE, McCullar FW, Heggeness L: Limb malformations following maternal use of haloperidol. JAMA 231:62, 1975
108. Koppe JG, Bosman W, Oppers VM et al: Epilepsie en aangeboren afwijkingen. Ned Tijdschr Geneesk 117:220, 1973
109. Kunstadter P: A study of herbicides and birth defects in the Republic of Vietnam: An analysis of hospital records. Natl Acad Press, 1982
110. Kurachi K, Aono T, Minagawa J, Miyake A: Congenital malformations of newborn infants after clomiphene-induced ovulation. Fertil Steril 40:187, 1983
111. Lamba PA, Sood NN: Congenital microphthalmus and colobomata in maternal vitamin A deficiency. J Pediatr Ophthalmol 5:115, 1968
112. Lammer EJ: Retinoic acid embryopathy: A neural crest migrational abnormality (abstr). Am Soc Hum Genet, 1984
113. Laurence KM, Miller M, Vowles M et al: Hormonal pregnancy tests and neural tube malformations. Nature 233:495, 1971
114. Lenz W: Kindliche Missbildungen nach Medikament-Einnahme wahrend der Graviditat. Dtsch Med Wochenschr 86:2555, 1961
115. Levin JN: Amphetamine ingestion with biliary atresia. J Pediatr 79:130, 1971
116. Levy EP, Cohen A, Fraser FC: Hormone treatment during pregnancy and congenital heart defects. Lancet 1:611, 1973
117. Lewis RB, Shulman JD: Influence of acetylsalicylic acid, an inhibitor prostaglandin synthesis, on the duration of human gestation and labour. Lancet 2:1159, 1973
118. Liban E, Abramovici A: Fetal membrane adhesions and congenital malformations. In Klingberg MA, Abramovici A, Chemke J (eds): Drugs and Fetal Development, p. 337. New York, Plenum Press, 1972
119. Long SY: Does LSD induce chromosomal damage and malformations? A review of the literature. Teratology 6:75, 1972
120. Lorber CA, Cassidy SB, Engel E: Is there an embryo-fetal exogenous sex steroid exposure syndrome (EFESSES)? Fertil Steril 31:21, 1979
121. Lowe CR: Congenital malformations among infants born to epileptic women. Lancet 1:9, 1973
122. Marynowski A, Sianoazecka E: Comparison of the incidence of congenital malformations in neonates from healthy mothers and from patients treated for tuberculosis. Ginekol Pol 43:713, 1972
123. Masland RL, Sarason SB, Gladwin T: Mental Subnormality. New York, Basic Books, 1958
124. Mast H, Quakernack K, Lenfers M et al: Der Einfluss des Geburtsverlaufes auf den ikterus neonatorum. Gebrutshilfe Frauerheilkd 31:443, 1971
125. Mastroiacovo P, Bertollini R, Morandini S, Segni G: Maternal epilepsy, valproate exposure, and birth defects. Lancet 2:1499, 1983
126. Mattingly RF, Stafl A: Cancer risk in diethystilbestrol-exposed offspring. Am J Obstet Gynecol 126:543, 1976
127. Mau G: Progestins during pregnancy and hypospadius. Teratology 24:285, 1981
128. McBride WG: Thalidomide and congenital abnormalities. Lancet 2:1358, 1961
129. McBride WG: Limb deformities associated with iminodibenzyl hydrochloride. Med J Aust 1:492, 1972
130. McCredie J, Kricker A, Elliott J, Forrest J: Congenital limb defects and the pill. Lancet 2:623, 1983

131. Meadow SR: Congenital abnormalities and anticonvulsant drugs. Proc R Soc Med 63:48, 1970
132. Mennuti MT, Shepard TH, Mellman WJ: Fetal renal malformation following treatment of Hodgkin's disease during pregnancy. Obstet Gynecol 46:194, 1975
133. Meyer MB, Tonascia JA: Maternal smoking, pregnancy complications and perinatal mortality. Am J Obstet Gynecol 128:494, 1977
134. Michaelis J, Michaelis H, Gluck E, Koller S: Prospective study of suspected associations between certain drugs administered during early pregnancy and congenital malformations. Teratology 27:57, 1983
135. Milham S Jr, Elledge W: Maternal methimazole and congenital defects in children. Teratology 5:125, 1972
136. Milkovich L, van den Berg BJ: Effects of prenatal meprobamate and chlordiazepoxide hydrochloride on human embryonic and fetal development. N Engl J Med 291:1268, 1974
137. Milkovich L, van den Berg BJ: An evaluation of the teratogenicity of certain antinauseant drugs. Am J Obstet Gynecol 125:244, 1976
138. Milkovich L, van den Berg BJ: Effects of the antenatal exposure to anorectic drugs. Am J Obstet Gynecol 129:637, 1977
139. Millar JHD, Nevin NC: Congenital malformations and anticonvulsant drugs. Lancet 1:328, 1973
140. Miller RW: Cola-colored babies: Chlorobiphenyl poisoning in Japan. Teratology 4:211, 1971
141. Milunsky A, Graef JW, Gaynor MF Jr: Methotrexate-induced congenital malformations, with a review of the literature. J Pediatr 72:790, 1968
142. Mitelman F, Hartley-Asp B, Ursing B: Chromosome aberrations and metronidazole. Lancet 2:802, 1976
143. Mjobnerod OK, Rasmussen K, Dommerud SA, Gjeruldsen ST: Congenital connective-tissue defect probably due to D-penicillamine treatment in pregnancy. Lancet 1:673, 1971
144. Monson RR, Rosenberg L, Hartz SC et al: Diphenylhydantoin and selected congenital malformations. N Engl J Med 289:1049, 1973
145. Morgan I: Metronidazole treatment in pregnancy. Int J Gynaecol Obstet 15:501, 1978
146. Morris N: Hexamethonium compounds in the treatment of pre-eclampsia and essential hypertension during pregnancy. Lancet 1:322, 1953
147. Mujtaba Q, Burrow GN: Treatment of hyperthyroidism in pregnancy with propylthiouracil and methimazole. Obstet Gynecol 46:282, 1975
148. Mulvihill JJ, Mulvihill CG, Neill CA: Congenital heart defects and prenatal sex hormones. Lancet 1:1168, 1974
149. Nelson N: Committee report: Hazards of mercury. Environ Res 4:1, 1971
150. Nelson MM, Forfar JO: Association between drugs administered during pregnancy and congenital abnormalities of the fetus. Brit Med J 1:523, 1971
151. Nicholson HO: Cytoxic drugs in pregnancy. Review of reported cases. J Obstet Gynaecol Br Commonw 75:307, 1968
152. Nishimura H, Tanimura T: Information in prenatal hazards of drugs. In Clinical Aspects of the Teratogenicity of Drugs, p. 106. Amsterdam, Excerpta Medica, 1976
153. Niswander JD, Wertelecki W: Congenital malformation among offspring of epileptic women. Lancet 1:1062, 1973
154. Nolan GH, Sweet RL, Laros RK, Rowe CA: Renal cadaver transplantation followed by successful pregnancies. Obstet Gynecol 43:732, 1974
155. Nora AH, Nora JJ: A syndrome of multiple congenital anomalies associated with teratogenic exposure. Arch Environ Health 30:17, 1975
156. Nora JJ, Nora AH: Birth defects and oral contraceptives. Lancet 1:941, 1973
157. Nora JJ, Nora AH, Perinchief AG et al: Congenital abnormalities and first-trimester exposure to progestagen/oestrogen. Lancet 1:313, 1976
158. Nora JJ, Vargo TA, Nora AH et al: Dexamphetamine: A possible environmental trigger in cardiovascular malformations. Lancet 1:1290, 1970
159. Oakley GP, Flynt JW: Increased prevalence of Down's syndrome (mongolism) among the offspring of women treated with ovulation-inducing agents (abstr). Teratology 5:264, 1972
160. Oakley GP, Flynt JW: Hormonal pregnancy tests and congenital malformations. Lancet 2:256, 1973
161. Pap AG, Tarakhovsky ML: Influences of certain drugs on the fetus. Akush Ginekol Moscow 43:10, 1967
162. Pauli RM, Hall, JG, Shaul WL: Spectrum of intrauterine effects of warfarin in Littlefield JW, Ebling FJG, Henderson IW (Eds): Fifth International Conference on Birth Defects,

abstracts of papers, p 68. Amsterdam-Oxford, Excerpta Medica, 1977
163. Peckham C, King R: A study of intercurrent conditions observed during pregnancy. Am J Obstet Gynecol 87:604, 1963
164. Penn I, Makowski E, Droegmueller W et al: Parenthood in renal homograft recipeints. JAMA 216:1755, 1971
165. Peterson F: Meclozine and congenital abnormalities. Lancet 1:675, 1964
166. Peterson WF, Stauch JE, Ryder CD: Metronidazole in pregnancy. Am J Obstet Gynecol 94:343, 1966
167. Pierog S, Chandavasu O, Wexler I: Withdrawal symptoms in infants with the fetal alcohol syndrome. J Pediatr 90:630, 1977
168. Pilotti G, Scorta A: Hypervitaminosis A during pregnancy and neonatal malformations of the urinary apparatus. Minerva Ginecol 17:1103, 1965
169. Potworowska M, Sianoazecke E, Szufladowicz R: Treatment with ethionamide in pregnancy. Gruzlica 34:341, 1966
170. Powell HR, Ekert H: Methotrexate-induced congenital malformations. Med J Aust 2:1076, 1971
171. Preblud SR, Stetler HC, Frank JA et al: Fetal risk associated with rubella vaccine. JAMA 246:1413, 1981
172. Quenneville G, Barton B, McDevitt E, Wright IS: The use of anticoagulants for thrombophlebitis during pregnancy. Am J Obstet Gynecol 77:1135, 1959
173. Rachelefsky GS, Flynt JW Jr, Ebbin AJ, Wilson MG: Possible teratogenicity of tricyclic antidepressants. Lancet 1:838, 1972
174. Rasmussen F: The oto-toxic effect of streptomycin and dihydrostreptomycin on the foetus. Scand J Respir Dis 50:61, 1969
175. Rayburn W, Wible-Kant J, Bledsoe P: Changing trends in drug use during pregnancy. J Reprod Med 27:569, 1982
176. Reddy AM, Harper RG, Stern G: Observations on heroin and methadone withdrawal in the newborn. Pediatrics 48:353, 1971
177. Richards IDG: Congenital malformations and environmental influences in pregnancy. Br J Prev Soc Med 23:218, 1969
178. Richards IDG: A retrospective inquiry into possible teratogenic effects of drugs in pregnancy. In Klingberg MA, Abramovici A, Chenuke J (eds): Drugs and Fetal Development, p 441. New York, Plenum Press, 1972
179. Robert E, Guibaud P: Maternal valproic acid and congenital neural tube defects. Lancet 2:937, 1982
180. Roberts JB: Does quinine, given a woman while pregnant, have any effect upon the fetus? Richmond Louisville Med J 10:238, 1970
181. Rodriguez SU, Leiken SL, Hiller MC: Neonatal thrombocytopenia associated with antepartum administration of thiazide drugs. N Engl J Med 270:881, 1964
182. Rosenberg L, Mitchell AA, Parsells JL et al: Lack of relation of oral clefts to diazepam use in pregnancy. N Engl J Med 309:1282, 1983
183. Rosett HL, Weiner L, Lee A et al: Patterns of alcohol consumption and fetal development. Obstet Gynecol 61:539, 1983
184. Rowe RD, Cooke RE: Vitamin D and craniofacial and dental anomalies of supravalvular stenosis. Pediatrics 43:1, 1969
185. Rumeau-Rouquette C, Goujard J, Huel G: Possible teratogenic effect of phenothiazines in human beings. Teratology 15:57, 1977
186. Rush D, Kass EH: Maternal smoking: A reassessment of the association with perinatal mortality. Am J Epidemiol 96:183, 1972
187. Safra MJ, Oakley GP: Association between cleft lip with or without cleft palate and prenatal exposure to diazepam. Lancet 2:478, 1975
188. Sarma V: Maternal vitamin deficiency and fetal microcephaly and anophthalmia. Obstet Gynecol 13:299, 1959
189. Saxen I: Cleft palate and maternal diphenhydramine intake. Lancet 1:407, 1974
190. Saxen I, Saxen L: Association between maternal intake of diazepam and oral clefts. Lancet 2:498, 1975
191. Saxen L: Association between oral clefts and drugs taken during pregnancy. Int J Epidemiol 4:37, 1975
192. Schenkel B, Vorherr H: Nonprescription drugs during pregnancy: Potential teratogenic and toxic effects upon embryo and fetus. J Reprod Med 12:27, 1974
193. Schienberg IH, Sternlieb I: Pregnancy in penicillamine-treated patients with Wilson's disease. N Engl J Med 293:1300, 1975
194. Schou M: What happened later to the lithium babies? A follow-up study of children born without malformations. Acta Pyschiatr Scand 54:193, 1976
195. Serment H, Ruf H: Les dangers pour le product de conception de medicaments admistres a la femme enciente. Bull Fed Soc Gynecol Obstet Lang Fr 20:69, 1968
196. Shapiro S, Heinonen OP, Siskind V et al: An-

tenatal exposure to doxylamine succinate and dicyclomine hydrochloride (Bendectin) in relation to congenital malformations, perinatal mortality rate, birth weight, and intelligence quotient score. Am J Obstet Gynecol 128:480, 1977
197. Shapiro S, Siskind V, Monson RR et al: Perinatal mortality and birth-weight in relation to aspirin taken during pregnancy. Lancet 1:1375, 1976
198. Shapiro S, Slone D, Hartz SC et al: Anticonvulsants and parental epilepsy in the development of birth defects. Lancet 1:272, 1976
199. Shaul ML, Hall JG: Multiple congenital anomalies associated with oral anticoagulants. Am J Obstet Gynecol 127:191, 1977
200. Shepard TH: Onset of function in the human fetal thyroid: Biochemical and radioautographic studies from organ culture. J Clin Endocrinol Metab 27:945, 1967
201. Sherman AI, Goldrath M, Berlin A et al: Cervical-vaginal adenosis after in utero exposure to synthetic estrogens. J Obstet Gynaecol Br Commonw 44:531, 1974
202. Shiono PH, Mills JL: Oral clefts and diazepam use during pregnancy. N Engl J Med 311:919, 1984
203. Shnider SM, Webster GM: Maternal and fetal hazards of surgery during pregnancy. Am J Obstet Gynecol 92:891, 1965
204. Shotten D, Monie IW: Possible teratogenic effect of chlorambucil on a human fetus. JAMA 186:74, 1963
205. Simpson JL: Review article: Relationship between congenital anomalies and contraception. Adv Contracept 1:3, 1985
206. Simpson WJA: A preliminary report on cigarette smoking and the incidence of prematurity. Am J Obstet Gynecol 73:808, 1957
207. Slone D, Siskind V, Heinonen OP et al: Aspirin and congenital malformations. Lancet 1:1373, 1976
208. Slone D, Siskind V, Heinonen OP et al: Antenatal exposure to the phenothiazines in relation to congenital malformations, perinatal mortality rate, birth weight, and intelligence quotient score. Am J Obstet Gynecol 128:486, 1977
209. Smith BE: Teratology in anesthesia. Clin Obstet Gynecol 17:145, 1974
210. Smithells RW, Chinn ER: Meclozine and foetal malformations: A prospective study. Br Med J 1:217, 1964
211. Smithells RW, Shepard S: Teratogenicity testing in humans: A method of demonstrating safety of Bendectin. Teratology 17:31, 1978
212. South J: Teratogenic effect of anticonvulsants. Lancet 2:1154, 1972
213. Speidel BD, Meadow SR: Maternal epilepsy and abnormalities of the fetus and newborn. Lancet 2:839, 1972
214. Steege JF, Caldwell DS: Renal agenesis after first trimester exposure to chlorambucil. South Med J 73:1313, 1980
215. Steen JSM, Stainton-Ellis DMS: Rifampin in pregnancy. Lancet 2:604, 1977
216. Steinbeck H, Neumann F: Aspects of steroidal influence on fetal development. In Klingberg MA, Abramovici A, Chemke J (eds): Drugs and Fetal Development, p 227. New York, Plenum Press, 1972
217. Stephens JD, Golbus MS, Miller TR et al: Multiple congenital anomalies in a fetus exposed to 5-fluorouracil during the first trimester. Am J Obstet Gynecol 137:747, 1980
218. Stillman RM, Chapa L, Stark ML et al: A ten year study of heparin therapy for thrombophlebitis in ambulatory patients. Surg Gynecol Obstet 145:193, 1977
219. Strandberg M, Sandback K, Axelson D, Sundell L: Spontaneous abortions among women in hospital laboratory. Lancet 1:384, 1978
220. Streissguth AP: The effects of moderate alcohol consumption during pregnancy on fetal growth and morphogenesis. In Littlefield JW, Ebling FJG, Henderson IW (eds): Fifth International Conference on Birth Defects, abstract of papers, Montreal, August 21–27, 1977. Amsterdam-Oxford, Excerpta Medica, 1977
221. Sweet DL, Kinzie J: Consequences of radiotherapy and antineoplastic therapy for the fetus. J Reprod Med 17:241, 1976
222. Tallent MB, Simmons RL, Najarian JS: Birth defects in child of male recipient of kidney transplant. JAMA 211:1854, 1970
223. Tanimura T: Effects on macaque embryos of drugs reported or suspected to be teratogenic to humans. Acta Endocrinol (Suppl) 166:293, 1972
224. Thiersch JB: Therapeutic abortions with a folic acid antagonist, 4-aminopteroylglutamic acid (4-amino PGA) administered by the oral route. Am J Obstet Gynecol 63:1298, 1952
225. Thiersch JB: The control of reproduction in rats with the aid of antimetabolites. Early experience with antimetabolites as abortifacient

agents in man. Acta Endocrinol (Suppl) 28:37, 1956
226. Toledo TM, Harper RC, Moses RH: Fetal effects during cyclophosphamide and irradiation therapy. Am Intern Med 74:87, 1971
227. Thomas PRM, Peckham MJ: The investigation and management of Hodgkin's disease in the pregnant patient. Cancer 38:1443, 1976
228. Tores CP, Milkovich L, Van den Berg BJ: The relationship between hormonal pregnancy tests and congenital anomalies: A prospective study. Am J Epidemiol 113:563, 1981
229. Totterman LE, Saxen L: Incorporation of tetracycline into human fetal bones after maternal drug administration. Acta Obstet Gynaecol Scand 48:542, 1969
230. Turner G, Collins E: Fetal effects of regular salicylate ingestion in pregnancy. Lancet 2:338, 1975
231. Udall V: Toxicology of sulphonamide-trimethoprim combinations. Postgrad Med J 45:42, 1969
232. Van Sydow G: Hypoprothrombinemia and cerebral injury in a newborn infant after dicoumarin treatment of the mother. Nord Med 34:1171, 1947
233. Van Waes A, Vande Velde E: Safety evaluation of haloperidol in the treatment of hyperemesis gravidarum. J Clin Pharmacol 9:224, 1969
234. Vevera J, Zatloukal F: Pfipad urozenych malformaet zpusobenyck pravdepodobne atebrinem, podavan-ym uranem tehotenstvi. Cs Pediatr 19:211, 1964
235. Walden PAM, Bagshawe KD: Pregnancies after chemotherapy for gestational trophoblastic tumors. Lancet 2:1241, 1979
236. Wallman IS, Hilton HB: Teeth pigmented by tetracycline. Lancet 1:827, 1962
237. Warkany J, Nelson RC: Appearance of skeletal abnormalities in the offspring of rats reared on a deficient diet. Science 92:383, 1940
238. Warkany J, Schraffenberger E: Congenital malformations induced in rats by roentgen rays. Am J Roentgenol Radium Ther 57:455, 1947
239. Watson GI: Meclozine (Ancoloxin) and foetal abnormalities. Br Med J 2:1446, 1962
240. Weinstein MR: Recent advances in clinical psycho-pharmacology. I. Lithium carbonate. Hosp Form 12:759, 1977
241. Williams JD, Brumfitt W, Condie AP, Reeves DS: The treatment of bacteriuria in pregnant women with sulphamethoxazole and trimethoprim. Postgrad Med J (Suppl) 45:71, 1969
242. Wilson JG: Environmental effects on development—Teratology. In Assali NS (ed): Pathophysiology of Gestation, vol. 2, pp 269–320. New York, Academic Press, 1972
243. Wilson JG: Environment and Birth Defects. New York, Academic Press, 1973
244. Wilson JG: Current status of teratology. In Wilson JG, Fraser FC (eds): Handbook of Teratology, vol. 1, p 61. New York, Plenum Press, 1977
245. Winckel CWF: Quinine and congenital injuries of the ear and eye of the foetus. J Trop Med Hyg 51:2, 1948
246. Wiseman R, Dodds-Smith IC: Cardiovascular birth defects and antenatal exposure to female sex hormones: A reevaluation of some base data. Teratology 30:359, 1984
247. Wolff J: Iodide goiter and the pharmacologic effects of excess iodide. Am J Med 47:101, 1969
248. Yerushalmy J, Milkovich L: Evaluation of the teratogenic effect of meclizine in man. Am J Obstet Gynecol 93:553, 1965
249. Zackai EH, Mellman WJ, Neiderer B, Hanson JW: The fetal trimethadione syndrome. J Pediatr 87:280, 1975
250. Zelson C, Rubio E, Wasserman E: Neonatal narcotic addiction: 10-year observations. Pediatrics 48:178, 1971
251. Zierski M: Effects of ethionamide on the development of the human fetus. Gruzlica 34:349, 1966
252. Zinkham WH, Childs B: A defect of glutathione metabolism in erythrocytes from patients with a naphthalene-induced hemolytic anemia. Pediatrics 22:461, 1958

SECTION 2: ALCOHOL

Ernest L. Abel and Robert J. Sokol

Alcohol is now widely recognized as a potential teratogen, capable of producing a wide spectrum of anomalies ranging from spontaneous abortion to subtle behavioral abnormalities in the absence of physical anomalies.

Current appreciation of the role of alcohol during pregnancy was brought about by seminal articles by Jones and Smith and their co-workers in 1973[25,26] and their coining of the term *fetal alcohol syndrome*, describing what they considered to be a distinctive pattern of anomalies occurring in children born to alcoholic women. Subsequently, the Fetal Alcohol Study Group of the Research Society on Alcoholism[53] proposed three specific criteria for diagnosis of fetal alcohol syndrome (FAS):

1. Pre- or postnatal growth retardation, or both
2. Facial anomalies, including microcephaly, indistinct or absent philtrum, low-set unparallel ears, flattened nasal bridge
3. Indications of central nervous system dysfunction, including varying degrees of mental retardation.

To merit a diagnosis of FAS, the patient must exhibit traits from each of these three categories. There is no single pathognomonic physical or behavioral characteristic. The presence of only one or two of the three diagnostic criteria, with or without other anomalies, has been referred to as *partial fetal alcohol syndrome, fetal alcohol effects,* or alcohol-related birth defects. (For a full list of anomalies associated with FAS, see reference 4).

Supported, in part by grants from the National Institute on Alcoholism and Alcohol Abuse (AA 05631), (AA 06999) and (P50 AA 07606)

INCIDENCE AND COST

Cases of FAS have now been noted worldwide, with reports from Australia, Belgium, Brazil, Canada, Chile, Czechoslavakia, France, Germany, Hungary, Ireland, Italy, Japan, Scotland, South Africa, Spain, Switzerland and the United States.[4] Despite such widespread occurrence, no unequivocal prevalence data are available as yet.

Current estimates of incidence vary with the locale and population studied, and range from 0.4 per 1000 in Cleveland[62] to 1.3 per 1000 in Seattle[18] to 3.1 per 1000 in Boston.[43] In Sweden, the incidence has been estimated at 1.6 per 1000[42] in France at 2.9 per 1000.[12] On the basis of total births, the average minimal incidence appears to be about 1 to 3 per 1000.

In contrast to the variability in estimates based on total population, estimates for the incidence of FAS in children born to women identified as problem drinkers are consistent and range from 23 to 29 per 1000.[18,49,62]

Estimates for alcohol-related birth defects are highly variable. Based on several epidemiologic studies, Abel[4] estimated the average minimal incidence at about 3.1 per 1000 for the total population and 90 per 1000 for alcohol-abusing women.

Sokol[63] has estimated that about 5% of all congenital anomalies may be due to in utero alcohol exposure. If substantiated, a considerable number of birth defects, previously attributed to "unknown origin," would ironically be due to one of the most commonly used substances in the world.

In 1980, Russell estimated a lifetime cost of $155 million for those born in New York State in a given year with FAS and fetal alcohol effects. More recently, the South Dakota Department of Health conducted a similar cost analysis and estimated the lifetime cost for caring for similar patients born in South Dakota at $21.6 to $64.8 million.

PROBLEMS IN ASSESSING THE RISK

Dose-Response Relations

A major problem in identifying possible threshold levels for FAS lies in the methods used in obtaining alcohol consumption data. In all studies of drinking during pregnancy, information regarding consumption is obtained from patient self-report. The difficulty with using such information in general, and specifically with respect to inferring dose-response relations, is that detailed recall of drinking behavior is likely to be inaccurate. This is especially true in the case of heavy drinkers who may under report their drinking or be unable to recall drinking patterns accurately. Estimates of alcohol consumption may vary from 1 to 8 ounces, depending on how the questions regarding drinking behavior are posed.[49]

In addition, there is the difficult problem of trying to summarize drinking throughout pregnancy by means of some simple statistics, such as number of ounces of absolute alcohol per day. If drinking does not occur every day, the actual amount of "drinks per drinking day" will be considerably higher than the average drinks per day; for example, if a woman drinks every other day, she would consume four drinks per drinking day, but only an average of two drinks per day. Likewise, a binge drinker who drank only once per week could be considered to drink only two drinks per day, but this drinking would represent 14 drinks per drinking day. While two drinks per day may be considered benign, 14 drinks per occasion could be potentially much more dangerous to a conceptus. Because of this variability and possible obfuscation of drinking histories, assessment of dose response relations is fraught with difficulties.

Studies in animals,[2,45,46] in contrast, have clearly demonstrated dose-related decreases in birth weight, physical anomalies, and behavioral anomalies associated with alcohol exposure during pregnancy.

Genetic Contributions to FAS

Although fraternal twins are presumably exposed to the same level and duration of alcohol, clinical reports show that one twin may be more severely affected than the other by prenatal alcohol exposure.[11,56] Such reports demonstrate that genetically-determined differences in prenatal susceptibility to alcoholism exist in the human.

Chernoff[10] reported that fetal anomalies in different strains of mice were not directly related to the amount of alcohol consumed by pregnant mice, but rather to the blood alcohol levels attained. The latter depends not only on the amount of alcohol consumed, but also on genetically determined rates of absorption, metabolism, and elimination. Although this has not been directly measured in the human, it is possible that two women might consume the same amount of alcohol but develop very different blood alcohol levels, leading to very different levels of exposure of their conceptuses.

Estimating Incidence of Behavioral Anomalies

A major difficulty in assessing the incidence of behavioral anomalies due to exposure to specific agents during pregnancy is the age at which such anomalies first become evident. In the case of children with malformations, earlier ascertainment is likely for every level of mental retardation, from profound to borderline. For example, Baird and Sadovnick[7] reported that children with profound mental retardation could be identified at age 2 if characterized by other disabilities, and at age 3 if not; for children with borderline mental retardation, identification occurred at age 8, and if no other disabilities presented, age 10.

Estimations of the incidence of behavioral anomalies, such as attention deficit syndrome due to prenatal exposure to agents such as alcohol, must consider the baseline incidence. However, baseline incidences for mental retardation or attention deficit syndrome have only rarely been reported in the context of epidemiologic studies of FAS. Therefore, it is not possible to estimate whether in utero alcohol exposure is indeed a risk factor in the etiology of mental retardation, attention deficit syndrome, or other disabilities.

In a recent large population-based study conducted in British Columbia, Baird and Sadovnick[7] estimated minimum prevalence of mental retardation at 9.3 per 1000 live births. For those with IQs of less than 50, the etiology was "nonspecific" for 74% of the cases.[21] If, on the one hand, there is a correlation between physical anomalies associated with prenatal alcohol exposure and degree of mental retardation, as has been suggested,[38,69] it could be expected that physical examination of subjects would lead to the attribution of a proportion of these "nonspecific" etiologies to alcohol. On the other hand, it is possible that prenatal alcohol exposure accounts for a very low percentage of cases of profound mental retardation. As a corollary to this last conclusion, one might expect that in the absence of physical anomalies related to alcohol exposure, estimations of the increase in mental retardation or other behavioral anomalies due to excessive alcohol intake would be very tenuous at present.

ALCOHOL-RELATED DISORDERS

Specific Adverse Pregnancy Outcomes

Excessive consumption of alcohol by pregnant women is associated with a number of adverse pregnancy outcomes. These effects have been described in detail by others, and only a brief summary will be presented here.

Spontaneous Abortion and Stillbirth

The risk of spontaneous abortion is considerably increased by maternal drinking during pregnancy. Some studies report as much as a twofold increase.[29] While this may be true only for women who are heavy drinkers,[64] in animal studies pregnant monkeys[5] and dogs[14] also tend to abort more frequently after being given alcohol.

Low doses of alcohol may indeed be abortigenic. Evidence that stillbirth rates are also increased by maternal drinking remains unclear.[27,28]

Physical Anomalies

Physical anomalies in children born to alcoholic women include facial disfigurement, heart and kidney disorders, urogenital abnormalities, limb and joint anomalies, and other disorders.[4] Virtually all these anomalies have been seen in animals exposed prenatally to alcohol but, in general, blood alcohol levels must be 100 mg/dl or higher for these to occur.[44] Timing of exposure to alcohol is also an important factor in determining the type of anomalies occurring in connection with alcohol exposure.[3,13,35]

Lowered Birth Weight and Failure to Thrive

The most consistent effect of prenatal alcohol exposure is decreased birth weight. Average birth weight of children born with FAS is about 2000 g,[4] compared to a median birth weight of 3300 g for all infants in the United States.[71] Lowered birth weight (<2500 g), in particular, intrauterine growth retardation, is of concern because it is generally associated with an increased risk of neurologic abnormalities.[32]

Decreases in birth weight due to prenatal alcohol exposure may occur in the absence of FAS. Little[33] reported that such decreases were alcohol dose-related. However, alcohol abusers in Little's study could have accounted for most of the observed relationship.[1] Kuzma and Sokol[30] found that consumption of 1.5 drinks per day did not result in a statistically significant decrease in birth weight. Examination of the contribution of various beverages suggested that a small proportion (3%) of beer drinkers who were frequent drinkers gave birth to children with reduced birth weight. At present, the effects of moderate drinking on birth weight is still not known.

Associated with the decrease in birth weight caused by prenatal alcohol exposure is a failure to exhibit catch-up growth postnatally.[53] Studies in animals suggest that the likelihood for catch-up growth is dependent on the amount of prenatal alcohol exposure.[4]

One reason for the failure to thrive in

children born to alcoholics may be a problem with feeding[23,73] caused by a weak sucking reflex,[40] which lasts up to 6 to 7 months of age in some cases. Sucking anomalies have also been noted in animals prenatally exposed to alcohol.[47] Other reasons for the failure to show catch-up growth may be an overall decrease in cell numbers in the body,[20] which would restrict the potential for both birth weight and postnatal development.

A recent study in which animals were exposed to alcohol in utero and postnatally through maternal milk also implicates decreased development of $_1$adrenergic receptors in hepatic plasma membranes as responsible for the alcohol's effects on pre- and postnatal growth.[54] Such a decrease results in reduced perinephrine-induced stimulation of glycogen phosphorylase activity.[55] During fetal development, relatively high levels of glycogen are stored in the liver to support postnatal growth while gluconeogenic enzymes are being induced.[15] Since glucose is the main oxidative substrate for fetal and newborn development,[58] this effect on hepatic $_1$adrenergic receptors could interfere with carbohydrate metabolism and result in growth inhibition.

Neurologic Disorders

Sleep Problems and Electroencephalographic Anomalies

Sleep problems are not uncommon in children born to heavy drinkers or alcoholic women.[48] Computerized electroencephalogram (EEG) analysis performed during quiet, intermediate, and active sleep indicated that these children have higher brain electrical amplitude than control children. Havlicek and co-workers[19] found the EEG hypersynchrony so prominent in the delta and theta frequencies that they were able to identify 20 out of 22 infants born to alcoholic mothers on the basis of EEG patterns alone. Chernick and co-workers[9] have also noted that "this increase in [EEG] amplitude was in several instances of such magnitude that amplification had to be reduced by half" (p 44).

Because neonates born to alcoholic women are often irritable and tremulous, some of these hypersynchronous EEGs may be indicative of acute withdrawal. To examine this possibility, Ioffe and associates[22] measured EEGs in alcohol-exposed preterm and control preterm infants at 4 to 6 weeks after birth when infants were at postconceptual term. Even long after alcohol exposure, power EEG in alcohol-exposed infants was 162%, 183%, and 188% higher during quiet, intermediate, and rapid eye movement sleep. Such hypersynchronous EEG patterns have also been noted by Majewski and colleagues[37] and represent a possible means for early detection of neural damage in FAS children, which would otherwise go undetected until the children were ages 8 to 10, as stated earlier.

Behavioral Disorders

Hyperactivity has frequently been noted in children with FAS[4] and in physically unremarkable children born to alcoholic women.[57] However, most of these children were raised by alcoholic mothers and, therefore, the environmental contributions to their behavior cannot be dismissed. Possible paternal contribution to this disorder is not indicated in these clinical or epidemiologic reports; however, the incidence of hyperactivity in male children has been reported to be increased by paternal alcohol abuse.[39]

Since hyperactivity associated with FAS may be similar to hyperactivity associated with attention deficit syndrome, Ulug and Riley[72] administered methylphenidate to 19 day-old rats prenatally exposed to alcohol. Methylphenidate is currently among the more widely used pharmacologic agents used to treat hyperactive children.[74] If the hyperactivity associated with FAS is indeed similar to that associated with attention deficit syndrome, animals so treated ought to be less active than controls. Although prenatal alcohol exposure did result in increased postnatal activity, methylphenidate did not reduce this increased activity. Based on this observation, the authors concluded that methylphenidate "would not be the treatment of choice for hyperactivity related to prenatal alcohol exposure" (p 38).

Neurobehavioral development was evaluated prospectively in 12 infants characterized by physical anomalies consistent with FAS and whose mothers had a history of alcohol abuse. These infants were compared to 12 control infants for age, sex, and race. Mental and motor scores for the alcohol-exposed infants were 20 points lower than for controls.[16] A similar negative correlation between maternal drinking and decreased performance on Bayley Mental Scores has been reported.[17]

Mental Retardation and Cerebral Palsy

Mental retardation in offspring is considered to be the most serious consequence of maternal drinking during pregnancy. Of 31 children diagnosed as having FAS in Scotland, 7 were severely retarded, 2 were moderately retarded, and 19 exhibited mild developmental delay. Only 3 children had normal IQ scores but, of these 3, one was characterized by "gross hyperactivity," one was hyperactive, and the third suffered from seizures.[8] As noted above, however, there are no normative data given against which to assess these findings.

Although the first trimester of pregnancy is the critical period for physical anomalies, mounting evidence suggests that the last trimester may be equally as critical as far as behavioral anomalies produced by alcohol are concerned.[13]

A recent evaluation of the long-term effects of ethanol infusion to arrest labor[59] is also suggestive. Until recently, alcohol was widely used to arrest preterm labor, but has largely been replaced by ritodrine hydrochloride. Sisenwein et al[59] compared 25 children, ages 4 to 7, born to women given ethanol infusions, with a comparable group matched for age, sex, birth weight, route of delivery, and institution of delivery. Evaluation was done blindly and involved physical, neurologic, and psychological testing. The children did not differ in growth. However, children born within 15 hours of termination of alcohol infusion had a significantly higher incidence of hyperactivity, significantly lower IQ scores and significantly more visual-motor integration problems than controls. Ethanol infusion during labor resembles binge drinking, in that it produced a rapid and high blood alcohol level over a short period of time. While further studies of outcome after therapeutic alcohol infusion are needed, this single available study is of considerable interest, since it documents a deleterious effect of alcohol resulting from a single large exposure to alcohol occurring at the very end of pregnancy, rather than during the first trimester (regarded as the most critical period for most teratogens to affect the conceptus).

The incidence of cerebral palsy has also been found to be increased 40-fold as a result of in utero alcohol exposure. In Sweden, the overall incidence of this disorder is 0.02%, whereas among children born with FAS the incidence was found to be 8.3%.[42]

PREVENTION

The Physician's Role

On the heels of the worldwide attention that has been focused on FAS has come the perennial question of whether there is any safe level for drinking. In July 1981, the Surgeon General advised "women who are pregnant or considering pregnancy not to drink alcoholic beverages. . . ."[70] A similar warning has since been voiced in England by the Royal College of Psychiatrists.[6]

These warnings presumed a dose-response relationship between maternal alcohol consumption and adverse fetal outcome and were intended as reasonable and conservative advice to pregnant women. However, the intention of this warning may have been misguided.[1] In a recent study, Jones and co-workers[24] found that binge drinking one to three times during the first trimester did not increase the risk of FAS, spontaneous abortion, or low birth weight; however, these anomalies were all increased by prolonged heavy drinking during this period. In another study, Majewski and colleagues[36] were unable to correlate severity of patient symptoms and maternal drinking. Likewise, Sokol and co-workers[62] found that only 5 infants with FAS were born to alcoholic women in their study, although 204 out of 12,127 women (1.7%) received diagnoses of maternal alcohol abuse.

Such findings raise difficult questions as to what advice physicians should offer their patients. Studies in animals also show that low to moderate amounts of alcohol exposure resulting in blood alcohol levels below 100 mg/dl produce minimal or no detectable effects.[4,14]

As previously noted, reports suggesting that limited alcohol intake is related to lowered birth weight,[33] abnormal neurobehavioral development,[67] and spontaneous abortion[29] may be due primarily to the contribution of only 1% to 10% of the women sampled in these studies.[53,63] In this regard, those who counsel women about their drinking would do well to consider that, in all likelihood, more than 50% of all Americans alive today were probably exposed to moderate amounts of alcohol in utero. If only about 0.2% to 0.3% of those pregnancies complicated by heavy alcohol use result in FAS, it is very unlikely that moderate alcohol consumption during pregnancy will result in such grave danger as to justify complete abstinence as suggested by the Surgeon General. From the point of view dose-response relations, there is no unequivocal information to be conveyed to patients on what is a safe level of drinking. The prudent physician must temper concern for the impact of alcohol on the conceptus with the possible impact of alarmist warnings on the overwhelming majority of women.[31]

Preventive Measures

The most rational and cost-effective approach in dealing with the potential teratogenic effect of alcohol is prevention. About 30% of adult American women do not drink alcoholic beverages or drink so infrequently as to be considered abstinent. Of the remaining 70%, the large majority drink occasionally; and most of these will not realize they are pregnant until well into their first trimester. While it is beneficial to discuss drinking habits during prenatal visits, it would be even more beneficial to alert women who are intending to become pregnant of the potential dangers of alcohol consumption. Indeed, if one waits to discuss these problems until pregnancy, one is faced with the problem that some women at risk may not be present for prenatal care at all.

Broad media coverage on the dangers of drinking has proven successful from an information standpoint, but has failed to have the desired impact. For example, in one survey, 90% of those questioned showed an awareness of the harm that drinking during pregnancy could do to their babies, but 75% considered three or more drinks per day to be still without danger for their developing infants.[34] Other studies have shown that the proportion of women drinking an average of at least two drinks per day has remained relatively constant over the last 6 years.[67] This group very probably represents the most vulnerable population for the development of fetal alcohol effects; if so, mass media efforts to warn women of the dangers of drinking during pregnancy have, for the most part, been preaching to the converted.

A viable alternative for prevention is to raise the issue in the clinic or physician's office[51] and to attempt to help patients decrease alcohol consumption during pregnancy. This has already been implemented in a number of cities and hopefully will improve pregnancy outcomes for many women.[51,52,60] A major difficulty with this approach is the need to educate and train health care personnel to identify alcohol abuse in their patients. Sokol[41,60,61] has provided one strategy for such determinations.[51] This involves indirectly probing for alcohol use and related problems by imbedding pertinent questions in the overall history-taking, rather than pointedly asking the patient questions about volume and frequency of drinking, an approach often frustrated by patient denial, especially when there is a drinking problem.

When patients indicate that they can consume three or more drinks at a time without feeling "high," the physician should be alerted to the possibility of tolerance. If the patient becomes irritable or defensive when questioned about drinking behavior, this is also suggestive of underlying alcohol abuse. In both cases, a more detailed history-taking is warranted. If it appears that the patient does indeed have an alcohol problem, repeating the suggestion during later prenatal visits to stop, or at least decrease drinking, along with follow-up questions about drinking, may help her to attain abstinence, or at least to significantly cut down on her drinking during pregnancy. This appears to be an effective way of aiding women whose fetuses may be at risk.

In evaluating the possibility of patient alcohol abuse, the health care professional may be guided in his or her diagnosis and intervention by these considerations:

- From the late teenage years to the early thirties, the large majority (about 90%) of women drink alcoholic beverages no more than twice a week and, when they do drink, seldom have over three drinks. Most women will begin to feel "high" after two to three drinks.
- If a woman gives a history of drinking more frequently than twice a week on the average, if she admits to typically more than two or three drinks per occasion, or if she does not feel "high" after two or three drinks, the possibility that she may be developing an alcohol problem should be a concern to the health care professional.

The health care professional should attempt to obtain a more detailed history concerning the types of occasions on which the patient drinks and any possible alcohol-related problems that may be experienced by the patient. Such alcohol-related problems might include arrest for driving while intoxicated, concern that she may not be a normal drinker, blackouts (not being able to remember events during the time she was drinking heavily), worry about her drinking among significant others (parents, boyfriends, husbands). None of these problems, in our experience, is rare among women who appear to be developing significant alcohol problems and should act as a warning sign to the health care professional.

- It is important for health care professionals to recognize that a glass of wine (4 oz) has the same amount of absolute alcohol as a can of beer (12 ozs) or mixed drink (1 jigger, 45 ml). Each of these has 0.5 ounce of absolute alcohol. Wine drinking does not rule out the development of a drinking problem.
- If a woman is planning pregnancy, it is certainly reasonable to recommend to her either limitation of her drinking or abstinence as a reasonable approach.
- During pregnancy it is certainly reasonable to recommend that drinking should be distinctly limited and inebriation avoided. This recommendation is based on animal studies, which have been previously cited in this chapter.
- If a woman presenting for prenatal care reports that she has had an occasional drink prior to pregnancy recognition, the clinician should reassure her that it is unlikely that this constitutes a significant risk to the embryo/fetus and that this should not be a source of concern to the patient.
- Very limited drinking or abstinence during pregnancy can help women to have healthier babies and contributes toward improved pregnancy outcomes.

REFERENCES

1. Abel E: Fetal Alcohol Effects: Advice to the Advisors. Alcohol and Alcoholism, 20:189, 1985
2. Abel EL, Dintcheff BA: Effects of alcohol exposure on growth and development in rats. J Pharmacol Exp Ther 207:916, 1978
3. Abel EL: Effects of ethanol exposure during different gestation weeks of pregnancy on maternal weight gain and intrauterine growth retardation in the rat. Neurobehav Toxicol Teratol 1:145, 1979

4. Abel EL: Fetal Alcohol Syndrome and Fetal Alcohol Effects. New York, Plenum Press, 1984
5. Altshuler HL, Shippenberg TS: A subhuman primate model for fetal alcohol syndrome research. Neurobehav Toxicol Teratol 3:121, 1981
6. Anonymous: New advice about alcohol and pregnancy. Lancet 1:636, 1982
7. Baird PA, Sadovnick AD: Mental retardation in over half-a-million consecutive livebirths: An epidemiological study. Am J Ment Defic 89:323, 1985
8. Beattie JO, Day RE, Cockburn F, Garg RA: Alcohol and the fetus in the west of Scotland. Br Med J 287:17, 1983
9. Chernick V, Childiaeva R, Isoffe S: Effects of maternal alcohol intake and smoking on neonatal electroencephalogram and anthropometric measurements. Am J Obstet Gynecol 146:41, 1983
10. Chernoff GF: The fetal alcohol syndrome in mice: Maternal variables. Teratology 22:71, 1980
11. Christoffel KK, Salafsky I: Fetal alcohol syndrome in dizygotic twins. J Pediatr 87:963, 1975
12. Dehaene PH, Samaille-Villette CH, Samaille P-P et al: Le syndrome d'alcoolisme foetal dans le nord de la France. (The fetal alcohol syndrome in the north of France.) Revue de l'Alcoolisme 23:145, 1977
13. Driscoll CD, Chen J, Riley EP: Passive avoidance performance in rats prenatally exposed to alcohol during various periods of gestation. Neurobehav Toxicol Teratol 4:99, 1982
14. Ellis FW, Pick JR: An animal model of the fetal alcohol syndrome in beagles. Alc Clin Exp Res 4:123, 1980
15. Girard JR, Guillet I, Marty J, Marliss EB: Plasma amino acid levels and development of hepatic gluconeogenesis in the newborn rat. Am J Physiol 229:446, 1975
16. Golden NL, Sokol RJ, Kuhnert BR, Bottoms SF: Maternal alcohol use and infant development. Pediatrics 70:931, 1982
17. Gusella JL, Fried PA: Effects of maternal social drinking and smoking on offspring at 13 months. Neurobehav Toxicol Teratol 6:13, 1984
18. Hanson JW, Streissguth AP, Smith DW: The effects of moderate alcohol consumption during pregnancy on fetal growth and morphogenesis. J Pediatr 92:457, 1978
19. Havlicek V, Childiaeva R, Chernick V: EEG frequency spectrum characteristics of sleep rates in infants of alcoholic mothers. Neuropaediatrie 8:360, 1977
20. Henderson GI, Hoyumpa AM, Rothschild MA, Schenker S: Effect of ethanol and ethanol-induced hypothermia on protein synthesis in pregnant and fetal rats. Alc Clin Exp Res 4:165, 1980
21. Herbst DS, Baird PA: Nonspecific mental retardation in British Columbia as ascertained through a registry. Am J Ment Defic 87:506, 1983
22. Ioffe S, Childiaeva R, Chernick V: Prolonged effects of maternal alcohol ingestion on the neonatal electroencephalogram. Pediatrics 74:330, 1984
23. Iosub S, Fuchs M, Bingol N, Gromisch DS: Fetal alcohol syndrome revisited. Pediatrics 68:475, 1981
24. Jones KL, Chernoff GF, Kelley CD: Outcome of pregnancy in women who binge drink during the first trimester of pregnancy. Clin Res 32:114A, 1984
25. Jones KL, Smith DW, Streissguth AP, Marianthopoulos NC: Patterns of malformation in offspring of chronic alcoholic women. Lancet 1:1267, 1973
26. Jones KL, Smith DW: Recognition of the fetal alcohol syndrome in early infancy. Lancet 2:999, 1973
27. Kaminski M, Franc M, Lebouvier M et al: Moderate alcohol use and pregnancy outcome. Neurobehav Toxicol Teratol 3:173, 1981
28. Kaminski M, Ruimeau-Rouquette C, Schwartz D: Alcohol consumption in pregnant women and the outcome of pregnancy. Alc Clin Exp Res 2:155, 1978
29. Kline J, Shrout P, Stein Z et al: Drinking during pregnancy and spontaneous abortion. Lancet 2:176, 1980
30. Kuzma JW, Sokol RJ: Maternal drinking behavior and decreased intrauterine growth. Alc Clin Exp Res 6:396, 1982
31. Leak AM: Alcohol and the fetus. Lancet 1:984, 1983
32. Lipper E, Kwang-sum L, Gartner LM, Grellong B: Determinants of neurobehavioral outcome in low-birth-weight infants. Pediatrics 67:502, 1981
33. Little R: Moderate alcohol use during pregnancy and decreased infant birthweight. Am J Pub Hlth 67:1154, 1977
34. Little RE, Grathwohl HL, Streissguth AP, McIntyre C: Public awareness and knowledge about the risks of drinking during pregnancy in Multhomah County, Oregon. Am J Public Health 71:312, 1981

35. Lochry EA, Randall CL, Goldsmith AA et al: Effects of acute alcohol exposure during selected days of gestation in C3H mice. Neurobehav Toxicol Teratol 4:15, 1982
36. Majewski F, Bierich JR, Loser H et al: Clinical aspects and pathogenesis of alcohol embryopathy: A report of 68 cases. Munchemer Medizinische Wochensschrift 118:1635, 1976
37. Majewski F, Bierich JR, Seidenberg J: On the frequency and pathology of alcohol embryopathy. Monatsschr Kinderheilkd 126:284, 1978
38. Majewski F: Alcohol embryopathy: Some facts and speculations about pathogenesis. Neurobehav Toxicol Teratol 3:129, 1981
39. Manshadi M, Lippmann S, O'Daniel RG, Blackman A: Alcohol abuse and attention deficit disorder. J Clin Psychiatry 44:379, 1983
40. Martin DC, Martin JC, Streissguth AP, Lung CA: Sucking frequency and amplitude in newborns as a function of maternal drinking and smoking. In Galanter M (ed): Currents in Alcoholism, Vol 5, pp 359–366. New York, Grune and Stratton, 1979
41. Miller SI, Collins B, Sokol RJ: Pregnancy, childbirth, and parenthood. In Ahmed P (ed): Alcohol Abuse and Alcoholism in Pregnancy, pp 115–137. New York, Elsevier, 1981
42. Olegard R, Sabel KG, Aronsson M et al: Effects on the child of alcohol abuse during pregnancy. Acta Pediatr Scand Suppl 275:112, 1979
43. Oulette EM, Rosett HL, Rosman NP, Weiner L: Adverse effects on offspring of maternal alcohol abuse during pregnancy. New Engl J Med 297:528, 1977
44. Randall CL: Alcohol as a teratogen in animals. In National Institute on Alcohol Abuse and Alcoholism: Biomedical Processes and Consequences of Alcohol Use. Alcohol and Health Monograph No. 2, DHHS Publication Number (ADM) 82-1191, pp 291–307. Washington, US Government Printing Office, 1982
45. Randall CL, Taylor WJ, Walker DW: Ethanol-induced malformations in mice. Alc Clin Exp Res 1:219, 1977
46. Riley EP, Lochry EA, Shapiro NR: Lack of response inhibition in rats prenatally exposed to alcohol. Psychopharmacology 62:47, 1979
47. Riley EP, Rockwood G, Estreich S: Alterations in feeding behavior in rat pups exposed to alcohol prenatally. Alc Clin Exp Res 7:119, 1983
48. Rosett HL, Snyder P, Sander LW et al: Effects of maternal drinking on neonate state regulation. Dev Med Child Neurol 21:464, 1979
49. Rosett HL, Weiner L, Lee A et al: Patterns of alcohol consumption and fetal development. Obstet Gynecol 61:539, 1983
50. Rosett HL, Weiner L: Alcohol and the Fetus. New York, Oxford University Press, 1984
51. Rosett HL, Weiner L: Identifying and treating pregnant patients at risk from alcohol. Can Med Assoc J 125:149, 1981
52. Rosett HL, Weiner L: Reduction of alcohol consumption during pregnancy with benefits to the newborn. Alc Clin Exp Res (Abstract) 2:202, 1978
53. Rosett HL: A clinical perspective of the fetal alcohol syndrome. Alc Clin Exp Res 4:119, 1980
54. Rovinski B, Hosein EA, Lee H: Effect of maternal ethanol ingestion during pregnancy and lactation on the structure and function of the postnatal rat liver plasma membrane. Biochem Pharmacol 33:311, 1984
55. Rovinski B, Hosein EA: Chronic maternal ethanol administration in the rat decreases the stimulation by (−) epinephrine of glycogen phosphorylase a in the livers of the progeny during development. Sub Alc Actions/Misuse 5:77, 1984
56. Santolya JM, Martinez G, Gorostiza E et al: Alcoholismo fetal. Drogalcohol 3:183, 1978
57. Shaywitz SE, Cohen DJ, Shaywitz BA: Behavior and learning difficulties in children of normal intelligence born to alcoholic mothers. J Pediatr 96:978, 1980
58. Silver M: Fetal energy metabolism. In Beard RW, Nathanielsz PW (eds): Fetal Physiology and Medicine, pp 173–193. Philadelphia, WB Saunders, 1976
59. Sisenwein FE, Tejani NA, Boxer HS, DiGiuseppe R: Effects of maternal ethanol infusion during pregnancy on the growth and development of children at four to seven years of age. Am J Obstet Gynecol 147:52, 1983
60. Sokol RJ, Judge NE: Alcohol abuse in pregnancy. In Quilligan EJ (ed): Current Therapy in Obstetrics and Gynecology, 2, pp 77–82. Philadelphia, WB Saunders, 1983
61. Sokol RJ, Miller SI, Martier S: Preventing fetal alcohol effects: A practical guide for ob/gyn physicians and nurses. NIAAA National Clearinghouse for Alcohol Information. Rockville, Maryland, 1981
62. Sokol RJ, Miller SI, Reed G: Alcohol abuse during pregnancy: An epidemiologic study. Alc Clin Exper Res 4:135, 1980
63. Sokol RJ: Alcohol and abnormal outcomes of pregnancy. Can Med Assoc J 125:143, 1981

64. Sokol RJ: Alcohol and spontaneous abortion. Lancet 2:1079, 1980
65. Sokol RJ: The effects of alcohol on pregnancy outcome. In Fifth Special Report to the US Congress on Alcohol and Health, pp 69–82. Rockville, MD, National Institute on Alcohol Abuse and Alcoholism, 1983
66. Stanage WF, Gregg JB, Massa LJ: Fetal alcohol syndrome—intrauterine child abuse. SD J Med 36:35, 1983
67. Streissguth AP, Barr HM, Martin DC, Herrman CS: Effects of maternal alcohol, nicotine and caffeine use during pregnancy on infant mental and motor development at 8 months. Alc Clin Exp Res 4:152, 1980
68. Streissguth AP, Darby BD, Barr HM et al: Comparison of drinking and smoking patterns during pregnancy over a six-year period. Alc Clin Exp Res 6:154, 1982
69. Streissguth AP, Herman CS, Smith DW: Intelligence, behavior and dysmorphogenesis in the fetal alcohol syndrome: A report on 20 clinical cases. J Pediatr 92:363, 1978
70. Surgeon General's Advisory Committee on Alcohol and Pregnancy: Report. FDS Drug Bull 11:9, 1981
71. US Department of Health and Human Services: Monthly vital statistics report: Annual summary for the United States, 1979. Hyattsville, MD, National Center for Health Statistics, 1980
72. Ulug S, Riley EP: The effects of methylphenidate on overactivity in rats prenatally exposed to alcohol. Neurobehav Toxicol Teratol 5:35, 1983
73. Van Dyke DC, Mackay L, Ziaylek EN: Management of severe feeding dysfunction in children with fetal alcohol syndrome. Clin Pediatr 21:336, 1982
74. Wender PH: Diagnosis and management of minimal brain dysfunction, in Shader RI (ed): Manual of Psychomotor Therapeutics, Practical Psychopharmacology and Psychiatry, pp 163–169. Boston, Little, Brown, 1975

SECTION 3: OCCUPATIONAL EXPOSURES AND FEMALE REPRODUCTION

Ellen K. Silbergeld, Donald R. Mattison, and Joan E. Bertin

Women of childbearing age are increasingly among the employed in the United States. As of 1981, over 50% of women between the ages of 18 and 64 were employed outside the home. While only 8% of female workers are pregnant at any given time, many women continue working during pregnancy, and return to the work force soon after delivery.

As the presence of women in the work force has expanded, so also has the range of women's employment. Traditionally women have been exposed to reproductive hazards at home, such as cleaning solvents, infection, and tasks requiring heavy lifting; farm women have had the added risks of pesticides and hazardous machinery. The range of women's employment has changed so that women's occupations now involve exposure to such toxic substances as heavy metals, organic solvents, aromatic hydrocarbons, anesthetics, drugs, and radionuclides. Moreover, while women's employment remains concentrated in many industries not usually considered chemical-intensive nor concerned with relatively large amounts of hazardous materials, many of these so-called clean industries in fact use substances which are reproductive toxins. For instance, the microelectronics industries use toluene, acetone, trichloroethane, and other solvents as well as highly toxic metals like gallium and arsenes; dry cleaning establishments use 1,1,1-trichloroethylene and tetrachloroethylene. Nurses are exposed to drugs and radiation, and both nurses and school teachers are at risk of infection.

These demographic developments suggest an increased opportunity for reproductive risk, including impaired fertility and fetal and neonatal exposure during pregnancy and lactation, as well as secondary exposures through contamination of worker's clothing, particularly with respect to reproductive toxicity.[5,79,84] All of these factors obligate the obstetrician and gynecologist to be increasingly aware of potentially hazardous conditions in the workplace for women's reproductive health.

If, however, only fertility and fecundity remain the primary indicators of reproductive toxicity in human populations, we risk ignoring other significant effects on sexual function, hormonal regulation, and the like, particularly when, as at present, fertility is deliberately limited by most women. Our actions to prevent toxic exposure will be mostly after the fact of damage, rather than at the early—and possibly reversible—stages of intoxication.

ASSESSMENT OF OCCUPATIONAL HAZARDS

Problem of Inadequate Data

Unfortunately, the detection of occupational effects on human reproduction is difficult, in large part because of the continuing lack of adequate background data.[5] Occupational data for the individual, spouse, or parent is often incomplete in medical histories, and reproductive outcomes are not uniformly assessed. In the United States, there is no national registry or other systematic collection of data on birth defects or other reproductive outcomes. Despite recent attempts, normative data on fertility and other reproductive end points remain poor.[32,42,49,102] Because of this lack of accessible data, the concerned clinician cannot easily determine the significance of observed effects and their possible association with drug, occupational, or environmental exposures.

Other variables such as the intentional use of reversible or irreversible contraception confound the detection of some reproductive effects, even in cases of exposure to well defined reproductive toxins. Work itself (*i.e.*, physical exertion) may have other effects on reproduction aside from those related to the specific exposure and occupation.[13,19,32,55] For example, Hemminki and co-workers[34] found that the rate of clinically detected spontaneous abortions is higher in women employed outside the home in any occupation during pregnancy than in women who are not. In contrast, other studies suggest that employment may yield "financial, sociological and medical benefits" which offset any possible adverse effects.[83] Moreover, unemployment itself has been identified as a hazard to health in general. One study has found that increases in unemployment associated with economic recession correlate with decreases in physical and mental health. Overall mortality, mortality from cardiovascular disease, mortality from cirrhosis, mental hospital admission rates, arrest and assault rates, suicide rates, and infant mortality all increase with unemployment.[10]

All of these factors must be considered in evaluating the significance of a purported occupational exposure on any reproductive end point or any category of workers. Thus, any epidemiologic study must consider the background rate for employed women in order to determine the significance of a purported occupational exposure on reproduction. Alcohol, smoking,[57] nutrition, age, race, and socioeconomic status[2,5] are all factors, although some may be difficult to separate from occupation in certain populations at risk; for instance, women of low socioeconomic status with inadequate nutrition may work under harsher conditions and experience greater exposures to toxic substances than women in higher income categories.

Paternal Risk Factor

It is particularly important for obstetricians and gynecologists to consider both partners in the procreative process. More than 70% of working women are married to working men who may be subjected to occupational reproductive risks. Reproduction in women who do not work outside the home can be affected adversely by their spouses' occupational exposures. Further, such factors as drug and alcohol use, smoking, and age may also affect male aspects of reproduction. The significant additive effect of combined parental exposures on reproductive outcome has been discussed by Hemminki and associates[33] in their review of studies of smelter and textile workers in Finland, where the highest rate of spontaneous abortion was found in couples of whom both were employed in industries where reproductive toxins were present. Also, many families live near places of employment, and are subject to general environmental contamination from the industry.[73,74]

Failure to consider the possible effects of paternal influences on reproductive outcomes complicates the interpretation of some data. For example, environmental and other studies examine maternal activities and exposures during pregnancy and correlate adverse reproductive outcome with such things as contaminated drinking water, alcohol consumption, living near or working in a smelter, and the like. In many or most instances, the fathers also drank contaminated water, consumed alcohol, and lived near or worked in a smelter. Since paternal exposures can result in infertility, miscarriage, and genetic consequences for offspring, studies which fail to control for paternal factors are of limited use. Any conclusions relating to maternally mediated effects may or may not be valid. For purposes of documenting a sex-specific effect, such research is critically flawed. Similarly, the absence or relative dearth of data about male reproductive risk may create a false impression of female or fetal hypersusceptibility. Although such a body of research may create the illusion that women or the fetus are at greater risk, it in fact proves only that women have been examined more intensively.[84]

Although it may be logical to assume that pregnant women and those considering pregnancy should leave their employment to avoid exposure to a potential reproductive health hazard, for most women, short- or long-term unemployment is not a viable option. The same problem may be relevant to men who work around suspected reproductive toxins. These individuals and couples need meaningful data correlating exposure levels, timing of exposures, and effects in order to make reasoned decisions.[8] Employment modifications such as job rotation or other schedule adjustments, biologic or environmental monitoring, material substitution, and personal protective equipment may significantly reduce occupational risks to reproduction.

Employer Health Policies

The obstetrician and gynecologist may be required to consider another important factor in addressing occupational reproductive health hazards, namely the employer's medical and industrial hygiene policies. If the employer's policy is receptive to the employee's individual medical needs and welcomes the participation of the private treating physician, problems rarely arise. However, if an employer's practices are coercive or punitive, the patient may be unable to accept sound medical advice and may be placed under intolerable stress. For example, corporate policies, dubbed "fetal protection" policies, sometimes require women to choose between their fertility and their employment.[8] Such policies prohibit or restrict the employment of women of childbearing age or capacity in an ostensible effort to prevent exposure to chemicals or conditions that might be hazardous to a fetus. Some women have been so threatened by the prospect of unemployment that they have submitted unwillingly to sterilization simply to ensure continuation in their jobs.[15] Although such policies have been disapproved by most courts (except under limited circumstances),[8] they continue to exist.

The private physician may be a woman worker's only persuasive ally in such a situation and may need to be sensitive to her need or desire to retain employment. The issue of sex discrimination in employment (especially with regard to the evaluation of health risks and the implementation of medical policies) may arise; or the pregnant worker or prospective parent may need detailed and specific information about risk, or reassurance in the absence of risk. Effective treatment may thus involve advocacy on the patient's behalf to the employer and interaction with state and federal health agencies to enlist their assistance and alert them to the needs of women workers.

Legal Standards

To a significant extent, the law already defines the rights and obligations of employers and employees with regard to occupational hazards to reproductive health. These issues are addressed primarily by two federal laws, and many states also have laws which mirror or complement the federal laws. The Occupational Safety and Health Act (OSH Act) promises "every working man and woman" a "safe and healthful workplace" and requires employers to maintain a workplace "free from recognized hazards that are causing or are likely to cause death or serious physical harm." The OSH Act contemplates that workplace protection will be achieved primarily through occupational exposure standards which must ensure, to the extent feasible, that "no employee will suffer material impairment of health or functional capacity." In United Steelworkers of America v. Marshall,[99] a federal appeals court has held that this statutory language permits, and may compel, the Occupational Safety and Health Administration (OSHA) to protect against occupational reproductive risk to women and men workers, including workplace hazards to a fetus.

In setting standards, OSHA may set permissible chemical exposure limits, it may require biologic and environmental monitoring, and it may prescribe medical surveillance procedures including medical removal with opportunity for job reassignment with no loss of pay or benefits, or, if no alternate employment exists, leave with pay. To date, OSHA has regulated occupational exposures to dibromochloropropane (DBCP), lead, and ethylene oxide because they potentially cause reproductive injury.[75]

Many women workers are also protected against discrimination on the basis of sex, including pregnancy, childbirth, and related medical conditions, as a result of Title VII of the federal Civil Rights Act and some state fair-employment laws. Discrimination is generally defined as any form of different treatment, regardless of motive. Thus, employer health policies that single out fertile or pregnant women would be discriminatory, even if adopted for apparently beneficial purposes. Employers who do have sex-specific health or medical policies could justify them, according to two federal courts of appeals, only by proving that: women workers face a significant or unreasonable risk, not just a speculative or hypothetical risk; that a hazardous exposure or event is likely to occur; that male workers face no similar risks; and that the policy is supported by a "substantial body of expert opinion in relevant fields" such that "an informed employer could not responsibly fail to act." Even an otherwise justifiable policy would be unlawful if there is an alternative that would provide protection without discrimination.[8]

Taken in conjunction, these laws suggest that women (and men) are entitled to a work environment that does not endanger their reproductive ability, and that they are entitled to work under nondiscriminatory conditions. Even if the law did not provide these rights, however, they are still reasonable goals to ensure that employment does not compromise either the ability to procreate or the health of future generations.

TYPES OF REPRODUCTIVE TOXICITY

The failure to produce viable offspring is often considered the significant end point for reproductive toxicity; other effects are only considered insofar as they may impair conception. However, fetal wastage is more appropriately considered as one of the most extreme forms of reproductive toxicity. There are many other physiologic and functional

Table 6-1. Events in Female Reproductive System

Prefertilization
   Reproduction system development
   Sexual maturation
   Ovulation-meiosis-corpus luteum
   Hormonal effects
   Ovum transport
   Sperm transport
Fertilization to implantation
   Sperm-egg recognition
   Sperm penetration
   Sperm nuclear decondensation
   Pronuclear interaction
   Conceptus transport
   Conceptus-endometrium interaction
Placentation to parturition
   Endometrial development
   Cytotrophoblast-syncytiotrophoblast
   Placental growth-maturation
   Fetal organogenesis
   Fetal growth-maturation
   Maternal metabolic alteration
   Fetal-placental-maternal interaction
Parturition
   Fetal-maternal interaction
   Uterine electrical and muscular activity
   Cervical relaxation
   Birth canal
Postnatal
   Placental delivery
   Uterine involution
   Fetal adaptation
   Lactation
   Maternal metabolic adaptation
Reproductive senescence
   Hypothalmic-pituitary failure
   Ovarian failure
   Uterine failure

(Mattison DR, Nightingale MS, Shiromizu K: Effects of toxic substances on female reproduction. Environ Health Perspect 48:43–52, 1983)

manifestations of toxicity to the female reproductive system.

The range of effects related to female reproduction is extensive (Table 6-1). In addition, because of delays between exposure and expression of toxicity (latency) and the fixation of certain aspects of reproductive function early on, adverse effects on female reproductive function may present at times far distant from fertile years or time of a pregnancy (*e.g.*, early menopause). The reproductive system is comprised of several organs—gonads, uterus, fallopian tubes, and the central nervous system (CNS)—all of which are potential structural targets for toxic action. During pregnancy, the placenta and fetus are also subject to intoxication. The following list has been proposed[9] as a summary of findings of epidemiologic surveys evaluating effects on reproductive function:

Sexual behavior or libido
Subfecundity
Structural abnormalities in the female reproductive system
Abnormal pubertal development
Amenorrhea and other menstrual abnormalities
Delays in conception
Early fetal loss (first trimester)
Late fetal loss
Neonatal death
Decreased birthweight
Change in gestational age at delivery
Altered sex ratio
Multiple births
Birth defects
Chromosomal abnormalities
Infant death
Neonatal morbidity
Childhood malignancies
Earlier menopause

Some xenobiotics associated with impairment of these functional end points are listed in Table 6-2.

Prenatal Development

The entire life span of the female, from the prenatal period through sexual maturation to reproductive senescence, represents periods of differing and often highly specific vulnerability to adverse effects.[97] Formation of the female reproductive system begins and ends prenatally. In early gametogenesis, primordial germ cells migrate to the urogenital

Table 6-2. Examples of Xenobiotics Associated with Reproductive Toxicity in Humans

Examples of Chemical	Effect
Dioxins, styrene, alpha-methyldopa	Sexual desire, potency
Kepone	Hormonal function
Dibromochloropropane (DBCP), lead, diethylstilbestrol (DES)	Sperm aberrations; number, motility, shape
Halothane, ether, lead, PCBs, 2,4,5-T, vinyl chloride, ethylene oxide	Fetal death; miscarriage
Synthetic sex hormones	Multiple births
Thalidomide, alkylating agents, ethanol, sodium valproate, phenytoin	Birth defects
Lead	Birthweight, morbidity, infant death
Hexachlorophene	Early childhood morbidity & death
Lead (?), DES, dilantin	Transplacental carcinogens
Warfarin, lead, PCBs, dioxin	Behavioral teratology

ridge, proliferate, and differentiate into oogonia. The development of the follicle complex (oocyte, granulosa cells, basement membrane, and thecal cells) is critical, since oocytes which do not associate with granulosa cells degenerate. Approximately 85% percent of the oocytes formed are lost at this early developmental stage. At birth, the normal human ovary contains approximately one million oocytes, and over the reproductive life span, this number declines to zero. However, only about 400 oocytes are actually ovulated during the period of a female's fertility. The large majority are lost by a nonovulatory process called atresia. Substances such as cyclophosphamide and certain polycyclic aromatic hydrocarbons (PAHs) can greatly decrease the length of reproductive life span in women or experimental animals by destroying oocytes or follicles or by increasing the rate of atresia.[94]

The vagina, cervix, uterus, and fallopian tubes also develop prenatally. Any disturbance at this phase of development can have a major impact on subsequent reproductive capacity, as has been observed in women exposed prenatally to the synthetic hormone diethylstilbestrol (DES). DES-induced malformations of the müllerian system appear to interfere with successful pregnancy in these women.[34,58,64,88]

Postnatal Effects

During puberty, the complex process of sexual maturation occurs. Much of this appears to be controlled by the CNS at or above the level of the hypothalamus. Substances that exert feedback influence on the hypothalamus—such as synthetic sex steroids or endogenous releasing factors, neuropeptides, or transmitter agonists or antagonists (specifically dopaminergic drugs, which regulate prolactin release)—can affect this level of control.[22,27] Compounds that affect gonadal receptor-mediated responses to circulating gonadotropins will also alter sexual maturation. Compounds that bind to the cytosolic estrogen receptor, such as the insecticides DDT and lindane,[43] can affect these aspects of development and have produced precocious puberty in experimental animals.[58]

During reproduction, CNS-gonadal-uterine interactions are critical for success. Ovulation depends upon proper release of gonadal hormones, gonadotropins, and releasing factors; implantation of the fertilized ova is dependent upon timing of changes in progesterone-estrogen interrelationships. Chemicals like the barbiturates which modify release of gonadotropins or gonadal release of estrogen may produce defective oocytes and abnormal fetuses.[2,12] Hyperprolactinemia, which can result from certain antipsychotics (haloperidol) may reduce fertility.[22] Lead appears to inhibit implantation by blocking progesterone surges.[16,38,101]

During fertilization and early blastocyst

Table 6-3. Relative Timing of Certain Malformations

Malformation	Cause Prior to
Anencephaly	26 days
Meningomyelocele	28 days
Cleft lip	36 days
Cleft palate	8 to 9 weeks
Esophageal atresia plus tracheoesophageal fistula	30 days
Rectal atresia with fistula	6 weeks
Duodenal atresia	7 to 8 weeks
Omphalocele	10 weeks
Diaphragmatic hernia	6 weeks
Extroversion of bladder	30 days
Biocornuate uterus	10 weeks
Hypospadias	12 weeks
Cryptorchidism	7 to 9 months
Transposition of great vessels	34 days
Ventricular septal defect	6 weeks
Aplasia of radius	38 days
Syndactyly, severe	6 weeks
Sirenomelus ("mermaid")	23 days

(Arena JM: Drug and chemical effects on mother and child. Pediatr Ann 8:690–697, 1979)

development, the karyotypic state of the oocyte is a major determinant of reproductive success. The most common type of chromosomal abnormality, which may be associated with perinatal mortality, embryolethality, or birth defects, involves nondisjunctional events at the time of meiosis which produce aneuploidy (excess or missing chromosomes).[72] A number of chemicals have been reported to induce aneuploidy.[9,20] Chromosomal and cytogenetic errors acquired during oogenesis and subsequent meiosis are major causes of pregnancy loss. Between 20% and 60% of all fertilized ova are estimated to fail to reach live birth; of this figure, nearly half are probably lost at or shortly after implantation.[23,42] In clinically recognized miscarriages, which occur later in pregnancy, about one-half were observed to have abnormal numbers of chromosomes.[9] This is the stage at which mutagenic effects (acquired by ova or sperm before fertilization) may be expressed.

Such effects may be the human parallel to the dominant lethal assay used in rodents.

Embryogenesis, when rapid cell division and the timed differentiation of primordial cells into organ systems occurs, is another period of increased vulnerability to toxic effects. This is the period when teratogens act. The expression of teratogenicity varies with dose and with timing of exposure during gestation (Table 6-3). Teratogenicity may be overtly detectable (in such conditions as phocomelia or neural tube defects), or it may be more difficult to discern, if, for example, the toxic effect involves disruption of neurologic function, with or without dysmorphogenesis, as caused by the heavy metals and other behavioral teratogens (Table 6-4).[12,67,68,103]

Another postnatal expression of prenatal toxicity is childhood cancer (with the exception of leukemia, most cancers in prepubertal

Table 6-4. Environmental Agents (Nondrugs) Reported to Be Perinatal Behavioral Toxins in Animals and/or Humans

Allura red AC
Aspartame
Brominated vegetable oil
Butylated hydroxyanisole
Butylated hydroxytoluene
Cadmium
Caffeine
Carbofuran
Carbon disulfide
Carbon monoxide
Chloroform
Diazinon
Ethanol
Excess iron
Lead
Methylazoxymethanol
Methyl mercury
Microwaves
Monosodium glutamate
Perchloroethylene
Polychlorinated biphenyls
X-irradiation

(Miller RK: Perinatal toxicology: Its recognition and fundamentals. Am J Med 4:205–244, 1983)

Table 6-5. Transplacental Carcinogens

Substance	Main Tumor Site	Species
Direct Acting		
n-Butylnitrosourea	Nervous system	Rat
1-3-bis(2-chloroethyl) 1-nitrosourea	Nervous system	Rat
Diethylsulphate	Nervous system	Rat
Dimethylsulphate	Nervous system	Rat
Ethylnitrosobiuret	Nervous system	Rat
Ethylnitrosourea (ENU)	Nervous system	Rat
	Lung, liver	Mouse
	Nervous system	Hamster
	Kidney	Rabbit
	Sweat glands/skin	Pig
Methylazoxymethanol	Nervous system	Rat
	Lungs	Rat
	Lungs	Mice
Methylmethanesulphonate	Nervous system	Rat
Methylnitrosourea (MNU)	Nervous system	Rat
	Kidney	Rat
	Mammary gland	Rat
Methylnitrosourethane (MNUt)	Various	Rat
	Lung	Mouse
Phosphate (P-32)	Nervous system	Rat
Propane sulfone	Nervous system	Rat
n-Propylnitrosourea	Nervous system	Rat
	Renal	Rat
Enzymatically Activated		
Aflatoxin B_1	Liver	Rat
Azoethane	Nervous system	Rat
Azoxyethane	Kidney	Rat
Benzo(a)pyrene (BaP)	Lung, skin	Mouse
Cholesteryl-14-methylhexadecanoate	Lung	Mouse
Cycasis (methylazoxymethyl-B-D-glucoside)	Brain, jejunum	Rat
Dibutylnitrosamine	Respiratory tract	Hamster
p,p'-Dichlorodiphenyltrichloroethane (DDT)	Lung	Mouse
3,3'-Dichlorobenzidine	Mammary	Mouse
	Lung, lymphoid	Mouse
1,2-Diethylhydrazine	Nervous system	Rat
Diethylnitrosamine (DEN)	Lung, liver	Mouse
	Mammary, kidney	Rat
	Respiratory tract	Hamster
Diethylstilbestrol (DES)	Vagina	Mouse
	Vagina	Hamster
	Vagina	Human
	Cervix	Human
Diethyltriazene	Nervous system	Rat

(Continued)

Table 6-5. Transplacental Carcinogens (*Continued*)

Substance	Main Tumor Site	Species
7,12-Dimethylbenza(a)-anthracene (DMBA)	Lymphoid	Mouse
	Ovary, lung	Mouse
	Various	Rat
4-Diemethylaminoazobenzol	Lung, liver	Mouse
	Mammary	
1,2-Dimethylhydrazine	Kidney	Rat
Dimethylnitrosamine	Kidney	Rat
Dipropylnitrosamine	Digestive, endocrine	Hamster
Ethylvinylnitrosamine	Kidney	Rat
	Olfactory bulb	Rat
Furylfuramide	Lung	Rat
3-Hydroxyxanthine	Liver	Rat
Isopropopyl-a-2-(methylhydrazine-p-tolumid (procarbazine)	Nervous system	Rat
1-Methyl-2-benzylhydrazine	Nervous system	Rat
Methylbutylnitrosamine	Olfactory bulb	Rat
3-Methylcholanthrene (3-MC)	Lung	Mouse
	Lymphoid	Mouse
	Lung, mammary	Rat
4-Nitroquinoline 1-oxide	Lung	Mouse
Nitrosohexamethyleneimine	Respiratory tract	Hamster
Nitrosopiperidine	Digestive, urogenital	Hamster
Orthoaminoazotoluene	Lung, liver	Mouse
Orthotoluidine	Lung, lymphoid mammary	Mouse
1-Phenyl-3,3-diethyltriazene	Nervous system	Rat
1-Phenyl-3,3-dimethyltriazene	Nervous system	Rat
1-(3-Pyridyl)-3,3-diethyltriazene	Nervous system	Rat
1-(3-Pyridyl)-3,3-dimethyltriazene	Nervous system	Rat
Urethane (ethyl carbamate)	Lung	Mouse
	Heart, liver	Rat

(Manson J, George JD, York PC: Reproductive toxicology. In National Institute of Occupational Safety and Health, USPHS, CDC: The Industrial Environment: Its Evaluation and Control. Cincinnati, NIOSH [in press])

children are thought to result from prenatal exposure of the fetus or pregestational exposure of the parents).[40,69,78] Of the transplacental carcinogens identified in animals studies (Table 6-5), only DES has been shown to be carcinogenic in humans exposed prenatally.[58,64] Several epidemiologic studies have reported associations between parental exposures to solvents and metals and increased incidence of specific tumors.[41,78]

Prematurity or reduced size for gestational age—both easily determined parameters—may also represent postnatal expression of reproductive toxicity. Elevated levels of organochlorine insecticides have been reported in the placenta of premature infants.[87] Reduced gestational length has also been correlated with relatively small increases in maternal blood lead concentrations.[21,65]

In the immediate neonatal period, occupational exposure may continue to affect the infant through the nursing mother who can transmit lipophilic compounds and metals in her milk in concentrations greater than those in her blood.[104] As shown in Table 6-6, women exposed occupationally and environ-

Table 6-6. Ratio of Chemical Concentration in Breast Milk (WHOLE BASIS) to that in Maternal Blood (M/P Ratio)

Chemical	M/P Ratio
Salicylate	0.35
Lithium	0.40
Caffeine	0.50
Theobromine	0.80
Theophylline	0.70
Phenobarbital	0.70
Methadone	0.80
Ethanol	0.80–1
Antipyrine	1
Mercury	
United States	0.90
Japan	0.10
Iran (organic)	0.03
Lead	≤1
Tetrachlorethylene	~3
Polybrominated biphenyls (PBB)	~3
Polychlorinated biphenyls (PCB)	4–10
Dieldrin	~6
Benzine hexachloride (BHC)	4–5
DDT residues	6–7

(Wolff MS: Occupationally derived chemicals in breast milk. Am J Ind Med 4:259–281, 1983)

mentally secrete significant amounts of organochlorine insecticides and polychlorinated or polybrominated biphenyls in their breast milk. In some cases, substances stored in maternal bone and fat may be mobilized and excreted in milk, increasing the risk to the neonate.[93,95]

DETECTION OF TOXIC EFFECTS

It is difficult to predict the types of adverse outcomes which may be associated with exposure to a specific agent. Effects are dependent both upon dose and time of exposure. The severity of an effect in terms of outcome may also vary considerably. Mutation, for instance, may be expressed as fetal death (dominant lethal effects), birth defects in a surviving infant, or altered karyotype with no adverse effect detected.[9,72] The toxicity of some agents may only be expressed when exposure occurs during a highly limited time period of fetal development. Nitrofen, an insecticide which appears to act by interfering with thyroxine-triiodothyronine–dependent development, is a teratogen in rodents only during those time periods when these hormones control the morphologic development of the heart. Exposure to nitrofen at the appropriate time produced defects in rodents comparable to the human syndrome of tetralogy of Fallot.[52]

Some agents which affect fetal development may only be detectable, in terms of effects, at later stages in postnatal development, and it may be difficult to separate prenatal or even preconception effects from postnatal effects.[67] This is particularly true for the neurotoxic metal lead, and possibly cadmium, which produced a decrease in infant cognitive development detectable at 6 and 12 months.[7] Because pediatrics and obstetrics are separate medical disciplines, this delay in detectable expression of reproductive toxicity may obscure important clinical associations in determining etiology.

Many aspects of reproductive function are inaccessible to measurement. Monitoring the hypothalamic-pituitary-gonadal axis (or early pregnancy), for instance, requires sensitive radioimmunoassay of hormones and gonadotropins (such as follicle-stimulating and luteinizing hormones, human chorionic gonadotropin-β, progesterone, and estrogen). This type of comprehensive assessment is rarely done except in cases of reported reproductive dysfunction when etiologic factors in infertility are being actively sought. Detection of early fetal loss is poor; some studies indicate that as many as 70% of all pregnancies abort spontaneously[42]; however, less than half of these are clinically noted.[21,102] Since early fetal loss may be caused by mechanisms substantially different from those causing later or clinically recognized miscarriages, failure to detect the former suggests that a major end point of reproductive toxicity may have been missed.

Information on menstrual abnormalities

is also infrequently collected, although there are reports in the Russian literature of such effects in women working with solvents, plastics, and pesticides.[84] Chromosomal or karyotypic data are not routinely collected and the bias of self-selection may affect those that are available.[36] That is, amniocentesis is usually performed on women with a familial or personal history of heritable birth defects, or on women over age 35. Gonadal effects are difficult to detect in the absence of significant effects on fecundity and fertility; the female gonads are not readily accessible and sampling of ova requires biopsy or collection for in vitro fertilization.

Much of what may appear to be adverse reproductive effects associated with the increasing entry of women into the work force may instead reflect increased case ascertainment or refinement in diagnostic criteria. These changes reduce the reliability of studies that use retrospective cohort analysis and other epidemiologic studies dependent on so-called background rates collected nonconcurrently.

TOXIC AGENTS

In general, reproductive toxins may be directly active, through chemical reactivity (such as alkylation) or through structural similarity to hormones. Or they may act indirectly after metabolic activation (see Table 6-5 for examples of direct- or indirect-acting transplacental carcinogens) or through disruptions in enzymes or other biologic processes.[54]

Heavy Metals

Heavy metals that adversely affect reproduction and development include lead, cadmium, mercury, chromium, nickel, selenium, lithium, copper, arsenic, and plutonium.[16] Occupational exposure to these metals occurs not only in the primary mining and smelting industries, but also in battery plants (lead, cadmium, nickel), microelectronics, electrical fabrication, including wiring and soldering (cadmium, copper, arsenic, lithium, mercury), medicinal chemistry (selenium, arsenic, copper), pigments manufacture (lead, mercury, cadmium), and plastics manufacture (lead, arsenic).

Some of the female reproductive effects which have been reported for these metals are listed in Table 6-7.[56,60] The target organs cover the entire spectrum of the reproductive system in females. Lead, cadmium, mercury, and lithium are also fetotoxic and, in the case of mercury, teratogenic. In addition, lead and cadmium are gonadotoxic and gametotoxic to males[3,6,16,18,46,79,90]; thus the spectrum of reproductive toxicity for these two metals includes both parents as well as the placenta and fetus.

Lead

Lead has been suggested to be an abortifacient since the late 19th century. Lead exposure in women pottery workers has long been associated with decreased fertility.[76] Lead affects reproduction through actions on several components of the reproductive system, including hypothalamic function, sex steroid receptors, decreased progesterone production following fertilization, and fetal viability and survival.

The possibility that lead is a teratogen or fetotoxin has been investigated in several clinical studies.[41,86] A retrospective case-control study reported higher blood lead levels and inhibition of the enzyme aminolevulinic acid dehydrase in the blood of newborn infants later diagnosed as mentally retarded.[70] An extensive prospective study recently reported a dose-related decrease in infant intelligence, at 6 months and one year, associated with cord-blood lead concentrations in excess of 12 mcg/100 ml, but it should be noted that this study did not control for paternal exposures.[7]

While the median blood levels for American women of childbearing age is between 10 and 15 mcg/100 ml, levels in workers are in the range of 30 to 50 mcg/100 ml.[50] Both OSHA and the World Health Organization recommend a medical removal policy for per-

Table 6-7. Effects of Metals on Female Reproduction

Site of Action	Lead	Cadmium	Lithium	Mercury	Chromium	Nickel	Selenium	Copper
Experimental Animals								
Developing reproductive system	+	+	0	+	0	0	+	0
Puberty/sexual maturation	+	+	0	0	0	0	0	0
Mature reproductive system								
Hypothalamus-pituitary	+	+	0	+	0	+	0	+
Ovary	+	+	+	+	0	+	0	+
Uterus	+	+	0	+	0	+	+	+
Preimplantation events	+	+	0	+	0	+	0	+
Implantation	+	±	0	−	0	+	0	+
Resorption/Embryonic death	+	±	+	+	+	+	+	+
Human Epidemiology								
Fertility, spontaneous abortion	+	+	+	+	0	0	+	+

(+, report of adverse effect; −, report of no effect; ±, both positive and negative effects reported; 0, no data)

(Mattison DR, Gates AH, Leonard A et al: Female reproductive system. In Clarkson T, Nordberg G, Sager PR (eds): Reproductive and Developmental Toxicity of Metals, pp 41–91. New York, Plenum, 1983)

sons planning to have children in order to keep blood lead levels below 30 mcg/100 ml.

Lead is reported to be mutagenic, and altered cytogenetics have been found in lymphocytes of male workers exposed to lead.[90] Abnormal sperm morphology and oligospermia was also reported in workers exposed to lead in a battery factory.[3,46] Altered endocrine function has also been found in lead-exposed workers.[18] Mutagenic effects occur in female gonads, or whether the effects observed on sperm morphology are of significance in reproductive outcome, has not been determined.

There is some evidence that lead may be a heritable carcinogen; in a study of children with Wilms' tumor it was noted that there was an association with paternal exposure to lead.[40] No studies exist to suggest transplacental carcinogenicity or maternally transmitted mutation due to lead exposure.

Mercury

Organic mercury is a human teratogen. Pregnant women who ate mercury-contaminated fish in Minimata, Japan, delivered babies with major birth defects; moreover, of these infants, even those without detectable defects at birth were reported to have profound behavioral deficits at postnatal follow-up.[16,49] Another episode of organomercurial intoxification occurred in Iraq, where over 6000 people were exposed by eating grain treated with fungicide, and has confirmed these findings. The children of exposed pregnant women, had a massive incidence of birth defects, primarily involving destruction of the cerebellum. Consequent palsylike abnormalities in movement and cognition have been described in this population.[4] In the United States a similar incident of prenatal exposure to methyl mercury resulted in severe neurologic deficits, including seizures and blindness.[76]

Cadmium

Cadmium is known to cause testicular toxicity, birth defects, and fetal death in experimental animals,[5,6,16] but no data exist for humans. Pihl and Parks[82] have described high levels of cadmium in hair samples taken from retarded children, but the association of this with maternal exposure is as yet unclear.

Other Metals

The association between exposure to copper, arsenic, and other metals and reproductive toxicity is primarily based on epidemiologic studies that associate increases in rates of clinically recognized spontaneous abortion in women living near a smelter,[74] but the effect of exposure of both parents remains unclear.

Solvents

Solvents and degreasing agents such as hexane, ketones, ethers, acetone, toluene, and butanol are widely used in the chemical and manufacturing industry. A major source of occupational solvent exposure for women is in the cleaning and electronics industries. The latter industry uses these chemicals to clean, and in some cases, to fabricate printed circuit boards. Tetrachlorethylene and trichloroethane are cleaning agents used in dry cleaning and equipment maintenance in the so-called service sector, in which women's employment is concentrated.

In a study of CNS defects in 120 cases out of 130,497 live births in Finland from 1976 to 1978, organic solvent exposure was more common in case mothers than matched controls. Anencephaly was the most commonly reported defect; styrene, toluene, and aliphatic hydrocarbon mixtures (of 7 to 9 carbons) were the most commonly noted chemicals.[35] As shown in Table 6-8, significant increases in the rate of spontaneous abortion were observed in Finnish women employed in these industries, with the greatest effects in women working with styrene, a monomeric precursor in plastics manufacture.[32]

In addition, attention has been focused on the potential teratogenic and fetotoxic effects of 1,1,1-trichloroethane (methyl chloroform or TCA), trichloroethylene (TCE), formaldehyde, and ethoxyethanol. Ethoxy-

Table 6-8. Spontaneous Abortions (SA) in Women Employed in Chemical Industries

Employment Status	Number of SA	Number per 100 Pregnancies	Number per 100 Births
All Finnish Women (1973–1976)	15,482	5.52	7.98
Chemical workers	52	8.54*	15.57†
Plastics	21	8.94*	17.80‡
Styrene	6	15.00†	31.59‡
Viscose rayon	9	11.25*	22.50‡
Dry cleaning	7	10.14	16.67*
Pharmaceuticals	5	10.20	22.72*

* $p < 0.05$
† $p < 0.01$
‡ $p < 0.0001$

(Hemminki K, Franssila E, Vainio H: Spontaneous abortions among female chemical workers in England. Int Arch Occup Environ Health 45:123–126, 1980)

ethanol, a solvent widely used in the textile industries, is a behavioral teratogen in experimental animals and a reproductive toxin for males.[29]

Polycyclic Aromatic and Halogenated Hydrocarbons

Polycyclic aromatic and halogenated hydrocarbons—organic chemicals that are ubiquitous in the environment— have been studied for their reproductive effects. There is clinical evidence to support experimental data for the following xenobiotics: benzo(a)pyrene (BaP), kepone, 2,3,7,8-tetrachlorodibenzo-p-dioxin (TCDD), and the polyhalogenated biphenyls (PCBs and PBBs). The observed effects of these compounds raise the likelihood that other related compounds may have similar activity, although doses required for such effects may vary.

Many of these compounds are inducers of the mixed function microsomal cytochrome P-450 dependent monooxygenases. Some of these compounds are also able to destroy oocytes[55,57,61-63,96] and block ovulation. Such PAHs as BaP, 3-methylcholanthrene, and 7,12-dimethylbenz[a]anthracene destroy oocytes in mice at relatively low (sub-lethal) doses. Corroborative clinical evidence exists for BaP, a constituent of cigarette smoke and a contaminant from many industrial processes, including coke oven emissions, and iron and steel smelting. The consequence of this ovotoxic action appears to be primarily manifested as a lowering of the age of menopause. Women who smoke a pack of cigarettes or more per day have significantly earlier onset of menopause than do nonsmoking women.[57]

Children who were exposed in utero and postnatally through mother's milk to dioxins or dibenzofurans (structurally related compounds) in two incidents involving ingestion of PCB-laden oil (also containing dioxins and dibenzofurans) showed darkening of the skin, hirsutism, and abnormal dental and skeletal development.[44] Reproductive function has not yet been assessed in either mature women or in females exposed pre- or postnatally by their mother's ingestion of contaminated oil.

The widespread contamination in Michigan resulting from substitution of polybrominated biphenyls (PBBs) for food additives for cattle has been followed prospectively for several years. A recent report suggests behavioral teratology in children exposed in utero to PBBs and whose parents were both exposed to PBBs prior to conception.[91]

The most described episodes of human exposure to reproductive toxins of this type involve male-mediated effects, the sterilizing effects of kepone, ethylene dibromide, and dibromochloropropane (DBCP) in men exposed during manufacture of these pesticides.[5,48,100] Kepone possesses significant estrogenic action and was associated with suppressed spermatogenesis in exposed men.[43] While in many cases the wives of kepone workers also had high blood levels of kepone (presumably through contaminated clothing), there are no studies of hormonal or other reproductive function in these women.

Chemical Mutagens

Mutagenic compounds can affect reproduction if they act on the gonads or gametes of men or women or on the conceptus. In spite of the potential consequences resulting from gamete mutation, most mutagenesis assays have focused on somatic cells in human populations[21] (Table 6-9). This is due to the difficulty in measuring mutations or chromosome aberrations in gametes.[11] In human populations it is thought that the expression of mu-

Table 6-9. Chromosome Studies of Persons Exposed to Industrial Chemicals

Substance	Study Size	Cell System	Sister Chromatid Exchange
Vinylchloride	>500	L	(+)
Epichlorohydrin	128	L	(+)
Chloroprene	>56	L	(+)
Styrene oxide	26	L	+/−
Chloromethyl ether	12	L	+
Trichloroethylene	28	L	(+)
Acrylonitril	15	L	−
Dialkylcarbamoylchloride	10	L	−
o-Phthalodinitrile	20	L	−
Spray adhesives	40	L	−
Benzene	>190	L, BM	+
Toluene	56	L	−
Lead	>250	L	(+)
Lead + cadmium	47	L	(+)
Cadmium	40	L	−
Chromium	Not given	L	+
Mercury	71	L	+/−
Arsenic	33	L	(+)
Organophosphates	>180	L	(+)
Benomyl	20	L	−
DDT	33	L	−
Zineb	15	L	+
Ziram	9	L	+

(L, lymphocytes; BM, bone marrow; +, positive; −, negative; (+), weakly positive; +/−, results equivocal)

(Gebhart ERE: The epidemiological approach: Chromosome aberrations in persons exposed to chemical mutagens. In Hsu TC (ed): Cytogenic Assays of Environmental Mutagens. Totowa, NJ, Allenheld, Osmun, 1982)

tagenic events can be in the form of infertility, birth defects, or cancer. Birth defects may be lethal, in which case detection must be based on an increased rate of spontaneous abortion or infertility. This may be the mechanism behind observations of increased rates of spontaneous abortion in women exposed to vinyl chloride.[37] Transplacental cancer has been described in humans only for DES, although data from experimental animals suggest that an entire range of other chemicals may be suspect.[20,51,68]

The best studied example of a mutagenic reproductive toxin in humans is ionizing radiation, which, in doses of sufficient intensity, can destroy or interrupt ongoing meiotic activity of oocytes and spermatogenesis. The impact of gamma radiation on fetal development has been estimated to be as much as 6 major birth defects per 10,000 live births ex-

Table 6-10. Cytogenetic Effects of Chemical Substances on the Meiotic Chromosomes of Mammalian Oocytes

	Mechanism of Action	Species	Mode of Treatment	Structural Abberations	Numerical Abberations
Streptonigrin	Direct	Mouse	In vitro	++	
			In vivo	++	
Sulfur dioxide	Direct	Mouse	In vitro	−	
			In vivo	−	−
		Cow	In vitro	+++	+
		Ewe	In vitro	+	+
Sodium fluoride	Unknown	Mouse	In vitro	+++	+
			In vivo	+++	
		Cow	In vitro	++	+
		Ewe	In vitro	+	−
Mercury	Unknown	Mouse	In vitro	−	+
			In vivo	−	−
Actinomycin D	Direct	Mouse	In vitro	+++	−
			In vivo	−	
Meprobamate	Unknown	Mouse	In vitro	−	−
			In vivo	−	−
LSD-25	Indirect	Mouse	In vitro	−	−
			In vivo	−	−
Caffeine	Indirect	Mouse	In vitro	−	−
			In vivo	−	−
Phleomycin	Direct	Mouse	In vitro	+++	
			In vivo	++	
Triethylenemelamine	Indirect	Mouse	In vivo	+	
Methylmethane sulfonate	Indirect	Mouse	In vivo	−	
Triaziquone	Indirect	Chinese Hamster	In vivo	++	+
		Mouse	In vivo	++	+
Cyclophosphamide	Indirect	Mouse	In vivo	++	+
Methotrexate	Indirect	Mouse	In vivo	++	+
Cadmium	Unknown	Mouse	In vivo		++
Oral contraceptives	Unknown	Several	In vitro		+

(+, some association; −, no association; ++, moderate association; +++, strong association)
(Brewen JG, Preston RJ: Cytogenic analysis of mammalian oocytes in Mutagenicity studies. In Hsu TC (ed): Cytogenic Assays of Environmental Mutagens. Totowa, NJ, Allenheld, Osmun, 1982)

posed to 100 mrem/year.[71] Radiation can also be cytotoxic to developing organ systems. One recent report suggests an increased incidence of microcephaly and reduced IQ in children subjected to gamma radiation in utero between 8 and 15 weeks gestation, but this study has certain statistical limitations which make extrapolations to low exposure levels difficult and which limit the conclusions that can be drawn.[89] Nonetheless, some corroborative evidence has been found in animals.[39]

In addition to radiation, many chemicals have been demonstrated to be mutagenic, primarily on the basis of bacterial revertant assays. Some of these chemicals are also reported to cause chromosomal abnormalities or increase the frequency of sister chromatid exchange (SCE) in humans, on the basis of cytogenetic analysis of lymphocytes taken from exposed persons. As shown in Table 6-9, increased incidence of SCE has been found in lymphocytes of workers who were exposed to some of these chemicals.[25] None of these assays is directly indicative of ovarian mutagenic activity, although, as shown in Table 6-10, some xenobiotics have also been tested in mammalian oocytes.[11] Such effects

Table 6-11. Correlation of Genotoxicity Between Experimental and Epidemiologic Findings

Effect/Exposure	Cigarette smoke	Hair dyes (synthetic)	Anesthetic agents (halothane, nitrous oxide)	Alkylating cytostatic drugs	Ethylene oxide
Genotoxicity of the Exposing Agent					
Mutagenicity in bacteria	+	+	−	+	+
Eucaryotes	+	+	+	+	+
SCEs in mammals	+	+	−	+	+
Chromosome aberations in vitro	+	+	..	+	+
Carcinogenicity in animals	+	+	..	+	+
Studies on Exposed Populations					
Determination of the chemical(s) in body fluids	+	+	+	+	+
Thioethers in urine	+	..	..	+	..
Mutagenicity of urine	+	..	±	+	..
Covalent adducts:					
Hemoglobin alkylation	..	..	..	..	+
DNA adducts	..	..	..	..	..
Cytogenetic parameters:					
Structural chromosome aberrations	+	+	..	+	+
SCEs	+	−	−	+	+
Micronuclei	+	..	..	+	+
Epidemiologic outcome					
Spontaneous abortions	+	..	+	..	(+)
Malformations	±	..	±	+	..
Malignancies	+	±	±	+	(+)

(+, positive data; (+), suggestive data; ±, contradictory data; −, negative data; .., no data)
(Bloom AD [ed]: Guidelines for studies of human populations exposed to mutagenic and reproductive hazards. New York, March of Dimes Birth Defects Foundation, 1981)

may not necessarily lead to infertility or birth defects because damaged oocytes may not be ovulated or fertilized, and because genetic repair mechanisms exist in male and female germ cells.[26,47,53,77] The few existing correlations of genotoxicity between experimental and epidemiologic data are shown in Table 6-11.

Anesthetics and Drugs

Specific drugs are associated with reproductive toxicity.[2] Many of the examples cited below were detected in patients treated during pregnancy; by extrapolation, toxic effects may be anticipated in women in the health care professions or pharmaceutical industry who are exposed occupationally to significant amounts of the same agents. Mutagenic substances have been reported in urine of workers exposed to drugs and chemicals, which suggests that the gametes of these individuals may also be exposed (Table 6-12). Drugs as diverse as antineoplastic agents[85] and antianxiety drugs are toxic to reproduction.[66,92] The antineoplastic cancer chemotherapeutic agents are designed to target the proliferating tumor, and as such are selectively toxic to rapidly dividing cells.[14] The ongoing meiotic activity of oocytes and spermatogenesis and mitosis of the conceptus renders these cells highly susceptible to such agents.

It is instructive to examine the mechanism of action of a representative, well-studied antineoplastic agent, cyclophosphamide. The evidence for gonadotoxicity of cyclophosphamide has been collected on women receiving this agent in chemotherapy.[52,58,59] Under these conditions, cyclophosphamide can produce ovarian dysfunction or complete ovarian failure and infertility.[14,92] At lower doses, reversible reproductive dysfunction results in both sexes, including irregular menses, impaired spermatogenesis, or reduced fertility. At higher doses, however, complete sterility is produced in both sexes. Cyclophosphamide is metabolized by microsomal monooxygenases into a more toxic reactive metabolite, which is then capable of reacting with gonadal cells and destroying oocytes. However, hepatic metabolism may not be the determining factor in degree of ovotoxicity after exposure to cyclophosphamide, because metabolism can take place in the ovary itself which contains these transforming enzymes. Moreover, the exact nature of cyclophosphamide ovotoxicity is not well understood. It may involve an increased rate of atresia (loss of oocytes) or specific cytotoxicity, possibly during periods of in-

Table 6-12. Examples of Human Monitoring Using Urine Analysis

POPULATION	EXPOSURE	RESPONSE*
Patients	Cyclophosphamide therapy	+
Patients	Metronidazole therapy	+
Patients	Niridazole	+
General	Cigarette smoking	+
Nurses	Cytostatic drugs	+
Workmen	Styrene production	−
Workmen	Rubber manufacturing	+
Workmen	Coke production	−
Workmen	Epichlorohydrin	+

* Microbial target cells were employed in all studies. (+, urine mutagenic; −, urine not mutagenic)

(Bloom AD [ed]: Guidelines for studies of human populations exposed to mutagenic and reproductive hazards. New York, March of Dimes Birth Defects Foundation, 1981)

Table 6-13. Reproductive Effects in Women Occupationally Exposed to Norethindrone

Job	Total Number	Number with Intermenstrual Bleeding
Processing	1	1
Quality assurance	5	1
Production	18	10
Office staff (no exposure)	5	0

(Harrington JM, Stein GF, Rivera RO, de Morales AV: The occupational hazards of formulating oral contraceptives—A survey of plant employees. Arch Environ Health 33:12–15, 1978)

higher rate of miscarriage, higher perinatal death rate, and higher rate of major malformations.[28] Increased rates of spontaneous abortions were also found in a similar study of women in the pharmaceutical industry in Finland.[98] Female workers in a plant formulating the synthetic hormone contraceptive norethindrone showed evidence of reproductive pathology, with a fourfold increase in intermenstrual bleeding as compared to controls (Table 6–13); men in the same plant had gynecomastia.[30] These workers were exposed to airborne concentrations of norethindrone up to 43.2 $\mu g/m^3$.

A study undertaken by NIOSH and the American Dental Association[1,17] reported that exposure to dental anesthetics increased the rate of spontaneous abortion and congenital abnormalities of the musculoskeletal system in female chair-side assistants (Table 6–14). Significant increases in congenital abnormalities were seen in association with either nitrous oxide or nitrous oxide and halothane; significant increases in spontaneous abortion were seen for the combined mixture. Possibly a more sensitive indicator of adverse affect is decreased birth weight (Table 6–15). For women anesthetists, median birth weight

creased vulnerability during the resumption of oocyte meiosis in the periovulatory interval and granulosa cell mitosis which occurs in maturing follicles.

Women exposed occupationally in the drug industry to cytostatic agents, synthetic sex steroids, and other pharmaceuticals also appear to be at risk for adverse reproductive effects. However, few studies have been done. In a survey of three pharmaceutical laboratories in Sweden, female workers had a

Table 6-14. Effects of Occupational Exposure to Anesthetic Gases in Female Dental Assistances*

	No Exposure	Light	Heavy
Spontaneous abortions	8.1 ± 0.5 (3184)	14.2 ± 1.7‡ (407)	19.1 ± 2.0‡ (400)
Congenital abnormalities per 100 pregnancies (no. of pregnancies)	3.6 ± 0.3 (2882)	5.7 ± 1.2§ (341)	5.2 ± 1.2 (316)
Musculoskeletal abnormalities per 100 pregnancies (no. of pregnancies)	1.15 ± 0.2	2.47 ± 0.61‡	
Cancer of the cervix per 100 respondents (no.)	0.12 ± 0.04 (6765)	0.24 ± 0.05 (10,104)	0.29 ± 0.10‖ (2692)

* Adjusted for age and smoking
† Data grouped for both light and heavy exposure
‡ $p < 0.01$, compared to no exposure
§ $p < 0.02$
‖ $p < 0.04$

(Pharoah POD, Alberman E, Doyle P, Chamberlain G: Outcome of pregnancy among women in anesthetic practice. Lancet 1:34–36, 1977)

Table 6-15. Effects of Exposure to Anesthetics on Birth Weight

	\multicolumn{3}{c}{MOTHER'S OCCUPATION}		
	Anesthesiologist	Other Medical Professions	Nonmedical
Mean birth ± SD	3347 ± 524	3388 ± 503	3430 ± 491
Number of births	541	5180	1649
Percent of births ≤ 2500 g	6.2%	4.0%	3.7%

(Pharoah POD, Alberman E, Doyle P, Chamberlain G: Outcome of pregnancy among women in ansthetic practice. Lancet 1:34–36, 1977)

was not significantly lower, but a larger proportion of their infants were less than 2500 g, particularly when compared to women not employed in medicine.[24,80] A recent Scandinavian study has observed that women exposed to ethylene oxide have a higher frequency of spontaneous abortion than non-exposed hospital personnel.[31]

REFERENCES

1. American Society of Anesthesiologists: Anesthesiology: Report of the adhoc committee on the effect of trace anesthetics on the health of operating room personnel. Anesthesiology, 41:321–340, 1974
2. Arena JM: Drug and chemical effects on mother and child. Pediatr Ann 8:690–697, 1979
3. Assemato G, Paci C, Baser ME et al: Sperm count supression without endocrine dysfunction in lead-exposed men. Arch Environ Health 41:387–390, 1986
4. Bakir F, Damluji SF, Amin-Zaki L et al: Methylmercury poisoning in Iraq. Science 181:230–241, 1973
5. Barlow S, Sullivan F: Reproductive Hazards of Industrial Chemicals. London, Academic Press, 1983
6. Barr M: The teratogenicity of cadmium chloride in two stocks of Wistar rats. Teratol 7:237–242, 1973
7. Bellinger D, Leviton A, Needleman, HL, et al: Low-level lead exposure and infant development in the first year. Neurobehav Toxicol Teratol 8:151–161, 1986
8. Bertin JE: Reproduction, women, and the workplace: Legal issues. In Stein 2, Hatch M (eds): Occupational Medicine State of the Art Reviews: Reproductive Problems in the Workplace, pp 497–507. Philadelphia, Hanley & Belfus, 1986
9. Bloom AD (ed): Guidelines for studies of human populations exposed to mutagenic and reproduction hazards. New York, March of Dimes Birth Defects Foundation, 1981
10. Brenner MH: Estimating the Effects of Economic Change on National Health and Social Well-Being. Washington, DC, US Government Printing Office, 1985
11. Brewen JG, Preston RJ: Cytogenetic analysis of mammalian oocytes in Mutagenicity studies. In: Hsu TC (ed): Cytogenetic Assays of Environmental Mutagens. Totowa, NJ, Allenheld, Osmun, 1982
12. Butcher RL, Page RD: Environmental endogenous hazards to the female reproductive system. Environ Health Perspect 38:35–37, 1981
13. Chamberlain G, Garcia J: Pregnant women at work. Lancet 1:228–230, 1983
14. Chapman RM: Gonadal injury resulting from chemotherapy. Am J Ind Med 4:149–161, 1983
15. *Christman, et al. v. American Cyanamid Co.* Civil Action No. 80–0024 P (N.D.W.Va.), Second Amended Complaint (1980)
16. Clarkson TW, Nordberg G, Sager PR (eds): Reproductive and Development Toxicity of Metals. New York, Plenum, 1983
17. Cohen EN, Brown BW, Wu ML et al: Occupational disease in dentistry and chronic exposure to trace anesthetic gases. J Am Dent Assoc 101:21–31, 1980
18. Cullen MR, Kayne RD, Robins JM: Endocrine and reproductive dysfunction in men associated with occupational inorganic lead intoxication. Arch Environ Health 39:431–440, 1984
19. Cumming DC, Rebar RW: Exercise and reproductive function in women. Am J Indust Med 4:113–126, 1983
20. Dellarco V, Mavournin KH, Waters MD, Rogers ET (eds): Aneuploidy: Methodology

and test data review. Mutat Res 167:1–188, 1986
21. Dietrich KN, Kraft KM, Shukla R et al: Postnatal lead exposure and early sensorimotor development. Environ Res 38:130–136, 1985
22. Dohanich G, Nock B, McEwen BS: Steroid hormones, receptors and neutotransmitters. In Mondgil UK (ed): Molecular Mechanisms of Steroid Hormone Action, pp 701–732. Berlin, deGruyter, 1985
23. Edmonds DK, Lindsay KS, Miller JF et al: Early embryonic mortality in women. Fertil Steril 38:447–453, 1982
24. Ericson A, Kallen B. Survey of infants born in 1973 or 1975 to Swedish women working in operating rooms during their pregnancy. Scand J Work Envir 58:302–305, 1979
25. Gebhart ERE: The epidemiological approach: Chromosome aberrations in persons exposed to chemical mutagens. In Hsu TC (ed): Cytogenetic Assays of Environmental Mutagens. Totowa, NJ, Allenheld, Osmun, 1982
26. Generosa W, Cain K, Krishner M, and Huff SW: Genetic lesions induced by chemicals in spermatozoa and spermatids of mice are repaired in the egg. Proc Natl Acad Sci USA 76:435–437, 1979
27. Gorski RA: Gonadal hormones and the perinatal development of neuroendocrine function. In Martini C, Ganong WF (eds): Frontiers in Neuroendocrinology, p 237. New York, Oxford University, 1971
28. Hansson E, Jansa S, Wande H et al: Pregnancy outcome for women working in laboratories in some of the pharmaceutical industries in Sweden. Scand J Work Envir Health 6:131–134, 1980
29. Hardin BD, Goad PT, Burg JR: Developmental toxicity of four glycol ethers applied cutaneously to rats. Environ Health Perspect 57:69–74, 1984
30. Harrington JM, Stein GF, Rivera RO, deMorales AV. The occupational hazards of formulating oral contraceptives—A survey of plant employees. Arch Environ Health 33:12–15, 1978
31. Hemminki K, Axelson O, Niemi M-L, Ahlborg G: Assessment of methods and results of reproductive occupational epidemiology: Spontaneous abortions and malformations in the offspring of working women. Am J Ind Med 4:293–307, 1983
32. Hemminki K, Franssila E, Vainio H: Spontaneous abortions among female chemical workers in Finland. Int Arch Occup Environ Health 45:123–126, 1980
33. Hemminki K, Kyyronen P, Niemi M-L et al: Spontaneous abortions in an industrialized community in Finland. Am J Public Health 73:32–37, 1983
34. Herbst AL, Hubby NM, Blough RR, Azizi F: A comparison of pregnancy experience in DES-exposed and DES-unexposed daughters. J Reprod Med 24:62, 1980
35. Holmberg PC: CNS defects in children born to mothers exposed to organic solvent during pregnancy. Lancet 2:177–179, 1979
36. Hook EB, Schreinemachers DM: Trends in utilization of prenatal cytogenetic diagnosis by New York State residents in 1979 and 1980. Am J Public Health 73:198–202, 1983
37. Infante PF, Wagoner JK, McMichael AJ et al: Genetic risks of vinyl chloride. Lancet 1:734–735, 1976
38. Jacquet P: Influence de la progesterone et de l'estradiol exogenes sur le processus de l'implantation embryonnaire, chez la souris femelle intoxiquee par le plomb. CR Soc Biol 172:1027–1040, 1978
39. Jensh RP, Brent RL: The effects of low level prenatal x-irradiation on postnatal development in the Wistar rat. Proc Soc Exp Biol Med 184:256–263, 1987
40. Kantor AF, Curnen MGM, Meigs JW, Flannery JT: Occupations of fathers of patients with Wilms' tumor. J Epidemiol Community Health 33:253–256, 1979
41. Khera AK, Wibberly DG, Dathan JG: Placental and still birth tissue lead concentrations in occupationally exposed women. Br J Ind Med 37:394–396, 1980
42. Kline JK: Maternal occupation: effects on spontaneous abortions and malformations. In Stein ZA, Hatch MC (eds): Reproductive Problems in the Workplace, pp 381–404. Hanley and Belfus, Philadelphia, 1986
43. Kupfer D: Effects of pesticides and related compounds on steroid metabolism and function. Crit Rev Toxicol 4:83–124, 1975
44. Kuratsume M, Yoshimura T, Matsuzaka J, Yamaguchi A: Epidemiologic study on Yusho, a poisoning caused by ingestion of rice oil contaminated with a commercial brand of polychlorinated biphenyls. Envir Health Perspect 1:119–128, 1972
45. Kurzel RB, Cetrulo CL: The effect of environmental pollutants on human reproduction, including birth defects. Environ Sci Technol 15:626–640, 1981
46. Lancranjan I: Reproductive ability of workmen exposed occupationally to lead. Arch Environ Health 30:396, 1975

47. Lee IP: Adaptive biochemical repair response toward germ cell DNA repair. Am J Ind Med 4:135–147, 1983
48. Levine RJ, Blunden PB, Dalcorso RD et al: Superiority of reproductive histories to sperm counts in detecting infertility at a dibromochloropropane manufacturing plant. J Occup Med 25:591–597, 1983
49. Longo LD: Environmental pollution and pregnancy: Risks and uncertainties for the fetus and infant. Am J Obstet Gynecol 137:162–173, 1980
50. Mahaffey KR, Annest JL, Roberts J, Murphy RS: National estimates of blood lead levels: U.S. 1976–1980; association with selected demographic and socioeconomic factors. N Engl J Med 307:575–579, 1982
51. Manson J, George JD, York PC: Reproductive toxicology. In National Institute of Occupational Safety and Health, USPHS, CDC: The Industrial Environment: Its Evaluation and Control. Cincinnati, NIOSH (in press)
52. Manson JM: Mechanism of nitrogen teratogenesis. Environ Health Perspect 70:137–147, 1986
53. Masui Y, Pederson R: Ultraviolet light induced DNA synthesis in mouse oocytes during meiotic maturation. Nature (London) 257:705–707, 1975
54. Mattison DR: The mechanisms of action of reproductive toxins. Am J Ind Med 4:65–79, 1983
55. Mattison DR (ed): Reproductive Toxicology. New York, Alan R. Liss, 1983
56. Mattison DR: Female reproductive system: Gametogenesis to implantation. In Clarkson T, Nordberg G, Sager PR (eds): Reproductive and Developmental Toxicity of Metals, pp 317–342. New York, Plenum, 1983
57. Mattison DR: The effects of smoking on reproduction from gametogenesis to implantation. Environ Res 28:410–433, 1982
58. Mattison DR: Effects of biological foreign compounds on reproduction. In Abdul-Karim RA (ed): Drugs During Pregnancy: Clinical Perspectives, pp 101–125. Philadelphia, Stickley, 1981
59. Mattison DR: Drugs, xenobiotics and the adolescent: Implications for reproduction. In Soyka LF, Redmord GP (eds): Drug Metabolism in the Immature Human. pp 129–143. New York, Raven Press, 1981
60. Mattison DR, Gates AH, Leonard A et al: Female reproductive system. In Clarkson T, Nordberg G, Sager PR (eds): Reproductive and Developmental Toxicity of Metals, pp 41–91. New York, Plenum, 1983
61. Mattison DR, Nightingale MS, Takizawa K et al: Benzo(a)pyrene reproductive toxicity and ovarian metabolism. In: Rydstrom J, Montelius J, Bengtsson M (eds): Extrahepatic Drug Metabolism and Chemical Carcinogenesis. pp 337–350. New York, Elsevier, 1983
62. Mattison DR, Nightingale MS, Shiromizu K: Effects of toxic substances on female reproduction. Environ Health Perspect 48:43–52, 1983
63. Mattison DR, Shiromizu K, Nightingale MS: Oocyte destruction by polycyclic aromatic hydrocarbons. Am J Ind Med 4:191–202, 1983
64. McLachlin JA, Newbold RR, Korach KS et al: Transplacental toxicology: Prenatal factors influencing postnatal fertility. In Kimmel C, Buelke-Sam J (eds): Developmental Toxicology, pp 213–221. New York, Raven Press, 1981
65. McMichael AJ, Vimpani GV, Robertson EG et al: The Port Pirie Short Study: Maternal blood lead and pregnancy outcome. J Epidemiol Community Health 40:18–25, 1986
66. Milkovich L, Van den Berg BJ: Effects of prenatal meprobamate and chlordiazepoxide hydrochloride on human embryonic and fetal development. N Engl J Med 291:1268–1271, 1974
67. Miller RK: Perinatal toxicology: Its recognition and fundamentals. Am J Med 4:205–244, 1983
68. Miller RK, Mattison DR, Filler RS et al: In Eskes TKAB, Finster M (eds): Drug Therapy During Pregnancy, pp 215–224. London, Butterworths, 1985
69. Miller RW: Environmental causes of cancer in childhood. Adv Pediatr 25:97, 1978
70. Moore MR, Meredith PA, Goldberg A: A retrospective analysis of blood-lead in mentally retarded children. Lancet 1(8014):717–719, 1977
71. National Research Council, Advisory Committee on Biological Effects of Ionizing Radiations: Effects on Populations of Exposure to Low Levels of Ionizing Radiation. Washington, National Academy of Sciences Press, 1980
72. Neel JV: Mutation and disease in man. Can J Genetics Cytology 20:295–306, 1978
73. Nordenson I, Beckman G, Beckman L, Nordstrom S: Occupational and environmental risks in and around a smelter in Northern Sweden. IV. Chromosomal aberrations in workers exposed to lead. Hereditas 88:263–267, 1978

74. Nordstrom S, Beckman L, Nordenson I: Occupational and environmental risks in and around a smelter in Northern Sweden. III. Frequency of spontaneous abortion. Hereditas 88:51–54, 1978
75. Office of Technology Assessment: Reproductive Health Hazards in the Workplace. Washington, DC, US Government Printing Office, 1985
76. Oliver, T: Lead poisoning and the race. Br Med J 1:1096–1098, 1911
77. Pederson R, Mangia F: Ultraviolet light induced unscheduled DNA synthesis by nesting and growing mouse oocytes. Mutat Res 49:425–429, 1978
78. Peters JM, Preston-Martin S, Yu MC: Brain tumors in children and occupational exposure of parents. Science 213:235–237, 1981
79. Petrusz P, Weaver CM, Grant LD et al: Lead poisoning and reproduction: Effects on pituitary and serum gonadotropins in neonatal rats. Environ Res 19:383–391, 1979
80. Pharoah POD, Alberman E, Doyle P, Chamberlain G: Outcome of pregnancy among women in anaesthetic practice. Lancet 1:34–36, 1977
81. Pierce PE, Thompson JF, Likosky W et al: Alkyl mercury poisoning in humans. JAMA 220:1439–1442, 1972
82. Pihl RO, Parkes M: Hair element content in learning disabled children. Science 198:204–206, 1977
83. Pritchard JA, McDonald PC, Gant NF: Williams' Obstetrics, p 257. Norwalk, CT, Appleton-Century-Crofts, 1985
84. Pruett JG, Winslow SG: Health effects of environmental chemicals on human reproduction. A selected bibliography with abstracts, 1963–1981. National Library of Medicine/Toxicology Information Reference Center 82/1, 1982
85. Ross GT: Congenital anomalies among children born of mothers receiving chemotherapy for gestational trophoblastic neoplasms. Cancer 37(Suppl):1043–1047, 1976
86. Routh DK, Mushak P, Boone L: A new syndrome of elevated blood lead and microcephaly. J Pediatr Psychol 4:67–76, 1979
87. Saxena MC, Siddiqui M, Bhargava AK et al: Role of chlorinated hydrocarbon pesticides in abortions and premature labor. Toxicology 17:323–331, 1981
88. Schmidt G, Fowler WC, Talbert LM, Edelman DA: Reproductive history of women exposed to diethylstilbestrol in utero. Fertil Steril 33:21–24, 1980
89. Schull WJ, Otake M: Developmental effects of irradiation on the brain of the embryo and fetus. In Castellani A (ed): Epidemiology and the Quantitation of Environmental Risk in Humans from Radiation and Other Agents, pp 515–536. New York, Plenum, 1985
90. Schwanitz G, Lehlnert G, Gebhart E: Chromosomal injury due to occupational lead poisoning. Dtsch Med Wochenschr 95:1636–1641, 1970
91. Seagull EAW: Developmental abilities of children exposed to polybrominated biphenyls (PPB). Am J Public Health 73:281–285, 1983
92. Sieber SM, Adamson RH: Toxicity of antineoplastic agents in man: chromosomal aberrations, antifertility effects, congenital malformations and carcinogenic potential. Adv Cancer Res 22:57–155, 1975
93. Silbergeld EK: Maternally mediated exposure of the fetus: In utero exposure to lead and other toxins. Neurotoxicology 7:557–568, 1986
94. Silbergeld EK, Nightingale MR, Godlove K et al: Reproductive toxicity of policyclic aromatic hydrocarbons. Pharmacol 1983
95. Silbergeld EK, Schwartz J: Mobilization of bone lead in women. Pharmacology 28:230, 1986
96. Swartz WJ, Mattison DR: Benzo(a)pyrene inhibits ovulation in C57B1/6N mice. Anat Rec 216:268–276, 1985
97. Takizawa K, Mattison DR: Female reproduction. Am J Ind Med 465–480, 1983
98. Taskinen H, Lindbohm ML, Hemminki K: Spontaneous abortions among women working in the pharmaceutical industry. Br J Ind Med 43:199–205, 1986
99. *United Steelworkers of America v. Marshall*, 647 F.2d 1189 (D. C. Cir. 1980), cert. denied sub nom. Lead Industries Ass'n Inc. v. Donovan, 453 U.S. 913 (1981)
100. Whorton D, Krauss RM, Marshall S et al: Infertility in male pesticide workers. Lancet 2:1259–1261, 1977
101. Wide M: Interference of lead with implantation in the mouse: effect of exogenous oestradical and progesterone. Teratology 21:187–191, 1980
102. Wilcox AJ: Surveillance of pregnancy loss in human populations. Am J Ind Med 4:385–391, 1983
103. Wilson, JG: Environment and Birth Defects. New York, Academic Press, 1973
104. Wolff MS: Occupationally derived chemicals in breast milk. Am J Ind Med 4:259–281, 1983

7

Controversies Surrounding Antepartum Rh Immune Globulin Prophylaxis

James H. Beeson

HISTORICAL BACKGROUND

Nearly 30 years have elapsed since the discovery that passive administration of Rh immune globulin (RhIg) to Rh-negative women could prevent Rh isoimmunization.[13,14] In that time postpartum and postabortal administration of RhIg has become the standard of obstetric practice, and the indications for usage and means of appropriate dosage calculation have been clearly enunciated.[19] This means of prophylaxis is so well accepted and undisputed that failure to offer it may be considered malpractice.

In spite of the success of the postpartum prophylaxis program, Rh isoimmunization has been far from eradicated. The most frequent reasons for failure can be collectively classed as underutilization of RhIg, and include the following:

Failure to accurately identify Rh-negative women. Such failures include both laboratory error and transcription error

Failure to administer RhIg after invasive procedures such as second trimester genetic amniocentesis

Failure to administer RhIg after a spontaneous abortion or ectopic pregnancy

Failure to recognize large fetomaternal hemorrhages for which a single 300-μg dose of RhIg is inadequate

In spite of a well-conceived and well-executed postpartum and postabortal prophylaxis program, a certain number of women become sensitized prior to delivery. The usual cause of this sensitization is presumed to be occult transfer of a sufficient number of fetal cells to the maternal circulation during gestation, which produces demonstrable antibodies during pregnancy or within three days of delivery.[8] These observations have led to empiric trials in which RhIg was administered to the Rh-negative mother during the third trimester of pregnancy.[8] The results of these trials were reported as having an overall protective efficiency of greater than 90%.

Since the initial enthusiastic reports of

172

antenatal prophylaxis appeared in about 1978, many large centers have instituted such prophylaxis programs. In November 1983, the American College of Obstetricians and Gynecologists in a technical bulletin update noted that

> the Food and Drug Administration has approved antepartum prophylaxis as an indication for the use of RhIg. In addition, there is evidence of the efficacy of antenatal prophylaxis as well as its cost effectiveness from a public health point of view. Based on careful and extensive consideration of these issues, the establishment of RhIg antenatal prophylaxis program is now recommended.[1]

This statement was followed by a technical bulletin in August 1984 on the prevention of Rho(D) isoimmunization. This bulletin stated that "the current recommendation is that the patient received 300 µg RhIg at approximately 28 weeks gestation and again postpartum."[2] Because these statements by the American College have effectively made antenatal prophylaxis the standard of care in the United States, it would seem to the casual observer that such a program would involve few controversies. Yet, this is not the case. Since 1978, the debate has raged in the obstetric literature in the form of both articles and letters to the editor. Even the data regarding the protection afforded by an antepartum RhIg prophylaxis program are disputed, so that ethical issues that arise are not easily resolved.

RATIONALE FOR ANTEPARTUM PROPHYLAXIS

Incidence of Antenatal Sensitization

There appears to be no general agreement as to the incidence of sensitization occurring prior to delivery. The lowest incidence appears in Finland, where sensitization is reported to occur in 0.7% of over 15,000 patients.[22] Bowman has reported a rate of 1.8% in 3532 deliveries in Manitoba, Canada.[5] Although some of these differences may be related to methodology, there may actually be genetic population differences in responsiveness. Based upon available data, 1% to 2% of pregnancies at risk would seem to be a reasonable figure for Rh isoimmunization prior to delivery.

Mechanism of Antenatal Sensitization

The entire antenatal prophylaxis program is based upon the assumption that sensitization occurs directly as a result of an occult fetomaternal transfusion. This leakage of fetal cells into the maternal circulation is occult in the sense that it may not be detectable by routine screening methodology, such as the Kleier-Betke test. Such an explanation is certainly plausible, since as little as 0.01 ml of Rh-positive cells is sufficient to produce Rh isoimmunization and ample evidence exists for leakage on this order of magnitude.[18]

Data regarding the incidence of sensitization by this mechanism must rely on a set of assumptions. The result of this set of assumptions is that the patient at risk must not have been sensitized, even with undetectable antibody titers, prior to the index pregnancy. Included in this set of assumptions is that the Rh-negative woman has received adequate RhIg after abortion, after ectopic pregnancy, after amniocentesis, and after delivery. It must also be assumed that she has not received a mismatched blood transfusion or been sensitized as a result of a subclinical abortion. Finally, it must be assumed that she was not sensitized as a result of having been born to an Rh-positive mother (the grandmother theory).

The grandmother theory refers to the situation in which an Rh-negative woman receives sufficient Rh-positive cells from her mother during gestation or delivery to develop an antibody response. Bowen gave some support to this theory in 1976 when he reported that 7 of 63 (11%) blood samples collected from infants between 1 and 9 months of age had detectable Rh(D) titers.[4] This antibody could be demonstrated only by the autoanalyzer technique, however. A subsequent study of 237 Rh-negative babies born of Rh-positive mothers failed to confirm these results.[16] In a retrospective review of 22 Rh-isoimmunized primigravidas collected from two hospitals, Scott and colleagues concluded that while in utero sensitization is a possibility, antepartum fetal to maternal bleeding appears to be the usual cause of Rh isoimmunization in primigravidas.[26]

Data from Prophylaxis Trials

Trials of antepartum administration of RhIg were started in Canada in 1968, and subsequently in several other centers around the world. Protocols for administration of the immune globulin have varied, but since previous studies indicated that only 8% of gravidas demonstrated antibodies prior to 28 weeks' gestation, most current protocols consist of the administration of 300 µg of RhIg at 28 weeks gestation.[5] Normal postpartum screening for the quantity of fetomaternal hemorrhage and RhIg administration are subsequently performed with all parturients delivering Rh-positive babies.

The results of three trials are detailed in Table 7-1. Bowman's data have been divided into two groups. The first group represents overall composite data. A second subgroup consists of patients who were followed up to 6 months postpartum with no evidence of sensitization at delivery. The data of Davey[11] and Zipurski[32] include follow-ups on all patients and concurrent controls. Two measurements of efficacy are given. The difference in percent sensitization is simply the difference between percent sensitization in control and prophylaxis groups. The percent protective efficacy is computed by subtracting the actual number of sensitizations from those expected, based on the percentage in the control group, and dividing this by the expected number.

Immediate differences between the studies are apparent from Table 7-1. The incidence of sensitization runs from 0.6% in Davey's study to 2.39% in Zipurski's study. These differences could arise from any of three sources: (1) They could represent an ascertainment bias due to the laboratory techniques used for the detection of anti-D antibodies. (2) The differences could be the result of true population differences. (3) The differences could be a reflection of the care with which the control groups were managed during their pregnancy (e.g., administration of RhIg at the time of amniocentesis, trauma, or hemorrhage). Regardless of the differences in sensitization rates of the control group, all three studies demonstrate protective efficacies on the order of 80% to 90%. These data form the basis for the current recommendations by the American College of Obstetricians and Gynecologists.

THE CONTROVERSY

With claims of 90% efficacy for antepartum prophylaxis programs, little dissent would be expected. This has not been the case, and arguments have raged in both the British and American literature challenging everything from the data themselves to the cost-benefit ratio of an antenatal prophylaxis program. Each area of controversy will be discussed individually.

The Efficacy of the Antenatal Prophylaxis Program

Hensleigh[17] has stated that the potential benefits of antenatal Rh prophylaxis are extremely limited, citing the 0.6% lower sensitization incidence in the Davey study.[11] He further calculates that to show that this difference is statistically significant at the 5% level with a power of 80% would require comparison of study and control groups with 2600 patients in each group, and that these controls be contemporary and randomly selected. The data of Table 7-1 clearly fail to meet these criteria. The largest single series (Bowman) used retrospective rather than concurrent controls, and the sample size in the two studies with concurrent controls is also less than that calculated by Hensleigh.

Table 7-1. Efficacy of Antepartum Administration of RhIg

AUTHOR	ASCERTAINMENT PERIOD	YEAR	PROPHYLAXIS GROUP			CONTROL GROUP			Difference In Percentage Sensitization	EFFICACY			Percentage of Protection
			Number	Sensitized	%	Number	Sensitized	Percentage		Expected	Actual	
Davey[11]	6 mos postpartum	1979	1616	1	0.06	3022*	18	0.6	0.54	10	1	90
Bowman[5]	Delivery	1978	1799	2	0.11	2768†	45	1.62	1.51	29	2	93
	6 mos postpartum	1978	803	1	0.12	2768†	45	1.62	1.50	13	1	92
Zipurski[32]	6 mos postpartum	1977	364	2	0.55	292*	7	2.39	1.85	9	2	78

* Concurrent
† Retrospective

175

Although no single study to date satisfies the rigid criteria for statistical validation, one cannot escape the overall impression that the procedure is efficacious. The challenge is in the underlying assumptions used to calculate the degree of efficacy, and this cannot be completely resolved on the basis of existing data.

Risks to the Fetus

The most frequent concern about the antenatal prophylaxis program expressed by both physicians and patients is that of iatrogenically induced hemolytic disease. The mechanism of concern is the transplacental passage of RhIg given to the mother, which causes hemolysis of fetal blood much as Rh isoimmunization does. Typically, injection of immune globulin usually produces anti-D titers of 1:1 or 1:2. Although a small percentage of newborns are weakly Coombs' positive, the infants are virtually never anemic.[5,15]

Hensleigh[17] cites possible adverse effects of gamma globulin in the immature fetal immune system.[24] These allusions as to yet unknown effects tend to raise the practitioner's blood pressure because they resemble the legalese typically found in malpractice complaints, and no one has forgotten the diethylstilbestrol story. As evidence, he cites the report by Durandy, Fisher, and Griscelli[12] of dysfunction of pokeweed mitogen T- and B-lymphocyte stimulation in children ranging from 4 to 12 years of age who were treated with gamma globulin for repeated respiratory tract infections. Proponents of antenatal Rh immune globulin prophylaxis point out that mitogen stimulation of lymphocytes *in vitro* is an artificial system that may have no clinical relevance. It is also frequently noted that the fetus receives quantitatively far more immunoglobulin G (IgG) from placental transfer of maternal immunoglobulin than could conceivably be received indirectly from RhIg transferred to the mother. This is generally considered to be a normal protective mechanism for the fetus, and no long-term ill effects have been noted.[7,9]

Hensleigh also cites the failure of clinical trials to collect data on fetal losses, birth weights, neonatal morbidity and mortality, neonatal immunologic status, or childhood illnesses.[17] To this, Bowman replies simply that the Canadian experience has seen no evidence of harm in the tens of thousands of infants delivered after maternal antenatal Rh prophylaxis. Tabsh, Lebherz, and Crandall have reported a retrospective study of 321 gravidas who received RhIg after second trimester amniocentesis.[27] They included 321 Rh-positive women undergoing second trimester amniocentesis as controls. These data are tabulated in Table 7-2. The authors concluded that no significant differences were seen between the groups, but, of course, they suggested that prospective studies need to be performed to confirm the safety of RhIg administration in the second trimester.

Risks to the Mother

An antenatal prophylaxis program doubles the number of doses of RhIg given to the mother of an Rh-positive baby, and in 40% of pregnancies with Rh-negative infants, they receive immune globulin that they do not need. Intramuscular administration of RhIg is quite common, and reactions are very rare. In fact, crossmatching of units of RhIg is no longer required. The rare reaction to the injection of RhIg seems to be confined to patients with a congenital IgA deficiency who have developed an anti-IgA. One case of an anaphylactic reaction has been reported in such a patient.[23] This type of reaction occurs because immune globulin prepared by the Cohn alcohol fractionation method contains IgA and other foreign proteins. By using ion exchange methods for preparation of the immune globulin, this rare problem may be completely circumvented.

A second potential problem is the production of nonspecific antiglobulins in mothers receiving intramuscular RhIg. The prevalence of these antibodies may be on the order of 25%, but the clinical significance of the finding is unknown.[30]

Table 7-2. Comparison of Rh-Negative and Rh-Positive Patients Receiving RhIg After Second Trimester Genetic Amniocentesis

	RH-NEGATIVE PATIENTS	RH-POSITIVE CONTROLS
Number	321	321
Intrauterine fetal death	7	3
Post-dates	3	Not stated
Placenta previa	1	Not stated
Spontaneous abortion	1	3
Total pregnancy loss	9	6
Congenital anomalies	3	4
Mean birth weight 1 ± SE	3420 ± 29	3435 ± 33 g
Prematurity rate	2.5%	1.6%

There is no known risk of hepatitis to the mother who is treated with RhIg produced by the Cohn method now in use.

A crucial issue to the Rh immune globulin recipient is the risk of transmission of the human immunodeficiency virus (HIV), the etiologic agent of acquired immunodeficiency syndrome (AIDS). Rh immune globulin *appears* safe based upon two lines of evidence. The first involved additions of known quantities of the retrovirus to serum, which was then processed by the Cohn fractionation method. The resulting virus concentration was 1×10^{-15} of the starting concentration.[20,31] These results were considered reassuring regarding the safety of immune globulin.

The second line of evidence involves clinical follow-up of hepatitis immune globulin recipients. Before testing was performed on donors, a number of batches of hepatitis immune globulin contained high titer antibody to HIV. In no case has confirmed transmission of HIV occurred in recipients of these batches of immune globulin.[10] HIV positive donors are no longer used, and with current testing practices for plasma donors, the risk should be very small indeed, but one must ponder whether any risk of a uniformly fatal disease is justified by a marginal decrease in fetal morbidity.

A social risk to recipients of immune globulin has been the false-positive HIV antibody test due to the passively acquired antibody. Since HIV antibody positive donors are no longer used, this should not be a problem.

Problems of Production and Supply

Critics of antenatal prophylaxis programs frequently note that such programs increase the use of immune globulin two- to threefold. This globulin is produced only in humans, and sources include women immunized by pregnancy as well as immunized male volunteers. Plasma is then harvested by plasmapheresis. The risks to these donors include the risk of transfusion necessary for immunization (hepatitis, AIDS, immunization to leukocyte and platelet antigens, and immunization to non-Rh[D] antigens), as well as the inherent dangers of plasmapheresis.[21]

In reply to these criticisms, it has been stated that 200 donors in the United States would produce about 6000 kg of Rh plasma per year, which would adequately meet the United States' needs, including antenatal prophylaxis. It is also noted that donor risks can be minimized by carefully screening immunizing cells for hepatitis and compatibility with regard to non-Rh antigens.[7,23] Risks of plasmapheresis have been said to be minimal in skilled hands.[6]

A Swiss study of RhIg requirements found that substantial reserves of anti-D globulin were found in naturally immunized female donors. They estimated that this source alone would serve the Swiss needs until the year 2000.[25]

Cost-Benefit Ratios

The cost of antenatal prophylaxis is the most frequently used argument against its use. As seen in Table 7-3, the cost-benefit ratios which have been determined vary widely and are highly dependent upon definitions and assumptions. In these publications, it is frequently unclear whether one is preventing Rh(D) isoimmunization or hemolytic disease of the newborn (HDN), which increases neonatal morbidity and mortality. There is clearly no consensus on the cost-benefit ratio of Rh prophylaxis. Adams, Marks, and Koplan conclude that the benefits of such a program *might* exceed its cost if the program were restricted to primiparous women at high risk of antepartum Rh sensitization.[3] Some have advocated limiting the Rh prophylaxis program to primigravidas in order to ensure each woman of one or two healthy children.[29]

Analysis of simple cost-benefit ratios must surely seem callous to anyone who has been confronted with a sensitized Rh-negative gravida in whom heroic measures such as intrauterine transfusion failed to provide a living child. Simplistic answers such as "stop getting pregnant" or "consider artificial insemination" may result in emotional problems in place of medical ones. Nevertheless, as medical technology evolves, the cost of medical care inevitably increases. As the cost of medical care becomes a larger proportion of our real gross national product, many future decisions will need to be based upon true cost-benefit ratios, and the needs of the individual will need to be balanced against the welfare of the population as a whole.

ALTERNATIVES TO ANTENATAL PROPHYLAXIS PROGRAMS

Mass antenatal prophylaxis has never been considered the ideal strategy for elimination of Rh isoimmunization. A more pleasing approach is to identify and treat only those pregnancies at risk. In the 40% of pregnancies in which the infant is Rh-negative, antenatal prophylaxis has no benefit. In addition, in the review of 22 cases of antenatal sensitization, males were overrepresented (19), most all were ABO compatible (21), and maternal blood type O was significantly underrepresented (2). Unfortunately, the data necessary to define pregnancies at low risk are not readily available (e.g., an ABO-incompatible female fetus whose mother's blood is

Table 7-3. Costs of Rh Prophylaxis

Reference	Date	Cost/Sensitization Avoided	Treatment Cost
Hensleigh[16]	1983	$41,000	$2,400
Tovey[26]	1980	$ 7,900	Not given
Kochenhour[18]	1982	$ 1,300	$2,800
Bowman[7]	1984	$ 3,500	Not given
Adams[3]	1984	$27,000*	$1,170 (Mild)
			$6,454 (Moderate to severe)

* Per case of HDN avoided

type O).[26] The known risks and costs of obtaining such fetal information clearly exceed those inherent in the antenatal prophylaxis program.

An alternative is to carefully screen maternal blood throughout gestation for evidence of small fetomaternal hemorrhages. If one is to believe that doses as small as 0.01 ml of Rh-positive blood are sufficient to cause isoimmunization, then a useful test would be required to identify one Rh-positive cell among 200,000 Rh-negative cells.[18,24] This is clearly beyond the capabilities of currently used laboratory techniques. While fluorescence-activated cell sorting (FACS) techniques have the ability to make such a determination, the instruments are expensive and not commonly available. In addition, the cost of repetitive screening with a FACS instrument is likely to be excessive. Consequently, there is no viable alternative to antepartum prophylaxis if we are to achieve the irreducible Rh immunization rate, calculated by Bowman to be 2 to 4 per 10,000 pregnancies.

RECOMMENDATIONS

The controversy surrounding the antepartum use of Rh immune globulin has been presented in as much detail as possible. Few experts deny that the administration of RhIg in the antepartum period is efficacious in preventing Rh isoimmunization. The biggest remaining arguments concern the magnitude of the benefits and cost-benefit ratios. Although there are many misgivings in the obstetric community about this program, the American College of Obstetricians and Gynecologists have stated that failure to offer antenatal prophylaxis to the Rh-negative gravida is tantamount to malpractice. Still, it would seem wise to obtain informed consent from each patient by giving her a description of the cost of the treatment, the expected benefits, and possible risks either real or theoretical. Each patient could then make her own decision on the basis of her own reproductive expectations.

REFERENCES

1. American College of Obstetricians and Gynecologists: Tech Bull 61, 1983
2. American College of Obstetricians and Gynecologists: Tech Bull 79, 1984
3. Adams MM, Marks JS, Koplan JP: Cost implications of routine antenatal administration of Rh immune globulin. Am J Obstet Gynecol 149:633, 1984
4. Bowen FW, Renfield M: The detection of anti-D in Rh (D)-negative infants born of Rh_o(D)-positive mothers. Pediatr Res 10:213, 1976
5. Bowman JM: Suppression of Rh isoimmunization. Obstet Gynecol 52:385, 1978
6. Bowman JM: Antepartum Rh immunoprophylaxis. N Engl J Med 304:425, 1981
7. Bowman JM: Letter. Am J Obstet Gynecol 148:1151, 1984
8. Bowman JM, Chown B, Lewis M, Pollack JM: Rh isoimmunization during pregnancy: Antenatal prophylaxis. Can Med Assoc J 118:623, 1978
9. Candle MR: Letter. Am J Obstet Gynecol 148:1152, 1984
10. Centers for Disease Control: Current Trends. Safety of therapeutic immune globulin preparations with respect to transmission of human T-lymphotrophic virus type III/lymphadenopathy-associated virus infection. MMWR 35:231, 1986
11. Davey MG: The prevention of rhesus isoimmunization. Clin Obstet Gynecol 6:509, 1979
12. Durandy A, Fisher A, Griscelli C: Dysfunctions of pokeweed mitogen-stimulated T and B lymphocyte responses induced by gamma globulin therapy. J Clin Invest 67:867, 1981
13. Finn R, Clark CA, Donohoe WTA et al: Experimental studies on the prevention of Rh haemolytic disease. Br Med J 1:1486, 1961
14. Freda VJ, Gorman JG: Antepartum management of Rh haemolytic disease. Bull Sloane Hosp Women 8:147, 1962
15. Hahn N, Gallasch EH, Smaluhn W, Luthje D: Zur Problematik der Anwendung der IgG-anti-D-Gabe in der Schwangerschaft. Zbl Gynak 96:897, 1984
16. Hattevig G, Jonsson M, Kjellman B et al: Screening of Rh-antibodies in Rh-negative female infants with Rh-positive mothers. Acta Paediatr Scand 70:541, 1981
17. Hensleigh PA: Preventing rhesus isoimmunization: Antepartum Rh immune globulin versus a sensitive test for risk identification. Am J Obstet Gynecol 146:749, 1983

18. Jokobowicz R, Williams L, Silverman F: Immunization of Rh negative volunteers by repeated injections of very small volumes of Rh positive blood. Vox Sang 23:376, 1972
19. Kochenour NK, Beeson JH: The use of Rh-immune globulin. Clin Obstet Gynecol 25:283–291, 1982
20. Mitra G, Wong MF, Mozen MM et al.: Elimination of infectious retroviruses during preparation of immunoglobulins. Transfusion 26:394, 1986
21. Nubcaher J, Bove JR: Sounding boards: Rh immunoprophylaxis: Is antepartum therapy desirable? N Engl J Med 303:935, 1980
22. Proceedings of McMaster conference on prevention of Rh isoimmunization. Vox Sang 36:50, 1979
23. Rivat L, Parent M, Rivat C: Accident servenu apre injection de gamma-globuline anti-Rh du la presence D/anti-corp anti-OA. Presse Med 7:2072, 1970
24. Ryan KJ: Ethical considerations of antenatal prophylaxis for Rh hemolytic disease. In Frigoletto FD, Jewett JF, Konugres AA (eds): Rh Hemolytic Disease: New Strategy for Eradication, pp 177–184. Boston, GK Hall, 1982
25. Scher V, Frey-Wettstein M: Anti-D hyperimmunoglobulin: A study of Swiss requirements. Schweiz Med Wochenschr 109:22, 1979
26. Scott JR, Beer AE, Guy AR et al: Pathogenesis of Rh immunization in primigravidas. Obstet Gynecol 49:9–14, 1977
27. Tabsh KM, Lebherz TB, Crandall BF: Risks of prophylactic anti-D immunoglobulin after second trimester amniocentesis. Am J Obstet Gynecol 149:225, 1984
28. Tovey GH: Should anti-D immunoglobulin be given antenatally? Lancet 2:466, 1980
29. Tovey LAD: Antenatal anti-D prophylaxis. Lancet 1:269, 1981
30. Vos GH, Shapiro M, Burgess BJ, Vos D: A comparative study of antiglobulin antibodies and residual anti-D between recipients of intramuscular anti-D immunoglobulin and intravenous plasma anti-D. Vox Sang 24:33, 1973
31. Wells MA, Wittek AE, Epstein JS: Inactivation and partition of human T-cell lymphotrophic virus, type III, during ethanol fractionation of plasma. Transfusion 26:210, 1986
32. Zipurski A: Rh hemolytic disease of the newborn—The disease eradicated by immunology. Clin Obstet Gynecol 20:579–772, 1977

PART IV:
OBSTETRIC MANAGEMENT

8

New Technology

SECTION I: Evolution of the Oxytocin Challenge Test as a Diagnostic Tool

Gregory L. Glover and Alfred G. Robichaux

The gradual evolution of any technology is a complex of scientific advancements, publications or patents, reevaluation, continual skepticism, and finally general acceptance. The shift from being considered experimental to standard may vary by years from institution to institution, occasionally catalyzed by the intrusion of external forces such as malpractice litigation over the use of a new technology. In this chapter, we will explore the evolution of a now-accepted technology, the oxytocin challenge test.

MEDICAL APPLICATIONS

A pyramiding of information followed the introduction of the initial concept of the oxytocin challenge test (OCT) which eventually led to its widespread acceptance. In 1966, Hammacher first suggested that the fetal heart rate pattern response to Syntocinon-induced contractions might be a valuable method for predicting the capability of the fetus to withstand the stresses of labor.[14] In 1968, Hon published the first atlas of fetal heart rate patterns with descriptions and illustrations of the classic early, variable, and late decelerations.[16]

In 1969, Kubli and associates began to research the physiologic basis of fetal heart rate patterns.[19] They described placental function as having two components, nutritive and respiratory. Placental nutritive insufficiency was postulated as a mechanism for development of intrauterine growth retardation with chronic maternal disease. Placental respiratory function as a prediction of fetal hypoxia in late pregnancy was evaluated by measuring the response of the fetal heart to oxytocin-induced contractions. The results of this testing were compared to other measures of chronic placental insufficiency; the authors found the OCT to be useful in evaluating the "respiratory" function of the placenta. In the same year, Pose and colleagues gave oxytocin to patients at risk for placental insufficiency and correlated the appearance of late decelerations with poor fetal prognosis.[20] The term *Uteroplacental insufficiency* was coined in their report.

In 1969 in the British literature, Huntingford and Pendelton classified fetal heart tracings as either benign, pathologic, or possibly pathologic.[17] Pathologic tracings included marked bradycardia of less than or equal to 99 beats per minute, loss of baseline fetal heart irregularity, or late decelerations. The possibly pathologic category included moderate and marked baseline tachycardia, decreased baseline fetal heart rate, any deceleration, or loss of baseline fetal heart rate with fetal movement or external stimulation.

In 1971, Spurrett reported the use of Syntocinon stress testing for "possibly pathological" heart tracings.[23] His procedure was to obtain a baseline tracing which was followed by 10 minutes of stimulation with Syntocinon or stimulation until pathology was seen. The stimulation was increased until the contractions were "painful," with 90-second intervals between contractions. The test was continued for another 10 minutes if no pathology was found. Spurrett felt that this test was useful for rapid evaluation of fetal well-being. He also felt that the test was useful to confirm the validity of low serum estriols and also to triage patients for induction of labor or elective cesarean section. The Syntocinon stress test was thought to be a useful adjunct in monitoring high-risk pregnancies, especially when used in conjunction with serum estriol measurements. Spurrett also reported that the stress testing resulted in no cases of premature labor.

In 1972, Ray and co-workers[21] published the hallmark paper for the clinical use of the OCT. This paper discussed 43 high-risk patients undergoing OCTs, 15 of whom had positive OCTs; within this group three fetal deaths occurred within 48 to 72 hours of the positive OCT. No deaths or decreases in serial 24-hour estriol levels within one week of negative tests were reported. It was also reported that one patient had a positive OCT 22 days prior to a fall in serum estriols.

Several conclusions in the study had an even greater impact on clinical obstetrics. First, it was postulated that oxytocin-induced contractions decreased intravillous blood flow, and this decrease in intravillous blood flow accounted for the clinically apparent late deceleration on fetal monitor tracings. Second, the flat beat-to-beat variability correlated with the likelihood of late deceleration. In cases where a positive OCT was accompanied by good beat-to-beat variability, the authors recommended bed rest and serial estriols. Measurement of estriols was still thought to be the standard of fetal well-being.

Although the literature up to this time had been favorable in evaluation of the OCT, publications over the next 2 years began to question its validity as a clinical tool. Schifrin postulated in 1972 that oxytocin-induced contractions were more likely than spontaneous contractions to produce late decelerations.[22] In 1974, two reports seriously questioned the OCT as a rapid and reliable method for evaluating fetal well-being. Christie and Cudmore conducted a study correlating OCTs with serum estriol measurements, fetal distress in labor, and Apgar scores in a group of 50 high-risk patients.[6] Out of this group there were 35 negative, 6 unsatisfactory, and 9 positive tests. The authors firmly concluded from the study that there was no correlation between a positive OCT and low estriols, Apgar scores, or fetal distress in labor; however, they did suggest that a negative OCT might allow some confidence in allowing a pregnancy to continue. At the same time, Boyd and co-workers published in the British literature a report of two fetal deaths following negative OCTs.[5] This report also included documentation of several pregnancies that had been followed expectantly after a positive OCT, but which resulted in normal outcomes. The authors reported that their study did not justify the OCT being used either once or serially as a measure of the placental capacity to withstand labor.

In 1974, Ewing and colleagues[8] described OCT testing in 58 patients, essentially agreeing with the thesis of Ray and associates that a positive oxytocin challenge test was indicative of an unfavorable fetal environment.[21] Later that year Boehm and Growdon,[4] in a letter to the American Journal of Obstetrics and Gynecology, took issue with the study of Christie and Cudmore,[6] pointing out that the late decelerations in their figure illustrating a positive OCT, in fact, illustrated variable decelerations. They suggested that the interpretation of the OCTs, rather than the test itself, might need reevaluation.

In 1975, Cooper and associates, in a large study of postdate pregnancies, championed their aggressive management with positive OCTs.[7] They described no fetal wastage in their series if infants were delivered within 24 hours of a positive OCT. They also noted a twofold increase in the incidence of meconium staining and a threefold increase in the incidence of postmature-dysmature infants in the groups with positive OCTs. The study also reported a large number of patients undergoing amniocentesis prior to testing, and aggressive use of intrauterine pressure catheters.

In February 1975, in his classic study of 1500 tests in 600 patients, Freeman[10] delineated stressed and nonstressed groups. He applied rigid criteria for the OCT, requiring three contractions per 10-minute interval and calling the test positive only if consistent, persistent late decelerations were recorded. Tests with inconsistent late decelerations were termed suspicious. Serum estriol measurements were still used as the standard method of determination. Delivery was implemented if the patient exhibited decreased serum estriols, a positive OCT and decreasing estriols, or a positive OCT with a mature lecithin/sphingomyelin (L/S) ratio.

Freeman concluded that negative weekly OCTs were reassuring; that a positive OCT was indicative of decreased placental reserve; that tests for suspicious OCTs or hyperstimulation should be repeated; that a positive OCT precedes a decrease in serum estriols; and that the nonstress test is a valid method of evaluating fetal well-being.

Several other papers in 1975 and 1976 fundamentally agreed with Freeman's conclusions.[2,3,11–13,23] The study by Christie and Cudmore was frequently referred to as a curiosity. Later that year, Hayden and co-workers in addressing the question of whether the OCT could serve as the primary standard for management of high-risk pregnancies concluded that this was, in fact, acceptable.[15] In 1976, Farahani and associates suggested that the OCT was a more sensitive test than urinary estriols as an indicator of fetal well-being.[9] They also took issue with the concept that false-positive OCTs tended to invalidate the test; they pointed out that although in a hand-picked, high-risk group of patients some favorable outcomes may be achieved by awaiting spontaneous labor and vaginal delivery, the overall risk for the group was too great for expectant management.

By this time the use of the OCT as a valid, easily applied test of fetal well-being was generally accepted. Still, however, several publications in 1975 and 1976 described single cases of poor fetal outcomes in patients with negative OCTs.[1,18]

It took approximately 10 years for the OCT to be accepted as a standard of care. Other tests, such as the biophysical profile, have been accepted more rapidly, perhaps because information was disseminated more expeditiously or because acceptance has been premature before adequate numbers and prospective randomized trials can be concluded. The danger of premature conclusions is that they ethically eliminate the ability of randomized trials to occur. If a test is accepted before scientifically proven, investigators may not wish to withhold management decisions in a blinded group.

Other technologies are in various stages of this process. Alpha-fetoprotein (AFP) testing for neural tube defects and aneuploidy and chorionic villus sampling are two technologies which are discussed at length in other chapters. They are mentioned here very briefly only to emphasize the continually evolving process of all new methods. It is clear that there exists a vast dichotomy in the availability of new technologies such as AFP in different areas of the country at different times. With increased scientific communication, the gap between initial report and multiple follow-up has decreased dramatically. Such a speed-up is not always desirable; the rush to be correct both scientifically or make new technologies standard before they have withstood any test of time can lead to significant problems.

We would suggest a protocol for any new idea that is to be assessed as a potential standard of care:

- Presentation of the idea in a well-designed format to a peer review process
- Confirmation of the study by independent groups
- Detailed analysis of confounding variables by a collaborative effort

No idea should be accepted on the basis of a single report.

REFERENCES

1. Baskett TF, Sandy E: Letter: False negative oxytocin challenge tests. Am J Obstet Gynecol 123(1):106, 1975
2. Bhakthavathsalan A, Mann LI, Tejani NA, Weiss RR: Correlation of the oxytocin challenge test with perinatal outcome. Obstet Gynecol 48(5):552–556, 1976
3. Boehm FH, Braun RD, Growdon JH Jr, Sherrell JW: The oxytocin challenge test. South Med J 69(7):884–886, 1976
4. Boehm FH, Growdon JH Jr: Letter: The oxytocin challenge test. Am J Obstet Gynecol 119(6):862–863, 1974
5. Boyd IE, Chamberlain GV, Fergusson IL: The oxytocin stress test and the isoxsuprine placental transfer test in the management of suspected placental insufficiency. Br J Obstet Gynaecol 81(2):120–125, 1974
6. Christie GB, Cudmore DW: The oxytocin challenge test. Am J Obstet Gynecol 118(3):327–330, 1974
7. Cooper JM, Soffronoff ED, Bolognese RJ: Oxytocin challenge test in monitoring high-risk pregnancies. Obstet Gynecol 45(1):27–33, 1975
8. Ewing DE, Farina JR, Otterson WN: Clinical application of the oxytocin challenge test. Obstet Gynecol 43(4):563–566, 1974
9. Farahani G, Vasudeva K, Petrie R, Fenton AN: Oxytocin challenge test in high-risk pregnancy. Obstet Gynecol 47(2):253–254, 1976
10. Freeman RK: The use of the oxytocin challenge test for antepartum clinical evaluation of uteroplacental respiratory function. Am J Obstet Gynecol 121(4):481–489, 1975
11. Freeman RK, Goebelsman UW, Nochimson D, Cetrulo C: An evaluation of the significance of positive oxytocin challenge test. Obstet Gynecol 47(1):8–13, 1976
12. Freeman RK, James J: Clinical experience with the oxytocin challenge test. II. An ominous atypical pattern. Obstet Gynecol 46(3):255–259, 1975
13. Gaziano EP, Hill DL, Freeman DW: The oxytocin challenge test in the management of high-risk pregnancies. Am J Obstet Gynecol 121(7):947–950, 1975
14. Hammacher K: Früher Kennung intrauterino Gefahrenzustände durch Electrophonocardiographie und Facographie. In Elert N, Huter KA (eds): Die Prophylaxie früh kindliche Hirnschaden, pp 120–131. Stuttgart, George Theime, 1966
15. Hayden BL, Simpson JL, Ewing DE, Otterson WN: Can the oxytocin challenge test serve as the primary method for managing high-risk pregnancies? Obstet Gynecol 46(3):251–254, 1975
16. Hon EH: An Atlas of Fetal Heart Rate Patterns. New Haven, Harty Press, 1968
17. Huntingford PJ, Pendelton HJ: The clinical application of cardiotocography. Br J Obstet Gynaecol 76:586–595, 1969
18. Klapholz H, Burke L: Intrauterine fetal demise with a negative oxytocin challenge test. J Reprod Med 15(4):169–170, 1975
19. Kubli FW, Kaeser O, Hinselmann M: Diagnostic management of chronic placental insufficiency. In Pecile A, Fenzi C (eds): The Foeto-Placental Unit, pp 323–339. Amsterdam, Excerpta Medica Foundation, 1969
20. Pose SV, Costello JB, Mora Rojas ET et al: Test of fetal tolerance to induced uterine contractions for the diagnosis of chronic stress. In Perinatal Factors Affecting Human Development, pp 96–104. Washington, DC, Pan American Health Organization, 1969
21. Ray M, Freeman RK, Pine S, Hesselgesser R:

Clinical experience with the oxytocin challenge test. Am J Obstet Gynecol 114(1):1–9, 1972
22. Schifrin B: Fetal heart rate patterns following epidural anesthesia and oxytocin infusion during labor. Br J Obstet Gynaecol 79:332–339, 1972
23. Spurrett B: Stressed cardiotocography in late pregnancy. Br J Obstet Gynaecol 79:894–900, 1971

SECTION 2: Technology Assessment and Reimbursement: Implications for Fetal Diagnosis and Therapy

Wayne I. Roe

Technology creates momentum and is irreversible. Nothing can be uninvented. . . . While any device can be made obsolete, no device can be forgotten, or erased from the arsenal of technology. . . . Our inability to uninvent will prove ever more troublesome as our technology proliferates and refines more and more unimagined, seemingly irrelevant wants.[2]

Few observers of America's health care system would argue that our virtually limitless capacity to innovate has helped create a dilemma of major proportions for those whose job it is to keep medical care inflation within socially tolerable limits. We are a public diagnosed with medical technology "schizophrenia,"[1] at once wishing for more spending directed at medical research breakthroughs, while simultaneously feeling we are spending far too much on health care. In addition, modern medical marvels have raised equally profound ethical, legal, and social questions regarding such issues as the right to die and the ability to conceive children outside the body.

No area of health care has been more affected by the development of technology and its attendant policy problems than fetal diagnosis and therapy. In the 1970s and 1980s, advances in in vitro fertilization, neonatal intensive care units (NICU), fetal monitoring, diagnostic ultrasound, cesarean delivery, and various prenatal screening tests have dramatically increased our ability to successfully attain, manage, and complete a pregnancy. Simultaneously, these advances have contributed significant economic costs (several thousands of dollars per day for NICU, for example) and multiple other spillovers, ranging from claims of unnecessary cesareans and fetal ultrasound examinations to rising abortion rates.

To date our medical system has not successfully developed a public or private sector technology policymaking process to manage these conflicts. In fact, recent efforts to erect both a federally directed technology assessment process and a public-private technology policy consortium have been uneventful. It is hard to imagine that this situation can be permanent, and there are several major developments in both the public and private sectors that signal more systematic technology management. Fetal diagnosis and therapy will inevitably be drawn into this managerial network, and physicians, hospitals, patients, and technology developers must be prepared.

DEVELOPMENTS IN HEALTH CARE DELIVERY

The organization and financing of the health care system in the United States through the sixties and seventies remained extremely accepting of new developments in fetal diagnosis and treatment. The financing system was structured around principles of cost-based payment for hospital care and charge-based reimbursement for physicians services. Medicare, Medicaid, and private insurers paid relatively little attention to bills for new medical services, so that fetal monitoring during labor, ultrasound during pregnancy, amniocentesis, and related technologies diffused rapidly through the health care system.

During this period, national health expenditures as a proportion of national income rose from 5.5% to almost 10% annually, which led to federal efforts at regulatory health planning and hospital utilization review. However, the passive attitude of health care payers fueled the growth of health care institutions, service providers, and technology developments. This overwhelmed regulatory hurdles and contributed to new medical expenditures. The public, of course, benefited tremendously from the growth in access to technology. In the area of fetal diagnosis and treatment, there were proportionately fewer complications at birth, increased survival of premature infants, and a greater ability to help couples with fertility problems.

Major public and private insurers fund 90% of all hospital care and two-thirds of all physicians services. Despite the benefits brought by medical advances, payers began in the 1980s to consider ways to inject more economic discipline into decisions about the use of medical resources. In particular, they have begun to ask more questions about the actual costs, risks, and benefits of medical interventions, as well as to establish payment mechanisms that force doctors and patients to do likewise.

Many financing and organizational changes have been developed to accomplish this task. The most prominent, of course, is the Medicare Prospective Payment System (PPS) for the elderly and disabled. This revolutionary approach reimburses institutions a fixed payment determined in advance for 470 mutually exclusive disease conditions (e.g., $3000 for a case of pneumonia). The prospective payments are based on average costs for all patients with that condition. Under this system hospitals are placed at financial risk for applying new diagnostic or therapeutic tools inappropriately, but rewarded for cost-effective use.

Because the diagnosis-related group system applies only to elderly and disabled patients, it has few direct implications for fetal diagnosis and therapy. However, it is a bellwether for future payer efforts at managing costs. In particular, health maintenance organizations (HMOs), which bundle payments for all medical services into a fixed annual capitated amount, and preferred provider organizations (PPOs), which negotiate fee discounts with efficient health care doctors and hospitals, provide similar incentives for economical use of technologies for generally younger patients. These systems now cover almost one-quarter of the United States population and will likely begin to influence the use of fetal-oriented technologies, because they recognize that without incentives for provider prudence they will be unable to compete in an increasingly cost-conscious market. Furthermore, they increasingly recognize that "managed care insurance" efforts to influence physician behavior may help avoid many socially undesirable outcomes, as noted in *Newsweek:*

> Processing equipment creates a psychological disposition to run tests and a legal imperative as well since failing to run a test may be grounds for a lawsuit. . . . A fellow obstetrician gave a new examination called an alpha-fetoprotein (AFP) test to one of his patients. The AFP is reasonably, though not completely, effective at predicting whether a baby will be born with a defect such as spina bifida, which often, though not always, causes profound retardation. The drawback is the test sometimes appears to find defects that aren't really there. The obstetrician administered a second AFP, also positive. Next he performed a sonogram. This sound-wave viewing of the womb can determine the exact stage of pregnancy, which has bearing on interpreting AFP results. But the sonogram was inconclusive. The doctor moved on to an amniocentesis. The procedure accurately predicts birth defects but also may lead to spontaneous stillbirth. This is an effect doctors do not know how to control, and it happened to the woman in question. Her baby, now lost, was revealed to have been perfectly normal all along.[3]

Major public and private insurers recognize that, in many ways, the generosity of past systems created too many of these unfortunate situations. The managed care revolution in payment insists on a stronger test of medical necessity in the application of AFP and other technologies. The potential savings in both personal suffering and economic costs are great, and systems are being developed to perform more technology evaluations. In the words of one leading-edge payer, "it is necessary to evaluate the impact of new technology. . . . Over the past decade decisionmaking has become more structured and technology assessment has begun to emerge as a discipline"* to inform reimbursement and regulatory decisions about medical advances. Both the quality of clinical medicine and its cost-effectiveness may improve as a result.

PRESSING NEEDS AND PAST POLICIES

Attempts to manage fetal technologies in the past through technology assessment and reimbursement policy met with little success. In the late seventies, an organization known as the National Center for Health Care Technology (NCHCT) was established within the United States Public Health Service to advise the Secretary of Health and Human Services (HHS) and other key government agencies on the economic, social, ethical, legal, and other consequences of new medical innovations. Among its duties, the center was directed to establish a target list of emerging medical technologies as an "early warning system"[6b] for items that might be assessed before they diffused rapidly into the medical market. Furthermore, the NCHCT was directed to advise both the Medicare program and, by disseminating information, other public and private insurers about "the impacts of particular health care technologies . . . as well as develop exemplary standards, norms, and criteria concerning the use of a particular technology".[6a]

One of the first and most controversial issues to be managed by the NCHCT process was the release of AFP testing. The Federal Drug Administration (FDA), Centers for Disease Control (CDC), NCHCT, and several other HHS agencies collaborated in an effort to examine "a wide-range of medical and scientific, ethical, legal, economic and other considerations" before the reagents were released to the market. In particular, because of the relatively high false-positive and false-negative rates from AFP testing, the NCHCT felt that screening without follow-up ultrasonography and genetic counseling could lead to unnecessary patient anxiety, abortions, and medical costs. There were also legal questions raised about AFP testing, particularly suggestions "that as such screening becomes more standard, those bearing children with open neural tube defects may well win lawsuits against physicians failing to inform them of the AFP test's availability".[4] The NCHCT's deliberations on AFP were designed to limit its diffusion as a screening tool to "well-integrated programs encompassing such components as laboratory facilities, education and counseling resources for follow-up of those with positive AFP levels, mechanisms of payment, and quality control".[4]

Despite a significant amount of publicity generated on AFP by the NCHCT, and some near-term success in slowing the release of test kits by the FDA, the effort to manage this emerging fetal diagnostic test ultimately proved unsuccessful. In 1981 the Reagan administration defunded the NCHCT based on concerns raised by organized medicine that it was too regulatory and duplicative of other government agencies. However, AFP diagnostic test kits were released by the FDA until 1983, and the notion of national regulatory norms for AFP screening was abandoned. The concept was readdressed in 1983 by the President's Commission for the Study of Ethical Problems in Medicine and Biomedical and Behavioral Research. This panel recommended that genetic screening programs not be initiated without a full range of prescreening and follow-up services available. How-

---

* R. Schaffarizk, vice president, Blue Shield of California. Personal communication.

ever, no formal HHS regulatory management of AFP is on the horizon.

Since the NCHCT was defunded, there have been other efforts to establish centralized technology assessment processes to deal with the multifaceted effects of medical technologies like AFP. Most notably, in 1986 the Institute of Medicine (IOM), National Academy of Sciences, established a Council on Health Care Technology to examine the appropriate use of both medical technology and the methods used to evaluate it. This new effort is jointly funded by federal and private sector contributions. It clearly reveals the ongoing political recognition of the policy concerns that technologies like those in fetal diagnosis and testing brings before society. The ethical, economic, legal, and other controversies are well recognized by even the most casual observers of health care technological development.

However the IOM group has also found, as did the NCHCT, that listing the issues associated with technologies, and even analyzing the size and distribution of their impacts, is much easier than developing and enforcing a consensus on the use of any particular innovation. Many medical technologies, particularly those associated with the unborn, raise too many issues for centralized technology management. Just as the NCHCT was unable to define the use of AFP screening, so too is the IOM finding it difficult to build a private market consensus on the appropriate applications of or constraints on technologies.

While public and private insurers would like very much for a single technology assessment group to provide them with definitive and legally enforceable guidelines for use of specific technologies, the IOM has yet to fill that void. There are two reasons for this. First, the state of clinical research rarely provides conclusive direction on the use of medical technologies. Second, individuals providing recommendations on standards of medical practice subject themselves to legal risks and public attacks. Until progress can be made on both fronts, the IOM will likely serve principally as a clearinghouse and public educational body for technology studies generated by multiple private and public organizations.[5]

FUTURE DIRECTIONS

Our failure to develop a centralized technology evaluation process in the face of explosive growth of fetal and other technologies reflects "our current inability to make and enforce decisions about what medical services we need and can afford.

> These are essentially social decisions, and in the face of the forces that promote the acquisition and use of medical technologies, they must be made in the context of a political consensus concerning both medical care priorities and resource allocation.[5]

Given our lack of progress in developing social consensus during the past 10 years, it seems unlikely that a broad-based national fetal technology assessment and reimbursement program will evolve in the next decade. However, this does not mean that manufacturers, geneticists, physicians, patients, and institutions will have unfettered access to the resources needed to develop and use advances in fetal and genetic technologies. Rather, the economic pressures created by our ability to do more are stimulating an array of decentralized responses to manage the cost of care, and with it, these technologies. These managed care pressures will grow with public awareness and demand for fertility technology, the malpractice-induced demand for expensive genetic diagnostics, and hospital interests in marketing state-of-the-art medical services.

The forces pressing for economic management of medical interventions are different among public and private payers, but both point in the same direction. For public payers, the dominant forces are the potential shortfalls in health insurance program budgets, the pressures of overall government deficits, and the divisiveness among provider organizations on important policy issues. In the first case, despite major program reforms in Medicare, Medicaid, Maternal and Child

Health programs, and other federal, state, and local health care initiatives, medical expenditures continue to rise faster than the national income. Since 1983, when Medicare's PPS and numerous state medicaid program reforms took effect, health spending as a percentage of national income grew from 10% to 11%. This growth put enormous pressures on federal and state budget deficits. Health programs, the third largest component of the federal budget, helped fuel federal budget deficits to an average of more than $150 billion since 1984. Added to this financial pressure is a health care provider industry which is finding it more difficult to unite against policy thrusts. Hospitals, physicians specialty groups, manufacturers, and others appear to be focused on policies that benefit them individually, thus providing federal and state authorities the opportunity to play one organization against the other.

On the private insurance side, concerns about rising medical expenditures are also bringing calls for technology management. Employers, the ultimate payers for much of privately financed care, are heavily engaged in health benefits management. Many employers have significantly altered benefits in recent years to increase patient co-payments, institute utilization review programs, offer HMO options, and expand coverage to low-cost treatment settings in an effort to economize on services. Furthermore, most large corporations have coupled benefits changes with a move to self-insurance, which has prompted traditional third-party payers to develop cost management programs, multiple option policies, and other innovations with the potential to influence technology use. Additionally, a number of national hospital chains have been experimenting with integrated insurance-hospital systems. These organizations provide even more direct opportunities for third-party payment incentives to dictate the use of fetal diagnostics and therapies.

The pressures on public and private payers to moderate health expenditure growth in the coming years will undoubtedly continue to grow. Many of the easy changes in medical care have already been made, such as reducing hospital admissions for outpatient care and shortening lengths of stay. Many feel that cost management in the future must begin to reduce marginally beneficial diagnostic and therapeutic interventions. Public and private payers are developing technology evaluation mechanisms of varying degrees of sophistication to provide a clinical foundation for technology management. The tools for this management will involve benefits coverage prescriptions, reimbursement limits to discourage proliferation of new services, and shifting of financial risk to providers to make them economically responsible for ordering new services.

Whether payers will be successful in constraining technology use is unclear. For example, the Harvard Community Health Plan (HCHP), a well respected HMO in Boston, waged a multiyear policy debate regarding coverage of in vitro fertilization. One important concern behind this policy noncoverage was the high cost of this technology (up to $5000 per intervention), and the low probability (24%–50%) of success in each attempt at fertilization. Many plan beneficiaries raised concerns about the HCHP policy, particularly because the plan simultaneously provided coverage for a number of high-cost, low frequency organ transplants. This kind of opposition to technology management recently was resolved in technology's favor at Kaiser Health Plans, a California HMO corporation. They first settled a legal dispute over their denial of coverage for in vitro fertilization for California subscribers, and now cover the technology for plan beneficiaries.

To stand up to the pressures of patients, providers, and the courts, technology management in the future must have its roots firmly grounded in peer-reviewed research and formal empirical analysis. A model for this approach has recently been established in the Technology Evaluation and Coverage (TEC) program of the Blue Cross and Blue Shield Association of America. This program provides guidance to member plans on the coverage, reimbursement, and management of new medical diagnostics and therapies.

For example, in 1986, such fetal diagnostic and therapy technologies as chorionic villus sampling, in vitro fertilization, and sperm penetration assays were considered by TEC.

To manage decisions regarding these controversial interventions, TEC is designed to "provide an objective, reproducible basis for evaluating the clinical utility of medical technologies." A technology that meets all five of the following criteria is considered eligible for coverage.

1. The technology must have final approval from the appropriate government regulatory bodies.
2. The scientific evidence must permit conclusions concerning the effect of the technology on health outcomes.
3. The technology must improve the net health outcome.
4. The technology must be as beneficial as any established alternatives.
5. The improvement must be attainable outside the investigational settings.[8]

The TEC program staff employs a rigorous process of literature review, expert consultant deliberations, and economic modeling to develop program policy recommendations. Member plans receive advisories on all phases of technology management including coverage, conditions for use, payment and pricing of services, and benefits design. Many feel that this program has the requisite and resource base and analytic rigor necessary to effectively shape future Blue Cross technology policy development.

The aggressiveness of HCHP, Kaiser, and Blue Cross and Blue Shield in challenging traditional policy norms that allow providers and patients access to whatever technologies they believe are appropriate represents a major shift in approach to fetal diagnosis and therapy. Federal and state authorities are also likely to challenge "automatic payment" for new services through targeted coverage and reimbursement reviews. It is impossible to predict the precise form and impact which these evolving technology assessment and reimbursement hurdles will take. Some question whether they will be effective in light of public demands for new advances and the legal liability attendant in fetal medicine. One thing is certain, however, and that is that efforts will be made to manage these new innovations. Those involved in the mainstream of fetal diagnosis and therapy must take the challenges seriously.

REFERENCES

1. Altman D, Blendon R: Public attitudes about health care costs: A lesson in national schizophrenia. N Engl J Med 311:616, 1974
2. Boorstin DJ: The Republic of Technology: Reflections on Our Future Community. New York, Harper & Row, 1978
3. Easterbrook G: The revolution in modern medicine. Newsweek, 109:68, January 26, 1987
4. MSAFP: Issues in the prenatal screening and diagnosis of neural tube defects. Draft conference summary, pp 7–8. Washington, DC, National Center for Health Care Technology, July 28, 1980.
5. Newletter. Council on Health Care Technology, Institute of Medicine, vol 1, November 4, 1987
6. Policy and Program. Draft HHS document, pp 8(a), 15(b). Washington, DC, National Center for Health Care Technology, June 28, 1979
7. TEC program description. Blue Cross and Blue Shield Association of America, 1987

SECTION 3: Liability and Emerging Technology

Frederic M. Rosen

The proliferation of malpractice actions, although generally viewed negatively by the medical profession, has generated some salutary effects, namely, upgrading the delivery of health care in certain fields and effecting the removal of grossly incompetent physicians from the scene. Less clearly understood is the situation wherein the generally competent physician is alleged to have committed a specific act of negligence causing physical damage to the patient.

Medicolegal issues are defined and shaped by the technology available to the ordinary (average) practitioner. Problems invariably arise along the continuum from conceptualization to accepted mode of care. To the lawyer, either proper care is rendered or it is not and this is clearly defined by the "standard in the industry." To the physician, medicine is an art and should rarely be subjected to finite (i.e., legal) examination and deliberation. It is this inherently dichotomous divergence which blocks interprofessional understanding and communication.

In this chapter we shall use the data base of Chapter 8, Section 1 and explore how deviations from accepted standards could be approached medicolegally at various points during technological development.

STANDARD OF CARE

Standard of care, like many terms in the medicolegal arena, is not capable of constant, singular definition; it is often a dynamic, changing concept formulated and molded by the advances in science, medical technology, and the continuing computer mechanization prevalent in modern society. In actuality, the evolving standard mirrors and reflects the expectations of our society.

From the attorney's perspective, standard of care has little mystical connotation: the operative word is *standard*—what the normally trained, competent physician would do in same or similar circumstances. For example, the State of Michigan (where the author practices as a plaintiff's negligence attorney) has now codified the developing common law as construed by its judiciary, Michigan Complied Law Annotated 600. 2912, provides as follows:

In an action alleging malpractice the Plaintiff shall have the burden of proving that *in light of the State of the art existing at the time* then of the alleged malpractices:

a) The defendant, if a general practitioner, failed to provide the Plaintiff the *recognized standard of acceptable professional practice in the community in which the Defendant practices or in a similar community*, and that as a proximate result of the Defendant failing to provide that standard, the Plaintiff suffered an injury.

b) The Defendant, if a specialist, failed to provide the recognized standard of care *within that speciality as reasonably applied in light of the facilities available in the community* or *other facilities reasonably available under the circumstances*, and as a proximate result of the Defendant failing to provide that standard, the Plaintiff suffered the injury. [Emphasis added.]

Although a physician in Michigan is not held to the high standards of a physician on the cutting edge of technologic innovation, he or she is required to use all reasonable modes of diagnostic tools and treatment which are reasonably available.

The above-quoted statute does not, in essence, change the history of the law in this particular area. In the case of *Ballance v. Dunnington* (1928),[1] the court clearly enunciated the obligations of both parties in a medical negligence suit:

Plaintiff had the burden of showing that he suffered an x-ray burn occasioned by an overdosage or exposure of his foot, and that such happened *because Defendant failed to exercise the reasonable and ordinary care, skill and diligence possessed by others in the same line of practice and work in similar localities.*

With mass dissemination of knowledge and information available to all practitioners, the exclusivity of the Locality Rule has been abrogated and the standards made to include practice in all *similar* communities. This interpretation will help ensure competent medical care and treatment for all similarly situated patients throughout the United States.

Although excellence and creative genius is appreciated and applauded in any field, they are *not* relevant when presenting the applicable standard of care. Perfection never has been the relevant standard in any state. However, modern medical practice (through the initial physical examination, testing, clinical diagnosis, and treatment) is being shaped by the development, expectations, and growth of the modern consumer society. We have come to expect a reasonable standard whether buying a car, dinner at a luxurious restaurant, or undergoing bypass surgery. It is this expectation and search for competency that drives the consumer's search for expertise and quality. Every physician, attorney, or clergyman must be responsive and diligent; if not, every patient, client or penitent is a potential adversary and rightfully so.

Empirically, the demand for competent, standardized service translates into better products and services for all. It is the 20th century equivalent of the utilitarian principle espoused by Jeremy Bentham ("The greater good for the greater number"). Both the legal and medical professions are producing consumer-oriented products. When the consumer is wronged he seeks the appropriate redress. From the very beginning, the doctor-patient relationship has been predicated upon an innate trust on the part of the patient. Once this bond of trust has been severely impaired or destroyed, the patient feels distress, disappointment, and despair. Logically, the wronged consumer seeks the appropriate redress. If a patient or his family feels aggrieved, they may contact a personal injury attorney for advice, who has the responsibility, much like a physician, to obtain the appropriate history, obtain the involved medical records, obtain expert assistance, and render his "diagnosis." In doing so, the concept of standard of care is accorded primacy.

APPLICATION TO OBSTETRIC PRACTICE

No other area of medicine has been placed under closer scrutiny than obstetric practice, for three primary reasons. First, the physician is dealing with the hopes, aspirations, heart, soul, and future of the patient—her children. Second, there are certain prenatal and perinatal signs which clearly exhibit potential trouble or complications (e.g., postmaturity, high maternal blood pressure, preeclampsia, meconicum staining). Third, many complications can now be identified by such standardized tests as fetal monitoring, systematic measurement of fundal height and weight, ultrasound, and early genetic determination.

In order to demonstrate the deductive reasoning which develops over time to evoke the applicable standard in obstetric care, we will use the events presented in Section 1 ("Evolution of the oxytocin challenge tests as a diagnostic tool") from concept to the legal articulation of standard of care. We will analyze from inception, through development and, ultimately, birth.

In 1966, Hammacher[9] conceived the possible correlation between Syntocinon-induced contractions and the capability of the fetus to withstand labor. The germination of this concept led directly to the next logical step, empirical testing, of whether Syntocinon would be harmful to the mother or fetus (always the paramount question).

In 1969, Kubli and associates[11] conducted research into the physiologic basis of fetal heart rate patterns relative to the prediction of insufficient fetal oxygenation. Their statement, "Placental respiratory function as a prediction of fetal hypoxia in late pregnancy was evaluated by measuring the response of the fetal heart to oxytocin-induced contractions," and others were precursors of the evolutionary development of the applicable standard of care in this particular area. These and other tests conducted during the same year added a clinical, statistical measure to support the use of oxytocin (OCT) as an indicator of potential fetal respiratory and neurologic damage. Also in 1969, Huntingford and Pendelton[11] further refined the basic premise and classified fetal heart tracings into categories of benign, pathologic, or possibly pathologic.

In 1971, the research conducted by Spurrett[15] provided invaluable information into the areas of feasibility and lack of deliterious side-effects. Within 20 minutes of administration (assuming no evidence of pathology), this particular test "was useful for rapid evaluation of fetal well being." In the hourly life span of labor and delivery, the ability to conduct tests with rapidity and attach integrity to the results is clearly beneficial and essential. Concurrently, and of equal importance, Spurrett's studies indicated no induction of premature labor which could, of course, open up a Pandora's box of additional, potential complications. However, Spurrett's conclusion would *clearly not* reach the level of standard of care:

> The Syntocinon stress test was thought to be a useful adjunct in monitoring high-risk pregnancies, especially when used in conjunction with serum estriol measurement.[15]

Nevertheless, the diligent physician was now aware of the benefits of OCT testing; the previous studies had provided a printed and documented *caveat emptor:* Let the obstetrician be aware that additional research was being conducted and there was a reasonable probability that this test would soon be an accepted (additional) measure and of potential use in determining the viability of the fetus relative to the rigors and duress of labor.

At this point we can visualize the growth of the concept and attach to it substantive clinical significance. Although it had yet to be fully documented and refined into a definable standard disseminated to physicians at large, the physician was still obligated to avail himself of all available data. A conscientious plaintiff's attorney handling a birth trauma case arising at or about that time would ask the attending physician if he was *familiar* with these studies. Again, this would not establish the breach of any standard (since it had yet to be established), but would indicate the degree of the physician's diligence and concern for the well-being of the mother and fetus. Considering the above information along with the studies conducted by Pose[13] (who correlated the appearance of late decelerations with fetal prognosis), the beginning stage for the development of an additional standard for fetal care was evident.

Perhaps the prudent obstetrician in 1971 would basically agree with the above premise, but would hesitate to routinely administer and rely on said tests, due to the lack of substantial, controlled testing. In 1972, Ray,[14] produced statistics from a considerable sample (43 high-risk patients) which clearly indicated the correlation between the administration of OCT and the prediction of fetal damage or demise. Still, no standard had yet to be enunciated; the measurement of estriols was still considered to be the gold standard for determination of fetal well-being.

At this point, the ingredients for standard of care are in place. We know what the test is, how it is administered, the purpose, and the lack of apparent adverse risks (assuming proper administration and observation). By now, the observant physician should be aware of the state of the art and seriously consider practical application within his practice. To do less would be to rob the expectant mother of a valid birthing alternative, which may be crucial to the difference between a healthy baby and an abnormal baby. From the publications to date, 1972, the obstetrician knew, or with due diligence should have known, of the benefits of OCT testing and its applicability to practice. This imputed knowledge is no different from the general standard we all live by—that we should never, by commission or omission, injure another. If our acts of misfeasance or malfeasance are the proximate cause of injuries, we are legally responsible for the natural and probable consequences. Why should a mother in the final stages of conception and her fetus be entitled to less?

Concepts such as standard of care are not static, but change as quickly as research, technological application, and professional acceptance will allow. A plaintiff's attorney handling a medical malpractice case in 1973 could (with expert corroboration) postulate the premise that OCT testing had, in fact, become the standard of care for identified high-risk obstetrical patients. This is only a hypothetical postulation, because there is no evidence that this was, in fact, "the recognized standard of acceptable professional practice in the community in which the Defendant practices or in a similar community." Moreover, the obstetrician specialist is *not* required to administer any tests or provide care which has not become widely accepted within his specialty. To require as much would be an unfair burden and is recognized as such in the legal community. One does not have to be the best obstetrician, but only equal to the majority of his or her peers.

As the reader is certainly aware, it would have been most unusual if all the research and testing in this particular area had proceeded without negative, critical evaluation. In 1974, two reports began to question the reliability of OCT in the evaluation of fetal well-being. Just as the concept of OCT testing for high-risk maternal patients was about to crown, a misstep occurred. Christie and Cudmore[4] concluded from their study of 50 high-risk patients "that there was no correlation between a positive OCT and low-estriols, APGAR scores, or fetal distress in labor." Additionally, Boyd[3] (in an unsubstantiated sample) reported two fetal deaths following negative OCTs. Assuming that obstetricians were not generally using OCT testing on high-risk patients in 1974, a challenged physician could point not only to the lack of mass professional acceptance, but to the above skeptical studies as well. However, such reliance would certainly have been misplaced and, at best, short-lived.

In 1974, the crowning of the concept finally occurred. Ewing[6] (using a larger sample) essentially agreed with Ray "that a positive oxytocin challenge test was indicative of an unfavorable fetal environment." Interestingly, Boehm and colleagues[2] suggested that the prior (negative) findings by Christie and Cudmore[4] were based upon the subjective interpretation of the OCTs, rather than the substantive test itself and, therefore, should be called into question. The following year Cooper[5] carried the process even further by strategically pointing out the obvious benefits of OCT testing and its accurate prediction of potential fetal insult. The final push to accept OCT testing was initiated by Freeman[8] in 1975. His indisputable study of 1500 tests in 600 patients clearly demonstrated the benefit of OCT administration, that a positive test was indicative of decreased placental function. Serum estriol measurements were still considered to be the gold standard, but not for long.

Probably the only basis for claiming that OCT testing was *not* the standard of care relative to the evaluation of high-risk maternal patients was the pronouncements by researchers in the field. Late in 1975, the concept was actually born in a two-pronged announcement. First Hayden[10] directly concluded that OCT was the primary standard for management of high-risk pregnancies. Then, in 1976, Farahani[7] made the ultimate statement that "OCT was a more sensitive test than urinary estriols as an indicator of fetal well-being."

By tedious, documented detail, research had clearly indicated that modern obstetric practice *needed* OCT testing in order to avoid unnecessary complications of high-risk pregnancies. By 1976, there had been sufficient, scientific, randomized testing in trials to validate OCT testing. Clearly, at this point, the applicable standard of care had been realized and any physician who failed to consider or implement OCT testing in the appropriate circumstances was acting below standard and was subject to legal consequences. In this particular area, the law allows the medical community to set its own standards. Standard of care becomes a synonym for "acceptable professional practice" and should be considered as a realistic, viable standard by which all professionals should live; the consumer society will expect and accept no less.

To return to our original example, a judge in Michigan at the conclusion of the trial would instruct the jury as follows:

When I use the words "professional negligence" or "malpractice" with respect to the Defendant's conduct, I mean the failure to do something which a physician of ordinary learning, judgment or skill in (this community or a similar one) practicing obstetrics would do or the doing of something which a physician of ordinary learning, judgment or skill would not do, under the same or similar circumstances you find to exist in this case.

It is for you to decide, based upon the evidence, what the ordinary physician of ordinary learning, judgment or skill would do or would not do under the same or similar circumstances. (Michigan Standard Jury Instructions—Civil. Second Edition, Vol. I.)

The operative word is *ordinary*. Again, our hypothetical physician is held to a standard of reasonable, acceptable, and obtainable competency. Contrary to the conventional wisdom, a bad result does not automatically indicate a breach of the applicable standard of care or a large jury verdict. Unless the nexus between the physician's negligence (breach of duty) and the plaintiff's damages can be reached through the concept of proximate cause, there is no recovery.

The interrelationship between medical technological advance and the legal concept of standard of care can often be a dynamic process subject to reevaluation on a periodic basis. In the case of OCT testing, if every physician in the country was immediately aware of the experiments, tests, and research as soon as each was accomplished, we would have the ultimate mass dissemination of information. It is quite possible that some practicing obstetricians considered the administration of OCT testing an indispensable adjunct to be used for all high-risk pregnancies *prior* to 1976. (It appears that the feasibility and applicability of OCT was accepted by virtually all obstetricians at that time.)

In order to show deviation from the applicable standard of care, the plaintiff's counsel would have to prove by a preponderance of the evidence that (1) OCT testing was necessitated by a particular case, and (2) that the failure to administer said test was a direct and proximate cause of the plaintiff's damages. It is apparent that an argument can be made that the prudent obstetrician should have been administering OCT testing in the early seventies, in particular after the 1972 study by Ray and co-workers correlated the relationship between OCT and prediction of fetal damage or demise.[14] If the plaintiff could produce expert testimony that the ordinary, prudent obstetrician in 1972 relied upon this test as a predictor of fetal well-being, then the jury must determine whether the defendant physician violated this standard and, if so, whether there was a proximate connection with the damages sustained by the fetus.

In reality, acceptable professional behavior is established by our peers. Like all professionals, physicians can only provide a better product if each and every member produces to the best of his ability based upon the accumulated knowledge available through continuing understanding, education, and vocational enlightenment.

REFERENCES

1. Ballance v. Dunnington, 241 Mich. Reports, 383, 1928.
2. Boehm FH, Braum RD, Growdon JH Jr, Sherrell JW: The oxytocin challenge test. South Med J 69(7):884–886, 1976
3. Boyd IE, Chamberlain GV, Fergusson IL: The oxytocin stress test and the isoxsuprine placental transfer test in the management of suspected placental insufficiency. J Obstet Gynaecol Br Commonw 81:120, 1974
4. Christie GB, Cudmore DW: The oxytocin challenge test. Am J Obstet Gynecol 118(3):327–330, 1974
5. Cooper JM, Soffronoff ED, Bolognese RJ: Oxytocin challenge test in monitoring high-risk pregnancies. Obstet Gynecol 45(1):27–33, 1975
6. Ewing DE, Farina JR, Otterson WN: Clinical application of the oxytocin challenge test. Obstet Gynecol 43(4):563–566, 1974
7. Farahani G, Vasudeva K, Petrie R, Fenton AN: Oxytocin challenge test in high-risk pregnancy. Obstet Gynecol 47(2):253–254, 1976
8. Freeman RK: The use of the oxytocin challenge test for antepartum clinical evaluation of uteroplacental respiratory function. Am J Obstet Gynecol 121:481, 1975
9. Hammacher K: Früher Kennung intrauterine Gefahrenzustände durch Electrophonocardi-

ographie und Facographie. In Elert N, Huter KA (eds): Die Prophylaxie früh kindliche Hirnschaden, pp 120–131. Stuttgart, George Theime, 1966
10. Hayden BL, Simpson JL, Ewing DE, Otterson WN: Can the oxytocin challenge test serve as the primary method for managing high-risk pregnancies? Obstet Gynecol 46(3):251–254, 1975
11. Huntingford PJ, Pendelton HJ: The clinical application of cariotocography. Br J Obstet Gynaecol 76:586–595, 1969
12. Kubli FW, Kaeser O, Hinselmann M: Diagnostic management of chronic placental insufficiency. In Pecile A, Fenzi C (eds): The Foeto-Placental Unit, pp 323–339. Amsterdam, Excerpta Medica Foundation, 1969
13. Pose SV, Costello JB, Mona-Rohas ET et al: Test of fetal tolerance to induced uterine contractions for the diagnosis of chronic stress. In Perinatal Factors Affecting Human Development, pp 96–104. Washington DC, Pan American Health Organization, 1969
14. Ray M, Freeman RK, Pine S, Hesselgesser R: Clinical experience with the oxytocin challenge test. Am J Obstet Gynecol 114(1):1–9, 1972
15. Spurrett B: Stressed cardiotocography in late pregnancy. Br J Obstet Gynaecol 79:894–900, 1971

9

High-Risk Situations: The Very Low Birth Weight Fetus

SECTION 1: Medical Considerations in Obstetric Management

Chin-Chu Lin

Successful perinatal outcome for very low birth weight (VLBW) fetuses depends upon continuous, meticulous effort throughout the antepartum, intrapartum, and neonatal periods. However, the decision-making required during the antepartum period is the most difficult and its impact on fetal outcome is usually profound. The obstetrician must always keep in mind that consideration of the risk-benefit ratio in each given case in deciding when and how to deliver the baby is the most important factor related to fetal outcome. In order to reach a decision, as much information as possible about the status of the fetus and the condition of a mother should be gathered.

The discussion in this chapter is concerned with the VLBW infant, those infants with birth weights between 500 and 1500 g. From an obstetric point of view, the fetus threatened with labor and delivery between 25 and 32 weeks gestation raises various questions concerning obstetric management such as:

- Will the infant survive?
- What types of immediate neonatal complications and long-term handicaps can be anticipated?
- Is the fetus associated with a major congenital anomaly and/or intrauterine growth retardation (IUGR)?
- Should labor be stopped?
- How should premature rupture of membranes (PROM) be managed during this period of gestation?
- What methods should be used to evaluate the fetus in terms of fetal size, fetal maturity, and fetal well-being?
- When delivery is inevitable, which route

of delivery should be chosen? Will cesarean section reduce perinatal mortality or neonatal morbidity?
- Will maternal transport to a tertiary care center improve fetal outcome?

This group of infants is particularly vulnerable to perinatal hypoxia, acidosis, and birth trauma. Thus, their long-term prognosis for mental and intellectual development, neurobehavioral handicaps, somatic growth retardation, and major organ system disorders must be carefully evaluated. The guiding concept in perinatal care for this extremely high-risk pregnancy is to provide a continuous team effort through the entire course of pregnancy, and during labor, delivery, and the neonatal period. The team should include not only the obstetricians and neonatologists, but also obstetric and intensive care nursery nurses, ultrasound experts, laboratory technicians, patient educators, and consultants from various medical specialties. Only a well coordinated, multidisciplinary action can further improve the prognosis for VLBW infants.

SURVIVAL RATES IN RELATION TO BIRTH WEIGHT, GESTATIONAL AGE, AND OTHER FACTORS

Preterm labor and delivery have been a significant cause of perinatal morbidity and mortality for centuries. Although the incidence of preterm labor varies from country to country, the impact of preterm delivery on perinatal mortality is always higher than any other single factor. In one report from the United States, 8% of deliveries that occurred preterm accounted for 75% of perinatal deaths.[82] A similar result was reported from England where 85% of neonatal deaths not due to lethal congenital anomalies occurred in infants born between 22 and 37 weeks gestation.[221] Prior to 1970, the survival expectation for infants between 1000 g to 1500 g was approximately 50%, while that for 500-g to 1000-g infants was only 10%.[164] Long-term follow-up studies of those infants of less than 1500 g at birth report that up to 70% of them manifest moderate to severe neurologic handicaps by age 10.[163] These discouraging data led to suggestions that obstetricians adopt a nonaggressive approach in treating VLBW fetuses born before 30 weeks of gestation.[105]

With the recent advances in intensive nursery care of VLBW newborns and more sophisticated obstetric management of pregnant women at risk of preterm delivery between 25 and 30 weeks gestation, the outlook for VLBW infants has been vastly improved.

The survival rate of the 500-g to 1000-g infant has increased from less than 10%[9,164] prior to 1970 to greater than 40%; since the late 1970s, the survival rate of the 1000-g to 1500-g infant has risen from 40%[9,164] to greater than 70%.[69,71,96,105,122,140,142,156,209,210,224]

Many factors interact to determine survival rate and the degree of long-term handicaps in VLBW infants. Birth weight, however, appears to be the single most important factor with respect to survival rate. Table 9-1 shows the survival rates for different weight groups of VLBW infants which were reported by various investigators in England, Belgium, Canada, and the United States between 1970 and 1985. Data from the Chicago Lying-In Hospital, University of Chicago,[156] are consistent with many recent reports. Roughly, the survival rate for the 500-g to 749-g birth weight group is 20% to 25%, while the rates for the 750-g to 999-g, 1000-g to 1249-g, and 1250-g to 1499-g groups are 50%, 75%, and 87% to 89%, respectively. Survival rates increase steadily with each increment in birth weight.

The gestational age of the newborn is second only to birth weight in its impact on the survival rate of VLBW infants. To facilitate analysis of neonatal mortality and morbidity, Battaglia and Lubchenco[19] divided newborn infants into nine subgroups classified by gestational age and birth weight. The value of using both birth weight and gestational age together to predict the neonatal

Table 9-1. Comparison of Neonatal Survival Rate in Infants Less Than 1500 g*

			Birth Weight (g)							
		500–749		750–999		1000–1249		1250–1499		
Author	Place (Years)	Births	Survival %	Births	Survival %	Births	Survival %	Births	Survival %
1. Fairweather[71]	London (1971–1977)	32	25	118	45	176	65	164	80
2. Saigal et al.[224]	Hamilton, Canada (1973–1978)	51	10	65	49	76	75	102	88
3. Knobloch et al.[140]	Albany (1975–1979)	44	0	74	32	211			
4. Hack et al.[105]	Cleveland (1976–1978)	44	20	119	56	139	73	165	87
5. Koops et al.[142]	Colorado (1974–1980)	82	27	108	55	196	79	152	89
6. Goldenberg et al.[96]	Alabama (1971–1980)				35.8				70.7
7. Gerara et al.[94]	Belgium (1976–1980)	127			22	172	65	205	70
8. Hoskins et al.[122]	Toronto (1979–1980)	39	49	67	79				
9. Lin[156]	Chicago (1981–1985)	127	19	89	47	135	78	107	89

* Reports were made after 1970 from one or multiple centers, except report no. 6, which was from the state of Alabama.

mortality rate has proven useful. For example, in a recent Colorado study,[142] the neonatal mortality rate of the 1000-g to 1499-g birth weight group was 16.4%, while mortality for the group with gestational ages of 29 to 31 weeks was 15.6%. Those infants with a birth weight of 500 g to 999 g had a mortality rate of 57.4%, compared to a mortality rate of 45% for those infants born at 26 to 28 weeks. The mortality rate for infants with a gestational age of less than 26 weeks or a birth weight of less than 500 g was virtually 100%. It appears obvious that the current lower limit for infant survival is 26 weeks. When delivery occurs before the 26th week of pregnancy, the fetus cannot survive outside the uterus no matter how aggressively intensive care is delivered.[142,227] Similarly, the survival of a less-than-700-g appropriate for gestational age (AGA) infant may be viewed as a rare exception.

An analysis of the survival rates of VLBW infants would be better done with separation between the AGA and the small for gestational age (SGA) neonate. Because IUGR and prematurity occur together in a substantial portion of low birth weight cases, however, the process of separating the two groups can often be complicated, misleading, and even impossible. Many of the high-risk factors which cause IUGR, such as preeclampsia, hypertension, multifetal pregnancy, maternal smoking, and sickle cell anemia, can also cause preterm delivery. Galbraith and colleagues[88] reported an incidence of 11% IUGR among 314 preterm infants. At the Chicago Lying-In Hospital from January 1979 to May 1981 there were 426 IUGR infants among a total of 7177 deliveries (approximately 6%). Breaking these cases down into gestational age subgroups revealed a higher incidence of IUGR in the earlier preterm gestations. The incidence of IUGR was 13.1% for 28 to 30 weeks of gestation, 9.4% for 31 to 33 weeks, 7.4% for 34 to 36 weeks, and 5.5% for those born after 37 weeks of gestation.[157] The prognosis for preterm IUGR infants is extremely serious. For a review of neonatal mortality in Colorado from 1974 to 1980, Koops and co-workers[142] reported a neonatal mortality rate of 71% for infants born between 26 and 29 weeks gestation who were preterm SGA versus 37% for AGA infants of the same gestational age. Between 29 and 32 weeks, the specific neonatal mortality rates for infants weighing less than 1500 g were 21% for SGA and 15% for AGA.

Other factors which are associated with a higher neonatal mortality rate are also secondary to an increased risk of delivering VLBW infants. Such factors include a nonwhite race,[69,171,179] a male infant,[171] a maternal age of 17 years or less,[173] and substandard medical care.[151,152] However, a high neonatal mortality rate in an industrialized community is primarily caused by the high birth rate of VLBW infants in such a population.[151]

CAUSES OF LOW BIRTH WEIGHT

The physiologic and biochemical events that initiate human labor, either prematurely or at term, are not well understood. Recent investigators have produced important new clues about the role of hormonal factors in the process of parturition.[39,42,91] Various risk factors appear to cause changes in the hormonal environment and the metabolic state of the uterus and cervix. These changes probably result from complex interactions involving progesterone, estrogen, prostaglandins, oxytocin, relaxin, calcium ions, catecholamines, adrenergic receptors, enzymes, myometrial gap junctions, and uteroplacental blood flow. Unfortunately, a detailed discussion of the mechanism of parturition is beyond the scope of this chapter.

Twenty years ago, Abramowicz and Kass[1] observed that 10% to 15% of preterm births resulted from obstetric intervention secondary to complications of pregnancy. These complications include preeclampsia, hypertension, placenta previa, abruptio placentae, diabetes mellitus, and Rh sensitization. In addition, relationships between preterm birth and various risk factors such as nutrition, anemia, smoking, high altitude, work during pregnancy, prenatal care, and bacteriuria among others have been intensively studied. A decade ago, Lubchenco[162] discussed possible correlations between preterm delivery and maternal or fetal conditions, including uterine malformations, incompatible blood groups, incompetent cervical os, multiple gestation, urinary tract infection, acute maternal systemic infections, PROM, low socioeconomic status, the very young mother, the black mother, and antepartum hemorrhage. Today most of these factors remain as high-risk factors for the preterm delivery. Table 9-2 summarizes the principal risk factors for low birth weight infants which were published in 1985 by the Committee to Study the Prevention of Low Birthweight.[46]

IUGR can be caused by both genetic and environmental factors that interact with cell proliferation, organ differentiation, and metabolic development in the process of fetal growth. These influences may be associated with a decreased growth potential of the fetus (type-I IUGR) or with restriction of fetal growth by a decrease in the supply of oxygen

Table 9-2. Principal Risk Factors for Low Birth Weight Infants

I. Demographic Risks
   A. Age (less than 17; over 34)
   B. Race (black)
   C. Low socioeconomic status
   D. Unmarried
   E. Low level of education

II. Medical Risks Predating Pregnancy
   A. Parity (0 or more than 4)
   B. Low weight for height
   C. Genitourinary anomalies/surgery
   D. Selected diseases such as diabetes, chronic hypertension
   E. Nonimmune status for selected infections such as rubella
   F. Poor obstetric history including previous low birth weight infant, multiple spontaneous abortions
   G. Maternal genetic factors (such as low maternal weight at own birth)

III. Medical Risks in Current Pregnancy
   A. Multiple pregnancy
   B. Poor weight gain
   C. Short interpregnancy interval
   D. Hypotension
   E. Hypertension/preeclampsia/toxemia
   F. Selected infections such as symptomatic bacteriuria, rubella, and cytomegalovirus
   G. 1st or 2nd trimester bleeding
   H. Placental problems such as placenta previa, abruptio placentae
   I. Hyperemesis
   J. Oligohydramnios
   K. Anemia/abnormal hemoglobin
   L. Isoimmunization
   M. Fetal anomalies
   N. Incompetent cervix
   O. Spontaneous premature rupture of membranes

(Continued)

Table 9-2. Principal Risk Factors for Low Birth Weight Infants (*Continued*)

IV. Behavioral and Environmental Risks
    A. Smoking
    B. Poor nutritional status
    C. Alcohol and other substance abuse
    D. DES exposure and other toxic exposures, including occupational hazards
    E. High altitude

V. Health Care Risks
    A. Absent or inadequate prenatal care
    B. Iatrogenic prematurity

VI. Evolving Concepts of Risk
    A. Stress (physical and psychosocial)
    B. Uterine irritability
    C. Events triggering uterine contractions
    D. Cervical changes detected before onset of labor
    E. Selected infections such as mycoplasma and *Chlamydia trachomatis*
    F. Inadequate plasma volume expansion
    G. Progesterone deficiency

(Adapted from Committee to Study the Prevention of Low Birthweight. Division of Health Promotion and Disease Prevention. Washington, DC, Institute of Medicine, National Academy Press, 1985)[46]

and nutrients from the mother to the fetus (type-II IUGR).[155,158] The possible causes of IUGR are many, but they can be divided into intrinsic and extrinsic factors. Some may be intrinsic to the fetus or placenta, while others may be extrinsic but act directly on the fetus, on both the fetus and the placenta, or on the placenta primarily and the fetus only secondarily. Examples of intrinsic causes of IUGR include such chromosomal abnormalities as trisomy 18 and Turner's syndrome. Intrauterine rubella infection in early pregnancy is a classic example of an extrinsic factor that produces IUGR by affecting both the fetus and the placenta. The most common extrinsic factors, affecting primarily the placenta during the second half of pregnancy, are related to reduced uteroplacental blood flow, or so-called uteroplacental insufficiency. When preeclampsia occurs in combination with IUGR, the incidence of vascular lesions found in placentas is high.[6,104,222] These placental lesions from IUGR pregnancies are also seen in placentas from normal newborn infants, indicating that the lesion is not specific for IUGR. It is probably the extent of placental damage, rather than the type of lesion, which is causally related to IUGR. Furthermore, the most important negative maternal influence on fetal growth is restriction of the supply of oxygen and nutrients to the fetus. Examples of these maternal complications and behavioral risk factors are preeclampsia, hypertension, multifetal gestation, sickle cell anemia, smoking, and chronic alcohol and drug abuse.

The timing of the interaction between etiologic factors and the stage of gestation plays an important role in determining whether type-I or type-II IUGR will occur in human pregnancies.[155,158] In the case of IUGR associated with genetic abnormalities or intrauterine TORCH* infections, the effect on fetal development occurs during the first trimester of gestation, interfering with hyperplastic cellular growth and organogenesis.

* Toxoplasmosis, other viruses, rubella, cytomegalovirus, herpes simplex viruses.

The result is a type-I IUGR infant with multiple organ system anomalies. On the other hand, the typical type-II IUGR infant is characterized by a disproportionately large head, small abdominal viscera, and a lack of subcutaneous fat tissue. However, no congenital anomalies are associated with type-II IUGR.

When birth weight is less than 1500 g, a large proportion of IUGR fetuses have congenital anomalies. The great majority of type-II IUGR infants have a birth weight between 1500 g and 2500 g,[106] indicating that the two major sources of VLBW-SGA infants are either type I IUGR or type-II IUGR resulting from severe maternal medical complications.

Clinical conditions such as an early onset of severe preeclampsia, chronic hypertension superimposed with severe preeclampsia,[11,159] sickle cell crisis,[74] active systemic lupus erythematosus,[60] recurrent pancreatitis,[262] and serious cardiopulmonary diseases[250,264] may require termination of pregnancy far before term. Many of these infants will turn out to be a preterm SGA. Nevertheless, careful antenatal evaluation for the presence or absence of gross congenital anomalies should be an important consideration in dealing with pregnancies at high risk for preterm SGA fetuses. An example of a preterm severe SGA infant is shown in Figure 9-1.

NEONATAL COMPLICATIONS

Of major concern in the care of VLBW newborn infants is the immaturity of their organ systems. As a result of this organ immaturity, various complications may occur during the neonatal period. These include problems affecting the pulmonary (apnea, respiratory distress), cardiovascular (hypotension, bleeding, persistent fetal circulation), metabolic (acidosis, hypoglycemia, hypocalcemia), gastrointestinal (poor feeding, enterocolitis), renal (anuria, renal failure), and central nervous (intracranial hemorrhage, hypothermia, seizure) systems. It should be noted that perinatal asphyxia is the common denominator for many of the neonatal complications listed.

There is abundant evidence correlating respiratory distress syndrome (RDS) and intraventricular hemorrhage (IVH)—two major causes of neonatal mortality in VLBW infants—to intrapartum asphyxia, particularly if the course of labor and delivery has been abnormal.[72,128,135,205,243,258,267] Worthington and group[267] analyzed factors influencing survival and morbidity in 214 VLBW infants. They found that RDS was the most common serious morbidity, occurring in 114 infants (62%), while IVH was diagnosed in 38 (21%) of the infants. Therefore, the prevention of

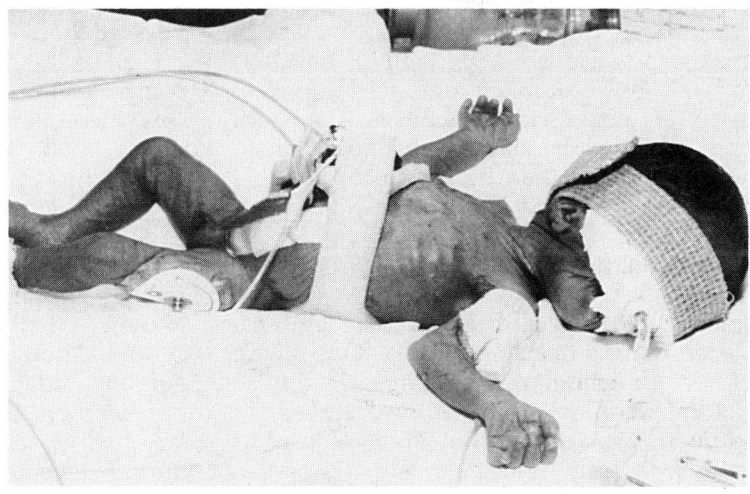

FIGURE 9-1. An example of a preterm severe SGA male infant, 580 g at 32 weeks, born to a mother with hypertension and superimposed severe preeclampsia. The baby survived for 6 days and died of cardiac failure secondary to RDS, patent ductus arteriosus, and sepsis.

perinatal asphyxia and its sequelae is the most important task for the obstetrician conducting labor and delivery of a VLBW fetus.

Perinatal Asphyxia

Fetal hypoxia refers to a decrease in the level of fetal oxygenation below a normal limit. Since fetal oxygenation is dependent on placental intervillous space blood flow, any factor which interrupts the maternal uteroplacental circulation will cause some degree of fetal hypoxia. Chronic reductions in uterine blood flow, as seen in cases of maternal hypertension, may result in persistently low fetal Po_2 levels. Similarly, in cases of severe maternal anemia, such as in sickle cell anemia, the decreased oxygen-carrying capacity of the maternal circulation prevents an adequate supply of oxygen from reaching the fetus. Maternal smoking is associated with a reduction in both uteroplacental blood flow and in the oxygen-carrying capacity of the maternal red blood cells.[215] Labor also represents a serious challenge to the preterm fetus. When labor contractions increase in frequency and intensity, blood flow within the intervillous space decreases, with a concomitant decrease in maternal-fetal oxygen transfer.[103] At some point a fetus subjected to these conditions becomes hypoxic, leading to myocardial depression and the appearance of late decelerations on fetal heart rate (FHR) tracings.[120] With progressive fetal hypoxia, a state of metabolic acidosis gradually develops through the accumulation of lactate, a product of the anaerobic metabolism of glucose. This condition is followed by an enlarged base deficit and then by a drop in the fetal blood pH.[161,231] This hypoxic-acidotic insult may lead to intrauterine meconium aspiration or fetal death.[175,241]

Because of the conservative, expectant approach which has been adopted by most obstetricians in managing VLBW fetuses with PROM, umbilical cord compression due to oligohydramnios is frequently observed. In addition, prolapse of the umbilical cord is more frequently associated with the small-size preterm fetus than with the term fetus, especially when the fetus is in a transverse lie or breech presentation. Perinatal asphyxia can also result from this type of prolonged, severe umbilical cord compression.

Both preterm and IUGR fetuses are more susceptible than the term fetus to intrauterine asphyxia.[155] Acute intrauterine partial and total asphyxia have been induced using animal models in order to study the pathogenesis of perinatal brain damage secondary to intrauterine asphyxia. Total asphyxia in the human fetus can be produced only by complete cord occlusion (true knot of the umbilical cord) or complete separation of the placenta (total abruptio placentae); fetal life ceases very shortly after the onset of either of these events. The majority of human fetuses associated with intrauterine asphyxia resemble the experimental model of partial asphyxia developed in the rhesus monkey.[33,34] Brain damage secondary to perinatal asphyxia may lead to postasphyxial seizures and cerebral palsy.

Respiratory Distress Syndrome

Neonatal RDS continues to be the most significant cause of neonatal death[72,128] despite the advanced techniques of respiratory care which were introduced during the early 1970s.[101] Estimates of the incidence of RDS range from a low of 14% at 35 weeks of gestation to 60% at 28 weeks of gestation.[135] As a larger percentage of infants with RDS survive, the incidence of permanent serious sequelae of the disorder itself or its associated complications continues to increase.[135] For this reason, it is important to explore the various methods which may prevent or reduce RDS in the VLBW fetus.

For newborn infants, the presence of adequate amounts of surface-active material in the alveolar space and adequate surface area for gas exchange across the alveolar membrane are the two prerequisites for adequate postnatal lung adaptation and extrauterine survival. Adequate gas diffusion implies the development of a sufficient pulmonary capillary bed in contact with an alveolar surface area covered by type-I epithelial cells.

According to Stahlman,[240] inadequate quantities of surface-active phospholipids (surfactant) in the neonatal lungs may result from several causes:

1. Extreme immaturity of the alveolar cells
2. Diminished or impaired production of surfactant secondary to transient fetal or early neonatal stress
3. Impairment of the release mechanism for surfactant from the type-II alveolar cells
4. Death of a significant number of type-II cells.

Biochemical and histologic evidence suggest that the first and the third mechanisms probably account for the inability of the very early fetus to survive extrauterine life. Mortality among newborn infants associated with severe hyaline membrane disease is probably caused by the fourth mechanism, while transient, mild respiratory distress is more likely related to the second mechanism.

Immature lungs have a higher percentage of undifferentiated cuboidal cells lining the potential airways. With inadequate numbers of type-II alveolar cells, production of surfactant is too low to ensure adequate lung stability in the very immature baby. In addition, the more immature the lung, the greater the risk that the nutritional blood supply to the developing lung cells may be compromised by fetal hypoxia and hypotension. Acute hypoxia is a powerful pulmonary vasoconstrictor in the fetus; its effect is further potentiated by a low blood pH. As long as fetal pathways for shunting blood away from the lung are open, pulmonary hypertension may critically reduce the nutritional blood supply to those pulmonary cells with a high metabolic requirement for survival. This mechanism, as well as hypovolemia, uncorrected metabolic acidosis, and extreme hypothermia, may lead to a progressive loss of lung compliance secondary to the death of type-II alveolar cells and to the cessation of surfactant production. The prevention of both preterm delivery using tocolytic agents and of RDS by the antenatal administration of corticosteroids has proven effective in reducing neonatal death due to RDS during the last decade. These methods will be discussed later in this section.

In recent years, pediatricians have used artificial surfactant to treat or to prevent hyaline membrane disease (HMD) with some success.[68,85] Since the underlying process of HMD is believed to be a deficiency of alveolar surfactant, the most direct form of treatment theoretically is to administer surfactant by aerosol through the airways. In animal experiments, both natural and artificial surfactants have been delivered to the lungs of preterm fetal animals before the onset of breathing in order to compensate for a deficiency of endogenous alveolar surfactant; the method appears to be effective in improving pulmonary function.[2,66,86,87] Artificial surfactant consists of a mixture of the naturally occurring surfactant phospholipids (extracted from calf lung lavage) and synthetic phospholipids which contain dipalmityl lecithin and phosphatidyl glycerol. In human preterm infants, Fujiwara and associates[85] observed a significant improvement in alveolar-arterial oxygen gradients, level of FiO_2 required, neonatal acidosis, and systemic hypotension in ten severely ill preterm infants with HMD after endotracheal instillation of artificial surfactant. Enhorning and co-workers[68] reported that surfactant supplementation prior to the first breath is of value as a preventive measure against HMD after a randomized clinical trial on 72 human preterm infants born at a gestational age of less than 30 weeks. It appears possible that the combined administration of antenatal corticosteroids and postnatal surfactant will effectively reduce the incidence of HMD in VLBW infants.

Another new development in pediatric intensive care is the use of extracorporeal membrane oxygenation (ECMO) to treat infants with intractable respiratory failure.[17,18,138] This technique was initially used to manage the larger infant with a birth weight of greater than 2000 g. However, it has recently been suggested that the method be used to treat VLBW infants with severe RDS.[62] The benefits of extracorporeal circulation for VLBW newborns could be due to conditioning of the extremely premature lung during a short period of bypass, after which ventilation at nontraumatic pressures and nontoxic oxygen concentrations become possible.

Intraventricular Hemorrhage

Germinal matrix hemorrhage and IVH occur in approximately 40% to 50% of preterm infants weighing less than 1500 g at birth.[47,205,258] Prior to the advent of computerized tomography (CT), IVH was commonly thought to be a fatal condition, but it is now known that the majority of cases of IVH survive and that many of them may be clinically silent.

A major advance in the diagnosis of neonatal periventricular-intraventricular hemorrhage is the use of ultrasound scanning with portable instruments, including real-time B-scan, gray scale image, and sector scanner.[4,22,133,202,245] Although CT scanning is an excellent tool for identifying IVH, it has been largely replaced by portable ultrasound because of the inconvenience of using CT and the possible long-term effects of the radiation exposure from multiple studies. Diagnosis of IVH must begin with the clinician's suspicion, and, in view of the high incidence of the hemorrhage in VLBW preterm infants, all such infants should be considered at high risk for this complication. The accuracy of ultrasound diagnosis reaches 85% in infants with germinal layer hemorrhage, 92% in those with IVH, and 97% in those with intracerebral hemorrhage.[245]

There is a definite correlation between the severity of hemorrhage and the prognosis of this complication.[258] IVH has been classified into four grades with progressive increases in severity:

Grade 1: Confined to germinal layer or subependymal hemorrhage
Grade 2: Intraventricular hemorrhage without ventricular dilatation
Grade 3: Intraventricular hemorrhage with ventricular dilatation
Grade 4: Intraventricular hemorrhage with parenchymal hemorrhage

Grade 1 and 2 lesions tend to resolve spontaneously, and both the mortality rate and the incidence of posthemorrhage progressive ventricular dilatation are relatively low. With grade 3 and 4 lesions, the majority of affected infants die, and progressive ventricular dilatation develops in most of the survivors.[205,258]

The pathogenesis of periventricular-intraventricular hemorrhage is related to several factors concerned with the distribution and regulation of cerebral blood flow, intravascular pressure, vascular integrity, and the extravascular environment.[258] Before 32 to 34 weeks of gestation, the relative prominence of the vascular supply to the subependymal germinal matrix and the deep regions of the cerebrum suggests that a disproportionate amount of the total cerebral blood flow enters these areas. In preterm infants, autoregulation of cerebral blood flow is impaired and blood flow to the periventricular region is exquisitely sensitive to changes in arterial blood pressure. Thus, elevation of arterial blood pressure or cerebral blood flow, or both, have been observed in infants in the first few minutes after delivery in association with motor activities, colloid infusion/exchange transfusion, seizures, apneic spells, and asphyxia.

Increased cerebral blood flow can be caused by three factors associated with perinatal asphyxia: hypercapnea, the preferential shunting of blood to the brain, and arterial hypertension. Elevated venous pressure may occur in infants with perinatal asphyxia along with myocardial failure, which will in turn cause elevations of pressure within the periventricular capillary bed; this capillary bed may be vulnerable to rupture. Cooke and colleagues[47] in an IVH case study observed a positive association between IVH and several clinical factors such as respiratory distress, ventilator therapy, metabolic acidosis, and hypercapnea, which tends to support the role of these factors in the pathogenesis of periventricular hemorrhage. In one study of 220 infants with birth weights of less than 1500 g, 56% of infants with RDS (112 cases) versus 31% of infants without RDS (108 cases) developed IVH during their early neonatal lives (p < 0.001).[90]

The long-term outcome of IVH depends upon a number of factors, most of which correlate with the severity of the original hemorrhage.[143,205] Severe motor and intellectual deficits are mostly associated with infants suffering from marked hemorrhages and are rare in those with mild lesions.[258] Prevention of IVH by minimizing perinatal asphyxia and reducing unfavorable postnatal events during the early hours of life is probably the most important consideration for both obstetricians and pediatricians.

PREVENTION OF PRETERM DELIVERY

The key to improved fetal outcome in VLBW fetuses with threatened preterm labor is delay of the delivery. The various drugs in use for the suppression of preterm labor are only partially successful. Furthermore, many patients with preterm labor are found to be in advanced labor, with PROM, antepartum hemorrhage, and the presence of fetal anomalies or severe fetal compromise. These conditions are associated with either imminent preterm delivery or represent a contraindication to long-term therapy to prevent preterm delivery. Prior to 1980 as few as 10% to 20% of patients with preterm labor were reported to be candidates for tocolytic therapy.[177,246,271]

If the preterm birth rate is to be reduced, every attempt must be made to maximize the number of patients whose preterm labor can be effectively prevented. Unfortunately, the symptoms of preterm labor are frequently so insidious that they are not recognized until labor is far advanced. The early symptoms of preterm labor are mild menstrual-like cramps, pelvic pressure, low backache, and a change in the amount and character of vaginal discharge, particularly if pink or mucoid.[52]

Two additional factors are also frequently involved with difficulty in stopping preterm labor. If the pregnant woman with intact membranes is in preterm labor and fetal breathing movements cannot be detected using real-time ultrasonography, the likelihood of early delivery is increased.[41] It has been postulated that fetal breathing movements may be inhibited by increasing concentrations of prostaglandin E_2 in the fetal blood.[41] The presence of subclinical infection of the intact amniotic membranes may also contribute to an inevitable preterm delivery.[28,181]

Prematurity Prevention Program

In the early 1980s Creasy and his associates[51,53,115] developed a program for the early detection of preterm labor. They reported that among patients at risk for preterm labor, it is possible to increase the proportion of preterm labor patients who are candidates for tocolysis to over 80%, with a corresponding 50% decrease in the incidence of preterm delivery.[51,115] Their program is based on weekly education and evaluation visits after 20 weeks of gestation for patients at high risk for preterm labor, with an emphasis on: patient and staff education as to the subtle symptoms of preterm labor; patient's self-detection for painless but regular uterine contractions; weekly evaluation of cervical changes; brief external tocographic evaluation for suspected preterm labor; patient's prompt report of regular uterine activity to the medical staff; and prompt treatment of preterm labor if it occurs.[52]

Several other investigators have attempted to identify prospectively those women most likely to have spontaneous preterm labor based on historical, social, and current medical factors. Intervention designed to prevent preterm births can then be selectively applied to these high-risk women. Papiernik was the first investigator to propose a high-risk scoring system and was able to predict up to 75% of spontaneous preterm labors.[203,204] Fredrick[79,80] developed a similar risk scoring system which can predict up to 45% of preterm births. Creasy and co-workers[53] developed a risk scoring system modified from the work of previous investigators (Table 9-3). Scoring is performed at the initial

Table 9-3. System for Determining Risk of Spontaneous Preterm Delivery

Points Assigned*	Socioeconomic Factors	Previous Medical History	Daily Habits	Aspects of Current Pregnancy
1	Two children at home Low socioeconomic status	Abortion × 1 Less than 1 year since last birth	Works outside home	Unusual fatigue
2	Maternal age <20 years or >40 years Single parent	Abortion × 2	Smokes more than 10 cigarettes per day	Gain of less than 5 kg by 32 weeks
3	Very low socioeconomic status Height <150 cm Weight <45 kg	Abortion × 3	Heavy or stressful work Long, tiring trip	Breech at 32 weeks Weight loss of 2 kg Head engaged at 32 weeks Febrile illness
4	Maternal age <18 years	Pyelonephritis		Bleeding after 12 weeks Effacement Dilation Uterine irritability
5		Uterine anomaly Second-trimester abortion DES exposure Cone biopsy		Placenta previa Hydramnios
10		Preterm delivery Repeated second-trimester abortion		Twins Abdominal surgery

* Score is computed by adding the number of points given any item. The score is computed at the first visit and again at 22 to 26 weeks gestation. A total score of 10 or more places patient at high risk of spontaneous preterm delivery.

(Adapted from Creasy RK, Gummer BA, Liggins GC: A system for predicting spontaneous preterm birth. Obstet Gynecol 55: 692, 1980)[53]

visit and repeated at 22 to 26 weeks of gestation. A total score of greater than or equal to 10 places the patient in the high-risk category for spontaneous preterm delivery. At the first office visit, a score of 10 or more on this screening survey corresponded to a 30% chance of preterm delivery. Repeating the risk assessment at 22 to 26 weeks gestation identified an additional group of women likely to be delivered prematurely. This system has been evaluated prospectively in a group of 966 patients,[52] in which it identified 64% of the patients who subsequently delivered preterm. However, only one-third of the patients with high-risk scores delivered preterm infants. The system so far has failed to identify at least one-third of the patients who will deliver spontaneously before 37 weeks of gestation.

Prematurity prevention programs have been reported as successful by some investigators,[115,204] but have been unsuccessful in the hands of others.[169,174] Since these prevention programs are designed to promote earlier intervention in women with idiopathic preterm labor, the relative risk of LBW and the success of the prevention program in different populations may differ. In a program undertaken in San Francisco,[115] the incidence of preterm birth was reduced from 6.8% to 2.4%. However, a prospective, randomized, controlled study of poor, inner city women with a 17% preterm delivery rate in Philadelphia[169] failed to demonstrate any significant difference in pregnancy outcome between the group in the prematurity prevention program and the controlled high-risk group. Likewise, implementation of a prematurity prevention program in North Carolina[174] failed to reduce the incidence of LBW births in a group of service patients. In a group of private patients, on the other hand, the program resulted in a decrease in newborns weighing less than 2500 g from 8.2% to 5.1%, and of those less than 1500 g from 2.6% to 0.8%.[174]

Incompetent Cervix and Cervical Cerclage

Incompetence of the uterine cervix is a known risk factor for recurrent pregnancy wastage, especially with respect to late abortion and early preterm birth. Most cases of cervical incompetence are caused by a previous traumatic delivery, an induced abortion, or cervical conization; cervical incompetence due to an inherent defect is quite rare.[226]

Cervical cerclage, by either vaginal or abdominal approach, appears to be effective in correcting the condition of incompetent cervix. The question of whether cervical cerclage is useful in the prevention of VLBW births remains controversial. Although many studies[54,107,197,199,200,229] indicate that cervical cerclage improves the ultimate outcome of pregnancy by reducing the incidence of late abortions and preterm births, two randomized, controlled studies[150,220] failed to demonstrate its efficacy. Nevertheless, we believe that cervical cerclage has a place in preventing immediate late abortion or preterm birth of VLBW infants in selected patients with a typical history of cervical incompetence, and in those women with evidence of cervical dilatation without preceding regular uterine activities.

Pharmacology Therapy

There is little evidence to support the use of sedatives or narcotics to inhibit preterm labor, and the use of several other compounds remains controversial. The hypothesis that preterm labor may be initiated by a deficiency of progesterone has generated several studies of the efficacy of giving progesterone compounds to patients at risk of preterm labor. Initial prophylactic use of 17α-hydroxyprogesterone caproate in patients at risk of preterm labor was reported to be promising.[131,132] However, in a recent prospective double-blind study,[112] active-duty military women who were at an increased risk of delivering LBW infants did not benefit from this agent. Thus, the usefulness of 17α-hydroxyprogesterone in preventing preterm labor is still not clear. The potential benefits of ethanol for the inhibition of preterm labor were intensively studied by several investigators.[83,84,273] Similarly, there are reports of the tocolytic efficacy of magnesium sulfate in the treatment of preterm labor.[180,239,242] However, none of these agents has ever become as popular as beta-sympathomimetic agents for inhibiting preterm labor.

Beta-sympathomimetic Agents

Since the late 1970s, beta-sympathomimetic agents such as isoxsuprine, salbutamol, ritodrine, and terbutaline have been the most widely used tocolytic agents in the United States and throughout the world. Ritodrine, however, is the only drug currently approved by the Federal Drug Administration (FDA) specifically for tocolysis of preterm labor.[195] Despite such potential side-effects as maternal tachycardia and hypotension, these agents are now the best means available for delaying delivery. A delay of only 7 to 14 days may enormously benefit the less-than-1500-g infant.[14]

Most studies[37,56,126,177,213,238] indicate that these drugs are effective in delaying delivery from 3 to 10 days in 80% of preterm labor patients, and for a longer period in at least 60% of these patients. In comparison to other tocolytic agents, betamimetic drugs may be as effective as intravenous magnesium sulfate[21,180] but distinctly superior to ethanol[36,148,237] in inhibiting preterm labor. Whether it would be more beneficial or more harmful to use magnesium sulfate and ritodrine in combination deserves further evaluation.[73,111]

Betamimetic agents can produce serious maternal complications or maternal death by the development of pulmonary edema,[136,183,211,259] cardiac disease, or myocardial ischemia.[25,136,249,268] To maximize the survival rate for the VLBW fetus, it is advisable to use betamimetic agents early and aggressively when the patient is suspected of preterm labor. At the same time, special precautions must be taken to avoid maternal side-effects. Dosage and the presence of underlying maternal disease appear to determine the occurrence and extent of these complications.

Other Agents

Recently, information has been reported about two other types of tocolytic agents, prostaglandin synthetase inhibitors and calcium channel blockers. Following the success of Zuckerman and co-workers[274] using indomethacin to inhibit preterm labor, many investigators[193,194,237,265] reported a success rate of 80% or higher in terms of complete inhibition of preterm labor for one week or longer. However, there have been reports from both animal and human experiments that prostaglandin synthetase inhibitors may promote closure of the fetal ductus arteriosus with resultant pulmonary hypertension, congestive heart failure, and death.[55,116,230] Recent studies have stated that some of the adverse effects reported in babies close to term have not been seen in smaller preterm fetuses if the drug is used for treatment courses of no more than 24 to 48 hours.[195] The ductus appears to resist closing at prior to 34 weeks of gestation.[63,195] The drug was found to be safe in a large European study when properly used.[137]

There are as yet no extensive controlled trials of calcium channel blockers in pregnant human subjects.[252] In the pregnant ewe, the tocolytic and hemodynamic effects of nifedipine seem to be comparable to those of ritodrine.[97] Orally administered nifedipine has been found to inhibit uterine contractions during the perimenstrual period,[225,251] following prostaglandin-induced uterine contractions in early pregnancy[8] and in the postpartum human uterus.[77] In two preliminary reports, oral nifedipine was found to effectively inhibit preterm labor with minimal maternal and no fetal side-effects.[8,58] Table 9-4 summarizes the mechanism of action, clinical efficacy, side-effects, and dosages of five different groups of tocolytic agents based upon a review of four articles in the literature.[8,52,58,217]

SPECIAL ISSUES IN ANTEPARTUM MANAGEMENT

The major obstetric complications of pregnancy that can lead to labor and delivery of the VLBW fetus include preeclampsia, third-trimester hemorrhage, PROM, and multifetal gestations. For most obstetric complications, with the exception of abruptio placentae, more concern has been focused upon the degree of maturity and well-being of the fetus than on the impact of these complications on the mother herself. This is particularly true for pregnancies between 26 and 32 weeks.

Expectant Management and Bed Rest

Several authors have suggested that bed rest may be useful in preventing preterm delivery,[24,141,208] but the issue is still considered controversial because of a lack of prospective controlled studies. Pregnant women who are managed with bed rest in the lateral recumbent position will have an increase in uterine blood flow and an increase in the transfer of oxygen and nutrients from the mother to the fetus.[12,102,160,170,178] It is reasonable to speculate that the benefit of long-term bed rest is due to an improvement in placental transfer that enhances fetal growth. Most of the reports concerning the value of bed rest in preventing preterm labor have dealt with multifetal gestations.[24,113,141,149,208] Besides the benefit of increased uteroplacental blood flow, bed rest may also act to reduce the physical force that might accelerate cervical dilatation secondary to overdistention of the uterus in twin gestation. However, Weekes and colleagues[261] failed to demonstrate a difference in fetal outcome with respect to birth weight and gestational age among three groups of patients with twin pregnancy: those who received no special treatment, those managed with bed rest, and those treated with cervical cerclage.

In the management of patients with placenta previa, a marked improvement in both maternal and perinatal mortality has been achieved over the past 40 years through the adoption of expectant management, adequate blood transfusion, and the liberal use of cesarean section.[130,165] Since the primary concern in placenta previa is fetal loss due to prematurity, a management protocol which includes prolonged bed rest in the hospital, correction of maternal anemia, and constant prenatal surveillance of fetal growth and development is the most reasonable approach to those cases remote from fetal maturity, unless the obstetrician is forced to deliver the patient because of massive hemorrhage, fetal distress, or active labor. In a study which compared 185 cases of placenta previa to 30,885 obstetric patients without placenta previa at the same institution and during the same period of time, no significant differences were found between the two groups with respect to mean fetal weight, placental weight, or fetal-to-placental weight ratios for each week of gestation.[35] However, an increased incidence of preterm infants and of infants with congenital anomalies remain the two major problems in placenta previa.[35] Today, the great majority of well managed cases of placenta previa are expected to carry the pregnancy to fetal maturity, or at least to a fetal weight of more than 1500 g, which is associated with a survival rate of 96% or higher.

Preeclampsia superimposed on chronic hypertension is the most common clinical entity associated with SGA infants.[11,159] The incidence of fetal growth retardation appears to correlate closely with the severity of maternal hypertension[43,147,159] and the extent of the plasma volume contraction.[10,166] We have studied fetal outcome in 157 hypertensive pregnant women and found that 22% of their infants were SGA and 40% were preterm.[159] Among 21 perinatal deaths in this series, nearly all were below the 50th percentile on the growth curve and were born before 30 weeks gestation. There were three categories of patients associated with an increased risk for delivering preterm SGA infants: those with glomerulonephritis, multiparous preeclampsia without preceding chronic hypertension, and chronic hypertension with superimposed preeclampsia. It is of interest to note that over 50% of the women in these three categories had both a prolonged period of hypertension (>4 weeks) and heavy proteinuria (>3.5 g/24 hours) during their pregnancies.

A difficult clinical situation is encoun-

Table 9-4. A Comparison of Five Tocolytic Agents

Representative Tocolytic Agents	Mechanism of Action	Clinical Efficacy	Side-effects	Dosage and Administration
Ritodrine	Beta$_2$-adrenergic effect on uterine smooth muscle	Suppresses uterine contractions Delays delivery 3 to 10 days in 80% patients Prolongs delivery in 60% patients	Myocardial ischemia Pulmonary edema Hyperglycemia Hypokalemia	IV 0.050–0.350 mg/min for 12 hours PO 10–20 mg q 2–4 hours
Terbutaline	Increased cyclic AMP preventing actin-myosin interaction		Contraindications: Cardiac disease, ? diabetes, twins	IV 0.010–0.080 mg/min for 12 hours PO 2.5–5 mg q 2–4 hours
Magnesium sulfate	Competitive antagonist with calcium Suppresses myometrial contractility	Delays delivery for 24 to 48 hrs in 70%, for more than 7 days in 45% patients	Respiratory depression and cardiac arrest with high level of 12–15 meq/dl Pulmonary edema	IV loading dose of 4 to 6 gm over 20 min followed by 1 to 3 g/hour for 24 hours
Ethanol	Alters neurohypophyseal release of oxytocin and antidiuretic hormone Directly inhibits myometrial contractility	Delays delivery for more than 3 days in 65% patients Inferior to beta-adrenergic drugs	Alcohol intoxication (headache, emesis, mental depression) Lactic acidosis	7.5 ml/kgBW of 10% ethanol IV for 2 hours followed by 1.5 ml/kgBW for 12 hours

Indomethacin	Acts on the cyclooxygenase enzyme, inhibiting the synthesis of all prostaglandins: PGE$_2$, PGF$_{2\alpha}$, PGI$_2$, and thromboxane A$_2$. Decreases myometrial contractility by inhibiting prostaglandin production	Prostaglandin synthetase inhibitors are perhaps the most effective agents to inhibit uterine activity. Delays delivery for more than 7 days in 80% patients	Affects fetal cardiovascular system by constriction of ductus arteriosus in utero and development of neonatal pulmonary hypertension, oligohydramnios	PO 50 mg initially followed by 25 mg q 4 hours for 24 hours
Nifedipine	Calcium channel blocker, prevents the entry of ionized calcium in the slow channels of the cell membrane and inhibits uterine smooth muscle contractions	Stops labor and prolongs pregnancy for 4 weeks in 6 out of 7 patients (88%)	Minimal maternal side-effect; facial flushing. No significant hypotension or tachycardia	PO 30 mg initially followed by 10–20 mg q 4 hours until total dose of 80 mg/day

(Anderson et al.,[8] Creasy RK,[52] D'Alton ME et al.,[58] Roberts JM[217])

tered if preeclampsia develops early in pregnancy when the fetus is immature and there are signs of maternal deterioration, fetal growth retardation, or fetal jeopardy. Under these circumstances, progressive deterioration of both maternal and fetal conditions is frequently observed, often necessitating termination of the pregnancy regardless of the gestational age of the fetus. However, if preventive measures and therapy are instituted early enough in the course of the disease process, severe preeclampsia or eclampsia are often preventable. Gant and associates[89] reported that hospitalization for bed rest of women with pregnancy-induced hypertension resulted in a marked reduction of perinatal morbidity and mortality. In most instances, the development of severe preeclampsia or eclampsia was delayed and a preterm delivery was prevented.

Premature Rupture of Membranes

Recently, several reports have suggested that subclinical infection plays a role in either initiating preterm labor, causing PROM, or decreasing the uterine response to tocolysis.[28,181,184] In a prospective study of the vaginal flora, *Trichomonas vaginalis* and bacteroides species were found to be associated with an increased risk of PROM, while *Ureaplasma urealyticum* was more frequently associated with preterm labor.[184] Similarly, in a retrospective study of 25,820 pregnancies, cervical instrumentation prior to pregnancy, incompetent cervix, and recent coitus were found to have a positive association with PROM.[76,190]

PROM occurs in as many as 38% of VLBW births.[187] PROM increases the risk of fetal sepsis, preterm labor, umbilical cord prolapse, and, on rare occasions, abruptio placentae. Each of these factors can lead to perinatal morbidity and mortality. Generally, because the risk of prematurity exceeds the risk of sepsis in pregnancies between 26 and 32 weeks with PROM, a conservative, expectant approach is warranted.[3,49,98,124] For example, RDS accounts for 50% to 70% of perinatal deaths, whereas neonatal infection is associated with 10% to 20% of perinatal deaths.[98] In addition, earlier delivery subjects the VLBW infant to such serious neonatal complications as IVH, persistent fetal circulation, pulmonary hemorrhage, enterocolitis, and the other complications of prematurity, as previously discussed.

When PROM occurs, the VLBW fetus is highly susceptible to compression or prolapse of the umbilical cord if an inadequate amount of amniotic fluid is present or if the fetus is in a breech presentation or transverse lie. Thus, frequent sonographic assessments of the amniotic fluid volume as well as of the fetal presentation are mandatory. If marked amniotic fluid leakage continues, it may be helpful to monitor the FHR periodically to detect the possibility of variable decelerations.[185] Furthermore, both the nonstress test (NST) and the biophysical profile can be used to predict the fetal condition and the presence of intrauterine infection. A nonreactive NST has been associated with clinical amnionitis and/or neonatal sepsis in preterm gestation with PROM.[256] The presence of fetal breathing is a good predictor of a noninfection outcome, but its absence does not necessarily indicate impending infection.[255] In preterm gestation between 25 to 32 weeks, PROM has been found to be associated with a higher incidence of reactive NSTs, the absence of fetal breathing movements, and reduced amniotic fluid volume.[254] However, the overall biophysical scoring of the healthy fetus is not significantly altered throughout gestation by the presence of ruptured membranes.[257]

Some small fetuses have mature lungs when PROM develops prior to 36 weeks gestation.[145] Analysis of amniotic fluid phospholipids obtained by amniocentesis or from the vaginal pool may provide a reliable guide for fetal pulmonary maturity.[32,49,167] The decision to deliver the under-1500-g fetus with close to mature phospholipid levels is a difficult one, because such a fetus may die from neonatal complications other than RDS.

Amniocentesis may also be used to identify bacteria-positive patients with PROM, since most of these patients subsequently develop clinical chorioamnionitis or preterm labor.[272] The risk of developing chorioamnionitis appears to increase with PROM of 24 hours or longer.[3] Because there is not a test which will consistently predict chorioamnionitis, attempts to identify fetuses at risk for infection and deliver them before amnionitis becomes established are often unsuccessful. Maternal and amniotic fluid leukocyte counts are frequently unreliable. C-reactive protein levels appear to be a more sensitive laboratory parameter for the detection of chorioamnionitis, but the specificity of this test is not high.[70,114,129,219] Therefore, the decision to deliver the VLBW fetus suspected of sepsis must be based upon such traditional clinical criteria as maternal fever, uterine tenderness, and fetal tachycardia, in addition to leukocytosis and elevated C-reactive protein levels.

For the majority of fetuses who develop fetal sepsis, aggressive treatment with antibiotics and an expeditious delivery are likely to provide the best fetal outcome. On the other hand, preterm gestation between 26 and 32 weeks with PROM, but with no signs of chorioamnionitis, should be managed conservatively. Vaginal examination should be avoided until delivery is planned within 24 hours, because vaginal examination after PROM promotes ascending infection.[228]

One disadvantage of prolonged conservative management of preterm gestation with PROM is the possible finding of pulmonary hypoplasia and positional deformities of the fetus. These fetal developmental abnormalities have been seen in patients whose membranes ruptured prior to 26 weeks gestation with a duration of rupture of more than 5 weeks.[196]

Effect of Corticosteroids on Lung Maturity

Since Liggins and Howie[154] reported in a controlled study that the antenatal administration of corticosteroids reduced the incidence of RDS, the use of these agents to enhance fetal lung maturity has become widespread. Their results indicated that if given adequate time ($\geq$24 hours), prenatally administered steroids were capable of reducing the incidence of RDS (56% in the control group v. 8.7% in the treated group). The complications and mortality which resulted from RDS in these infants were also significantly reduced.

By 1980, more than 25 published studies worldwide have attempted to duplicate Liggins and Howie's work. Almost all of these studies have shown a positive effect of exogenously administered steroids in reducing the incidence and severity of RDS, with improved neonatal outcome.[20] However, most of the controlled studies spanned a wide range of gestational age (26 to 35 weeks), and specific information regarding the effect of corticosteroids on lung maturity for VLBW babies is quite limited.[27,188] Moore and Resnik[187] summarized the results of seven placebo-controlled studies in which the effect of corticosteroids on RDS in the VLBW infant can be assessed separately. Although data for the total study population (26 to 36 weeks gestation) in all seven studies indicated a relative decrease in the incidence of RDS with corticosteroid therapy, only two of the seven studies[40,123] showed a statistically significant decrease.

The reason that glucocorticoids are less effective in the VLBW fetus is not clear. Possible explanations range from markedly immature bronchoalveolar development, insensitivity of the pulmonary tissue of the VLBW fetus to the induction of surfactant synthesis and release, or a study sample that was too small to establish statistical significance.

PROM has been shown to accelerate fetal lung maturity and lead to elevated phospholipid contents in amniotic fluid.[144,145,167] In preterm gestation with PROM, neither corticosteroids[44,92,125] nor betamimetic agents[57] showed any additive effect of RDS prevention compared to PROM alone. It has been recommended, however, that in the management of patients with PROM at less than 34 weeks gestation, delivery should be delayed for 24 to 48 hours, using betamimetic agents if necessary to allow sufficient time for improved lung maturity with or without the concomitant use of glucocorticoids.[198,244]

In view of the available data, it seems

reasonable to allow patients with PROM to labor and deliver without tocolysis or steroids. Steroids should be considered for the patient with intact membranes whose labor has been arrested if a delay of at least 48 hours between steroid therapy and delivery is anticipated. Amniocentesis for phospholipid analysis before the institution of steroid therapy will make it possible to omit those fetuses whose lungs are already mature. By excluding those fetuses with an estimated delivery time of less than 24 hours or more than 7 days, those with a mature L/S ratio, and those with other contraindications for steroid therapy, Depp and associates were able to obtain 47 candidates out of 439 patients (10.7%) for antenatal corticosteroid therapy.[59] These strict selective criteria are currently in use at the Chicago Lying-In Hospital. Thus, glucocorticoid therapy is given only to those patients with the potential for maximum benefit.

Fetal Evaluation

As mentioned previously, survival of VLBW infants depends upon both birth weight and fetal lung maturity. In our institution, the survival rate for infants under 700 g is approximately 10%; this figure increases to greater than 50% for infants between 900 and 1000 g and to over 80% for those weighing 1250 g or more. Determining estimated fetal weight (EFW) accurately before delivery is essential for predicting survival prospects and for selecting an appropriate delivery route. In the past, a significant number of potentially salvageable babies were incorrectly identified as "pre-viable" as a result of inaccurate clinical methods; passive management of these babies doubled the mortality rate for the overall VLBW population.[206] Fortunately, it is now possible to determine EFW with much greater accuracy by using the sophisticated ultrasound machines that are currently available.

Table 9-5 summarizes the different formulas for ultrasonic EFW developed by several investigators, some with an error of only 7% to 8% when compared to actual birth weight in those newborns born within a few days of obtaining EFW.[201,232,233,247,260] Careful estimation of fetal weight is the key step in the management of VLBW fetuses.

Antepartum FHR testing has been the most convenient method for evaluating fetal well-being when screening a large population of high-risk pregnancies. One of the handicaps of NST, however, is its inability to predict fetal outcome between 20 and 30 weeks gestation. Sorokin and associates[235] observed that 97% of fetuses at 20 to 22 weeks exhibited FHR decelerations with fetal movements. In a second group of fetuses between 28 and 30 weeks gestation, one-third exhibited FHR accelerations, one-third decelerations, and one third accelerations with decelerations in response to fetal movements. There was significantly more clustering of FHR changes associated with fetal movement at 28 to 30 weeks gestation than at 20 to 22 weeks gestation.[236] This phenomenon of a gradual evolution of FHR change and fetal body movements was also reported by Natale and group.[191] Their data suggested that there is a maturational aspect to the relationship between FHR and fetal body movements as gestational age increases from 24 to 32 weeks. Body movements in younger fetuses occur without recognizable accelerations (i.e., <15 bpm). As fetuses mature, the interaction between body movements and FHR becomes more evident and accelerations become more recognizable (i.e., >15 bpm). Therefore, the NST, as presently defined for older fetuses, is not valid for gestations below 32 weeks, unless new interpretive criteria can be established in the future.

Fetal biophysical scoring of the healthy fetus, on the other hand, does not change throughout gestation, regardless of the presence or absence of ruptured membranes.[257] The incidence of a fetal biophysical score of 8 or more was found to be similar among different gestational age groups: 25 to 28 weeks, 29 to 32 weeks, 33 to 36 weeks, and 37 to 40 weeks.[257] The predictability of infectious fetal outcome by analysis of fetal breathing movements in pregnant women with PROM was not different between those at less than or

Table 9-5. Accuracy of Estimated Fetal Weight by Ultrasound

AUTHOR	FORMULA FOR EFW*	R†	MEAN ERROR (%)‡
Warsof et al.[260] 1977	$Log_{10}(EFW) = 1.599 + 0.144(BPD) + 0.032(AC) - 0.111(BPD^2 \times AC)/1000$		11.0
Shepard et al.[232] 1982	$Log_{10}(EFW) = -1.7492 + 0.166(BPD) + 0.046(AC) - 2.646(AC \times BPD)/1000$		16.4
Ott[201] 1981	Warsof's formula	0.92	8.2
Thurnau et al.[247] 1983	$EFW = (BPD \times AC \times 9.337) - 299$	0.96	7.0
Shinozuka et al.[233] 1986	$EFW = 1.07 \times BPD^3 + 2.91 \times ATPD \times TTD \times LV$	0.90	10.2

* EFW, estimated fetal weight
† R, correlation coefficient
‡ Percentage of difference between EFW and actual birth weight

(BPD, biparietal diameter; AC, abdominal circumference; APTD, anteriopostorior trunk diameter; TTD, transverse trunk diameter; LV, length of vertebra)

equal to 30 weeks and those at greater than 30 weeks.[255] It seems advisable, therefore, that biophysical parameters other than NST alone should be used to evaluate the health of the VLBW fetus during the antepartum period.

Another important issue in fetal evaluation is the prenatal diagnosis of fetal anomalies. It is estimated that 10% to 20% of IUGR pregnancies involve congenital fetal anomalies.[153] A diagnosis of type-I IUGR can usually be made in the early stages of pregnancy by genetic amniocentesis, alpha-fetoprotein study, or TORCH screening.[146,168,253] The presence of major congenital malformations in the fetus can also be diagnosed by ultrasound[118,223] or fetoscopy.[67,218] Furthermore, the presence of polyhydramnios or oligohydramnios, which is readily detected by ultrasound, has been associated with a higher incidence of congenital malformations and poor fetal outcome.[16,176,212,214]

Maternal Transport to a Tertiary Care Center

Moore and Resnik[187] summarized the results of seven studies assessing neonatal mortality in the under-1500-g infant after maternal or neonatal transport to a tertiary care center. These seven centers were located in different regions of the United States and the studies were conducted from the late 1970s to the early 1980s.[7,48,108,109,153,182,186] While maternal transport accounts for only a modest improvement in survival, neonatal morbidity and the length of hospitalization are significantly decreased.[7,186] In one study, 1-minute Apgar scores were not different among inborn and outborn infants, but after 5 minutes of resuscitation, only 22% of outborn infants had Apgar scores above 7, compared with 57% of inborn infants.[48] These data indicate that initial resuscitation by a skilled team significantly reduces morbidity and mortality in the VLBW infants. If delivery is not imminent, every effort should be made to transport the mother, especially those bearing VLBW fetuses, to ensure adequate resuscitation by an experienced neonatologist and care in a nursery staffed and equipped for the high-risk infant.

A recent review of the regional perinatal statistics for the Women and Infant Hospital of Rhode Island in Providence indicated major changes in patterns of perinatal care, including an increasing proportion of low birth weight infants in the region being born at the tertiary care center, a decreasing number of neonatal transports in concert with an increasing number of maternal transports, and an increasing proportion of neonatal transports with birth weights of greater than or equal to 2500 g.[50] Eventually, all VLBW infants should be delivered at a tertiary care center.[216]

LABOR AND DELIVERY

Although VLBW fetuses will continue to gain weight and increase organ maturity with expectant management for preterm labor or PROM at a preterm gestation, it is unwise to delay delivery further if fetal-maternal compromise develops or tocolysis fails. At this time, the obstetrician has to decide on the optimal intrapartum care as well as a delivery route to minimize fetal trauma. This group of infants is particularly vulnerable to perinatal hypoxia, acidosis, birth trauma, RDS, and IVH. Some obstetricians suggest that labor per se may be harmful to the VLBW fetus, whether it is in a vertex or breech presentation[81] and whether it is delivered vaginally or by cesarean section after a period of active labor.[23,61] Therefore, intensive intrapartum fetal evaluation is critical for those patients with VLBW fetuses who are allowed to labor.

Intrapartum Fetal Evaluation

Today, any VLBW fetus in the weight range of 500 g to 1500 g or with a gestational age between 25 and 32 weeks must be considered viable. The obstetrician either has to provide the proper care or make sure that the patient has access to it. The primary care institution must either raise the level of its expertise or transfer the mother to a facility that can provide more intensive care.

Martin and co-workers[172] reported a positive correlation between ominous abnormal

FHR patterns (severe variable or late decelerations, decreased baseline variability) and the incidences of RDS or neonatal death from RDS in preterm infants weighing 2000 g or less. Similarly, both late decelerations and decreased FHR baseline variability were found to correlate with low fetal pH values in preterm deliveries.[270]

Braithwaite and associates[31] investigated the usefulness of intrapartum FHR patterns in the management of fetuses between 26 to 30 weeks gestation by a comparing 26 cases of neonatal death with 31 infants who survived. They found that a normal FHR pattern was associated with good fetal outcome. An abnormal FHR pattern (decreased variability, severe variable decelerations, late decelerations) predicted 90% of deaths; however, an abnormal FHR pattern was also found in 15 of 31 infants with no mortality or morbidity. They suggested that in addition to FHR patterns, other parameters must be evaluated in VLBW fetuses before the diagnosis of fetal distress can be made with certainty.

Myers and group[189] evaluated the importance of the one-minute Apgar score with respect to the survival rate of VLBW infants. Of 99 neonates weighing 600 g to 1499 g with 1-minute Apgar scores of 4 or more, the survival rate was 96%. Among VLBW infants in a comparable birth weight range with 1-minute Apgar scores of 3 or less, the survival rate was only 56%. These data suggest that the initial condition at birth substantially affects the survival of the VLBW infant. In a recent study of the survival of VLBW infants at the Chicago Lying-In Hospital,[117] both 1-minute and 5-minute Apgar scores correlated well with infant survival, but umbilical cord blood pH (both umbilical arterial and venous pH were studied) did not. Perkins and Papile[207] also found a poor correlation between cord blood gases and Apgar scores in VLBW infants. They argued that the depressed state of VLBW babies is associated with disturbed respiratory physiology rather than with asphyxia at birth.

Vintzileos and associates[254] assessed amniotic fluid volume by real-time ultrasound in a total of 90 patients with PROM prior to onset of labor. Fifty of the study patients were between 25 and 32 weeks gestation. In VLBW fetuses, the degree of oligohydramnios was found to be positively correlated with unfavorable fetal outcome. The incidences of umbilical cord compression FHR patterns, neonatal sepsis, depressed Apgar scores, and perinatal death were highest in the group associated with severe oligohydramnios, as compared to the groups with moderate or no oligohydramnios. Therefore, in the evaluation of labor and delivery of the VLBW fetus, information regarding estimated fetal weight, fetal presentation, and the degree of oligohydramnios are the three most important factors which should be used to guide obstetric management decisions.

Anencephaly is associated with no extrauterine survival. Now, pediatric surgery can offer a life of reasonable quality to some infants with hydrocephaly, hydronephrosis, omphalocele/gastroschisis, and tracheoesophageal fistula. However, in extremely severe cases of congenital malformation, such as hydrocephalus without demonstrable brain cortex, nonfunctioning polycystic kidneys, renal agenesis with hypoplastic lungs, or total evisceration with severe gastroschisis, the chances for neonatal survival are minimal. Ultrasound diagnosis of gross fetal malformations should be established in such cases long before the decision is made whether or not to deliver by cesarean section in the event of intrapartum fetal distress. In a study of FHR monitoring of 41 infants born with major congenital malformations, Garite and associates[93] found that there were no characteristic FHR patterns that would specifically identify major congenital malformations. However, 17 infants with major malformations were delivered by cesarean section because of fetal distress and 44% of these infants died neonatally.

Cesarean Section Versus Vaginal Delivery

For the VLBW fetus in vertex presentation, the best route of delivery remains debatable. Most investigators prefer vaginal delivery with intensive intrapartum fetal monitoring and the liberal use of cesarean section for fetal indications.[29,30,81,139] Bowes and colleagues[30] compared the outcome of cesarean and vaginal vertex VLBW deliveries and found no survival advantage for abdominal delivery. Similarly, Kitchen and co-workers[139] studied 326 infants born at 24 to 28 completed weeks of gestation and found that the survival rate of infants delivered by cesarean section (62.7%) was not significantly superior to that of infants delivered vaginally (50.9%). However, two other studies reported improved survival with cesarean section (56%) over vaginal delivery (38%), but only when the fetus in vertex presentation weighed less than 1000 g.[29,234]

For the VLBW breech, investigators have consistently reported that mortality is two to seven times higher after vaginal delivery than after cesarean section.[64,65,71,127,234] When vaginal and cesarean VLBW breech pairs are compared, birth trauma and IVH are five times more frequent with vaginal delivery.[64] Delivery by cesarean section in preterm breech significantly reduced the incidence of severe prolonged asphyxia (from 37.5% to 9.5%) and the incidence of neonatal mortality (from 14.6% to 4.8%).[127] There seems little doubt based upon these study results that the potentially salvageable VLBW breech fetus should undergo cesarean section. A generous vertical uterine incision will further reduce the risk of fetal trauma or asphyxia.[110]

Studies of abnormal FHR patterns and fetal acid-base balance in LBW infants have indicated that cesarean section produces better immediate fetal outcome.[119,172] It is difficult to conclude from these studies whether it was the cesarean section or the fact that the fetus was monitored and not dismissed as nonviable when abnormal FHR patterns were detected, which improved the outcome.

Two recent studies which used real-time ultrasound to detect IVH and periventricular hemorrhage compared the incidence of these types of central nervous system bleeding to the type of delivery.[23,61] One study found hemorrhage was more frequent in infants born after labor, suggesting that performing a cesarean section before the onset of labor is appropriate to prevent IVH.[23] The second study showed that cesarean section after the onset of labor, at any gestational age, probably had no effect on the risk of bleeding in preterm fetuses.[61] Two other studies[13,143] also attempted to evaluate obstetric events with respect to IVH but failed to provide clear-cut answers. Both groups of investigators noted that IVH correlated with the degree of prematurity but was not linked to the mode of delivery or other antenatal obstetric factors. However, if a cesarean section is indicated in the VLBW fetus, it seems advisable that the section be performed before the onset of labor, in order to protect against IVH in the VLBW infant.

The right of patients to be actively involved in decision-making in obstetric management is now widely accepted.[134] Fetal distress and breech presentation are two less controversial conditions for both the obstetrician and the patient to consider as a medical indication for cesarean section. However, in those cases where the fetus is believed to have a very low probability of survival (e.g., EFW of 500–700 g or gestational age of 24 to 26 weeks) and those cases with major malformations and/or documented chromosomal trisomies, the patient and her family's involvement in the decision-making process is very important. Obstetricians should try to diagnose the condition as early as possible, involve the patient and her family, and let the neonatologists or pediatric surgeons assist in the prediction of fetal outcome. (The ethical aspects of this problem are discussed in the next section.)

Resuscitation in the Delivery Room

Resuscitation of the newborn infant requires the combined efforts of the obstetrician and the pediatrician during labor, delivery, and the immediate neonatal period because the transition from intrauterine to extrauterine life involves considerable risk to the newborn infant. It is particularly difficult for the VLBW infant, because of the prematurity of its organ systems, to adapt to the sudden respiratory and circulatory changes involved. In addition, the delivery process itself usually leads to a progressive increase in fetal hypoxia, hypercapnea, and acidosis. Although only 10% of term infants fail to make the transition smoothly,[99] the incidence of 1-minute Apgar scores of less than 7 in VLBW neonates is in the range of 70% to 85%.[30,31,95,117,189]

For more than 10 years, we have practiced the three-code system—code pink, white, and blue—for requesting pediatric assistance for newborn resuscitation in the delivery room at the Chicago Lying-In Hospital. This system is established according to the level of resuscitation anticipated before the delivery actually takes place. Pediatricians are notified of a code pink if an elective cesarean section for an uncomplicated term pregnancy is performed. A junior pediatric resident or intern from the neonatology division will then be sent to the delivery room. Code white is associated with meconium-stained fluid, mild to moderate abnormal FHR patterns, or a term SGA delivery, and two pediatric residents (including one senior resident) participate in the newborn resuscitation. Code blue is associated with the delivery of a VLBW fetus, or fetuses with severe FHR patterns or acidosis, or with massive antepartum/intrapartum hemorrhage. Three pediatricians (including one attending or one neonatology fellow) are then involved with newborn resuscitation.

The delivery of VLBW fetuses is always attended by the most skillful and experienced neonatologists in newborn resuscitation at our institution.

The delivery room team should be prepared for complete resuscitation, including immediate endotracheal intubation. When meconium is present, it has been shown that deep suctioning of the nasopharynx before delivery of the thorax using a DeLee suction trap, together with tracheal suction under direct visualization after delivery, reduces the incidence of meconium aspiration syndrome and its complications,[38,100,248] including pneumothorax, persistent fetal circulation, and bacterial pneumonia.[266] Antibiotics are recommended to prevent secondary bacterial infection. HMD is common in the VLBW infant.[267] Prevention of both perinatal asphyxia and RDS have already been discussed. The prevention of the former and its sequelae remains the most important task for the obstetrician-neonatologist team in managing the labor and delivery of a VLBW fetus.

PROGNOSIS AND LONG-TERM FOLLOW-UP

In addition to the survival rate and immediate neonatal complications of the VLBW infant, the quality of life of those infants must also be considered. Although neurologic deficits remain a problem, improved obstetric and neonatal care during the last decade has sharply reduced the incidence and severity of these handicaps among VLBW babies. More than 80% of VLBW babies born today can expect to lead productive lives with minimal neurologic disabilities.[26,71,121,224,243,269]

Allen and Jones[5] have reviewed the literature on the long-term prognosis for the survival of VLBW infants. They found that the incidence of major handicaps (cerebral palsy and/or mental retardation) ranges from 7% to 16% for those with birth weights below 1500 g; 9% to 21% for those born below 1000 g; and 12% to 42% for those with birth weights below 800 g. The prevalence of the lesser morbidities, however, particularly learning disabilities, have been demonstrated in 20% to 36% of school-age children with birth weights below 1500 g, and up to 64% of those with birth weights below 1000 g. The reports subjected to this review include those dating from the mid-1960s.

However, data from the late seventies and early eighties show definite improvement. The best results were reported by Stewart and Reynolds.[243] Among 95 London children with birth weights between 501 g and 1500 g, 86 (90.5%) had no handicaps at age 5; 4 children (4.2%) had physical handicaps, and 5 children (5.3%) had mental handicaps. Saigal and associates[224] studied 294 VLBW infants (501–1500 g birth weight) from Canada and reported a 16.8% incidence of neurologic handicaps which included cerebral palsy, hydrocephalus, microcephaly, blindness, deafness, and mental retardation among 179 survivors. The incidence of neurologic handicaps was 30% among babies who received intermittent positive pressure ventilation (IPPV) versus 10% in those who did not. Ingermarsson and group[127] reported from Sweden that 24% of 42 preterm breeches delivered vaginally, compared to 2.5% of those delivered by cesarean section, had developmental or neurologic handicaps at the age of 12 months. Fairweather[71] reported an incidence of 11% handicaps among 376 VLBW infants at age 2.

For specific problems, Bergman and colleagues[26] found that bilateral hearing loss occurred in 9.7% of infants who survived VLBW, and in 28.6% of infants who survived both VLBW and neonatal seizures. Yu and co-workers[269] studied 294 VLBW infants over a 4-year period in Australia. By age 2, both major handicaps (27% v. 15%) and developmental delay (13% v. 4%) were significantly higher in survivors of VLBW with prolonged initial hospitalization compared to the group without prolonged hospitalization. Among all of the VLBW survivors, 34% were below the tenth percentile for weight and 39% were below the tenth percentile for height, but head circumferences were normal. Among VLBW infants, 10% to 20% are preterm SGA.[71,88,158,224] There are no specific data available for the long-term prognosis of SGA in the VLBW category. However, most investigators have reported that SGA infants tend to have lower IQs with an increased risk for learning and behavior disorders when compared to AGA infants of the same gestational age at birth.[15,45,75,78,192,263] Neligan and associates stated that it is better to be born too soon than too small, based on multivariate analysis of their long-term follow-up study of LBW infants.[192] It is reasonable to state that the preterm SGA infant has, relatively speaking, the worst prognosis of all of the VLBW infants.

REFERENCES

1. Abramowicz M, Kass EH: Pathogenesis and prematurity. N Engl J Med 275:878, 1966
2. Adams FH, Towers B, Osher AR et al: Effects of tracheal instillation of natural surfactant in premature lambs. Pediatr Res 12:841, 1978
3. Andreyko JL, Chen CP, Shennan AT et al: Results of conservative management of premature rupture of the membranes. Am J Obstet Gynecol 148:600, 1984
4. Allan WC, Roveio CA, Sawyer LR et al: Sector scan ultrasound imaging through the anterior fontanelle: Its use in diagnosing neonatal periventricular-intraventricular hemorrhage. Am J Dis Child 184:1225, 1980
5. Allen MC, Jones MD: Medical complications of prematurity. Obstet Gynecol 67:427, 1986
6. Altschuler G, Russel P: The human placental villitides: A review of chronic intrauterine infections. Curr Top Pathol 60:63, 1975
7. Anderson CL, Aladjem S, Ayote O et al: An analysis of maternal transport within a suburban metropolitan region. Am J Obstet Gynecol 140:499, 1981
8. Anderson KE, Forman A, Ulmsten U: Pharmacology of labor. Clin Obstet Gynecol 26:56, 1983
9. Apgar V, James LS: Further observations on the newborn scoring system. Am J Dis Child 104:133, 1962
10. Arias F: Expansion of intravascular volume and fetal outcome in patients with chronic hypertension and pregnancy. Am J Obstet Gynecol 123:610, 1975
11. Arias F: The diagnosis and management of intrauterine growth retardation. Obstet Gynecol 49:293, 1977
12. Assali NS, Bekey GA, Morrison LW: Fetal and neonatal circulation. In Assali NS (ed): Biology of Gestation: The Fetus and Neonate. New York, Academic Press, 1968
13. Bada HS, Korones SB, Magill HL et al: Influence of the mode of delivery on the occurrence of intraventricular hemorrhage. Pediatr Res 16:275A, 1982
14. Barden TP: Premature labor. In Queenan JT (ed): Management of High Risk Pregnancy. Hagerstown, MD, Harper and Row, 1984
15. Barker DJP: Low intelligence—Its relation to length of gestation and rate of foetal growth. Br J Prev Soc Med 20:58, 1966
16. Barss VA, Benacerraf BR, Frigoletto FD: Second trimester oligohydramnios, a predictor of poor fetal outcome. Obstet Gynecol 64:608, 1984
17. Bartlett RH, Andrews AF, Toomasian JM et al: Extracorporeal membrane oxygenation (ECMO) for newborn respiratory failure: 45 cases. Surgery 92:425, 1982

18. Bartlett RH, Roloff DW, Cornell RG et al: Extracorporeal circulation in neonatal respiratory failure: A prospective randomized study. Pediatrics 76:479, 1985
19. Battaglia FC, Lubchenco LO: A practical classification of newborn infants by weight and gestational age. J Pediatr 71:159, 1967
20. Bauer CR: Corticosteroids and lung maturity. In Sciarra JJ: Gynecology and Obstetrics, vol 3, chap 88, pp 1–15. Philadelphia, Harper & Row, 1981
21. Beall MH, Edgar BW, Paul RH et al: A comparison of ritodrine, terbutaline, and magnesium sulfate for the suppression of preterm labor. Am J Obstet Gynecol 153:854, 1985
22. Bejar R, Curbelo V, Coen RW et al: Diagnosis and follow-up of intraventricular and intracerebral hemorrhages by ultrasound studies of infant's brain through the fontanelles and sutures. Pediatrics 66:661, 1980
23. Bejar R, Curbelo V, Coen R et al: Large intraventricular hemorrhage and labor in infants greater than or equal to 1000 grams. Pediatr Res 15:649, 1981
24. Bender S: Twin pregnancy. A review of 472 cases. Br J Obstet Gynaecol 59:510, 1952
25. Benedetti TJ: Maternal complications of prenatal betasympathomimetic therapy for premature labor. Am J Obstet Gynecol 145:1, 1983
26. Bergman I, Hirsch RP, Fria TJ et al: Cause of hearing loss in the high risk premature infant. J Pediatr 106:95, 1985
27. Block M, King OR, Cosby WM: Antenatal glucocorticoid therapy for the prevention of the respiratory distress syndrome in the premature infant. Obstet Gynecol 50:186, 1977
28. Bobitt JR, Ledger WJ: Unrecognized amnionitis and prematurity: A preliminary report. J Reprod Med 19:8, 1977
29. Bowes WA: Delivery of the very low birth weight infant. Clin Perinatol 8:183, 1981
30. Bowes WA, Halgrimson M, Simons MA: Results of the intensive perinatal management of the very low birth weight infant (501–1500 grams). J Reprod Med 23:245, 1979
31. Braithwaite NDJ, Milligan JE, Shennan AT: Fetal heart rate monitoring and neonatal mortality in the very preterm infant. Am J Obstet Gynecol 154:250, 1986
32. Brame RG, MacKenna J: Vaginal pool phospholipids in the management of premature rupture of membranes. Obstet Gynecol 63:33, 1984
33. Brann AW, Myers RE: Central nervous system findings in the newborn monkey following severe in utero partial asphyxia. Neurology 25:327, 1975
34. Brann AW, Myers RE: Brain swelling and hemorrhagic cortical necrosis following perinatal asphyxia in monkeys. J Neuropathol Exp Neurol 28:178, 1978
35. Brenner WE, Edelman DA, Hendricks CH: Characteristics of patients with placenta previa and results of expectant management. Am J Obstet Gynecol 132:180, 1978
36. Caritis SN, Carson D, Greebon D et al: A comparison of terbutaline and ethanol in the treatment of preterm labor. Am J Obstet Gynecol 142:183, 1982
37. Caritis SN, Toig G, Heddinger LA et al: A double-blind study comparing ritodrine and terbutaline in the treatment of preterm labor. Am J Obstet Gynecol 150:7, 1984
38. Carson BS, Losey RW, Bowes WA et al: Combined obstetric and pediatric approach to prevent meconium aspiration syndrome. Am J Obstet Gynecol 126:712, 1976
39. Casey ML, MacDonald PC: Endocrinology of preterm birth. Clin Obstet Gynecol 27:562, 1984
40. Caspi E, Schreyer P, Weinraub Z et al: Dexamethasone for prevention of respiratory distress syndrome: Multiple perinatal factors. Obstet Gynecol 57:41, 1981
41. Castle BM, Turnbull AC: Presence or absence of fetal breathing movement predicts outcome of preterm labor. Lancet 2:471, 1983
42. Challis JRG: Characteristics of parturition. In Creasy RK, Resnik R (eds): Maternal Fetal Medicine: Principles and Practice, pp 401–414. Philadelphia, WB Saunders, 1984
43. Cibils LA: The placenta and newborn infant in hypertensive conditions. Am J Obstet Gynecol 118:256, 1974
44. Collaborative Group on Antenatal Steroid Therapy: Effect of antenatal dexamethasone administration on the prevention of respiratory distress syndrome. Am J Obstet Gynecol 141:276, 1981
45. Commey JOO, Fitzhardine PM: Handicap in the preterm small-for-gestational age infant. J Pediatr 94:779, 1979
46. Committee to Study the Prevention of Low Birthweight (Headed by Behrman RE): Preventing Low Birthweight. Washington, DC, Division of Health Promotion and Disease Prevention, Institute of Medicine, National Academy Press, 1985
47. Cooke RW: Factors associated with periventricular hemorrhage in very low birthweight infants. Arch Dis Childhood 56:425, 1981

48. Cordero L, Backes CR, Zuspan FP: Very low birth weight infant. I. Influence of place of birth on survival. Am J Obstet Gynecol 143:533, 1981
49. Cotton DB, Hill LM, Strassner HT et al: Use of amniocentesis in preterm gestation with ruptured membranes. Obstet Gynecol 63:38, 1984
50. Cowett RM, Coustan DR, Oh W: Effects of maternal transport on admission pattern at a tertiary care center. Am J Obstet Gynecol 154:1098, 1986
51. Creasy RK: Prevention of preterm birth. Birth Defects 19(5):97, 1983
52. Creasy RK: Preterm labor and delivery. In Creasy RK, Resnik R (eds): Maternal Fetal Medicine: Principles and Practice, pp 415–443. Philadelphia, WB Saunders, 1984
53. Creasy RK, Gummer BA, Liggins GC: A system for predicting spontaneous preterm birth. Obstet Gynecol 55:692, 1980
54. Crombleholme WR, Minkoff HL, Delke I et al: Cervical cerclage: An aggressive approach to threatened or recurrent pregnancy wastage. Am J Obstet Gynecol 146:168, 1983
55. Csaba IF, Sulyok E, Ertl T: Clinical note: Relationship of maternal treatment with indomethacin to persistent of fetal circulation syndrome. J Pediatr 92:484, 1978
56. Csapo AI, Herczeg J: Arrest of premature labor by isoxsuprine. Am J Obstet Gynecol 129:482, 1977
57. Curet LB, Rao AV, Zachman RD et al: Association between ruptured membranes, tocolytic therapy, and respiratory distress syndrome. Am J Obstet Gynecol 148:263, 1984
58. D'Alton ME, Hou S, Cetrulo CL: Treatment of premature labor with nifedipine: A preliminary report. The 4th Annual Scientific Meeting of the Society of Perinatal Obstetricians, San Antonio, abstract 162, 1984
59. Depp R, Boehm JJ, Nosek JA et al: Antenatal corticosteroids to prevent neonatal respiratory distress syndrome: Risk versus benefit considerations. Am J Obstet Gynecol 137:338, 1980
60. Devoe LD, Taylor RL: Systemic lupus erythematosus in pregnancy. Am J Obstet Gynecol 135:478, 1979
61. Driscoll JW: Personal communication. Cited by Leppert PC, Petrie RH: Delivering the preterm by cesarean. Contemp OB/GYN 19:116, 1982
62. Dudenhausen JW: Extracorporeal circulation for the newborn with lung immaturity. The 4th Asia-Oceania Congress of Perinatology, abstract PC 2–3, 1986
63. Dudley DKL, Hardie MJ: Fetal and neonatal effects on indomethacin used as a tocolytic agent. Am J Obstet Gynecol 151:181, 1985
64. Duenhoelter JH, Wells E, Reisch JS et al: A paired controlled study of vaginal and abdominal delivery of the low birth weight breech fetus. Obstet Gynecol 54:310, 1979
65. Efer SB, Saigal S, Rand C et al: Effect of delivery method on outcomes in the very low birth weight breech infant: Is improved survival related to cesarean section or other perinatal care maneuvers? Am J Obstet Gynecol 145:123, 1983
66. Egan EA, Notter RH, Kwong MS et al: Natural and artificial surfactant replacement therapy in premature lambs. J Appl Physiol 55(3):875, 1983
67. Elias E: Fetoscopy in prenatal diagnosis. Semin Perinatol 4:199, 1980
68. Enhorning G, Shennan A, Possmayer F et al: Prevention of neonatal respiratory distress syndrome by tracheal instillation of surfactant: A randomized clinical trial. Pediatrics 76:145, 1985
69. Erhardt CL, Joshi GB, Nelson FG et al: Influence of weight and gestation on perinatal and neonatal mortality by ethnic group. Am J Pub Health 54:1841, 1964
70. Evans MI, Hajj SN, Devoe LD et al: C-reactive protein as predictor of infectious morbidity with premature rupture of membranes. Am J Obstet Gynecol 138:648, 1980
71. Fairweather DVI: Obstetric management and follow-up of the very low birth weight infant. J Reprod Med 26:387, 1981
72. Farrell PM, Wood RM: Epidemiology of hayaline membrane disease: Analysis of national mortality statistics. Pediatrics 58:167, 1976
73. Ferguson JE, Hensleigh PA, Kredenster D: Adjunctive use of magnesium sulfate with ritodrine for preterm labor tocolysis. Am J Obstet Gynecol 148:166, 1984
74. Fiakpui EZ, Moran EM: Pregnancy in the sickle hemoglobinopathies. J Reprod Med 11:28, 1973
75. Fitzhardine PM, Steven EM: The small-fordate infant II. Neurological and intellectual sequelae. Pediatrics 50:50, 1972
76. Flood B, Naeye RL: Factors that predispose to premature rupture of the fetal membranes. JOGN Nurs 13:119, 1984
77. Forman A, Gandrup P, Anderson KE et al: Effect of nifedipine on spontaneous and methylergometrine-induced activity postpartum. Am J Obstet Gynecol 144:442, 1982

78. Francis-Williams J, Davies PA: Very low birth weight and later intelligence. Dev Med Child Neurol 16:709, 1974
79. Fredrick J: Antenatal identification of women at high risk of spontaneous preterm birth. Br J Obstet Gynecol 83:351, 1976
80. Fredrick J, Anderson ABM: Factors associated with spontaneous preterm birth. Br J Obstet Gynecol 83:342, 1976
81. Freeman RK, Gluck L, Hobbins JC, Petrie RH: Fetus at risk: Guide to salvageability. Contemp OB/GYN 19:89, 1982
82. Fuchs F: Prevention of prematurity. Am J Obstet Gynecol 126:809, 1976
83. Fuchs F: Ethanol for prevention of preterm birth. Semin Perinatol 5:263, 1981
84. Fuchs F, Fuchs A-R, Poblete VW Jr et al: Effect of alcohol on threatened premature labor. Am J Obstet Gynecol 99:627, 1967
85. Fujiwara T, Chida S, Watabe Y et al: Artificial surfactant therapy in hyaline membrane disease. Lancet 1:55, 1980
86. Fujiwara T, Maeta H, Chida S et al: Improved lung-thorax compliance and prevention of neonatal pulmonary lesion in prematurely delivered rabbit neonates subjected to IPPV after tracheal instillation of artificial surfactant. IRCS Med Sci 7:313, 1979
87. Fujiwara T, Maeta H, Chida S et al: Improved pulmonary pressure-volume characteristics in premature newborn rabbits after tracheal instillations of artificial surfactant. IRCS Med Sci 7:312, 1979
88. Galbraith RS, Karchmar EJ, Piercy WN et al: The clinical prediction of intrauterine growth retardation. Am J Obstet Gynecol 133:281, 1979
89. Gant NF, Worley RJ, Cunningham FG et al: Clinical management of pregnancy-induced hypertension. Clin Obstet Gynecol 21:397, 1978
90. Garcia-Prats JA, Procianoy RS, Adams JM et al: The hyaline membrane disease-intraventricular hemorrhage relationship in the very low birth weight infant: Perinatal aspects. Acta Paediatr Scand 71(1):79, 1982
91. Garfield RE: Control of myometrial function in preterm versus term labor. Clin Obstet Gynecol 27:572, 1984
92. Garite TJ, Freeman RK, Lingen EM: Prospective randomized study of corticosteroids in the management of premature rupture of the membranes and the premature gestation. Am J Obstet Gynecol 141:508, 1981
93. Garite TJ, Linzey M, Freeman RK et al: Fetal heart rate patterns and fetal distress in fetuses with congenital anomalies. Obstet Gynecol 53:716, 1979
94. Gerara P, Bachy A, Battisti O et al: Mortality in 504 infants weighing less than 1501 g at birth and treated in four neonatal intensive care units of South-Belgium between 1976 and 1980. Eur J Pediatr 144:219, 1985
95. Goldenberg RL, Huddleston JF, Nelson KG: Apgar scores and umbilical arterial pH in preterm newborn infants. Am J Obstet Gynecol 149:651, 1984
96. Goldenberg RL, Humphrey JL, Hale CB et al: Neonatal deaths in Alabama, 1970–1980: An analysis of birth weight and race-specific neonatal mortality rates. Am J Obstet Gynecol 145, 545, 1983
97. Golichowski AM, Hathaway DR, Fineberg N et al: Tocolytic and hemodynamic effects of nifedipine in the ewe. Am J Obstet Gynecol 151:1134, 1985
98. Graham RL, Gilstrap LC, Hauth JC et al: Conservative management of patients with premature rupture of fetal membranes. Obstet Gynecol 59:607, 1982
99. Gregory GA: Resuscitation of the newborn. Anesthesiology 43:225, 1975
100. Gregory GA, Gooding CA, Phibbs RH et al: Meconium aspiration in infants: A prospective study. J Pediatr 85:848, 1974
101. Gregory GA, Kitterman JA, Phibbs RH et al: Treatment of idiopathic respiratory distress syndrome with continuous positive airway pressure. N Engl J Med 284:1333, 1971
102. Greiss FC: Concepts of uterine blood flow. In Wynn RM (ed): Obstetrics and Gynecology Annual: 1973, pp 55–83. New York, Appleton-Century-Crofts, 1973
103. Greiss FC, Anderson SG: Uterine blood flow during labor. Clin Obstet Gynecol 11:95, 1968
104. Gruenwald P: Chronic fetal distress and placental insufficiency. Biol Neonate 5:215, 1963
105. Hack M, Faranoff AH, Merkatz IR: The low birthweight infant. Evolution of a changing outlook. N Engl J Med 301:1162, 1979
106. Hadlock FP, Deter RL, Harrist RB: Sonographic detection of abnormal fetal growth patterns. Clin Obstet Gynecol 27:342, 1984
107. Harger J: Comparison of success and morbidity in cervical cerclage procedures. Obstet Gynecol 56:543, 1980
108. Harris TR, Isaman J, Giles HR: Improved neonatal survival through maternal transport. Obstet Gynecol 52:294, 1978
109. Harris BA, Winschafter DD, Huddleson JF et al: Utero versus neonatal transport of high

risk perinates: A comparison. Obstet Gynecol 57:496, 1981
110. Hasselin HC, Goodlin RC: Delivery of the tiny newborn. Am J Obstet Gynecol 134:192, 1979
111. Hatjis CG, Nelson LH, Meis PL et al: Addition of magnesium sulfate improves effectiveness of ritodrine in preventing premature delivery. Am J Obstet Gynecol 150:142, 1984
112. Hauth JC, Gilstrap LC, Brekken AL et al: The effect of 17α-hydroxyprogesterone caproate on pregnancy outcome in an active-duty military population. Am J Obstet Gynecol 146:187, 1983
113. Hawrylyshyn PA, Barkin M, Bernstein A et al: Twin pregnancies—A continuing perinatal challenge. Obstet Gynecol 59:463, 1982
114. Hawrylyshun PA, Bernstein P, Milligan JE et al: Premature rupture of membranes: The role of C-reactive protein in the prediction of chorioamnionitis. Am J Obstet Gynecol 147:240, 1983
115. Herron M, Katz M, Creasy RK: Evaluation of a preterm birth prevention program: Preliminary report. Obstet Gynecol 59:452, 1982
116. Heymann MA, Rudolph AM: Effects of acetylsalicylic acid on the ductus arteriosus and circulation in fetal lambs in utero. Circ Res 38:418, 1976
117. Hibbard JU, Moawad AH: Umbilical cord blood pH values and Apgar scores in very low birth weight infants (unpublished data). Personal communication
118. Hobbins JC, Grannum PAT, Berkowitz RL: Ultrasound in the diagnosis of congenital anomalies. Am J Obstet Gynecol 134:331, 1979
119. Hobel CJ, Hyvarinen MC, Oh W: Abnormal fetal heart rate patterns and fetal acid-base balance in low birth weight infants in relationship to respiratory distress syndrome. Obstet Gynecol 39:83, 1972
120. Hon EH: The classification of fetal heart rate. Obstet Gynecol 22:137, 1963
121. Horwood SP, Boyle MH, Torrance GW et al: Mortality and morbidity of 500–1499 gram birth weight infants live-born to residents of a defined geographic region before and after neonatal intensive care. Pediatrics 69:613, 1982
122. Hoskins EM, Elliot E, Shennan AT et al: Outcome of very low birth weight infants born at a perinatal center. Am J Obstet Gynecol 145:135, 1983
123. Howie RN, Liggins GC: Clinical trial of antepartum betamethasone therapy in pre-term infants. Preceedings of Fifth Study Group Royal College of Obstetricians and Gynecology, p 281. October, 1977
124. Hurwitz A, Adoni A, Palti Z et al: Is conservative management of preterm rupture of membranes justified? Int J Gynaecol Obstet 22:131, 1984
125. Iams JD, Barrows H: Management of preterm prematurely ruptured membranes: A retrospective comparison of observation versus use of steroid and timed delivery. Am J Obstet Gynecol 150:977, 1984
126. Ingermarsson I: Effect of terbutaline on premature labor: A double blind placebo-controlled study. Am J Obstet Gynecol 125:520, 1976
127. Ingemarsson I, Westgren W, Svenningsen NW: Long-term follow-up of preterm infants in breech presentation delivered by cesarean section. Lancet 2:171, 1978
128. Inselman LS: Respiratory distress syndrome. Pediatr Ann 7:34, 1978
129. Ismail MA, Zinaman MJ, Lowensohn RI et al: The significance of C-reactive protein levels in women with premature rupture of membranes. Am J Obstet Gynecol 151:541, 1985
130. Johnson HW: The conservative management of some varieties of placenta previa. Am J Obstet Gynecol 50:248, 1945
131. Johnson JWC, Austin KL, Jones GS et al: Efficacy of 17α-hydroxyprogesterone caproate in the prevention of premature labor. N Engl J Med 293:675, 1975
132. Johnson JWC, Lee PA, Zachary AS et al: High-risk prematurity: Progestin treatment and steroid studies. Obstet Gynecol 86:913, 1979
133. Johnson ML, Mack LA, Rumack CM, et al: B-mode echoencephalography in the normal and high risk infant. Am J Radiol 133:375, 1979
134. Johnson SR, Elkins TE, Strong C et al: Obstetric decision-making: Responses to patients who request cesarean delivery. Obstet Gynecol 67:847, 1986
135. Kamper J: Long term prognosis of infants with severe idiopathic respiratory distress syndrome. I. Neurological and mental outcome. Acta Paediatr Scand 67:61, 1978
136. Katz M, Robertson PA, Creasy RK: Cardiovascular complications associated with terbutaline treatment for preterm labor. Am J Obstet Gynecol 139:605, 1981
137. Katz Z, Lancet M, Yemini M et al: Treatment of premature labor contractions with com-

bined ritodrine and indomethacin. Int J Gynaecol Obstet 21:337, 1983
138. Kirkpatrick BV, Krummel TM, Mueller DG et al: Use of extracorporeal membrane oxygenation for respiratory failure in term infants. Pediatrics 72:872, 1983
139. Kitchen W, Ford GW, Doyle LW et al: Cesarean section or vaginal delivery at 24 to 28 weeks gestation: Comparison of survival and neonatal and two year morbidity. Obstet Gynecol 66:149, 1985
140. Knobloch H, Malone A, Ellison PH et al: Considerations in evaluating changes in outcome for infants weighing less than 1501 grams. Pediatrics 69:285, 1982
141. Komaromy B, Lampe L: Value of bed rest in twin pregnancy. Int J Obstet Gynecol 14:262, 1977
142. Koops BL, Morgan LJ, Battaglia FC: Neonatal mortality risk in relation to birth weight and gestational age: Update. J Pediatr. 101:969, 1982
143. Krishamoorthy KS, Shannon DS, DeLong GR et al: Neurologic sequelae in the survivals of neonatal intraventricular hemorrhage. Pediatrics 64:233, 1979
144. Kuhn RJP, Speirs AL, Pepperell RJ et al: Bethamethasone, albuterol, and threatened premature delivery: Benefits and risks. Obstet Gynecol 60:403, 1982
145. Kulovich MV, Gluck L: The lung profile. II. Complicated pregnancy. Am J Obstet Gynecol 135:64, 1979
146. Larsen JW, Evans MI: Genetic causes of IUGR. In Lin CC, Evans MI (eds): Intrauterine Growth Retardation: Pathophysiology and Clinical Management, pp 81–97. New York, McGraw-Hill, 1984
147. Laudesman R, Holze E, Scherr L: Fetal mortality in essential hypertension. Obstet Gynecol 6:354, 1955
148. Lauersen NH, Merkatz IR, Tejani N et al: Inhibition of premature labor: A multicenter comparison of ritodrine and ethanol. Am J Obstet Gynecol 127:837, 1977
149. Laursen B: Twin pregnancy: The value of prophylactic rest in bed and the risk involved. Acta Obstet Gynecol Scand 52:367, 1973
150. Lazar P, Gueguen J, Dreyfus R et al: Multicentered controlled trial of cervical cerclage in women at moderate risk of preterm delivery. Br J Obstet Gynecol 91:731, 1984
151. Lee KS, Paneth N, Gartner LM: The very low birth weight rate: Principal predictor of neonatal mortality in industrialized populations. J Pediatr 97:759, 1980
152. Lee KS, Paneth N, Gartner LM et al: Neonatal mortality: An analysis of the recent improvement in the United States. Am J Public Health 70:15, 1980
153. Levy DL, Noelke K, Goldsmith JP: Maternal and infant transport program in Louisiana. Obstet Gynecol 57:500, 1981
154. Liggins GC, Howie RN: A controlled trial of antepartum glucocorticoid treatment for prevention of the respiratory distress syndrome in premature infants. Pediatrics 50:515, 1972
155. Lin CC: Intrauterine growth retardation. In Wynn RM (ed): Obstetrics and Gynecology Annual 1985, pp 127–221. Norwalk, CT, Appleton-Century-Crofts, 1985
156. Lin CC: Weight specific neonatal survival rates in very low birth weight infants at the University of Chicago, 1981–1985 (unpublished data), 1986
157. Lin CC, Evans MI: Diagnosis of IUGR. In Lin CC, Evans MI (eds): Intrauterine Growth Retardation: Pathophysiology and Clinical Management, pp 179–223. New York, McGraw-Hill, 1984
158. Lin CC, Evans MI: Introduction to IUGR. In Lin CC, Evans MI (eds): Intrauterine Growth Retardation: Pathophysiology and Clinical Management, pp 3–15. New York, McGraw-Hill, 1984
159. Lin CC, Lindheimer MD, River P et al: Fetal outcome in hypertensive disorder of pregnancy. Am J Obstet Gynecol 142:255, 1982
160. Longo LD: Placental transfer mechanism—An overview. In Wynn RM (ed): Obstetrics and Gynecology Annual: 1972, pp 103–138. New York, Appleton-Century-Crofts, 1972
161. Low JA, Pancham SR, Worthington D et al: The acid-base and biochemical characteristics of intrauterine fetal asphyxia. Am J Obstet Gynecol 121:446, 1975
162. Lubchenco LO: The preterm infant. In Lubchenco LO (ed): The High Risk Infant, pp 125–150. Philadelphia, WB Saunders, 1976
163. Lubchenco LO, Homer FA, Reed LH et al: Sequelae of premature birth. Am J Dis Child 106:105, 1973
164. Lubchenco LO, Searls DT, Brazie JV: Neonatal mortality rate: Relationship to birth weight and gestational age. J Pediatr 81:814, 1972
165. Macafee CHG: Placenta previa: A study of 174 cases. Br J Obstet Gynecol 52:313, 1945
166. MacGillivary I, Campbell DA: A prospective study of factors affecting intrauterine growth.

In Lindheimer MD, Katz AI, Zuspan FP (eds): Hypertension in Pregnancy, pp 23–29. New York, John Wiley & Sons, 1976
167. MacKenna J, Brame RG: Fetal lung maturity and phospholipids. In Wynn RM (ed): Obstetrics and Gynecology Annual 1985, pp 222–239. Norwalk, CT, Appleton-Century-Crofts, 1985
168. Macri J, Weiss RR: Prenatal diagnosis of neural tube defects. Semin Perinatol 4:207, 1980
169. Main DM, Gabbe SG, Richardson D et al: Can preterm deliveries be prevented? Am J Obstet Gynecol 151:892, 1985
170. Makowski EL, Meschia G, Droengemueller W et al: Distribution of uterine blood flow in the pregnant sheep. Am J Obstet Gynecol 101:409, 1968
171. Manniello RL, Farrell PM: Analysis of United States neonatal mortality statistics from 1968–1974, with specific reference to changing trends in major casualties. Am J Obstet Gynecol 129:667, 1977
172. Martin CB, Siassi B, Hon EH: Fetal heart rate patterns and neonatal death in low birthweight infants. Obstet Gynecol 44:503, 1974
173. McCormick MC, Shapiro S, Starfield: High risk young mothers: Infant mortality and morbidity in four areas in the United States, 1973–1978. Am J Public Health 74:18, 1984
174. Meis PJ, Ernest JM, Moore ML: Prematurity prevention—Success or failure? The Sixth Annual Meeting of the Society of Perinatal Obstetricians, San Antonio, abstract 103, 1986
175. Meis PJ, Hall M, Marshall JR et al: Meconium passage: A new classification for risk assessment during labor. Am J Obstet Gynecol 131:509, 1978
176. Mercer LJ, Brown LG: Fetal outcome with oligohydramnios in the second trimester. Obstet Gynecol 67:840, 1986
177. Merkatz IR, Peter JB, Barden TP: Ritodrine hydrochloride. A betamimetic agent for use in preterm labor. II. Evidence of efficacy. Obstet Gynecol 56:7, 1980
178. Meschia G: Supply of oxygen to the fetus. J Reprod Med 23:160, 1979
179. Miller HC, Hassanein K, Hensleigh PA: Maternal factors in the incidence of low birthweight infants among black and white mothers. Pediatr Res 12:1016, 1978
180. Miller JM, Keane MWD, Horger EO: A comparison of magnesium sulfate and terbutaline for the arrest of premature labor. J Reprod Med 27:348, 1982
181. Miller JM, Pupkin MJ, Hill GB: Bacterial colonization of amniotic fluid from intact fetal membranes. Am J Obstet Gynecol 136:796, 1980
182. Miller TC, Densberger M, Krogman J: Maternal transport and the perinatal denominator. Am J Obstet Gynecol 147:19, 1983
183. Milliez J, Blot P, Sureau C: A case report of maternal death associated with betamimetics and betamethasone administration in premature labor. Eur. J. Obstet Gynaecol Reprod Biol 11:95, 1980
184. Minkoff H, Grunebaum AN, Schwarz RH et al: Risk factors for prematurity and premature rupture of membranes: A prospective study of the vaginal flora in pregnancy. Am J Obstet Gynecol 150:965, 1984
185. Moberg LJ, Garite TJ, Freeman RK: Fetal heart rate patterns and fetal distress in patients with preterm premature rupture of membranes. Obstet Gynecol 64:60, 1984
186. Modanlou HD, Dorchester W, Freeman RK et al: Perinatal transport to a regional perinatal center in a metropolitan area: Maternal versus neonatal transport. Am J Obstet Gynecol 138:1157, 1980
187. Moore TR, Resnik R: Special problems of VLBW infants. Contemp OB/GYN 29:174, 1984
188. Morrison JC, Schneider JM, Whybrew WD et al: Effect of corticosteroids and fetomaternal disorders on the L/S ratio. Obstet Gynecol 56:583, 1980
189. Myers SA, Paton JB, Fisher DE: Neonatal survival of the tiny infant: The challenge. Proceedings of the 5th Annual Scientific Meeting of the Society of Perinatal Obstetricians, Las Vegas, abstract 17, 1985
190. Naeye RL: Coitus and associated amniotic fluid infections. N Engl J Med 301:1198, 1979
191. Natale R, Nasello C, Turliuk R: The relationship between movements and accelerations in fetal heart rate at twenty-four to thirty-two weeks' gestation. Am J Obstet Gynecol 148:591, 1984
192. Neligan GA, Kolvin I, Scott DM et al: Born Too Soon or Born Too Small. London, Heinemann, 1976
193. Niebyl JR: Prostaglandin synthetase inhibitors. Semin Perinatol 5:274, 1981
194. Niebyl JR, Blake DA, White RD et al: The inhibition of premature labor with indomethacin. Am J Obstet Gynecol 136:1014, 1980
195. Niebyl JR, Caritis SN, Lipshiz J et al: Toco-

lytics: When and how to use them. Contemp OB/GYN 27:146, 1986
196. Nimrod C, Varela-Gittings F, Machin G et al: The effect of very prolonged membrane rupture on fetal development. Am J Obstet Gynecol 148:540, 1984
197. Nnatu S: Value of cervical encirclarge in the treatment of mid-trimester abortion. Int J Gynaecol Obstet 21:469, 1983
198. Nochimson DJ, Petrie RH, Shah BL et al: Comparison of conservative and dynamic management of premature rupture of membranes/premature labor syndrome. Clin Perinatol 7:17, 1980
199. Novy MJ: Transabdominal cervicoisthmic cerclage for the management of repetitive abortion and premature delivery. Am J Obstet Gynecol 143:44, 1982
200. Olsen S, Tobiassen T: Transabdominal isthmic cerclage for the treatment of incompetent cervix. Acta Obstet Gynecol Scand 61:473, 1982
201. Ott WJ: Clinical application of fetal weight determination by real-time ultrasound. Obstet Gynecol 57:758, 1981
202. Pape KE, Blackwell RJ, Cusik G et al: Ultrasound detection of brain damage in premature infants. Lancet 1:1261, 1979
203. Papiernik E: Discussion. In Anderson A, Beard R, Brudenell JM, Dunn PM (eds): Pre-Term Labour. London, Royal College of Obstetrics & Gynecology, 1977
204. Papiernik E: Proposals for a programmed prevention policy of preterm birth. Clin Obstet Gynecol 27:614, 1984
205. Papile LA, Burstein J, Burstein R et al: Incidence and evolution of subependymal and intraventricular hemorrhage: A study of infants with birth weights less than 1,500 gm. J Pediatr 92:529, 1978
206. Paul RH, Koh KS, Monfred AH: Obstetric factors influencing outcome in infants weighing from 1001 to 1500 grams. Am J Obstet Gynecol 133:503, 1979
207. Perkins RP, Papile LA: The very low birth weight infant: Incidence and significance of low Apgar scores, "asphyxia," and morbidity. Am J Perinatol 2:108, 1985
208. Persson PH, Grennert L, Gennser G et al: An improved outcome in twin pregnancies. Acta Obstet Gynecol Scand 58:3, 1979
209. Pharoah POD, Alberman ED: Mortality of low birth weight infants in England and Wales 1953–1979. Arch Dis Child 56:86, 1981
210. Philip AGS, Little GA, Polivy DR et al: Neonatal mortality risk for the eighties: The importance of birth weight/gestational age groups. Pediatrics 58:122, 1981
211. Philipsen T, Eriksen PS, Lynggard F: Pulmonary edema following ritodrine-saline infusion in premature labor. Obstet Gynecol 58:304, 1981
212. Phillipson E, Sokol R, Williams T: Oligohydramnios: Clinical association and predictive value for intrauterine growth retardation. Am J Obstet Gynecol 146:271, 1983
213. Pincus R: Salbutamal infusion for premature labor—The Australian trials experience. Aust NZ J Obstet Gynecol 21:1, 1981
214. Pritchad JA, MacDonald PC: Williams Obstetrics, 16th ed, pp 578–581. New York, Appleton-Century-Crofts, 1984
215. Quigley ME, Sheehan KL, Wilkes MM et al: Effects of maternal smoking on circulating catecholamine levels and fetal heart rates. Am J Obstet Gynecol 133:685, 1979
216. Roberton NRC: Intensive care and the very low birth weight infant. Lancet 1:362, 1979
217. Roberts JM: Current understanding of pharmacologic mechanisms in the prevention of preterm birth. Clin Obstet Gynecol 27:592, 1984
218. Rodeck CH, Nicolaides KH: The use of fetoscopy for prenatal diagnosis and treatment. Semin Perinatol 7:118, 1983
219. Romem Y, Artal R: C-reactive protein as a predictor for chorioamnionitis in cases of premature rupture of the membranes. Am J Obstet Gynecol 150:546, 1984
220. Rush RW, Issacs S, McPherson K et al: A randomized controlled trial of cervical cerclage in women at high risk of spontaneous preterm delivery. Br J Obstet Gynecol 91:724, 1984
221. Rush RW, Keirse MJNC, Howat P et al: Contribution of preterm delivery to perinatal mortality. Br Med J 2:965, 1976
222. Russell P, Alkinson K, Krishnaw L: Recurrent reproductive failure due to severe placental villitis of unknown etiology. J Reprod Med 23:93, 1980
223. Sabbagha R, Shkolnik A: Ultrasound diagnosis of fetal abnormalities. Semin Perinatol 4:213, 1980
224. Saigal S, Rosenbaum P, Stopskopf B et al: Follow-up of infants 501 to 1,500 gm birth weight delivered to residents of a geographically defined region with perinatal intensive care facilities. J Pediatr 100:606, 1982
225. Sandahl B, Ulmsten U, Anderson KE: Trial of the calcium antagonist nifedipine in treatment

of primary dysmenorrhea. Arch Gynecol 227:147, 1979
226. Savarese MFR, Chang IW: Incompetent cervical os: A collective review of the literature with a report of thirty new cases. Obstet Gynecol Surv 19:201, 1964
227. Schechner S: For the 1980s: How small is too small? Clin Perinatol 7:135, 1980
228. Schutte MF, Treffers PE, Kloosterman GJ: Management of premature rupture of membranes: The risk of vaginal examination to the infant. Am J Obstet Gynecol 146:395, 1983
229. Seppala M, Vara P: Cervical cerclage in the treatment of incompetent cervix. Acta Obstet Gynecol Scand 49:343, 1970
230. Sharpe GL: Indomethacin and closure of the ductus arteriosus. Lancet 1:693, 1975
231. Shelley HJ: The metabolic response of the fetus to hypoxia. Br J Obstet Gynecol 76:1, 1969
232. Shepard MJ, Richards VA, Berkowitz RL et al: An evaluation of two equations for predicting fetal weight by ultrasound. Am J Obstet Gynecol 142:47, 1982
233. Shinozuka N, Kohzuma S, Mukubo M et al: A new formula for fetal weight estimation by ultrasonic measurement. Proceedings for the 4th Asia-Oceania Congress of Perinatology, Tokyo, Japan, abstract S1-5, 1986
234. Smith ML, Spence SA, Hull D: Mode of delivery and survival in babies under 2000 grams at birth. Br Med J 281:118, 1980
235. Sorokin Y, Bottoms SF, Dierker LJ et al: The clustering of fetal heart rate changes and fetal movements in pregnancies between 20 and 30 weeks of gestation. Am J Obstet Gynecol 143:952, 1982
236. Sorokin Y, Dierker LJ, Pillay SK et al: The association between fetal heart rate patterns and fetal movements in pregnancies between 20 and 30 weeks' gestation. Am J Obstet Gynecol 143:243, 1982
237. Spearing G: Alcohol, indomethacin, and salbutamol: A comparative trial of their use in preterm labor. Obstet Gynecol 53:171, 1979
238. Spellacy WN, Cruz AC, Birk SA et al: Treatment of premature labor with ritodrine: A randomized controlled study. Obstet Gynecol 54:220, 1980
239. Spisso KR, Harbert GM, Thiagoriajah S: The use of magnesium sulfate as the primary tocolytic agent to prevent premature delivery. Am J Obstet Gynecol 142:840, 1982
240. Stahlman MT: Acute respiratory disorders in the newborn. In Avery GB (ed): Neonatology: Pathophysiology and Management of the Newborn, pp 371–390. Philadelphia, JB Lippincott, 1986
241. Starks GC: Correlation of meconium stained amniotic fluid, early intrapartum fetal pH, and Apgar scores as predictors of perinatal outcome. Obstet Gynecol 56:604, 1980
242. Steer CM, Petrie RH: A comparison of magnesium sulfate and alcohol for the prevention of premature labor. Am J Obstet Gynecol 129:1, 1977
243. Stewart AL, Reynolds EOR: Improved prognosis for infants of very low birthweight. Pediatrics 54:724, 1974
244. Stubblefield PG, Heyl PS: Treatment of premature labor with subcutaneous terbutaline. Obstet Gynecol 59:457, 1982
245. Szymonowicz W, Schafler K, Cussen LJ et al: Ultrasound and necropsy study of periventricular haemorrhage in preterm infants. Arch Dis Child 59:637, 1984
246. Tejani NA, Verma UL: Effect of tocolysis on incidence of low birth weight. Obstet Gynecol 61:556, 1983
247. Thurnau G, Tamura R, Sabbagha RE et al: A simple estimated fetal weight equation based on real-time ultrasound of fetuses of less than 34 weeks gestation. Am J Obstet Gynecol 145:557, 1983
248. Ting P, Brady JP: Tracheal suction in meconium aspiration. Am J Obstet Gynecol 122:767, 1975
249. Tye KH, Dener KB, Benchimol A: Angina pectoris associated with use of terbutaline for premature labor. JAMA 244:692, 1980
250. Ueland K: Cardiovascular disease complicating pregnancy. Clin Obstet Gynecol 21:429, 1978
251. Ulmsten U, Anderson KE, Forman A: Relaxing effects of nifedipine on the nonpregnant human uterus in vitro and in vivo. Obstet Gynecol 52:436, 1978
252. Ulmsten U, Anderson KE, Wingerup L: Treatment of premature labor with the calcium antagonist nifedipine. Arch Gynecol 229:1, 1980
253. Verp MS: Antenatal diagnosis of chromosome abnormalities. In Sciarra JJ (ed): Gynecology and Obstetrics, vol 3, chap 102, pp 1–12. New York, Harper & Row, 1984
254. Vintzileos AM, Campbell WA, Nochimson DJ et al: Degree of oligohydramnios and pregnancy outcome in patients with premature rupture of the membranes. Obstet Gynecol 66:162, 1985
255. Vintzileos AM, Campbell WA, Nochimson DJ et al: Fetal breathing as a predictor of infection

255. in premature rupture of the membranes. Obstet Gynecol 67:813, 1986
256. Vintzileos AM, Campbell WA, Nochimson DJ et al: The use of the nonstress test in patients with premature rupture of the membranes. Am J Obstet Gynecol 155:149, 1986
257. Vintzileos AM, Feinstein S, Leodiero JG et al: Fetal biophysical profile and the effect of premature rupture of the membranes. Obstet Gynecol 67:818, 1986
258. Volpe JJ: Current concepts in neonatal medicine—Neonatal intraventricular hemorrhage. N Engl J Med 304:856, 1981
259. Wagner JM, Morton MJ, Johnson KA et al: Terbutaline and maternal cardiac function. JAMA 246:2697, 1981
260. Warsof SL, Gohari P, Berkowitz RL et al: The estimation of fetal weight by computer assisted analysis. Am J Obstet Gynecol 128:881, 1977
261. Weekes AR, Menzies DN, deBoer CH: The relative efficacy of bed rest, cervical suture, and no treatment in the management of twin pregnancy. Br J Obstet Gynecol 84:161, 1977
262. Weinberg RB, Sitrin MD, Adkins G et al: The treatment of hyperlipidemic pancreatitis in pregnancy with total parenteral nutrition. Gastroenterology 83:1300, 1982
263. Weiner G: The relationship of birth weight and length of gestation to intellectual development at age 8 to 10 years. J Pediatr 76:694, 1970
264. Weinstein AM, Dubin BD, Wojciech KP et al: Asthma and pregnancy. JAMA 24:1161, 1979
265. Wigvist N, Kjellmer I, Thiringer K et al: Treatment of premature labor by prostaglandin synthetase inhibitors. Acta Biol Med Ger 37:923, 1978
266. Woo D, Gartner LM: The small-for-gestational-age neonate. In Lin CC, Evans MI (eds): Intrauterine Growth Retardation: Pathophysiology and Clinical Management, pp 353–370. New York, McGraw-Hill, 1984
267. Worthington D, Davis LE, Grausz JP et al: Factors influencing survival and morbidity with very low birth weight delivery. Obstet Gynecol 62:550, 1983
268. Ying YK, Tejani NA: Angina pectoris as a complication of ritodrine hydrochloride therapy in premature labor. Obstet Gynecol 60:385, 1982
269. Yu VY, Kinlay S, Orgill AA et al: Outcome of very low birthweight infants who require prolonged hospitalization. Aust Pediatr J 20:293, 1984
270. Zanini B, Paul RH, Huey JR: Intrapartum fetal heart rate: Correlation with scalp pH in the preterm fetus. Am J Obstet Gynecol 136:43, 1980
271. Zlatnick FJ: The applicability of labor inhibition to the problem of prematurity. Am J Obstet Gynecol 13:704, 1972
272. Zlatnick FJ, Cruikshank DP, Petzold CR et al: Amniocentesis in the identification of inapparent infection in preterm patients with premature rupture of the membranes. J Reprod Med 29:656, 1984
273. Zlatnick FJ, Fuchs F: A controlled study of ethanol in threatened premature labor. Am J Obstet Gynecol 112:610, 1972
274. Zuckerman H, Reiss U, Rubinstein I: Inhibition of human labor by indomethacin. Am J Obstet Gynecol 44:787, 1974

SECTION 2:
Ethical Considerations in Obstetric Management

E. Haavi Morreim

This section is concerned with the ethical dimensions of a fairly specific situation: the use of cesarean delivery for the very low birth weight (VLBW) fetus in those cases where the fetus is believed to have a very low probability of survival (approximately 5% with cesarean delivery, and even less without it).

Low birth weight is the leading source of perinatal morbidity and mortality. It is most commonly due to prematurity or intrauterine growth retardation (IUGR), which may or may not lead to preterm labor and delivery.[3,16,17] The less common type-I IUGR (less than 20%) is characterized by a low potential for growth and may arise from genetic or from teratogenic causes, such as first trimester infection or medication side-effects. It results in a uniform restriction of growth, both in cell number and size, with no sparing of brain or other vital organs. Prognosis for survival is generally poor and those who do survive are often severely impaired.

In type-II IUGR growth potential is normal, but actual growth is restricted during the second and particularly the third trimesters. It is commonly associated with placental dysfunction, maternal malnutrition, medical disease, or multiple pregnancy.[16] Type-II IUGR is usually brain-sparing and carries a generally better prognosis than type-I. Therefore, type-II IUGR does not often mean a low probability of survival, except where it is also associated with prematurity. Like prematurity, its most prominent risk factors are social and economic: poverty, malnutrition and undernutrition, poor education, little or no prenatal care, young maternal age, race, smoking, drug and alcohol abuse.

Very low fetal weight is generally a strong indication for cesarean delivery. These fetuses usually have less tolerance for the stress of labor. They may have less fetal glycogen reserve, compromised placental function, increased risk of perinatal asphyxia, fetal acidosis, and meconium aspiration.[3,16] Furthermore, the "incidence of breech presentation, dystocia, hypertension (chronic and pregnancy-induced), diabetes, placenta previa, abruptio placentae, and prolapsed cord are all higher in this [low birthweight] population than in the normal population."[5] Systematic avoidance of cesarean delivery is seen only in the more unusual situations, as in type-I IUGR, in which the fetal prognosis is extremely poor even for those who survive delivery, or in which special maternal risk factors render cesarean delivery inadvisable (e.g., seriously compromised cardiac or pulmonary function).

Maternal risks in cesarean delivery have been considerably reduced in recent years. Nevertheless, the procedure still constitutes major surgery and, therefore, carries significant risks. In addition to a mortality rate of approximately two to four times that of vaginal delivery,[21] there is a wide range of morbidity risks (including aspiration, respiratory infection, wound infection, sepsis, antibiotic side-effects, trauma to other organs, thromboembolism, pulmonary embolus, bowel obstruction, urinary tract infection, hemorrhage, and hysterectomy in rare cases in which severe hemorrhaging cannot be otherwise controlled).[3,9] Maternal-infant bonding may be inhibited, as pain, weakness, and postpartum depression are increased.[3,9] In addition, the decision to perform one cesarean delivery has implied in the past a commitment to future cesareans, which in turn are associated with further maternal risks and an increase in subsequent low birth weight deliveries.[3] This practice is undergoing scrutiny and change within the medical profession, but continues to be a potentially important consideration.[10]

LEGAL CONSIDERATIONS

To begin the discussion of ethical issues with a discussion of legal considerations does not imply that legal prescriptions and proscriptions somehow dictate ethical obligations. Indeed, our ethical responsibilities often go beyond, and sometimes can actually conflict with, legal duties. However, physicians need to be aware of legal factors. Like other citizens, physicians are expected to abide by the rules which govern our society. And as professionals under threat of malpractice suits, they need to understand which actions can best minimize their risk of legal conflict. This requires that physicians know not only which actions are likely to produce trouble, but which actions will not. Ignorance or erroneous beliefs about the law can lead to needless constraints on the physician's options. Finally, there may be times when the physician would like to invoke the law's assistance, as for example to seek court orders to require treatment, and will need to know both the mechanics and the hazards of such procedures in order to determine their appropriateness.

Although there are no legal precedents that specifically address cesarean delivery of the VLBW fetus with poor survival prospects, it is possible to identify the key interests at stake and to address their relative weights.

The state has an interest in protecting the viable fetus; in the autonomy of competent, pregnant women; and in the health and safety of all pregnant women. Usually the interests of the pregnant woman and her developing fetus are in harmony, but in the cases under discussion conflicts can occur. The cesarean delivery, which usually secures the best chance for fetal survival, typically also brings an increased risk of morbidity and mortality for the woman. Therefore, we need not only to examine these interests individually, but to consider how the courts have balanced them against each other.

Protection of the Fetus

We begin by considering the welfare of the fetus. Broadly speaking, United States law has traditionally maintained a strong interest in protecting children. Child abuse and neglect are indictable offenses, and the law's usual reluctance to invade parental autonomy maybe suspended if a child's welfare is jeopardized.[8] This tenet is well established in such cases as *Prince v. Commonwealth of Massachusetts*, a case in which a Jehovah's Witness violated child labor laws by permitting the children in her custody to sell religious literature on the streets. Upholding the woman's conviction, the United States Supreme Court stated that although parents must normally be allowed to nurture their children without state interference, "neither the rights of religion nor rights of parenthood are beyond limitation. . . . Parents may be free to become martyrs themselves. But it does not follow they are free, in identical circumstances, to make martyrs of their children . . ."[22]

The legal status of the unborn is less clear. In the past the law has been quite willing to act prior to birth to protect future children. In *Hoener v. Bertinato*, a New Jersey court ordered that the as-yet unborn child of a Jehovah's Witness receive a blood transfusion immediately after birth to correct for anticipated erythroblastosis fetalis. Two previous children of this woman had died of the same problem, subsequent to her unchallenged refusal to permit blood transfusions for them.[11] Further, injuries done to a fetus before birth can sometimes be compensable, particularly if the fetus is viable.[4,24] And the unborn can have vested rights, such as inheritance. Normally these rights and recoveries are contingent upon live birth.[12,15] Nevertheless, there is no precedent granting full legal personhood to the fetus per se, and no direct protection is afforded to the pre-viable fetus.[25]

The viable fetus has, however, commanded some direct legal protection. In *Roe v. Wade*, the landmark abortion decision of 1973, the Supreme Court stated that once a fetus reaches viability—when it "presumably has the capacity of meaningful life outside the mother's womb"—the state's interest in protecting potential life can be sufficient to override the mother's acknowledged rights of autonomy (called "privacy" by the Court). States may then proscribe abortions, except when maternal life or health are endangered.[25,29]

Beyond this, there is some precedent for regarding those fetuses who are about to be born or who are in the actual process of birth as full persons. For these fetuses, the abdominal and uterine walls of the woman are, "quite literally, all that stand between them and full and immediate human life."[20,28]

State interest in this about-to-be-born status figures prominently in three cases in which women were ordered to undergo medical interventions for the benefit of their fetuses. In the first, *Raleigh Fitkin–Paul Morgan Memorial Hospital v. Anderson,* a Jehovah's Witness, 7 months pregnant and at high risk for severe hemorrhage, was ordered to undergo blood transfusions to save the lives of herself and her fetus should she actually begin to hemorrhage. The order was never carried out because the woman had already left the hospital against medical advice and the court did not authorize police to apprehend her. Nevertheless, the decision (issued in 1964, well before *Roe v. Wade*) did maintain that the "unborn child is entitled to the law's protection."[23]

More recently, several courts have ordered pregnant women to undergo cesarean delivery in order to save the lives of their endangered fetuses. In a 1980 Colorado case, a morbidly obese woman appeared at the hospital in labor, but was generally angry and uncooperative with physicians' efforts. Ninety minutes after admission, there were strong indications of fetal distress: the amniotic fluid was meconium stained, fetal heart rate showed late decelerations and a loss of baseline variability, and all of this was compounded by the high station of the presenting part, dystocia, and probable fetal hypoxia. The patient refused cesarean delivery, and urgent legal efforts by physicians and the hospital administration led to a bedside judicial hearing. After the judge declared the fetus to be a dependent and neglected child and ordered a cesarean delivery, the woman became more cooperative. The surgery, performed nearly 10 hours after the diagnosis of fetal distress, yielded a normal child with an Apgar score of 2 and 8 at 1 and 5 minutes; there were no maternal postoperative complications.[6]

In *Jefferson v. Griffin Spalding County Hospital Authority*,[13] physicians had diagnosed a complete placenta previa with a prognosis of 90% chance of fetal mortality and 50% chance of maternal mortality if cesarean delivery were not performed. With the cesarean, both mother and child stood a nearly 100% chance of healthy survival. The patient refused on religious grounds with the concurrence of her husband, who was minister for the Shiloh Sanctified Holiness Baptist Church in rural Georgia. The Superior Court of Butts County twice ordered, and the Supreme Court of Georgia upheld, that a cesarean delivery and any other medically necessary procedures should be performed for the benefit of the fetus. As in the case of *Raleigh Fitkin*, the initial Superior Court order was applicable only if the woman voluntarily presented herself for medical care. Even the second Superior Court order declined to authorize police to apprehend her, although it did specifically order her to report to the hospital of her choice for a sonogram and other necessary medical procedures. The late ultrasound revealed a rare reversal of the placenta previa (prompting some observers to question the original diagnosis), and the woman delivered a healthy infant vaginally.

Altogether, it has been recently reported that courts have ordered cesarean deliveries against a pregnant woman's wishes in at least 11 states. In two states courts ordered hospital detention for diabetic women in their third trimester who had refused therapy. In another case, an intrauterine transfusion was judicially mandated.[14] Most of these were unpublished decisions of lower court judges, not appealed to any higher court, and therefore lacked any force of precedent for other situations.[14] Nevertheless, such orders are judicially binding upon the particular individuals in each case.

Protection of the Mother

In contrast, and sometimes in opposition to its interest in protecting the lives of children and viable fetuses, the state also asserts strong interests in protecting the autonomy of pregnant women. *Roe v. Wade* clearly establishes the right of a woman to decide, at least during the first two trimesters of pregnancy, whether she wishes to carry her pregnancy to term. More generally, there are strong precedents throughout the common law allowing the competent adult to decide for him- or herself the extent to which he or she shall submit to medical care. "Every human being of adult years and sound mind has a right to determine what shall be done with his own body; and a surgeon who performs an operation without his patient's consent commits an assault, for which he is liable in damages."[27,7,18,19]

Similarly, the law has a strong interest in maternal health. As stipulated in *Roe v. Wade*, and reinforced in a more recent case,[29] states may not jeopardize maternal health or safety in their efforts to protect even third-trimester fetal life.[8,25] In general, the legal system does not expect parents to expose themselves to personal risk in order to benefit their children. They are not required to donate blood, bone marrow, kidneys, or other organs, for example, even to save their children's lives.[1,14,26]

Legal Intervention in Cesarean Deliveries

It is difficult to predict just how any court would resolve any particular case. On the one hand, important rulings of higher courts have favored maternal health and autonomy over fetal life. On the other hand, trial judges who have rushed to hospitals to answer urgent questions have felt relatively free to enforce cesarean delivery, hospital detention, or other measures in order to protect the near-term fetus. Few of these were appealed, and so it is uncertain whether they would have been upheld by higher courts.[14]

Whatever we may predict regarding what courts might in fact do, there are strong moral, medical, and even legal reasons why physicians should be loath to appeal for judicial determination in cases of cesarean delivery.

First, trial courts' decisions may rest on dubious legal grounds.[14] "When a judge arrives at the hospital in response to an emergency call, he or she is acting much more like a lay person than a jurist.

> Without time to analyze the issues, without representation for the pregnant woman, without briefing or thoughtful reflection on the situation, in almost total ignorance of the relevant law, and in an unfamiliar setting faced by a relatively calm physician and a woman who can easily be labeled 'hysterical,' the judge will almost always order whatever the doctor advises.[2]

While the physician may initially "win" these hasty decisions (often made in less than 6 hours[14]), those which ultimately are appealed may be decided very differently. In the end, physicians' liability may be increased if such interventionism leads to a new standard of care.[14]

Second, the proposed benefits to the fetus are not sufficiently certain. To justify intervention, there must be assurance that intrusion upon maternal autonomy would actually yield the hoped-for results. Without that, there is less ground for insisting upon intervention. In the case of the VLBW fetus with a poor chance for survival, the fruits of medical intervention are anything but certain. Cesarean section offers at best a 5% chance for fetal survival; and in cases in which vaginal delivery offers a survival prospect greater than zero, cesarean surgery offers only a slightly better chance over vaginal delivery.

It is interesting to note that even in the court cases just cited, the presumed benefits of medical intervention have not always been validated. A healthy *Jefferson* infant was delivered vaginally, despite the 90% prediction of mortality; the Colorado infant had an Apgar score of 8 at 5 minutes, despite 10 hours of legal maneuvering between the diagnosis of fetal distress and the delivery. Altogether, "in three of the first five cases in which court-ordered cesarean sections were sought, the women ultimately delivered vaginally and uneventfully."[2] Beyond this, of 15 recently reported court-ordered cesareans, three were required simply on grounds of previous cesarean section.[14] As previously noted, the grounds of justification for this criterion are uncertain, and have come increasingly under dispute in recent years. The intrinsic uncertainties of medicine can be exacerbated by the haste and confusion with which decisions must be made when a woman is in labor.

Third, in the case of the VLBW fetus, it is not always clear that survival would actually constitute a benefit to the child. Medical techniques for salvaging seriously ill newborns can themselves sometimes cause substantial iatrogenic harm. Further, where VLBW arises from serious underlying anomalies, as in cases of type-I IUGR, surviving fetuses may be severely impaired. These cases contrast with *Jefferson, Raleigh,* and the Colorado case, in which court-ordered interventions were expected to save the fetus for a normal, healthy life.

Fourth, in the case of cesarean delivery, meager and uncertain benefits to the fetus are ordinarily pitted against clear and serious risks to the mother, such as a mortality risk at least double that associated with vaginal delivery, and the assorted morbidities already discussed. In contrast, the courts in both *Jefferson* and in *Raleigh* took pains to note that the ordered medical care not only presented no major risk to the mother, but was expressly in her best interest.[13,23]

Fifth, the unavoidably adversarial character of legal proceedings can harm the physician-patient relationship. The trust which is so important to good health care can be seriously damaged when legal force is invoked to resolve disputes. When courts order that a particular treatment be rendered only if the woman voluntarily presents herself for medical care (as in *Raleigh Fitkin* and in the first *Jefferson* decision), the woman may feel driven away from medical care altogether. Indeed, if court-ordered intrusions upon pregnant women's autonomy became commonplace, there could be a serious overall chilling of women's willingness to seek prenatal care.[2,14]

Finally, even if such court interventions were desirable on their own merits, the invasiveness required to enforce such orders can present its own moral problems. While it might be desirable prima facie to require a pregnant woman to abstain from heavy smoking, drinking, and drug use, for example, it would be difficult to enforce such a requirement except by incarcerating the woman for the entire gestation period or by imposing some other equally burdensome penalty. Even when courts do order medical interventions, the practical force of these orders is mainly limited to the power of persuasion and the threat of subsequent punishment. It is both morally repugnant and medically dangerous to apprehend forcibly a pregnant woman and physically constrain her to submit to treatment. As noted in the Colorado case, "had the patient steadfastly refused [cesarean delivery even after the court order], it might not have been either safe or possible to administer anesthesia to a struggling, resistant woman who weighed in excess of 157.7 kg."[6] If the physician is thus limited to the powers of persuasion, then it should be the persuasive power of a solid, trusting relationship, rather than the punitive persuasion of court intervention. Court intervention into obstetric decisions may be morally, medically, and legally warranted on some occasions, but these cases should be relatively rare and based only on the most persuasive reasons. Arguably, the cases under discussion do not fit these requirements.

In sum, although courts are sometimes willing to override the decisions of pregnant women for the benefit of the fetus, they are less likely to subject women to the risks of cesarean delivery for a small chance of benefiting a VLBW fetus. More importantly, it is generally undesirable for physicians to seek such intervention. This is a matter best resolved informally between the physician and the woman. As the physician attempts to achieve this resolution, he needs to consider morally those same three factors in which the state is interested legally: the best interests of the fetus, the best interests of the mother, and the wishes of the mother.

MEDICAL CONSIDERATIONS

The Fetus

A cesarean delivery can maximize the fetus's chance of survival. In that case, the question of whether a cesarean delivery is in the fetus's best interests is, in effect, the question of whether life itself is in his best interests. The answer to this question will depend largely upon the condition of the fetus. It has been noted, for example, that in the case of type-I IUGR, those fetuses which survive usually suffer severe impairments in their short lives, such as trisomy 13, trisomy 18, and osteogenesis imperfecta type II. Extreme prematurity incompatible with survival may also be included in this category. If the physician is able to diagnose such conditions prenatally, there are usually reasonable grounds to believe that attempts to promote fetal survival are not in the fetus's best interests.

In many other cases, however, it is reasonable to assume that life would be a benefit to the fetus and that it is in his interest to maximize his survival prospects, as in the case of uncomplicated prematurity and many cases of type-II IUGR. To acknowledge that the pursuit of survival is in the fetus's interests, however, does not commit the physician to unlimited heroic efforts, such as endless postnatal intensive care support. It does imply that all reasonable measures to preserve his life must be taken until it becomes evident either that he is unlikely to survive or that continued medical interventions pose too great a burden to be warranted by the child's fading prospects.

Still remaining are the numerous cases in which the physician is simply unsure of the fetus's diagnosis or prognosis. Usually it is reasonable to assume that, in these cases, life would be in the fetus's best interests. Again, to make this prima facie assumption does not mean that life must be pursued at all costs, but only that it would be reasonable, other things being equal, at least to buy more time in which to assess further the fetus's condition and prospects.

Unfortunately, even when it can be clearly stated that cesarean delivery would be in the fetus's best interests, the moral challenge is not likely to be resolved. Potentially competing maternal interests must still be considered.

The Pregnant Woman

In some cases there are fairly clear medical indications for or against cesarean delivery, such as the complete placenta previa, on the one hand, or seriously compromised maternal cardiac or pulmonary function on the other. In many other cases, however, there is considerable room for legitimate disagreement among physicians. In these latter cases, either vaginal or cesarean delivery may be medically acceptable (Table 9-6).

In Table 9-6, the situations represented in possibilities 1, 2, 3, and 5 are relatively easy to resolve, at least medically. In 1, 3, and 5, the absence of any fetal interest in survival means that there is no conflict between maternal and fetal interests. In 2, cesarean delivery favors the best medical interests of both woman and fetus, so here, too, there is no conflict.

Important questions remain however. What should the physician recommend to the woman when maternal and fetal interests conflict, as seen in possibility 4? What should be recommended when medical indications are unclear (possibility 6)? And how should the physician respond when the woman opts for a course which contradicts clear medical indications, for example, refusing cesarean delivery in the situation represented by possibility 2 (as seen in the *Jefferson* case)? None of these questions can be answered without investigating the proper role of maternal autonomy.

INFORMED CONSENT

It is tempting to be simplistic and argue that morally the physician's only option is to explain the situation to the patient and to abide by her decision. The principle of autonomy states that every (competent) individual should be permitted to make his or her own decisions regarding his or her own medical care—at the least, to refuse treatment. Ob-

Table 9-6. Maternal v. Fetal Interests in Cesarean Delivery

| | Fetal Interests in Survival | |
Maternal Medical Interests	*Not Possible or Desirable*	*Possible and Desirable*
Cesarean clearly indicated	1	2
Cesarean contraindicated	3	4
No clear indications	5	6

stetric medicine raises some very important human value choices regarding the times and ways in which children should be brought into the world, about the risks which parents should bear for their children, about the value of a life which bodes to be seriously impaired. These values are deeply personal, and each couple will have their own beliefs. The physician must try to honor them, and it is unwarranted for either the law or the physician to override such important values in the name of protecting children or potential children in cases of VLBW fetuses.

The issue is more complex, however. Patient autonomy can be upheld only when the patient is actually capable of exercising autonomy, that is, when the patient is able to assimilate information, weigh the options and their implications, and to make a decision which reflects her values. Patients do not always have the ability or the opportunity to exercise this prerogative, nor do they always articulate their wishes and concerns clearly and straightforwardly.

In the specific case of the VLBW infant, there are serious obstacles to the patient's autonomous decision-making. Frequently the patient is in pain and may be partly sedated. There is little time for prolonged discussion and contemplation and, unless the fetus's condition was diagnosed and discussed prenatally, the mother may be unable to overcome the confusion and fear the situation is likely to generate. Furthermore, the physician and patient may be complete strangers, disparate in cultural, social, educational, and economic background. The very absence or inadequacy of prenatal care, which is especially likely to lead to prematurity or to growth retardation, almost inevitably ensures that physician and patient do not share that solid relationship which could help them to confront together the decisions they must make. At the same time, it is unlikely that patient autonomy can be adequately respected when the physician simply recites a list of facts and then defers to the patient's first response.

The physician's first responsibility is to make every effort to diagnose and discuss fetal and maternal risk factors in advance with the patient. This is simply a requirement of good medicine. But the physician should also discuss the choices and chances of pregnancy on a more general level. Even if there is no indication that a particular patient will require a cesarean delivery, he should discuss with each patient the values she attaches to the process and outcome of pregnancy. A strong preference for natural childbirth will generally mean a relatively high threshold before cesarean delivery is considered, while a strong desire to avoid prolonged labor pain would yield a somewhat lower threshold. Such conversations need not alarm the patient if carefully conducted, and can be of enormous value in guiding the prenatal relationship and delivery.

Although it is morally irresponsible to wait until the urgency of the delivery room to discuss important issues which could easily have been considered before, advance discussions are not always possible. Physician and patient may meet as strangers in the delivery room. This does not mean, however, that the physician is free to ignore the patient's wishes or that he or she cannot be prepared to encourage effective patient participation in the decision. A physician who serves a distinct cultural group can make an effort to learn about the views of medicine, health, and childbirth that are common in that culture. Plans can be made in advance for specific ways to simplify a complex medical situation for the patient who has little education or scientific background. The physician can also learn by talking with patients themselves, at leisure after delivery, about what was understood and how communication might have been more effective. Care must be taken not to view patients in terms of stereotypes or to adopt rigid formulas for communicating from a different cultural or social background. Each patient brings her own special beliefs, concerns, and values to the situation.

Good communication is no less important with the patient who asks the physician to make a decision on her behalf. Even when medical indications are clear, the physician must ensure that the patient understands as much as possible about her situation and about the reasons why a particular course of action is recommended.

When the medical indications are not decisive and the woman still wishes to entrust the decision to the physician, the physician is obligated to discuss the relevant values with her so far as time and circumstances permit. No reasonably competent patient will be utterly devoid of values and feelings regarding the key issues at stake:

Was the pregnancy wanted?
How does she feel about the prospect of raising an impaired child?
What are her fears about surgery?
What are her fears and feelings about "natural" vaginal delivery?
Does she have religious beliefs relevant to this situation?
Are there family members whose views she believes will or should play a role in her own thoughts and feelings?

Admittedly, there are limits to the depth and quality of discussion which can be carried out in delivery room. Yet the values at stake here are too personal and the consequences of the decision too great for the physician simply to look solely at the medical values or to introject personal values about the bearing and rearing of children, without an effort to discern whether these are values with which the patient can be satisfied.

ARRIVAL AT A PHYSICIAN-PATIENT DECISION

It is consoling a well as vexing to realize that in these situations there often is not a single, clearly correct resolution. Fetal life is precious, especially when that fetus is near term and near to full personhood. Morally, it is entirely acceptable for a woman to assume even a fairly serious level of risk to preserve that life. Reciprocally, there is nothing morally suspect about a woman's valuing her own personal life and health above a small prospect for fetal survival. And if either of these options represents a morally acceptable choice, surely it is acceptable for the physician to defer those choices to the patient. Only the (competent) woman herself can decide how she shall balance the nonmedical concerns, such as her religious beliefs and family values, against her medical interests.

Although we cannot state definitively WHAT decision should be made, there is considerable moral significance in HOW the decision is made. This should not be an adversarial, either/or question of who should make the decision, the woman OR the physician? Rather, the important question concerns how the two shall work together toward a mutually agreeable resolution.

The physician is best equipped to understand the medical situation and the outcomes to which each option is most likely to lead. Without his or her careful guidance, the woman has no real understanding of her options. The physician must also work within his or her own medical and moral standards of practice. The woman, in turn, is best qualified to evaluate the implications of each option for her own life, for it is she who must live with whatever decision is made. Neither physician nor patient can reach a satisfactory decision without the other.

Because in these particular cases the *process* of decision-making is morally more central than the *outcome,* the physician's chief moral task is to make a serious, honest effort. The physician must not only offer the best medical care and advice of which he or she is capable, but must strive to involve the woman in the decision-making as deeply as circumstances and her own willingness permit. This requires that the physician genuinely care about the values of the patient and that he or she strive to reach a decision with which this particular woman can feel comfortable.

REFERENCES

1. Annas GJ: Forced cesareans: The most unkindest cut of all. Hastings Cent Rep 12:16, 1982

2. Annas GJ: Protecting the liberty of pregnant patients. N Engl J Med 316:1213, 1987
3. Banta HD, Thacker SB: Assessing the costs and benefits of electronic fetal monitoring. Obstet Gynecol Surv 34:627, 1979
4. Bonbrest v. Kotz, 65 F. Suppl. 138, DDC, 1946)
5. Bottoms SF, Rosen G, Sokol RJ: The increase in the cesarean birth rate. N Engl J Med 302:559, 1980
6. Bowes WA, Selgestad B: Fetal versus maternal rights. Obstet Gynecol 58:209, 1981
7. Canturbury v. Spence, 464 F 2d 772 DCCA, 1972
8. Finamore E: Jefferson v. Griffin Spalding County Hospital Authority: Court-ordered surgery to protect the life of an unborn child. Am J Law Med 9:83, 1983
9. Gilfix MG: Electronic fetal monitoring: Physician liability and informed consent. Am J Law Med 10:31, 1984
10. Gleicher N: Cesarean section rates in the United States. JAMA 252:3273, 1984
11. Hoener v. Bertinato, 67 NJ Sup. 517, 171 A 2d 140, Juv Ct, 1961
12. In re Peabody, 158 NE 2d 841, 1959
13. Jefferson v. Griffin Spalding County Hospital Authority, 247 Ga 274 SE 2d 457, 1981
14. Kolder VEB, Gallagher J, Parsons MT: Court-ordered obstetrical interventions. N Engl J Med 5:1192, 1987
15. Lenow JL: The fetus as a patient. Am J Law Med 9:1, 1983
16. Lin CC, Evans MI: Intrauterine Growth Retardation. New York, McGraw-Hill, 1984
17. McCormick MC: The contribution of low birth weight to infant mortality and childhood morbidity. N Engl J Med 312:82, 1985
18. Natanson v. Kline, 186 Kan 393, 350 P 2d 1093, 1960; 187 Kan 186 354 P 2d 670, 1960
19. Pratt v Davis, 118 Ill. App. 161, 1905; Aff 224 Ill 300, /9 N.E. 562, 1906
20. People v Chavez, 77 Cal App 2d 621, 176 P 2d 92, Dist Ct App, 4th Dist, 1947
21. Petitti DB, Cefalo RC, Shapiro S, Whalley P: In-hospital maternal mortality in the United States: Time trends and relation to method of delivery. Obstet Gynecol 59:6, 1982
22. Prince v Commonwealth of Massachusetts, 321 US 158, 64 S Ct 438, 88L Ed 645, 1944; 88 L Ed 645, 1944
23. Raleigh Fitkin–Paul Morgan Memorial Hospital v Anderson, 42 NJ 421, 201 A 2d 537 NJ S Ct, 1964
24. Renslow v Mennonite Hospital, 367 NE 2d 1250, 1977
25. Roe v Wade, 410 US 113, 1973
26. Ruddick W, Wilcox W: Operating on the fetus. Hastings Cent Rep 12:10, 1982
27. Schloendorff v Society of New York Hospital, 211 NY 125, 105 NE 92, NY, 1914
28. Shriner TL: Maternal versus fetal rights. Obstet Gynecol 53:518, 1979
29. Thornburgh v American College of Obstetrics and Gynecologists, 106: S Ct 2169, 1986

SECTION 3:
Multiple Gestation

Richard A. Bronsteen and Mark I. Evans

The diagnosis of a twin gestation usually brings about a considerable emotional response on the part of both the future parents and the medical personnel caring for the pregnancy. Unfortunately, often overlooked is the fact that this pregnancy is not special solely because of the presence of multiple fetuses, but also because of an increased risk for a less than optimal outcome. Multiple gestation is a high-risk condition for both the mother and the developing fetuses. The following pregnancy complications are seen more often with multiple gestations[63]:

Pregnancy-induced hypertension
Anemia
Pyelonephritis
Postpartum hemorrhage
Preterm labor
Premature delivery
Intrauterine growth retardation
Hydramnios
Abnormal fetal presentation
Cord prolapse
Abnormal placentation
   Previa
   Abruption

Congenital malformations
Postpartum hemorrhage
Spontaneous abortion
Perinatal mortality

It is the goal of this section to review pertinent issues and recent progress in the care of multiple gestations. Epidemiology and etiologic aspects are not included as they are covered elsewhere.[12,13,46] The majority of our experience, both clinically as well as in the literature, is with twin pregnancies. Much of the discussion that follows is specific for twins, although the principles involved can be applied to all multiple gestations. At the end of this section we have addressed the higher order multiple gestations (triplets, quadruplets, etc.).

EARLY DIAGNOSIS

The cornerstone to appropriate care of twin pregnancies is diagnosis, and more importantly, early diagnosis. As the majority of twin morbidity and mortality occurs before 30 weeks, it is clear that any therapy aimed at improving outcome rests on diagnosis before this time. Antenatal diagnosis of twins also avoids the presence of an undiagnosed twin at delivery, with its increase in morbidity and mortality to the second twin. Early diagnosis by routine ultrasound has been associated with a decrease in fetal morbidity and mortality in Sweden, though this certainly was not the only factor responsible for the improved outcome.[121]

Findings that may make the obstetrician suspicious for the presence of a twin gestation include physical examination with size larger than dates or excessive number of fetal parts to palpation, increased weight gain, and elevated biochemical tests such as alpha-fetoprotein (AFP), human chorionic gonadotropin-beta, human placental lactogen, and pregnancy specific beta-1 glycoprotein. These have all been suggested as screening tests for multiple gestation. It is important to remember that these are screening tests and are not diagnostic of twins. There is little evidence that biochemical tests are more sensitive or specific than clinical examinations in identifying twins.[79] In recent studies, the median AFP value for twins was 2.5 multiples of median (MOM) of the singleton.[57] Thus, one-half of all twins would not be diagnosed by AFP screening, since 2.5 MOM is a commonly used point for an upper limit of normal.

The antenatal diagnosis of twins is best made by ultrasound examination. Prior to widespread availability of real-time ultrasound, approximately one-half of all twin gestations were undiagnosed prior to the onset of labor.[51] The earliest reported ultrasonic diagnosis of twins was made at 47 postmenstrual days.[149] An incorrect diagnosis of twins can be the result of retromembranous collections of blood and fluid, or of refraction of the ultrasound beam by the rectus muscles to give the impression of two gestational sacs.[124,134] A yolk sac may also be erroneously mistaken for a second twin. Current American statistics show over 90% of twins are detected before labor at a university medical center[29]; data from Sweden where routine ultrasound screening with either one or two ultrasounds detected 98% of twin gestations.[122]

ANTENATAL CONCERNS

The in utero environment in twin gestations may be a hostile one, as noted by the increased morbidity and mortality. The physician following a twin pregnancy needs to be aware of these complications so that appropriate antenatal care can be rendered.

Prematurity

The most important factor affecting perinatal morbidity and mortality is preterm delivery. As the number of fetuses increases, mean length of gestation decreases. Twins have a mean gestation length of 35 weeks, while that of triplets and quadruplets is 33 and 29 weeks, respectively.[24] Although early studies found low birth weight the most important factor in perinatal mortality, these studies did not distinguish between low birth weight because of prematurity and that caused by intrauterine growth retardation (IUGR). Prematurity is the best predictive factor for perinatal outcome, with IUGR increasingly more important as the pregnancy progresses into the third trimester. The majority of morbidity and mortality seen in multiple gestation occurs prior to the 30th week of pregnancy.[29,62]

Intrauterine Growth Retardation

IUGR is seen in increased frequency in twins, and may play a significant role in perinatal outcome. Individual twin growth curves are similar to singletons up until the early third trimester. However, studies from a variety of patient populations show that as the third trimester progresses, increasing differences in birth weight are found between twins and singletons.[9,15,90,102,109]

The importance of in utero growth on long-term fetal development has been shown in several studies. Drillien found higher IQs in the larger neonate in five of seven twin pregnancies.[44] Babson and co-workers also found a higher IQ and better speech and language variables in the heavier of the twin pair when the birth weight difference was at least 25%; the average follow-up was 8.5 years.[2] In nine pairs felt to be monozygotic by sex and blood type, intellectual differences were equal or greater than that noted for the whole group. In a follow-up looking specifically at these monozygotic twin pairs at age 18, physical differences including weight, height, and head circumference, as well as intellectual parameters all still favored the larger twin.[3] Other studies have confirmed the superior performance seen in the larger twin.[32,74] Although no intelligence differences were detected in one study of unequal birth weight twins, the definition of unequal weight (>15% difference) may have been too low.[54]

Intrauterine growth in multiple gestations is evaluated differently from a singleton gestation. One difference is a conceptual one, with the use of discordancy to describe twin growth. Fetal size is a comparison between the twins rather than to normalized standards. Another difference from singletons is the possibility of a twin-to-twin transfusion. Placental vascular anastomoses allow blood to be transferred from one fetus (donor) to its twin (recipient), with the potential for significant effects on both fetuses.

Discordancy

The concept of discordant twin growth or, more specifically, its in utero diagnosis by real-time ultrasound examinations has gained increasing attention in the literature over the past decade. Birth weight discordancy is defined as birth weight difference divided by the weight of the heavier twin, and has been shown to be a significant factor in the prediction of neonatal morbidity and mortality.[9] Exactly what constitutes significant discordancy has not been clearly delineated. A commonly used cutoff of a 25% birth weight difference is credited to Babson and co-workers.[2,3] In their studies this arbitrarily chosen value was associated with a poorer outcome in the smaller babies. Alternatively, others have used cutoff points of 15%[37] and 20%.[30]

Recent neonatal data are helpful to statistically define discordancy.[116] The mean twin birth weight difference was 11%. The 90th percentile cutoff for birth weight difference was 23%, and two standard deviations above the mean was 30%.

Twin-to-Twin Transfusion

A situation unique to multiple gestations is that of twin-to-twin transfusion, in which blood from a "donor" fetus passes through vascular anastomoses in the placenta to the opposite "recipient" fetus. These anastomoses can be artery-to-artery, artery-to-vein, or less commonly, vein-to-vein, and can result in a spectrum of clinical presentations. Placental studies have verified the presence of these vascular anastomoses in the majority of monochorionic placentas. Their sizes, number, and type are varied. Although, anastomoses in dichorionic placentas have been identified, they are quite rare.[11,16,152]

Sequelae of this disease can be seen in the fetuses, placentas, and amniotic fluid volumes. Placentas of the donor fetus are typically larger and pale in appearance with edematous trophoblastic tissue. The donor fetal capillaries are smaller and contain nucleated red blood cell precursors suggesting increased red cell synthesis. Donor fetuses appear to be smaller and pale with lower hematocrits. Their placentas are smaller with normal villi, and fetal capillaries are dilated and congested in appearance. Recipient fetuses, in general, are large and plethoric with polycythemia and cardiac hypertrophy.[108] Amniotic fluid abnormalities seen with twin-to-twin transfusion include recipient infants being surrounded by excess amniotic fluid and donor fetuses having decreased fluid. Figure 9-2 shows an example of twin-to-twin transfusion with unequal fetal sizes. The donor twin is held tightly to the anterior uterine wall by an amniotic sac with scant fluid, while its twin floats freely below it in a sac with excess fluid.

The differences in the fetuses are not solely the result of blood transfer. Neonatal IgG levels at birth, predominantly the result of maternal-fetal transfer, show significantly higher levels in the recipients. The donor-to-recipient gradient is not seen with other plasma proteins, since these are predominantly the result of fetal synthesis.[21] These findings, along with the placental findings already described indicate that a compromised maternal-to-fetal transfer of nutrients in the donor fetus also plays a role in the smaller donor size.

Diagnosis. The twin-to-twin transfusion syndrome can be subdivided into acute and chronic types. In reviewing cases from the literature, Klebe and Ingomar found that in most cases with evidence of "unidentical in utero nutrition" (defined as greater than 300-g birth weight difference), the donor fetus was uniformly smaller.[83] With equal in utero nutrition (less than 300-g birth weight difference), smaller size did not uniformly predict a donor role. They hypothesized that the transfusion seen in this latter group was acute and was due to blood transferred during labor and delivery, and possibly secondary to the timing of cord clamping. A follow-up study by Tan and co-workers found that when the birth weight difference was greater than 20%, the larger twin was uniformly the recipient, whereas only 16 of 26 recipients were larger when the birth weight difference between twins was less than 20%.[153] This cut-off of approximately 20% also holds for Klebe's and Ingomar's data (in which the equal nutrition group had less than a 17% birth weight difference). Further support for acute transfer of blood during labor and delivery is that reticulocytes (evidence of chronic anemia) were only seen in donor fetuses from the larger birth weight difference group.[153]

The clinical presentation of twin-to-twin transfusion is varied depending on the quan-

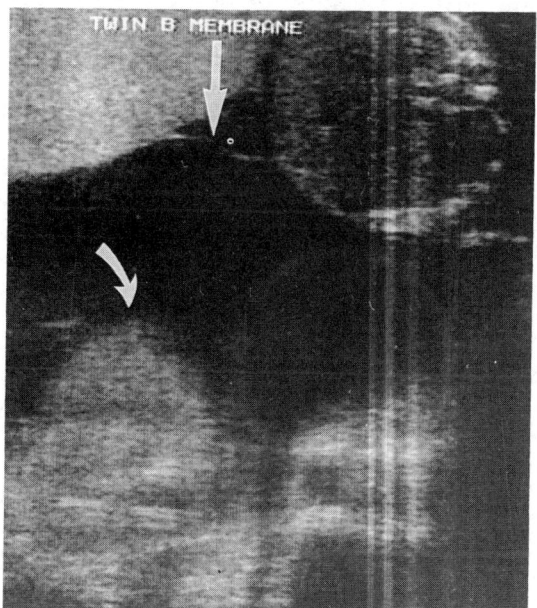

FIGURE 9-2. Twin-to-twin transfusion syndrome. The donor twin, shown in cross section, is trapped against the anterior uterine wall in a sac (separating membrane shown by *straight arrow*) with low fluid volume, while the recipient twin (tangential view shown by *curved arrow*) floats freely below.

tity of blood transferred. There is no set definition for diagnosis of twin-to-twin transfusion; most studies base the diagnosis on clinical impressions. Rausen and co-workers defined a hemoglobin difference of 5 g/dl as being diagnostic of twin-to-twin transfusion because it was greater than that seen in any of their dizygotic pregnancies.[131]

The frequency of twin-to-twin transfusions is difficult to estimate owing to the ubiquitous nature of vascular anastomoses in monochorionic placentas and the lack of either specific diagnostic criteria or a diagnostic test. Clinically obvious cases probably represent only the severe manifestations of this syndrome. Studies estimate that 15% of monochorionic twin pregnancies result in twin-to-twin transfusion syndrome.[131,150] Robertson and Neer report a slightly lower incidence of twin-to-twin transfusion of 5.5% in monochorionic placentas,[133] while Galea and colleagues found a 25% incidence.[55]

Clinically, the twin-to-twin transfusion syndrome is a high-risk situation with a very high perinatal mortality. It is usually detected in the second trimester. Diagnosis in utero can be inferred from ultrasound findings, mainly that of a single growth retarded twin.[160] Recent reports report treatment with digoxin or selected feticide.[39,161] These two methods should be recognized as experimental in nature and should not be taken as standard.

Management. When twin-to-twin transfusion is suspected on the basis of ultrasound, careful monitorings of both babies is imperative, including serial sonographic examinations and fetal heart rate monitoring. Plans for delivery should be based on the severity of the disease, its progression, and fetal gestational age. Perinatal mortality from twin-to-twin transfusion is reported to be near 100%.[158] One study reported on nine cases of twin-to-twin transfusion that were treated with bed rest, tocolytics, and serial amniocentesis to remove some excess fluid in an attempt to decrease the incidence of preterm delivery. Eight of the 18 fetuses survived.[140] Other small series have also shown success with serial amniocentesis.[19,20,52,105] Fluid should be withdrawn slowly to minimize the potential complication of premature separation of the placenta.[128,130,158] Decreased serum protein levels (7.2–5.3 g/dl) have been reported in a patient who had almost 8 liters of fluid removed over a 3-week period. Despite treating a manifestation of the disease and not its etiology, serial amniocentesis may be effective by decreasing uterine distention, resulting in a lower frequency of preterm labor and an increase in uterine blood flow. One must be cautious in accepting this as a standard therapy, since the literature may be biased by the reporting of only good results. Spontaneous resolution of fetal hydrops with no therapy has been noted in singletons.[97,104,125]

Single Fetal Demise

Another potential complication of twins is the in utero demise of one of the fetuses. Twin pregnancies suffer from a high rate of single fetal loss resulting in the delivery of only a single viable baby. This loss can occur at any time in gestation, but is most commonly seen early in the pregnancy.

Early ultrasounds that diagnose twins are often followed up by ultrasounds or the delivery of only one fetus. In a recent review of nine studies of ultrasounds before 14 weeks, a "vanishing twin" was found in frequencies ranging from 13% to 78% of twin pregnancies.[86] The higher loss rates were seen in those studies in which the initial ultrasound was done before 10 weeks. The vanished twin is usually not detected pathologically at the time of delivery and also does not appear to have any prognostic significance for adverse maternal or fetal outcome with the surviving singleton pregnancy. One study, though, did find that 92% (11 out of 12) of the pregnancies with a vanishing twin ultimately resulted in a spontaneous loss of the second fetus.[155] Otherwise, miscarriage rates of 7% to 37% are quoted.[86] The true incidence of this syndrome is unknown and its significance for the surviving twin is probably minimal.

Etiology. Causes for a single intrauterine demise after the first trimester include severe IUGR, twin-to-twin transfusion syndrome, cord accidents, and fetal abnormalities (malformations and genetic abnormalities). The incidence of a single antepartum death has been placed at between 0.5% and 6.8%.[47] Once a single in utero demise is documented, concern and attention turns towards the health of surviving fetus and the mother. Given the possibility that an suboptimal uterine environment was responsible for the first demise, the physician must be concerned that this hostile environment may also adversely affect the health of the surviving fetus. There is also evidence that toxic products from the deceased fetus may affect the surviving fetus with unfavorable consequences.

In 1944, Kindred reviewed 150 cases involving single fetal death. He felt that chronic maternal illness was responsible for most of the deaths. In addition, there was little effect on either the mother or the surviving fetus because of the death of the first baby.[82] More recent reports have also shown good outcomes of the surviving twin outside of complications of prematurity.[61,89] In a recent three-decade review, Enbom found the mortality rate of the surviving twin to be 18%, with a prematurity rate of 45%.[47]

In 1961, Benirschke reported a case of a liveborn twin from a monochorionic twin gestation with one stillbirth, who died at 62 hours of age. Autopsy of the baby revealed necrosis of the brain, renal cortex, and spleen, as well as the presence of numerous thrombi in many of the fetal vessels.[10] He hypothesized that tissue thromboplastin from the deceased twin transferred through vascular anastomoses in the placenta to cause intravascular thrombi in the surviving fetus. Further evidence for this process comes from Durkin and colleagues in a review of 281 infants with cerebral palsy.[45] Nineteen (6.8%) of these infants were the product of multiple gestation, a higher incidence than expected. Five of these were associated with a stillborn, suggesting that in utero coagulopathy could be responsible for cerebral palsy. However, prematurity was a large factor in the neurologic abnormalities seen. In reviewing the National Perinatal Collaborative Data, Melnick found seven cases of antenatal demise of one of the fetuses of a monozygotic twin pregnancy. Of the seven, two of the babies had long-term problems including one with central nervous system abnormalities, and the other with microcephaly but normal intellect; the other five babies were normal.[103] Fetal pathology on the basis of transfused factors from the deceased twin requires the presence of placental vascular anastomoses, so it is not surprising that the majority of cases reported are in monochorionic twins.[47] Others have also found similar evidence of altered intravascular coagulation and renal cortical necrosis, aplasia cutis congenita, and multicystic encephalomalacia in the surviving twin.[99,107,163]

Management. Appropriate antenatal care and timing of delivery when one twin dies in utero have not been well set out in the current literature. In Enbom's review, the prematurity rate was 45%, but survival of liveborn twins was 82%.[47] On follow-up, 54% were alive and well, whereas 46% either died after birth or suffered from major sequelae. These figures may be artificially pessimistic because they are based on case reports present in the literature. The author could not find any evidence that early delivery after documentation of the first demise would cut down on the incidence of morbid sequelae in the survivor. The data also do not show whether early delivery would affect not just the incidence, but also the severity of sequelae that develop. Unfortunately, most of the articles reviewed were case reports with limited numbers of patients.

In a larger series published at the same time and not included in Enbom's review, 15 cases were reported in which all but one of the fetuses survived. The management protocol had consisted of delivery immediately if the patient was at term or upon documentation of pulmonic maturity by amniocentesis. In those cases that were immature or amniotic fluid was not available, steroids were given and delivery was done 48 hours later.

One of the survivors was diagnosed in the neonatal period to have multicystic encephalomalacia, indicating the possibility of transferred toxins from the dead fetus. Of those 15 cases 9 involved twin gestation with documented monochorionic placentas (including the fetus that developed multicystic encephalomalacia). Seven of the remaining babies were normal on follow-up, which ranged from 6 months to 4 years. The final baby in this group was severely handicapped at age 2 due to an intraventricular hemorrhage felt to be the result of prematurity.[34]

In another series, Hagay and co-workers discussed their 15-year experience with 21 cases of multiple gestations complicated by a single intrauterine death.[60] In their series, 4 of the 21 deaths had monochorionic placentas, and in 2 of these 4 cases, the second twin died in utero within a short time of expiration of the first fetus. In the other 17 cases with dichorionic placentas, there were no deaths of the second fetus. All 21 cases were managed conservatively.

Unfortunately, current methods of fetal assessment, including biophysical profile and antenatal fetal heart rate testings, would probably not be helpful in predicting the presence of fetal morbidity due to transferred thromboplastic material from the dead fetus. Similarly, it is not felt that Doppler studies are able to predict this morbid outcome.

It appears that, although this is a high-risk situation, the outcome is not as pessimistic as one is lead to believe from the Enbom survey of case reports and literature. One should also be careful in drawing conclusions in favor of aggressive delivery in this group, since even with immediate delivery, the majority of the stillborn babies are already macerated, indicating they had been dead for at least several days before the diagnosis and delivery.

The in utero demise of one twin does not appear to lead to significant maternal complications. Unlike in utero demise in singleton pregnancies, maternal coagulopathy is extremely rare. Skelly and associates reported a single case of maternal consumptive coagulopathy following in utero demise of one of a pair of triplets.[146] Averback and Wigglesworth reported on a case of monochorionic monoamniotic twin gestation with one stillborn in which the mother experienced disseminated intravascular coagulation (DIC) postpartum and a cerebellar infarct. However, this patient was also preeclamptic, which could explain her postpartum morbidity.[1]

A logical and consistent approach should be taken towards the twin pregnancy with a single fetal demise. For those gestations at or near term, delivery is the appropriate choice. For those pregnancies that are preterm, an attempt should be made at establishing chorionicity of the placenta. If there is evidence for a dichorionic placenta, it is appropriate to follow the pregnancy conservatively with serial ultrasounds and antenatal fetal heart rate testings. However, if a dichorionic placenta cannot be proven, the obstetrician should consider delivering the surviving fetus early. The current literature certainly does not support the immediate delivery of the premature surviving fetus for this reason. However, it is possible that delivery once pulmonary maturity is reasonably ensured may decrease both the frequency and/or severity of sequelae in the surviving baby. Appropriate surveillance of the surviving fetus includes serial ultrasound exams and antenatal testing, which may indicate a need for early delivery.

Congenital Malformations: Acardia

A recent review of studies comparing twin and singleton births found varying ratios in the relative frequencies of congenital anomalies. Overall, however, it was felt to be increased in twin gestations. The increase seen with twins is felt to be due to an increase in monozygotic, not dizygotic, twins. The concordance rate for anomalies (both twins with the same anomaly) ranges from 3.6% to 18.8%. Thus, in the majority of twin pregnancies with an anomaly present, the anomaly is only in one of the two fetuses.[93] As with singletons, twin fetuses can experience a wide range of congenital anomalies. Anomalies such as syrinomelia and single umbilical artery are more common in twin gestations.[35,64] There are also suggestions in the literature that midline defects, such as anencephaly and congenital heart disease, are also increased in twins.[93]

One congenital malformation specific to multiple gestations is acardia. In acardia, one fetus is present without a well defined cardiac structure and is kept alive through placental vascular anastomoses by the viable fetus. This perfused fetus or, as it is sometimes called, *acardiac monster*, can range in appearance from an unrecognizable mass of tissue to a fairly complete and well formed fetus.[154] There are two possible etiologies for this anomaly. The first is congenital absence of the heart in one of the fetuses with circulation provided from early gestation from the other twin. The second possibility is hypoplastic formation of the heart due to hemodynamic influences from blood transfused from the opposite fetus. This condition can be described as an early type of the twin-to-twin transfusion syndrome. Due to the transfused blood, part of the hemodynamic work load in the recipient fetus is done by the heart of the donor fetus. The lessened work load on this heart results in atrophy of the remaining heart muscle. As this process continues, eventually all of the circulation in the recipient is provided through the donor heart. Animal embryo studies that show cardiac formation is controlled by mechanical hemodynamic factors support this theory.[137] Also supportive is the presence of more normal-appearing tissue at the distal end of the acardiac twin, where the fresh blood enters.

Since vascular anastomoses are needed to support the acardiac twin, the vast majority of these cases are monozygotic. In one case where the two fetuses were found to be of different sexes and one was an abnormal karyotype, fertilization of the polar body was hypothesized as the etiology.[110] Different genetic makeup of acardiac and normal twins has been found, with the abnormality uniformly appearing in the acardiac baby.[45] In one study, 50% of the acardiac twins were karyotypically abnormal, although no one consistent karyotypic abnormality was found to be present.[154] Forty percent of acardiac twins are also monoamniotic twins, and triplets are responsible for one-quarter of the cases.[71] Placental analyses in these pregnancies have found predominantly artery-to-artery and artery-to-vein anastomoses, and loss by the acardiac twin of all its direct vascular connections to its placenta.[154]

The risk to the normal fetus by the presence of an acardiac twin is significant. A recent study presented 14 cases of acardiac twins. The mortality rate in the "pump" (normal) twin was 50%, with IUGR and congestive failure being significant factors. Of the 5 survivors, 4 were normal. One survivor, however, born at 34 weeks gestation had severe IUGR; the neonatal period was complicated by respiratory difficulty and mild congestive failure. Unlike the single in utero monozygotic twin whose twin dies, there has been no evidence of embolic phenomena in the surviving fetus.[154]

Chromosomal Abnormality

Most known chromosomal anomalies have also been reported in twins.[93] In dizygotic twins they are usually discordant. Surprisingly, and of concern to those patients undergoing antenatal chromosomal analysis, discordancy as a result of postzygotic nondisjunction has been found among chromosomal anomalies in monozygotic twins. Thus, in patients undergoing second trimester amniocentesis for chromosomal analysis, an ultrasonic placental appearance diagnostic for monozygotic pregnancy should not dissuade the obstetrician from obtaining specimens from both sacs. Obviously, in cases where only one sac is present, (monoamniotic twins) only one sample can be obtained. Figure 9-3 contains an example of a twin gestation discordant for both karyotype and malformation. One fetus is normal, while its twin has trisomy 21, as well as fetal hydrops and a cystic hygroma. Chromosomal analysis had been done 3 weeks earlier when the malformation was discovered. In general, when significant malformations are detected we offer fetal genetic testing because of the

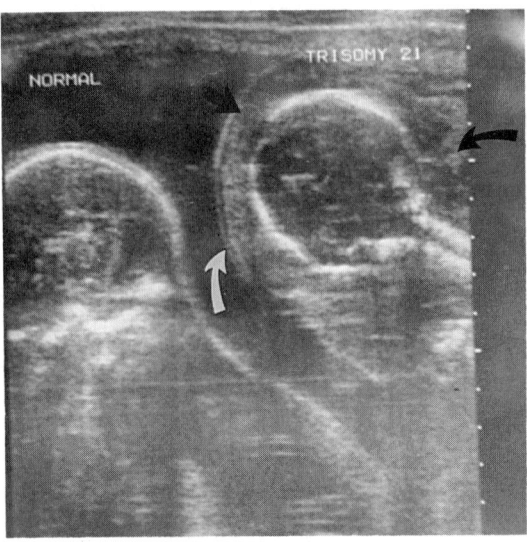

FIGURE 9-3. Twins discordant for karyotype and anomalies. Normal fetus and its twin with scalp edema (*straight black arrow*) cystic hygroma (*curved black arrow*). Separating membrane is shown by the white arrow.

increased incidence of chromosomal abnormalities.

ANTENATAL CARE

Because of the increase risk present, women with twin pregnancies should be seen at more frequent intervals by their physician. As with all pregnancies the mother should be checked for weight, blood pressure, fundal height measurement, and urine dip stick at each visit. Her blood count should be tested at regular intervals for anemia. Routine fetal evaluations should also be done, since fundal height measurement alone is not an adequate assessment of fetal health.

Ultrasound Examinations

Serial ultrasound examinations play an important role in the evaluation of twin pregnancies.[33] In early gestation ultrasound is helpful to confirm gestational age and fetal number, and to evaluate placentation and fetal growth.

Fetal Number and Placentation. Visualization of separate placental masses or opposite-sexed twins is consistent with a diagnosis of dichorionic placentation. However, the presence of a single placenta may represent a fused dichorionic placenta or a single monochorionic placenta, and thus is not definitive in differentiating chorionic types. By subjectively evaluating the placenta and separating membrane, Barss and co-workers were able to correctly identify the chorionic type of placentation in 33 out of 34 twin gestations studied prospectively.[6] Separate placentas were classified as dichorionic. Single fused placentas with a thin hair-like septum were classified as monochorionic, while those with a thicker septum were dichorionic. A second more recent study also found this type of ultrasound classification helpful in predicting placental type.[66] Both studies found that the difference in septum size was most notable early on in the pregnancy. A quantitative examination of the dividing septum may also help predict placental type. The presence of two layers in the septum is consistent with monochorionic placenta. Three or four layers in the septum suggest a dichorionic placenta.[4] Monoamniotic pregnancies are quite rare and difficult to diagnose in utero. Inability to visualize any dividing membranes is not diagnostic of a monoamniotic placenta, especially in the later stages of pregnancy when visualization of the membranes by ultrasound becomes more difficult.

The in utero diagnosis of twin-to-twin transfusion has been reported.[17,160] Key diagnostic features include second trimester onset; a larger, more active twin with increased fluid who is possibly hydropic; and a smaller fetus with decreased fluid and restricted activity. This situation must be differentiated from growth retardation of one of the twins, which usually presents in the third trimester with a normally growing twin surrounded by normal fluid, and a poorly growing twin with decreased fluid. These differences are listed in Table 9-7 and illustrated by Figure 9-2.

Fetal Growth. Studies detailing biparietal diameter (BPD) growth through pregnancy

Table 9-7. Ultrasonic Differentiation of Twin-to-Twin Transfusion from Single Fetal Growth Retardation

	Initial Detection	Sex	Placentas	Larger Twin	Smaller Twin
Twin-to-twin transfusion	2nd trimester	Same	Monochorionic	Increased fluid Active fetus Thick placenta Size ≥ dates Possibly hydropic	Decreased fluid Decreased fetal activity Thin placenta Size < dates
Single IUGR fetus	3rd trimester	Variable	Variable	Normal fluid Size = dates No hydrops	Decreased fluid Size < dates

have found varying results when comparing twins to singletons. Some report BPD progression to be consistent with that of singletons, whereas in other studies twin BPD size is noted to fall behind singleton values in the third trimester.[31,41,59,92,139,141,143] When unequal twin BPD measurements are present, the larger of the two BPDs has been found to be usually consistent with that for singletons of a similar gestational age, and only the smaller BPD lags behind.[68]

Several investigators have evaluated the significance of discordant ultrasound measurements. In an early publication, Dorros suggested discordancy was a sign of IUGR of the smaller twin, with the "naturally occurring internal control" (the normal twin) useful in assessing the adequacy of growth of the smaller infant.[43] In the first study looking specifically at divergent BPDs, as BPD discrepancy increased, the incidence of IUGR increased from 40% (with a 2–6 mm twin BPD difference) to 71% (when the BPD difference was greater than 6 mm).[67] Also when the BPD discrepancy was greater than 6 mm, a higher incidence of IUGR was found in both twins. Other studies have found twin BPD differences to be a suboptimal parameter to use for the diagnosis of IUGR. Divers and Hemsell found poor sensitivity and accuracy with divergent BPDs (BPD cutoff not specified) for the prediction of IUGR.[41] Of eight pregnancies with IUGR, an accurate diagnosis was only made in three and there were two false-positives. Others have found widely varying BPD differences (0–16 mm differences) despite a birth weight difference of at least 25%.[31,92] False-positive diagnoses of IUGR from large BPD differences have been attributed to fetal dolichocephaly. The use of head circumference in those cases with a significant BPD difference to distinguish discordancy from abnormal fetal head shape has been suggested.[31] Socol and co-workers analysed their data on twins with concordant birth weights.[148] BPDs were found to fall off the normal singleton curve at about 32 weeks gestation, while abdominal circumferences fell off the singleton curve at around 34 weeks gestation. Nineteen percent of the pregnancies had at least a 5-mm BPD difference noted. On newborn anthropometric data, only birth weight values were significantly below singleton values, while head circumference and length were within expected limits for singletons.

Other studies have also shown that the primary neonatal parameter lagging in twins is birth weight and not head size, suggesting asymmetric IUGR.[96,164] The experience of the Yale New Haven Hospital is similar; no significant mean BPD differences were found among groups of twins with no discrepancy (less than 10% birth weight difference), moderate discrepancy (10%–20% birth weight difference), and large discrepancy (greater than 20% birth weight difference).[4]

The summary in Table 9-8 shows that

Table 9-8. Accuracy of Twin BPD Differences in Predicting IUGR

Study	BPD Cutoff for Discordancy	IUGR Sensitivity	False-Positives
Divers & Hemsell[41]	>2 mm	38%	40%
Houlton[18]	>3 mm	59%	24%
	>6 mm	27%	14%
Crane et al.[31]	>5 mm	100%†	25%
Leveno et al.[92]	>5 mm	54%*	78%
Houlton et al.[69]	>3 mm	51%	50%
	>6 mm	13%	33%
Erkkola et al.[49]	>3 mm	35%†	77%
	>5 mm	9%†	71%
Barnea et al.[5]	>3 mm	55.5%	73%
	>6 mm	55.5%	37.5%

* SGA here defined as one S.D. below mean birthweight for twins
† For birth weight difference >25%

BPD difference is not an accurate method of detecting IUGR. Except for the Crane study, sensitivities are less than 60% and significant numbers of false-positives are seen.

In analyzing the use of ultrasound to diagnose IUGR in twins, Chitkara and associates found that the optimum accuracy in detecting both IUGR and discordant growth was obtained through the use of multiple parameters to estimate fetal weight.[30] Among single fetal parameters, abdominal circumference was the most accurate; however, accuracy was improved by the use of multiple parameters.

Neonatal data suggest that the concept of discordancy is a poor one as far as diagnosing IUGR. The mean twin birth weight difference is 11%, with 90% and two standard deviation (SD) cutoffs of 25% and 30% birth weight difference. Using the two-SD cutoff, only one-fifth of the IUGR fetuses were identified, and the positive predictive value was 70%. Decreasing the cutoff point to 15% of the birth weight difference (just above the mean value of 11%), the sensitivity increased to 70%, but positive predictive value dropped to 34%. The main reason for the inaccuracies was that in 9.4% of the twin pregnancies, both twins were growth retarded.[116]

The detection of inter-twin discordancy, although associated with a growth deficiency, is not an accurate measurement of IUGR. This should not come as a surprise, since even in singleton gestations, BPD is a poor predictor of fetal birth weight. In twin situations the BPD is further compromised by in utero crowding and an increase in malpresentation, which increases the likelihood of inaccurate or unobtainable BPD measurements.

In summarizing, discordancy is a marker for, but not diagnostic of, abnormal growth of one of the twins in utero. Using the normal control fetus by which to evaluate the abnormal one may be helpful in situations in which the patient's dates are unclear or the patient is not seen until late in the gestation. However, discordancy will not be helpful when both twins are small for gestational age (9% of the twin gestations). As the goal of doing serial ultrasound examinations is to evaluate fetal health as mirrored in fetal growth, it seems the most appropriate to interpret the ultrasound results for each fetus individually. Recent neonatal data from our population supports this. Classification of twins by individual birth weight for gestational age more closely correlated with morbidity than did classification by birth weight discordancy.[18] Serial ultrasound examinations should begin in the mid–second trimester and be repeated approximately every 3 weeks. Multiple parameters should be measured and fetal weights estimated. As there is little data to support the contention that twins are physiologically smaller than singletons, the use of nomograms constructed from singletons is recommended. Nomograms specific for twins will be a little less sensitive in detecting IUGR.

Fetal Assessments

Although serial ultrasound examinations late in the second trimester are helpful in detecting growth retardation, they are not sensitive to acute changes in fetal health and require several weeks between scans to accurately detect differences. Antenatal fetal heart rate testing has become the standard method of antenatal assessment. As with singletons, a reactive nonstress test is associated with a good outcome and a nonreactive test is associated with IUGR and increased perinatal morbidity.[4,14,40,88] The number of fetal heart rate accelerations in a 20-minute period is equal in singleton and twin gestations for any given gestational age. Knuppel and co-workers used a nonstress test (NST) backed up by an oxytocin challenge test (OCT) for nonreactive tests after 32 weeks to follow 90 twin pregnancies with no intrauterine demises.[84] Intervention was required in 6 of the pregnancies because of abnormal tracings. Weekly or biweekly NSTs appear to be an appropriate way to follow twin gestations.

More recently the biophysical profile, using a NST and ultrasonically evaluated parameters within the fetal placental unit, has become popular. Its usefulness has been shown in singleton gestations, but there has not yet been a large experience with twins. Lodeiro and co-workers reported that the biophysical profile was a good predictor of outcome in 49 twin gestations.[94] With their small numbers, the data did not show any benefit to using the full biophysical profile if the nonstress test was reactive.

Doppler is a new tool to evaluate fetal and maternal blood flow through the assessment of blood flow volume or velocity wave form analysis. It is still in its infancy and the significance of the results are encouraging but not yet clearly understood. Using the ratios of peak flow in systole and diastole, Giles and co-workers evaluated 76 twin pregnancies.[58] Fetuses with normal birth weights had systolic to diastolic velocity ratios within the normal range for singletons. In pairs in which one or both of the liveborn babies was growth retarded, 78% had at least one fetus with an abnormally elevated ratio. In half of the pregnancies, when a normal ratio was found in spite of a small-for-gestational-age fetus, the cause was not IUGR, but rather twin-to-twin transfusion. Thus, a small baby and an abnormal systolic to diastolic flow ratio was suggestive of IUGR, whereas a small baby but a normal ratio was more indicative of a twin-to-twin transfusion. It will be interesting to see if further data supports this conclusion, since placental changes in twin-to-twin transfusion presented above could be predicted to result in abnormal flows. Farmakides and co-workers used umbilical artery Doppler wave form analysis and found that twins of normal birth weight had a slightly but significantly greater ratio than that seen for appropriate-for-gestational-age singleton births.[50] The difference of flow ratios between twins was predictive of a birth weight difference, with flow differences of 0.4 or greater having a 73% sensitivity and 82% specificity for a twin-to-twin birth weight difference of greater than 349 g.

Several questions about wave form analysis remain. What is an appropriate frequency inbetween examinations? What is the significance and predictive value of abnormal-normal examinations? What is the appropriate next step once an abnormal examination is obtained? Data collection in this field is growing significantly.

PROPHYLACTIC THERAPY

Because of increased twin morbidity and mortality, various preventive therapies have been attempted. Of these therapies cervical cerclage, bed rest, and prophylactic tocolysis are the most commonly discussed.

Cervical Cerclage

The routine placement of a cervical cerclage has been attempted in an effort to decrease preterm delivery. In a nonrandomized study, Weekes and co-workers evaluated the effects of cervical cerclage compared to bed rest and no therapy on the outcome of twin gestations.[157] Patient care was dictated by physician preference. Approximately 25% of the patients received a cervical cerclage with the mean time of insertion being just over 29 weeks gestation. No significant differences in outcome between the three groups were seen. The study can be criticized for the late placement of the cerclage. Certainly in singletons it has been shown that placement after 18 weeks is associated with increased morbidity.[26] Any potential benefits gained by the cerclage may be overshadowed by detriments obtained by the late time of placement.

Zakut reported on the elective placement of a cervical cerclage early on in the course of 15 twin pregnancies. Both this group and a similar number of controlled twin pregnancies were taken from a larger group of women whose pregnancies followed ovulation induction. Cervical cerclage by McDonald procedure was selected for those women who, on early pelvic examination, had a uterine size that was felt to be at least two weeks larger than dates. The cerclage group showed a significant increase in duration of the pregnancy as well as decrease in perinatal mortality.[165] Other studies have been done with conflicting conclusions.[42,145] Until more data is presented, routine cervical cerclage for multiple gestation is not recommended. Certainly, if there is an indication either by history or early examination (either ultrasound or pelvic examination), then a cerclage should be placed.

Tocolysis

Prophylactic use of tocolytic agents before preterm labor is diagnosed has been evaluated in several twin studies. Unlike bed rest and cerclage, this method of treatment has been evaluated by double-blind controlled studies. Marivate and associates administered fenoterol or a placebo daily in a double-blind study to 23 twins of less than 33 weeks gestation. There were no significant differences for gestational age, number of growth retarded fetuses, or incidence of spontaneous labor.[100] O'Connor and co-workers in 1979 reported on 25 twin gestations treated with 40 mg of ritodrine daily in comparison to 24 controlled twin pregnancies.[118] The betamimetic agent was started at the time of diagnosis of the twin gestation, which ranged between 20 and 34 weeks. Although no significant increase in gestational age or birth weight was found, the increases of 1 week in gestational age and 200 g in birth weight in the treated group were suggestive of improved outcome (p value = .07). Because the sample sizes were too small to adequately detect a statistical significance in the noted differences, the results are more appropriately called inconclusive and do not support a lack of effect.[126]

O'Leary in 1986 treated twins with 2.5 mg of terbutaline every 6 hours with increases to higher doses if uterine activity was noted.[119] Here again, onset of therapy was started at the time of diagnosis, which ranged from 20 to 30 weeks. The tocolytics were continued until 35 weeks in 32 twin pregnancies. Although the study was done prospectively, no placebo was given to the 32 women in the control group. Bed rest was recommended for women in both groups and all patients were followed in a special twins outpatient clinic. It is not clear if the women in the two groups were randomized. Results showed a significant increase in gestational age and birth weight. A recent Swedish study also looked at the effectiveness of terbutaline.[147] Although a dose of only 15 mg/day was used, and sample sizes were small, a significant decrease in preterm labor compared with the control group was found. However, neither birth weight nor preterm delivery was significantly improved, possibly due to the fact that parenteral tocolysis was given to 15 of the 25 control patients. Though not completely supportive, this study suggests a beneficial effect from the prophylactic use of tocolytics.

Bed Rest

The final therapy in this group, bed rest, has received by far the majority of the attention in the literature. By having a patient with twins decrease her activity and remain at rest in a lateral decubitus position, it is hoped that maternal exertion is minimized and uterine blood flow is maximized in a noninvasive manner. Unfortunately the studies tend to be retrospective and observational, and not appropriate for true statistical comparison. Within each study there is no controlling for the time of starting the bed rest, stopping the bed rest, or electively delivering the patient. Certainly gains made by starting bed rest early in patients with twins may be negated in the final results by a more aggressive approach towards delivering the patient once the end of the third trimester is reached. Many studies contain too few patients to detect statistical differences between the groups. Despite the design deficits of most of the studies, many recent reviews and texts state that bed rest is most likely to result in an increase in birth weight. Table 9-9 compares recent studies of the effectiveness of bed rest; results were varied.

The importance of good, routine antenatal care cannot be underestimated and cannot be replaced by the above-mentioned therapies. Good pregnancy outcomes have been obtained through the use of a specialized outpatient clinic for twins.[117] Despite the lack of good data, we feel that bed rest can be both a benign form of therapy and helpful with twin gestations. To be helpful, however, it needs to be started before 30 weeks when the majority of morbidity and mortality in twins occurs.[62] Bed rest after this time, although possibly helpful in improving twin outcome, will have little effect on overall statistics, since the majority of untoward outcomes has already taken place. We do not feel that the literature supports the use of routine hospitalized bed rest. Certainly this form of therapy can be quite expensive if started in the second trimester and carried into fetal viability, and can be very difficult psychologically on both patient and family.

Recent interest has focused not only on preventing the complications, but also on diagnosing them earlier. Several studies have shown that excessive uterine activity may precede the development of preterm labor.[8,162] Over the last several years, the use of an ambulatory home monitor to detect uterine contractions has been examined.[7,76] Twin gestations have more contractions per hour

Table 9-9. Antenatal Effects of Bed Rest in Recent Studies

Study	Gestational Age	Birth Weight	Mortality
Jeffrey et al.[72]	−	+	+
Misenhimer & Kaltreider[106]	−	+	+
Weekes et al.[157]	−	−	−
Hawrylyshyn et al.[62]	+	−	−
Jouppilla et al.[73]	−	−	+
Persson & Grennert[120]	+	−	+
Sanders et al.[138]	−	−	−
Laursen[87]	+	+	+
Erkkola et al.[48]	−	−	+
Kappel et al.[75]	+	+	+

+ Improvement noted with bed rest
− No improvement with bed rest

than their singleton counterparts. Also the increase in uterine activity noted several weeks before term in singletons occurs at an even earlier gestational age in twins.[112] Certainly more clinical information is needed before this new technology can be put to use clinically. There are reports in the literature of patients with increased uterine activity without premature labor.[77]

LABOR AND DELIVERY

Fetal Lung Maturity

Amniocentesis with analysis of fluid for pulmonary maturity is a commonly accepted antecedent to elective, but preterm, delivery in singleton pregnancies. The situation also arises in twin gestations in which preterm delivery is contemplated but not mandatory. The question arises whether fluid should be obtained from one twin or both. The lecithin/sphingomyelin (L/S) values of twin fetuses have been found to be similar in studies by Spellacy and Sims and colleagues of 34 twin pairs.[144,151] Similarly, Norman and group found concordance in 24 twin pairs when amniocentesis was done prior to the onset of labor.[114] However, when labor preceded the amniocentesis (6 pregnancies), twin A had a higher L/S value than twin B. The presence of growth retardation had no effect on the L/S values obtained.

Leveno and colleagues found discordant L/S values (one twin with an L/S greater than 2:1, the other twin with an L/S of less than 2:1) in 5 of 42 twin pregnancies.[91] Only one of these infants developed respiratory distress syndrome. The authors also found that twin fetal lung maturation was independent of fetal sex, fetal zygosity, birth order, and fetal weight discordancy. The authors also found that fetal lung maturity is reached at an earlier gestational age in twins than is typically seen in singleton gestation. The mean gestational age for finding L/S values above 2 was approximately 31 to 32 weeks. Although the number of complicated twin gestations was small, the authors did not notice any further acceleration of fetal lung maturity by these complications.

Neonatal data show that when respiratory distress is seen in twin neonates, it is usually concordant. However, when only one fetus has respiratory insufficiency, it was usually twin B (70 of 85 cases).[111,135,156]

Although the reported experience is small, tapping one sac appears to be adequate to assess pulmonary maturity. If both amniotic sacs are easily accessible to do dual amniocentesis, or if any fetal complications are present, then dual amniocentesis may be desirable. If amniocentesis is considered when the patient presents in labor, the amniotic sac for twin B should be the one that is sampled. With dual amniocentesis small doses (3–5 ml) of either Evans Blue or Indigo Carmine dye can be injected into the first sac to help verify the appropriate sac for the second sample.

In the event of more advanced prematurity or pulmonary lung immaturity, can or should steroids be used to accelerate fetal lung development in twins? This question is often considered by obstetricians because of the high rate of preterm birth in twins. The recent National Institutes of Health Collaborative Study on the prevention of respiratory distress found steroids to be effective in decreasing the incidence of respiratory distress overall, with female infants responding more to this therapy than males.[127] Although a significant beneficial effect was not seen in twins, a similar trend to singletons was noted. In females of twin pairs given steroids, there was a suggestion that the incidence of respiratory distress was decreased, although the numbers were too small to be of statistical significance.[23] Cord blood levels of dexamethasone showed levels well below those considered therapeutic. It is possible that with either a higher maternal dose or increased frequency of steroid, and larger twin numbers, that this therapy could be effective in twins. Thus, consideration to the use of steroids in twin pregnancies should be based on the gestational age of the pregnancy, fetal sex, and possibly amniotic fluid maturity study.

Elective Timing

In the absence of specific indications to electively deliver twins, the optimal timing for the delivery of twins is not clearly set out in the literature. A large Swedish study showed an increase in perinatal mortality in twin infants born after 38 weeks, suggesting that elective delivery of twins at 38 weeks may improve outcome.[120] These data contradict another study which noted no such increase in mortality at term.[115] Two more recent studies have addressed this issue. Puissant and Leroy did find an increase in perinatal mortality when pregnancy went beyond 38 weeks, but the increase was statistically significant only for primiparous mothers.[129] The majority of the deaths after 38 weeks were antepartum (58%), and most of these babies were found to be macerated on delivery. Unfortunately, the data do not indicate when these fetuses died. It would be inappropriate to suggest elective termination based on this data, if a significant proportion of the post-38-week deaths actually died in utero several weeks earlier, but were not diagnosed or delivered until term.

Heluin and co-workers also found an increase in perinatal mortality in twins allowed to go into spontaneous labor at term, compared to a group electively delivered.[65] The inclusion of complicated cases in the "elective" delivery group (IUGR, preeclampsia, and polyhydramnios) make comparisons of morbidity difficult to assess, but no significant increases in low Apgar scores or neurologic damage were seen between the two groups. Elective induction of labor was associated with a slightly higher cesarean section rate (22% v. 16% for spontaneous labor), but given the inequality of the groups, the significance of this finding is not clear.

The current data is not sufficient to recommend elective delivery of all twin gestations not delivered by 38 weeks. However this data, together with the trend of increased lagging of fetal growth behind singleton levels and of growth retardation as the third trimester progresses,[102] serve as a caveat to those caring for twins. Potential problems do not stop once term is reached, and fetal monitoring should continue up until delivery.

Labor Management

The increased risk for twins does not end once labor commences. Potential intrapartum problems stem from risks of uteroplacental insufficiency, uterine distension resulting in increased maternal great vessel occlusion, incoordinate uterine contractions, malpresentations, and prematurity.

Several factors may affect labor duration. Increased cervical dilatation prior to the onset of labor can shorten labor, while malposition and uterine distension can have the opposite effect. Friedman and Sachtleben found increased prelabor dilatation and shorter latent phase but longer active phases with twins as compared to singleton gestations.[53] Bender and Garrett found no difference in the overall length of labor between singleton and twin gestations.[13,56] In general, twin gestations do not appear to have a significant overall effect on the duration of labor.

Intrapartum Risks

Several concerns should be addressed for appropriate intrapartum care. Both fetuses must be monitored throughout labor. In most hospitals this requires two separate monitors, though some of the newer fetal monitors are capable of monitoring uterine contractions and two fetal heart rates (one with a scalp electrode, the other with an external monitor) simultaneously. The position and estimated size of both babies should be known, and access to rapid delivery with appropriate anesthesia should be available.

A recent review of twin gestations by MacGillivray quotes over a dozen references showing a higher frequency of problems for twin B compared to twin A.[98] Published predominantly before 1970, they predate modern improvements in antepartum and intrapartum diagnosis and care of twins. Also, the effects of an undiagnosed second twin, fetal position, birth weight, and route of delivery on outcome are not evaluated.

More recently a poor outcome for twin B was again noted and a liberal use of cesarean section was recommended.[25] McCarthy and co-workers, however, found that the birth weight specific mortality was equal or better for twins as compared to singleton babies, implying that the poorer results seen with second twins may be due to lower birth weights.[101] Other recent studies found no difference in neonatal mortality between twin A and twin B, and although one study found differences in cord pH, the differences were small and found predominantly in umbilical venous but not arterial samples.[51,78,80]

Interlocking of twins can produce mechanical obstruction to delivery, resulting in a high incidence of morbidity and mortality in both twins. In a review of this topic, Nissan classified four types of mechanical twin-to-twin interaction[113]:

1. Collision: contact prevents engagement of both twins
2. Impaction: contact allows only partial engagement of both twins
3. Compaction: both twins engage, but their contact prevents further descent or disengagement
4. Interlocking, with chins of the two babies locking on delivery

The most dramatic of these interactions, interlocking, has been estimated to occur in one of every 1000 twin gestations.[81] The breech/vertex presentation is the most common setting for interlocking, but only 10% of twins present in this position, making interlocking a rare occurrence even with this presentation.

Route of Delivery

The optimal route of delivery, vaginal versus abdominal, has not been unequivocally demonstrated, though discussion of this issue can stir up a considerable amount of debate. A variety of factors are important in deciding on the route of delivery. Gestational age, absolute and relative fetal (estimated) weights, fetal positions, availability of anesthesia and ultrasound, and physician skill can all affect outcome.

The most uniformly agreed upon management concerns the most common presentation. Vertex-vertex twins (approximately 40% of twins) can safely be delivered vaginally.[63] The optimal route of delivery for breech babies is not as clear cut. Kelsick and Minkoff found that cesarean section improved the outcome of breech twins, although the improvement was primarily seen in those weighing in the 1- to 2-kg range.[80] Larger breech twins weighing between 2 kg and 3 kg had increased perinatal mortality when delivered by cesarean section. Lower Apgar scores were found in second twins, but this was irrespective of the route of delivery.

Data on the outcome of breech second twins suggests birth weight–specific effects with cesarean section. Chervenak and co-workers found there to be no significant difference for route of delivery in the outcome of nonvertex twin Bs in groups of babies weighing either less than 1500 g or more than 1500 g.[27,28] However, due to small numbers in the less-than-1500-g group, the increase in low Apgar scores (14.3% v. 55.6%) and neonatal morbidity (14.3% v. 36.8%) was not statistically significant. Because of small numbers in the low birth weight group it is appropriate to say that the data suggest improved outcome by cesarean section. The authors recommended vaginal delivery for twins presenting as vertex-nonvertex when the estimated weight of twin B was greater than 2000 g. When the estimated weight of the nonvertex baby B is less than 2000 g, they recommend attempting fetal version, and if successful, vaginal delivery. The authors chose the 2000 cutoff based on a neonatal cutoff of 1500 g plus a 10% standard deviation by ultrasound of estimated weight. Hayes and Smeltzer also recommended delivery based on an estimated fetal weight of 1500 g. Internal version was recommended for breech second twins weighing less than 1500 g, with cesarean delivery if unsuccessful.[63]

This data on birth weight–specific improvement in outcome with cesarean section, although limited, is consistent with that for singletons. But is there a difference between breech singletons and breech twins? A recent study addressed this issue looking at the outcome of 103 twin breeches in comparison to singleton breech deliveries.[22] Both groups were subdivided by birth weight (greater or less than 1500 g) and evaluated for Apgar scores and mortality. No significant differences were found between the various groups except for a decreased frequency of low 5-minute Apgar scores in first-born breech twins in comparison to singletons.

The appropriate route of delivery when twin A is presenting breech is also not settled. Based on singleton data[27,29] as well as data on nonvertex twin Bs, many authors recommend cesarean section when twin A presents as breech with an estimated fetal weight of less than 1500 g. For fetuses above 1500 g, there is a small possibility of interlocking twins. Our experience is that when patients present in labor with twin A breech at greater than 34 weeks gestation, the majority opt for delivery by cesarean section once the various risks and options are discussed. It is quite appropriate, especially given today's legal climate, to present patients with appropriate information and have them involved in the decision-making process.

In summary, recommended approaches for delivery of twins can be made, but the final decision must be individualized for the specific circumstances. For those pregnancies presenting vertex-vertex, irregardless of gestational age, vaginal delivery is the accepted route. As stated earlier, both babies should be monitored throughout labor and rapid access must be available for cesarean section for any problems that may develop during labor. For those babies presenting as breech for twin A, cesarean section is recommended if the estimated weight is less than 1500 g. For those greater than 1500 g, a vaginal delivery may be offered, but both obstetrician and patient should be aware of the potential of interlocking twins.

For twins that present breech-breech, the birth weight of twin B must be kept in mind also. Here again, for estimated weights of less than 1500 g to 2000 g, delivery should be considered by cesarean section. When twin A is vertex and twin B is nonvertex, vaginal delivery can be planned. For twins less than 1500 g, version of twin B after delivery of twin A is recommended. The use of sonography in the delivery room can be quite helpful. We prefer the use of conduction anesthesia. Although this can decrease maternal efforts in bearing down, this disadvantage is offset by the ease allowed for performing manipulations. If twin B is considerably larger than twin A, delivery by version and extraction may result in birth trauma and should not be attempted. Many obstetricians find this regimen undesirable in that it requires skill in the use of fetal version and may increase maternal morbidity by requiring a cesarean section after a full course of labor and delivery of a single infant. In a recent study in which this protocol was used, approximately 30% of the twins presenting as vertex-nonvertex required cesarean section for twin B after vaginal delivery of twin A.[27]

After vaginal delivery of twin A, no preset limits should be set for the delivery of twin B. Several authors have shown no correlation between the twin delivery interval and morbidity.[27,28,132] The second fetus should be monitored after twin A delivers and, if needed, pitocin can be given to augment contractions.

HIGHER ORDER MULTIPLE GESTATIONS

With the relatively recent increase in the use of ovulation induction agents, the number of multiple gestations is increasing. This increase is predominantly seen in twins, but increases have also been seen in triplets, quadruplets, and other higher order multiple gestations (HOMGs). The overall frequency of HOMGs is still low, even in large referral centers, so that most published studies on HOMGs either contain a small number of patients or are of long duration, encompassing significant changes in standard obstetric practice, neonatal skills, and technology.

The approximate incidence of non-iatrogenic HOMGs can be calculated from Hellins'

Law of $1:n^x$, in which n is the frequency of twins and x is one less than the number of fetuses. Thus, if the twinning rate is 1 in 90 livebirths, the frequency of triplets is 1:8100 births, and quadruplets can be predicted as 1:729,000 births.

Antenatal Care

As with twin gestations, early diagnosis is an important first step in the antenatal care of HOMGs, and is best done with an ultrasound examination. Because infertility patients undergoing ovulation induction cycles form a significant number of HOMGs, and they usually receive close medical supervision until a viable pregnancy is confirmed, they are an ideal patient population for this type of pregnancy. A recent study illustrates the importance of early diagnosis by showing that induced triplet pregnancies had a better outcome than spontaneous triplets.[67] Although not specifically evaluated, no doubt at least part of the improvement noted was the result of earlier diagnosis in this group.

Once diagnosed, HOMGs should receive antenatal care reflective of their high-risk status. HOMGs experience similar fetal and maternal complications as do twin gestations. However, the frequency of these complications can be expected to be higher than with twins due to the extra stresses placed upon mother and fetuses by the larger fetal load. It is not unexpected that one or several of the early fetuses seen will not survive, but rather undergo demise early in the pregnancy. In a recent review, preterm delivery was noted in 97% of triplets, with pregnancy-induced hypertension and anemia seen in 46% and 20% of pregnancies, respectively. As the number of fetuses increase, the gestational age at which birth weight first is found to lag behind singletons decreases. As the pregnancy progresses further into the third trimester, a larger difference is noted from mean singleton birth weight.[102] Perinatal morbidity and mortality is increased in HOMGs, with prematurity being the most significant factor.[85,123,136] Besides maternal parameters, which are routinely checked on antenatal visits, the fetus should receive similar evaluation as described for twins.

Ultrasound should play a central role in the evaluation of fetal health in HOMGs. Serial ultrasound examinations looking at growth (by multiple biometric parameters) should be done at approximately 3-week intervals. These scans should also evaluate for placental chorionicity by looking at fetal sex and membrane thickness. Fetal-fetal transfusions can take place between monochorionic twins, and growth retardation of any number of the fetuses may be detected. We prefer to assess fetal growth individually, using singleton growth curves. In addition, fetal health should also be evaluated by either fetal heart rate testing or biophysical profiles. We use biophysical testing instead of the NST and OCT to ensure that each fetus is tested.

As with twins, consideration has been given to the prophylactic use of bed rest, tocolytics, steroids, and cervical cerclages in an effort to prolong the pregnancy and improve outcome. Here, too, controlled evaluations are lacking. There is currently insufficient evidence that the benefit from empiric use of cerclages is greater than the risk of the procedure. Certainly though, if past history is consistent with the diagnosis of an incompetent cervix, the surgery should be performed.

Bed rest appears to be nearly uniformly accepted as appropriate therapy for women with HOMGs. Usually, maternal discomfort in ambulating during the latter half of pregnancy makes this form of therapy well accepted. To maximize its effectiveness, bed rest should be started in mid-gestation, prior to when most losses occur. The optimal location for bed rest should be individualized, with hospitalization preferred for the mother with a hectic home situation, and home bed rest considered for those with assistance at home (possibly visiting nurses) and minimal responsibilities.

Empiric use of steroids and tocolytics also appear to be not uncommon practice. This practice is based on the high rate of preterm delivery and not on studies showing significant improvement in outcome. These modalities are aimed at reducing the incidence of preterm birth, but there are no randomized control studies evaluating their effectiveness. Although many physicians favor empiric use of tocolytic agents due to the high frequency of preterm delivery, others prefer to await the onset of regular contractions. One must be aware of additive side-effects of a much increased maternal blood volume from the multiple gestation and the cardiac stimulating effects of betamimetics.

The small amount of data available on pulmonary maturity suggest a maturation process in HOMG similar to twins. The presenting fetus typically has been found to have the more mature pulmonic system than the babies that follow.[123,136] The discrepancy should be kept in mind when considering amniocentesis for fetal lung maturity before electively delivering a patient.

Delivery

As with twins, the optimal route of delivery for HOMGs is not clear. Several studies have reported lower perinatal mortality in baby A compared with succeeding births, and improvement of the outcome with cesarean section.[36,38,67,85] In other reports, cesarean section did not result in improved outcome, though these studies often stress the importance of skilled atraumatic and rapid vaginal delivery.[70,95,123,136]

A consistent effect of birth order has not been seen on neonatal outcome. As mentioned above, care must be taken in drawing conclusions from those studies in which a significant number of patients predate modern advances in fetal diagnosis and surveillance.

The timing and route of delivery must be individualized, taking into account maternal and fetal complications, fetal positions and estimated weights, skill of the physician at difficult vaginal deliveries, and availability of ultrasound and anesthesia during "off hours." The incidence of fetal malposition is increased in HOMGs, with a wide variety of combinations being seen, though the first fetus is most typically vertex. Many physicians now practice routine cesarean section for all HOMGs.

The issue of optimal route of delivery for HOMGs is a very sensitive one, especially given today's medical and legal climate in which a perfect outcome is often expected and demanded. The literature does not provide unequivocal support for one route of delivery over another. The data on triplets suggest that vaginal delivery can be safely performed without any increased morbidity and mortality to the babies, although few physicians are willing to deliver triplets vaginally. Despite the lack of supporting data, there does not seem to be any question that pregnancies of quadruplets or more should be delivered by cesarean section.

REFERENCES

1. Averback P, Wiglesworth F: Monochorionic, monamniotic double-battledore placenta with stillbirth and postpartum cerebellar syndrome. Am J Obstet Gynecol 128:697, 1977
2. Babson SG, Kangas J, Young N, Bramhall JL: Growth and development of twins of dissimilar size at birth. Pediatrics 33:327, 1964
3. Babson SG, Phillips DS: Growth and development of twins dissimilar in size at birth. N Engl J Med 289:937, 1973
4. Bailey D, Flynn AM, Kelly J: Antepartum fetal heart rate monitoring in multiple pregnancy. Br J Obstet Gynaecol 87:561, 1980
5. Barnea ER, Romero R, Scott D et al: The value of biparietal diameter and abdominal perimeter in the diagnosis of growth retardation in twin gestation. Am J Perinatol 2:221, 1985
6. Barss VA, Benacerraf BR, Frigoletto FD: Ultrasonographic determination of chorion type in twin gestation. Obstet Gynecol 66:779, 1985
7. Bell R: Measurement of spontaneous uterine activity in the antenatal patient. Am J Obstet Gynecol 140:713, 1981
8. Bell R: The prediction of preterm labor by recording spontaneous antenatal uterine activity. Br J Obstet Gynaecol 90:884, 1983
9. Bender S: Twin pregnancy. A review of 472 cases. J Obstet Gynecol BE 59:510, 1952
10. Benirschke K: Twin placenta in perinatal mortality. NY State J Med 61:1499, 1961
11. Benirschke K, Driscoll SG: In: The Pathology

of the Human Placenta. Berlin, Springer-Verlag, 1967
12. Benirschke K, Kim CK: Multiple pregnancy. N Engl J Med 288:1329, 1973
13. Benson MD, Keith LG, Keith DM: The etiology of twins. Curr Prob Obstet Gynecol VI:4, 1983
14. Blake GD, Knuppel RA, Ingardia CJ et al: Evaluation of nonstress fetal heart rate testing in multiple gestations. Obstet Gynecol 63:528, 1984
15. Bleker OP, Breur W, Huidekoper BL: A study of birthweight, placental weight, and mortality on twins as compared to singletons. Br J Obstet Gynaecol 86:111, 1979
16. Boyd JD, Hamilton MJ: The Human Placenta. Cambridge, MA, Hefber, 1970
17. Braat DDM, Bernardus RE, Arts NFT, Rajnherc JR: Twin pregnancy: Case reports illustrating variations in transfusion syndrome. Eur J Obstet Gynecol Reprod Biol 19:383, 1985
18. Bronsteen R, Goyert G, Bottoms S: Prediction of neonatal morbidity in twins: IUGR vs discordancy. Presented to Society of Perinatal Obstetricians, Buena Vista, FL, 1987
19. Brown GR: Letter to the editor. Br J Obstet Gynaecol 87:255, 1980
20. Brown GR, Macaskill S: Acute hydramnios with twins successfully treated by abdominal paracentesis. Br Med J 1:1739, 1961
21. Bryan E, Slavin B: Serum IgG levels in fetofetal transfusion syndrome. Arch Dis Child 49:908, 1974
22. Buekens P, Lagasse R, Puissant F, Leroy F: Do breech presentations in twins and singletons run different risks? Acta Genet Med Gamellol 34:207, 1985
23. Burkett G, Bauer C, Morrison JC, Curet LB: Effect of prenatal dexamethasone administration on prevention of respiratory distress syndrome in twin pregnancies. J Perinat 6:305, 1986
24. Caspi E, Ronen J, Schreyer P et al: The outcome of pregnancy after gonadotropin therapy. Br J Obstet Gynecol 83:967, 1976
25. Cetrulo CL, Ingardia CJ, Scarra AJ: Management of multiple gestation. Clin Obstet Gynecol 23:533, 1980
26. Charles D, Edwards WR: Infectious complications of cervical cerclage. Am J Obstet Gynecol 141:1065, 1981
27. Chervenak FA, Johnson RE, Berkowitz RL et al: Is routine cesarean section necessary for vertex-breech and vertex-transverse twin gestations? Am J Obstet Gynecol 148:1, 1984
28. Chervenak FA, Johnson RE, Youcha S: Intrapartum management of twin gestation. Obstet Gynecol 65:119, 1985
29. Chervenak FA, Youcha S, Johnson RE et al: Twin gestation: Antenatal diagnosis and perinatal outcome in a series of 385 consecutive twin pregnancies. J Reprod Med 29:727, 1984
30. Chitkara U, Berkowitz GS, Levine R et al: Twin pregnancy: Routine use of ultrasound examinations in the prenatal diagnosis of intrauterine growth retardation and discordant growth. Am J Perinatol 2:49, 1985
31. Crane JP, Tomich PG, Kopta M: Ultrasonic growth patterns in normal and discordant twins. Obstet Gynecol 55:683, 1980
32. Churchill JC: The relationship between intelligence and birth weight in twins. Neurology 15:341, 1965
33. D'Alton ME, Dudley DKL: Ultrasound in the antenatal management of twin gestation. Semin Perinatol 10:30, 1986
34. D'Alton ME, Newton ER, Cetrulo CL: Intrauterine fetal demise in multiple gestation. Acta Genet Med Gemellol 33:43, 1984
35. Davies J, Chazen E, Nance WE: Symmelia in one of monozygotic twins. Teratology 4:367, 1971
36. Daw E: Triplet pregnancy. Br J Obstet Gynecol 85:505, 1978
37. Daw E, Walker J: Growth differences in twin pregnancy. Br J Clin Pract 29:151, 1975
38. Deale CJC, Cronje HS: A review of 367 triplet pregnancies. S Afr Med J 66:92, 1984
39. DeLia JE, Emery MG, Sheafor SA, Jennison TA: Twin transfusion syndrome: Successful in utero treatment with digoxin. Int J Gynaecol Obstet 23:197, 1985
40. Devoe LD, Azor H: Simultaneous nonstress fetal heart rate testing in twin pregnancy. Obstet Gynecol 58:450, 1981
41. Divers WA, Hemsell DL: The use of ultrasound in multiple gestations. Obstet Gynecol 53:500, 1979
42. Dor J, Shalev S, Mashiach J et al: Elective cervical suture of twin pregnancies diagnosed ultrasonically in the first trimester following induced ovulation. Gynecol Obstet Invest 13:55, 1982
43. Dorros G: The prenatal diagnosis of intrauterine growth retardation in one fetus of a twin gestation. Obstet Gynecol 48:465, 1976
44. Drillien CM: The incidence of mental and physical handicaps in school-age children of very low birth weight. Pediatrics 27:452, 1961
45. Durkin MV, Kaveggia EG, Pendleton E et al:

Analysis of etiological factors in cerebral palsy with severe mental retardation. Eur J Pediatr 81:67, 1976
46. Ellis JW, Keith LG, Keith DM: The etiology of twins. Curr Probl Ob Gyn 6:8, 1983
47. Enbom JA: Twin pregnancy with intrauterine death of one twin. Am J Obstet Gynecol 152:424, 1985
48. Erkkola R, Ala-Mello S, Kero P, Sillanpaa M: Fetal growth and perinatal mortality in twin pregnancy—Effect of sick leave and hospitalization. Int J Gynaecol Obstet 23:115, 1985
49. Erkkola R, Ala-Mello S, Piiroinen O et al: Growth discordancy in twin pregnancies: A risk factor not detected by measurements of biparietal diameter. Obstet Gynecol 66:303, 1985
50. Farmakides G, Schulman H, Saldana LR et al: Surveillance of twin pregnancy with umbilical arterial velocimetry. Am J Obstet Gynecol 153:789, 1985
51. Farooqui MO, Grossman JH, Shannon RA: A review of twin pregnancy and perinatal mortality. Obstet Gynecol Surv 28;144, 1973
52. Feingold M, Cetrulo CL, Newton ER et al: Serial amniocentesis in the treatment of twin to twin transfusion complicated with acute polyhydramnios. Acta Genet Med Gemellol 35:107, 1986
53. Friedman EA, Sachtleben MR: The effect of uterine overdistension on labor. I. Multiple pregnancy. Obstet Gynecol 23:164, 1964
54. Fujikura T, Froehlich LA: Mental and motor development in monozygotic co-twins with dissimilar birth weights. Pediatrics 53:884, 1974
55. Galea P, Scott JM, Goel KM: Feto-fetal transfusion syndrome. Arch Dis Child 57:781, 1982
56. Garrett WJ: Uterine overdistension and the duration of labor. Med J Australia 47:376, 1960
57. Ghosh A, Woo JSK, Rawlinson HA, Ferguson-Smith MA: Prognostic significance of raised serum alpha-fetoprotein levels in twin pregnancies. Br J Obstet Gynaecol 89:817, 1982
58. Giles WB, Trudinger BJ, Cook CM: Fetal umbilical artery flow velocity-time waveforms in twin pregnancies. Br J Obstet Gynaecol 92:490, 1985
59. Grennert L, Persson PH, Gennser G: Intrauterine growth of twins judged by BPD measurements. Acta Obstet Gynecol Scand Suppl 78:28, 1978
60. Hagay ZJ, Mazor M, Leiberman JR: Multiple pregnancy complicated by a single intrauterine fetal death. Obstet Gynecol 66:837, 1985
61. Hanna J, Hill J: Single intrauterine fetal demise in multiple gestation. Obstet Gynecol 63:126, 1984
62. Hawrylyshyn PA, Barkin M, Bernstein A, Papsin FR: Twin pregnancies—A continuing perinatal challenge. Obstet Gynecol 59:463, 1982
63. Hays PM, Smeltzer JS: Multiple gestation. Clin Obstet Gynecol 29:264, 1986
64. Heifetz SA: Single umbilical artery. A statistical analysis of 237 autopsy cases and review of the literature. Perspect Pediatr Pathol 8:345, 1984
65. Heluin G, Papiernik E, Berardi JC, Frydman R: Delivery in twin pregnancy. Acta Genet Med Gemellol 28:361, 1979
66. Hertzberg BS, Kurtz AB, Choi HY et al: Significance of membrane thickness in the sonographic evaluation of twin gestations. AJR 148:151, 1987
67. Holcberg G, Biale Y, Lewenthal H, Insler V: Outcome of pregnancy in 31 triplet gestations. Obstet Gynecol 59:472, 1982
68. Houlton MCC: Divergent biparietal diameter growth rates in twin pregnancies. Obstet Gynecol 49:542, 1977
69. Houlton MCC, Murivate M, Philpott RH: The prediction of fetal growth retardation in twin pregnancy. Br J Obstet Gynaecol 88:264, 1981
70. Itzkow, D: A survey of 59 triplet pregnancies. Br J Obstet Gynaecol 86:23, 1979
71. James WH: A note on the epidemiology of acardiac monsters. Teratology 16:211, 1977
72. Jeffrey RL, Bowes WA, Delaney JJ: Role of bed rest in twin pregnancy. Obstet Gynecol 43:822, 1974
73. Jouppila P, Kauppila A, Koivisto M et al: Twin pregnancy: The role of active management during pregnancy and delivery. Acta Obstet Gynecol Scand 44:13, 1975
74. Kaelber CT, Pugh TF: Influence of intrauterine relations on the intelligence of twins. N Engl J Med 280;1030, 1969
75. Kappel B, Hansen KB, Moller J, Faaborg-Andersen J: Bed rest in twin pregnancy. Acta Genet Med Gemellol 34:67, 1985
76. Katz M, Gill PJ: Initial evaluation of an ambulatory system for home monitoring and transmission of uterine activity data. Obstet Gynecol 66:273, 1985
77. Katz M, Newman RB, Gill PJ: Home monitoring of uterine activity prior to the develop-

ment of preterm and term labor. Clin Res, 33:255, 1985
78. Keith L, Ellis R, Berger GS et al: The Northwestern University multihospital twin study. I. A description of 588 twin pregnancies and associated pregnancy loss, 1971 to 1975. Am J Obstet Gynecol 138:781, 1980
79. Keith LG, Newton WP: Twin gestation. In Sciarra (ed): Gynecology and Obstetrics, vol 2. Philadelphia, Harper & Row.
80. Kelsick F, Minkoff H: Management of the breech second twin. Am J Obstet Gynecol 144:783, 1982
81. Khunda S: Locked twins. Obstet Gynecol 39:453, 1972
82. Kindred JE: Twin pregnancies with one twin blighted. Am J Obstet Gynecol 48:642, 1944
83. Klebe JG, Ingomar CJ: The fetoplacental circulation during parturition illustrated by the inter-fetal transfusion syndrome. Pediatrics 49:112, 1972
84. Knuppel RA, Rattan PK, Scerbo JC, O'Brien WF: Intrauterine fetal death in twins after 32 weeks of gestation. Obstet Gynecol 65:172, 1985
85. Kurtz GR, Davis LL, and Loftus JB: Factors influencing the survival of triplets. Obstet Gynecol 12:504, 1958
86. Landy HJ, Keith L, Keith D: The vanishing twin. Acta Genet Med Gemellol 31:179, 1982
87. Laursen B: Twin pregnancy. The value of prophylactic rest in bed and the risk involved. Acta Obstet Gynecol Scand 52:367, 1973
88. Lenstrup C: Predictive value of antepartum nonstress test in multiple pregnancies. Acta Obstet Gynecol Scand 63:597, 1984
89. Leppert P, Wartel L, Lowman R: Fetus papyraceus causing dystocia: Inability to detect blighted twin antenatally. Obstet Gynecol 54:381, 1979
90. Leroy B, Lefort F, Neveu P et al: Intrauterine growth charts for twin fetuses. Acta Genet Med Gemellol 31:199, 1982
91. Leveno KJ, Quirk JG, Whalley PJ et al: Fetal lung maturation in twin gestation. Am J Obstet Gynecol 148:405, 1984
92. Leveno KJ, Santos-Ramos R, Duenholter JA et al: Sonar cephalometry in twins: A table of biparietal diameters for normal twin fetuses and a comparison with singletons. Am J Obstet Gynecol 135:727, 1979
93. Little J, Bryan E: Congenital anomalies in twins. Semin Perinatol 10:50, 1986
94. Lodeiro JG, Vintzileos AM, Feinstein SJ et al: Fetal biophysical profile in twin gestations. Obstet Gynecol 67:824, 1986
95. Loucopoulos A, Jewelewicz R: Management of multifetal pregnancies. Sixteen years' experience at the Sloane Hospital for Women, Am J Obstet Gynecol 143:902, 1982
96. Lubchenco LC: The High Risk Infant. Philadelphia, WB Saunders, 1976
97. Lubinsky M, Rapoport P: Transient fetal hydrops and "prune belly" in one identical female twin. N Engl J Med 308:256, 1983
98. MacGillivray I, Nylander PPS, Corney G: Human Multiple Reproduction. Philadelphia, WB Saunders, 1975
99. Mannino F, Jones KL, Benirschke K: Congenital skin defects and fetus papyraceus. J Pediatr 91:559, 1977
100. Marivate M, DeVilliers KO, Fairbrother P: Effect of outpatient administration of fensterol on the time of onset of spontaneous labor and fetal growth rate in twin pregnancy. Am J Obstet Gynecol 128:707, 1977
101. McCarthy BJ, Sachs BP, Layde PM et al: The epidemiology of neonatal death in twins. Am J Obstet Gynecol 141:252, 1981
102. McKeown T, Record RG: Observations on fetal growth in multiple pregnancies in man. J Endocrinol 8:386, 1952
103. Melnick M: Brain damage in survivor after in utero death of monozygous co-twin. Lancet 2:1287, 1977
104. Meuller-Heuback E, Mazer J: Sonographically documented disappearance of fetal ascites. Obstet Gynecol 61:253, 1983
105. Mills WG: Letter to the editor. Br J Obstet Gynaecol 87:256, 1980
106. Misenhimer HR, Kaltreider DF: Effects of decreased prenatal activity in patients with twin pregnancy. Obstet Gynecol 51:692, 1978
107. Moore C, McAdams AJ, Sutherland J: Intrauterine disseminated intravascular coagulation: A syndrome of multiple pregnancy with a dead twin fetus. J Pediatr 74:523, 1969
108. Naeye RL: Organ abnormalities in human parabiotic syndrome. Am J Pathol 46:829, 1965
109. Naeye RL, Benirschke K, Hagstrom JWC, Marcus CC: Intrauterine growth of twins as estimated from liveborn birth-weight data. Pediatrics 37:3, 1966
110. Nance WE: Malformations unique to the twinning process. Prog Clin Biol Res 69:123, 1981
111. Neligan G, Robson E, Hey F: Hyaline membrane disease in twins. Pediatrics 43:143, 1969
112. Newman RB, Gill PJ, Katz M: Uterine activity during pregnancy in ambulatory patients: Comparison of singleton and twin gestations. Am J Obstet Gynecol 154:530, 1986

113. Nissen ED: Twins: Collision, impaction, compaction, and interlocking. Obstet Gynecol 11:154, 1958
114. Norman RJ, Joubert SM, Marivate M: Amniotic fluid phospholipids and glucocorticoids in multiple pregnancy. Br J Obstet Gynaecol 90:51, 1983
115. Nylander PPS: Perinatal mortality in twins. Acta Genet Med Gemellol 28:363, 1979
116. O'Brien WF, Knuppel RA, Scerbo JC, Rattan PK: Birth weight in twins: An analysis of discordancy and growth retardation. Am College Obstet Gynecol 67:483, 1986
117. O'Connor MC, Arias E, Royston JP, Dalrymple IJ: The merits of special antenatal care for twin pregnancies. Br J Obstet Gynaecol 88:222, 1981
118. O'Connor MC, Murphy H, Dalrymple IJ: Double blind trial of ritodrine and placebo in twin pregnancy. Br J Obstet Gynaecol 86:706, 1979
119. O'Leary J: Prophylactic tocolysis of twins. Am J Obstet Gynecol 154:904, 1986
120. Persson PH, Grennert L: Diagnosis and treatment of twin pregnancy. Acta Genet Med Gemellol 28:311, 1979
121. Persson PH, Grennert L, Gennsen G, Kullander S: On improved outcome of twin pregnancies. Acta Obstet Gynecol Scand 58:3, 1979
122. Persson PH, Kullander S: Long-term experience of general ultrasound screening in pregnancy. Am J Obstet Gynecol 146:942, 1983
123. Pheiffer EL, Golan A: Triplet pregnancy—A 10 year review of cases at Baragwanath Hospital. S Afr Med J 55:843, 1979
124. Pierce G, Golding RH, Cooperberg PL: The effects of tissue velocity changes on acoustical interfaces. J Ultrasound Med 1:185, 1982
125. Platt LD, Collea JV, Joseph DM: Transitory fetal ascites: An ultrasound diagnosis. Am J Obstet Gynecol 132:906, 1978
126. Prescott P: Sensitivity of a double blind trial of ritodrine and placebo in twin pregnancy. Br J Obstet Gynaecol 87:393, 1980
127. Prevention of respiratory distress: Effect of antenatal dexamethasone administration. US Dept of Health and Human Services, NIH Publ 85-2695, August 1985
128. Pritchard JA, Mason R, Corley M, Pritchard S: Genesis of severe placental abruption. Am J Obstet Gynecol 108:22, 1970
129. Puissant F, Leroy F: A reappraisal of perinatal mortality factors in twins. Acta Genet Med Gemellol 31:213, 1982
130. Queenan JT, Gadow EC: Polyhydramnios chronic versus acute. Am J Obstet Gynecol 108:349, 1970
131. Rausen AR, Seki M, Strauss L: Twin transfusion syndrome. A review of 19 cases studied at one institution. J Pediatr 66:613, 1965
132. Rayburn WF, Lavin JP, Miodovnik M, Varner MW: Multiple gestation: Time interval between delivery of the first and second twins. Obstet Gynecol 63:502, 1984
133. Robertson EG, Neer KJ: Placental injection studies in twin gestation. Am J Obstet Gynecol 147:170, 1983
134. Robinson DE, Wilson LS, Kossoff G: Shadowing and enhancement in ultrasonic echograms by reflection and refraction. JCU 9:181, 1981
135. Rokos J, Valusorn O, Nachman R, Avery ME: Hyaline membrane disease in twins. Pediatrics 42:204, 1968
136. Ron-El R, Caspi E, Schreyer P et al.: Triplet and quadruplet pregnancies and management. Obstet Gynecol 57:458, 1981
137. Rychter Z: Experimental morphology of the aortic arches and the heart loop in chick embryos. Adv Teratol 2:333, 1962
138. Sanders MC, Dur JS, Brown IM et al: The effects of hospital admission for bed rest on the duration of twin pregnancy: A randomized trial. Lancet 2:793, 1985
139. Scheer K: Ultrasound in twin gestation. J Clin Ultrasound 2:197, 1974
140. Schneider KTM, Vetter K, Huch R, Huch A: Acute polyhydramnios complicating twin pregnancies. Acta Genet Med Gemellol 34:179, 1985
141. Schneider L, Bessis R, Tabaste JL et al: Echographic survey of twin fetal growth—A plea for specific charts for twins. In: Twin Research Clinical Studies, p 137. New York, Liss 1978
142. Scott JM, Ferguson-Smith MA: Heterokaryotypic monozygotic twins and the acardiac monster. Br J Obstet Gynaecol 80:52, 1973
143. Secher NJ, Kaern J, Hansen PK: Intrauterine growth in twin pregnancies: Prediction of fetal growth retardation. Obstet Gynecol 66:63, 1985
144. Sims CD, Cowan DB, Parkinson CE: The lecithin/sphingomyelin (L/S) ratio in twin pregnancies. Br J Obstet Gynaecol 83:447, 1976
145. Sinha DP, Nandakuman VC, Brough AK, BeeGeejann: Relative cervical incompetence in twin pregnancy. Assessment and efficacy of cervical suture. Acta Genet Med Gemellol 28:327, 1979
146. Skelly H, Marivata M, Norman R et al: Consumptive coagulopathy following fetal death

in a triplet pregnancy. Am J Obstet Gynecol 142:595, 1982
147. Skjaerris J, Aberg A: Prevention of prematurity in twin pregnancy by orally administered terbutaline. Acta Obstet Gynecol Scand Suppl 108:39, 1982
148. Socol ML, Tamura RK, Sabbagha RE et al: Diminished biparietal diameter and abdominal circumference growth in twins. Obstet Gynecol 64:235, 1984
149. Smith DH, Picker RH, Saunders DM: Twin pregnancy suspected before implantation. Obstet Gynecol 56:252, 1980
150. Smith JJ, Benjamin F: Post haemorrhagic anemia and shock in the newborn at birth. Obstet Gynecol 23:511, 1968
151. Spellacy WN, Cruz AC, Buhi WC, Birk SA: Amniotic fluid L/S ratio in twin gestation. Obstet Gynecol 50:68, 1977
152. Strong SJ, Corney G: The placenta in Twin Pregnancy. Oxford, Pergamon Press, 1967
153. Tan KL, Tan R, Tan SH, Tan AM: The twin transfusion syndrome. Clin Pediatr 18:111, 1979
154. Van Allen MI, Smith DW, Shepard TH: Twin reversed arterial perfusion (TRAP) sequence: A study of 14 twin pregnancies with acardius. Semin Perinatol 7:285, 1983
155. Varma TR: Ultrasound evidence of early pregnancy failure in patients with multiple conceptions. Br J Obstet Gynaecol 86:290, 1979
156. Verduzco R, Rosario R, Rigatto H: Hyaline membrane disease in twins. Am J Obstet Gynecol 125:668, 1976
157. Weekes ARL, Menzies DN, DeBoer CH: The relative efficacy of bed rest, cervical suture, and no treatment in the management of twin pregnancy. Br J Obstet Gynaecol 84:161, 1977
158. Weir PE, Ratten GJ, Beischer NA: Acute polyhydramnios—A complication of monozygous twin pregnancy. Br J Obstet Gynaecol 86:849, 1979
159. Wilson RS: Growth standards for twins from birth to four years. Ann Hum Biol 1:175, 1974
160. Wittmann BK, Baldwin VJ, Nichol B: Antenatal diagnosis of twin transfusion syndrome by ultrasound. Obstet Gynecol 58:123, 1981
161. Wittmann BK, Farquharson DF, Thomas WDL et al: The role of fetocide in the management of severe twin transfusion syndrome. Am J Obstet Gynecol 155:1023, 1986
162. Wood C, Bannerman RHO, Booth RT, Pinkerton JHM: The prediction of premature labor by observation of the cervix and external tocography. Am J Obstet Gynecol 91:396, 1965
163. Yoshioka H, Kadomoto Y, Mino M et al: Multicystic encephalomalacia in liveborn twin with a stillborn macerated co-twin. J Pediatr 95:798, 1979
164. Young BK, Suidan J, Antoine C et al: Differences in twins: The importance of birth order. Am J Obstet Gynecol 151:915, 1985
165. Zakut H, Insler V, Serr DM: Elective cervical suture in preventing premature delivery in multiple pregnancies. Israel J Med Sci 13:5, 1977

SECTION 4: Ethical Problems in Multiple Gestations: Selective Termination

Mark I. Evans, John C. Fletcher, and Charles Rodeck

Public fascination with multiple gestations is an age-old phenomenon. Buried in the fascination about the wonders of multiple births has been an ignorance of the increased reproductive risks inherent in the event. In this chapter we shall address some of the ethical issues that arise in which there is not only a potential conflict between the interests of mother and child but also among fetal siblings.

The ethical issues surrounding multiple gestations are posed in two situations: twin gestations in which one fetus is found to be abnormal, and multiple gestations in which the number of fetuses in and of itself threatens the ability of the mother to carry them far enough in pregnancy to survive.

ONE ABNORMAL TWIN

The Controversy

Prior to the 1980s, the diagnosis of multiple gestations was limited to auscultation of fetal heart beats, crude outlines on x-ray films, or limited ultrasound images. With increased diagnostic abilities have come fundamental ethical problems. By far the most common situation involving one abnormal fetus in a multiple gestation is that of one twin who is shown to be either dysmorphic by ultrasound or aneuploid by amniocentesis. Since the earliest report by Aberg[1] in 1978 who detailed cardiac puncture for one fetus of twins with Hurler's disease, the subject has always drawn criticism. In 1981, a published report from New York detailed a mid-trimester "selective feticide" of a Down's syndrome fetus when the other was normal.[10] The authors implied they were forced to attempt the procedure by the mother who threatened to abort both fetuses. Despite the disclaimers, they were criticized for intervening at risk to the normal twin.

Sentiment against risking a normal twin has continued in many forums such as the International Fetal Medicine & Surgery Society (see Chapter 15, Section 5). A set of guidelines for fetal therapy was devised in 1982, which included avoidance of experimental procedures when there was a normal twin.[8] We agree with others now in that society that such guidelines should be modified to permit experimental procedures on an abnormal twin prior to the viability of the normal twin. This view is more consistent with a mother's right to abortion prior to fetal viability than is the restraint of her rights because of the presence of the normal twin.

Over the past several years, despite the certainty of many diagnoses of one abnormal twin, very few publications have discussed outcomes involved with selective intervention on one fetus. Several such cases have not been published by physicians engaged in such procedures primarily because of the "heat" that would be generated. Furthermore, what to call the procedure evokes great emotional fervor. Possibilities have included selective abortion, selective feticide, selective reduction, selective birth, and selective termination. We favor selective termination because the term seems an appropriate compromise between *reduction*, which tends to mask the fate of the abnormal fetus or embryo, and *abortion* or *feticide* which masks the intended aim to preserve the potential life of the remaining one or more fetuses.

The incidence of abnormalities is higher in twin pregnancies than in singleton pregnancies. For dizygotic twins the risks are essentially the product of two singleton infants' risks. For example, the risk of a chromosome abnormality at age 35 is about 1 in 200 and the chance that one of a set of twins would be aneuploid is about 1 in 100. Overall, serious disorders are stated at 2% to 3% for singletons and 4% to 6% for twins. For monozygotic pairs, aneuploidy risk is for both or none and is identical to the singleton rate. Disorders of laterality and dysmorphology are higher than for singletons or dyzygotic twins. Thus, the chance of facing one abnormal twin is not rare.

With increasing diagnostic capabilities, diagnoses of one abnormal twin have moved from the nursery to the second or even first trimester and within the legal rights of the mother to consider termination of pregnancy. Couples facing the diagnosis of one abnormal twin must confront an excruciating dilemma either to continue the pregnancy with the birth of an abnormal child or abort both fetuses, including that which is normal. Such a choice transcends the traditional arguments about social abortion (which will not be reviewed here) and even those about abortion of a singleton abnormal fetus in a planned and wanted pregnancy.

Ethical Justification for Selective Termination

In assessing the ethical perspectives about twin selective termination, various arguments are possible. First, there are the traditional objections to aborting an abnormal pregnancy. However, the issues involved in selective termination are far more complex because of the presence of the normal twin. In our thinking, the overriding principle is one of trying to preserve the most good and doing the least harm. As with all new techniques, there is often much uncertainty as to the true risks and benefits of such procedures. As with any termination procedure, there are risks of infection, ruptured membranes, and premature delivery, all of which can cause death to the normal twin and pose maternal risks. Furthermore, retention of a dead fetus carries known risks of coagulopathies, such as disseminated intravascular coagulation, which could be life-threatening. There are data, however, which have suggested that earlier undetected twin pregnancy loss is much more common than generally realized, and that such losses can be tolerated.[7,11,23]

Nevertheless, it is understandable that for some couples the risks from selective termination would seem preferable to the alternatives. There are no good data on choices made by couples to either continue or terminate. We are aware of both options being chosen. Anecdotally, most couples who have chosen selective termination tended to be in the group that would have terminated both fetuses if that were their only option.

The approach to ethical reasoning about selective termination must be different from that for abortion per se and, therefore, requires a basic justification. By *basic* we mean our reasoning ought not to be derived from precedents that appear to be morally similar, but which on examination are not (i.e., arguments for social abortion). It is simplistic to argue that since society permits abortion of normal fetuses on request in the first trimester, selective termination must fall well within the sphere of permissible actions created by abortion practices. Such reasoning derives an ethical imperative, an *ought*, from an existing cultural situation that is still ethically controversial.

Any intentional action that could or does result in fetal harm or death requires a basic ethical justification. Otherwise, physicians would be liable to moral blame for destroying innocent human life without regard for the many ethical traditions which transmit respect for human life. For example, a basic ethical justification for fetal research, independent of arguments for and against abortion, was developed in the mid-1970s,[15] and even that process has evolved considerably (see Chapter 17).

Both abortion and selective termination cause fetuses to die and are similar in this consequence. But selective termination may enable the surviving fetus to have a better chance for life. Moreover, morally they differ because the intent or aim is different. In abortion, the woman wants to end the whole pregnancy and enlists a physician's help. In selective termination cases, the woman wants to continue a pregnancy.

In practice, selective mid-trimester termination in twins has been limited to centers that provide the technical expertise to carry out twin diagnoses, use methods of termination that carry minimal risk to the healthy twin, and manage the continuing pregnancy to avoid the potential dangers of a dead twin in the uterus, such as clotting, hemorrhagic diathesis, and shock.[19] Historically, concerns for these possible complications have served to limit intervention. To date, no case involving such adverse consequences has been reported, but no significant follow-up of these cases has been done. A serious deficit in knowledge about the consequences of this type of prenatal diagnosis and intervention has resulted because of fear of publishing such data.[6] Nevertheless, in our view, the option of selective termination meets the criteria of most good–least harm because it preserves the chance for couples to have a healthy child unburdened by abnormalities—the original intent of the pregnancy. An appropriate analogy would be an abortion of an abnormal child followed by a subsequent normal pregnancy. The intent is the same even if the methods are different and the risk to the normal twin is higher. To be certain the risks and benefits should be proportionate. However, early experiences suggest that selective termination can be a relatively safe procedure.

Despite our approval of the ethical probity of such procedures, we still hold concerns about the timing of the procedure and indications for it. We reaffirm our beliefs that such procedures can only be considered prior to viability and should not be performed for objectionable reasons such as sex selection or simply a desire for only one child.

The literature on the ethics of sex selection is expanding. We believe that "social" sex selection is inconsistent with an open and equal society and inherently creates inequalities between the sexes. Despite disclaimers to the contrary, the vast majority of sex selection requests are for boys. We do believe that sex selection can be appropriate but only for sex-linked diseases whose diagnoses are not possible or completely reliable. Until recently, Duchenne muscular dystrophy or hemophilia would have fit that category. Interestingly enough, in such cases the selection is against males.

The advent of increasingly sophisticated ultrasound has allowed diagnosis of abnormalities much earlier. In the next several years diagnosis of dysmorphic anomalies may be common in the first trimester. We believe that pressures against abortion may curtail the rights to abort late in the mid-trimester, which will in turn emphasize the need for earlier diagnosis and earlier intervention, making selective termination both technically easier and safer and more ethically accepted.

MULTIPLE PREGNANCIES

With a twin pregnancy, the obstetric outcome in uncomplicated cases is reasonably good. The only justifiable reason to consider selective termination in twins would be on the basis of an abnormality. In gestations of larger size, even perfectly normal fetuses may be at considerable risk from prematurity.

Rationale for Selective Termination

We previously have reported selective termination ending in twins in octuplet and quadruplet pregnancies in the first trimester for couples treated with drugs following long-term infertility.[5] When we first confronted these issues in 1986, such cases were not reported in the literature, and ethical precedents for such procedures were lacking. We debated as to the best course of action under such circumstances, recognizing that the use of fertility drugs such as human menopausal gonadotropin (HMG, Pergonal) in the treatment of infertility carried the risk of inducing multiple gestations.[20,21] Despite reduced occurrences and better understanding of the mechanisms of fertility drugs, the possibility for inducing multiple gestations still exists. With Pergonal, twin pregnancies occur in about 10% of patients. Higher numbers of conceptuses are seen in about 1% of patients.

The obstetric outcome of triplets (or more) is known to be significantly poorer than with singleton or even twin pregnancies.[13] The ability to carry four or more fetuses to viability is by no means ensured. A successful gestation of octuplets has never been substantiated. Thus, a couple faced with the prospect of an octuplet pregnancy has a very serious dilemma. In all likelihood, with no intervention, they would lose all the fetuses. In 1985, a case of septuplet births in California was highlighted in the national media.[16] In follow-up three years after birth, only three infants had survived. All have mental and physical handicaps, and malpractice litigation has been instituted.

In the case of multifetal pregnancies, one management alternative would be to abort the entire pregnancy and have the couple try to conceive again. Since conception cannot be guaranteed, another more attractive possibility would be to reduce the number of fetuses with the hope of increasing the probability of a good outcome for at least some of them. Selective termination in multiple pregnancy, usually of one abnormal twin, in the mid-trimester had been reported in the literature on a few occasions,[10,19] but literature on the ethics of selective termination was essentially nonexistent when we first had to make hard choices.

In our view, selective reduction in these patients was the only alternative available to achieve a reasonable chance of successful pregnancy outcome. In all instances, the couples understood the potential risks of the procedure and its experimental nature. Informed consent was obtained after thorough counseling. We stressed that any attempt to reduce the number of fetuses would be experimental and could result in miscarriage of the pregnancy. Infection, bleeding, and other unknown risks were possible. If successful, the attempt could theoretically result in damage to the remaining fetuses. All felt strongly, however, that because of their infertility history their current pregnancy might be their only or last opportunity to have children. Kanhai and associates, in their report of quintuplet selective termination, addressed some of the same concerns.[9]

The safety of the procedure to the remaining fetuses, of course, could not be accurately gauged. We felt that it was important not to significantly alter the total intrauterine volume by rapid removal of large amounts of amniotic fluid. Our first two cases, octuplets to twins and quadruplets to twins, were accomplished by transabdominal needle disruption of the embryos. Both were followed closely and went on to deliver normal fetuses at 35 to 37 weeks, although discordancy of birth weight between twins was observed in our first two cases. In a third case of quadruplet fetuses, the procedure was performed without difficulty by intrathoracic injection of potassium chloride. The change in protocol significantly reduced procedure time and, therefore, should make the procedure potentially less risky. Normal-appearing ultrasound pictures were observed before and after the procedure at 10 weeks. However, at 18 weeks one of the two remaining fetuses had no bladder and had probable renal agenesis. The mother suffered a spontaneous loss of that fetus at 19 weeks. In the process, the membranes of the other twin were ruptured, causing it to be delivered stillborn at 20 weeks. We do not believe the fetal anomalies were the result of the procedure, but it is impossible to be certain.

As of 1989 about 200 cases have been reported. The rate of subsequent live twin births appears to be about 75% and has improved with the use of transabdominal ultrasound guided potassium chloride intrathoracic injections.

Ethical Justification for Selective Termination

Clinical experiences with good outcomes has demonstrated the technical feasibility and possible safety of first trimester selective terminations even in grand multiple pregnancies. We recognized from the outset, however, that selective termination in multiple pregnancies would be an inherently controversial topic and would require a thorough prior ethical reflection.

First, we recognized as with selective termination for one abnormal twin that a basic ethical justification was required. Second, we recognized that our reasoning should not be limited to cases of multiple pregnancies following iatrogenic effects of infertility treatment. We must be and are willing to reason similarly in cases in which the pregnant woman's health and the survival of any infants are endangered by a grand multiple pregnancy, regardless of cause.

Selective termination in a grand multiple pregnancy raises ethical issues different from those for one abnormal twin. In grand multiple pregnancy, childbearing has been endangered by multiple fetuses, all of which may be normal. The patient may or may not regard this pregnancy as her final chance to have a child. She enlists a physician's help to facilitate the continuation of the pregnancy.

As noted earlier in this chapter, termination of one genetically abnormal twin is, in some respects, similar to cases of termination in grand multiple pregnancies. In both instances the woman desires to complete the pregnancy. The harms and dangers of severe genetic disease and prematurity of multiple newborns can be similar in expected morbidity and mortality, the major difference being between a diagnosis of a congenital anomaly and a history of infertility. The chance of a subsequent normal pregnancy following abortion for genetic disorders is more likely than in cases that involve infertility.

Despite generally good anecdotal outcomes in twin cases, we were reluctant to rely on mid-trimester precedents because, at the time, the outcomes of mid-trimester terminations of an affected twin and selective birth of a healthy surviving twin had not been adequately studied. Recent work by Rodeck has documented acceptable risks for such patients.[18] Without reliable knowledge of long-term beneficial consequences, the value of the precedent was dubious, even though ethical reasoning about the two problems might be similar.

In our particular cases, we began from the premise that a pregnancy that has been finally achieved, particularly in the face of previous infertility, is a basic human good worth preserving. To what lengths is it ethically acceptable to go to achieve and preserve a pregnancy? Some, such as Tiefel[22] or the Vatican 1987 document, challenge the ethical acceptability of methods of fertility treatment (including in vitro fertilization [IVF]). Tiefel views the anxiety that brought these women into fertility treatment as caused by "dehumanizing socialization" in which "having a child is the ultimate need and in which infertility is seen as personal failure and a sign of worthlessness."[22] Had they only come to terms with these (supposed) feelings, they would never have found themselves in this situation. We doubt whether "dehumanizing socialization" is the basic cause of the despair of infertile couples. Furthermore, we find it impossible to accept the Vatican's position that attempts to treat infertility involving anything beyond marital coitus are immoral.

There are straightforward biologic causes of infertility that can be remedied by a number of methods, including IVF. We do not accept the posture of passive resignation in the face of biologic problems of infertility. If something can be done about infertility, we believe there is a strong moral obligation to do it, because infertility is a significant form of human suffering. However, we agree with the Vatican report that one is not ethically permitted to do simply anything to achieve or preserve pregnancy.

How should the human need for a child be evaluated on ethical grounds? Is there a moral duty to have a child of one's own? Is there a right to have a child, as some parents have argued? Tiefel makes a case, with which we agree, that there is no moral or legal right to have children in a positive or enabling sense. Society is not obligated to meet an entitlement of a child, in the same sense that rights to life, freedom of speech, and protection from enemies are entitlements. On the other hand, the Vatican not withstanding, there is a negative duty not to be restrained or prevented from childbearing. In our society we believe that right is guarded by the legal right to privacy.[22] Once having obtained help in becoming pregnant, women in this situation deserve help to achieve their aim, as long as the means used are proportionate to the ends sought.

A proportionate relationship between means and ends entails two criteria. First, there must be no other way to achieve the end, in this instance, preservation of a viable and desired pregnancy. Secondly, in choosing among the means available, the chosen one must be the one that results in least harm and results in the most good for all involved.[14]

In our cases of grand multiple pregnancies, there were only three real alternatives. We recognized that any of the three could lead to harm. First, the pregnancy could be electively aborted, causing death to all fetuses and possibly not succeeded by any future pregnancy. A second possibility was to do nothing and risk the birth of multiple premature infants, many of whom might die or be significantly impaired.[12] In such a choice, there was also a very high likelihood of a spontaneous loss of the entire pregnancy. The third alternative was selective termination. Negative outcomes included the deaths of multiple fetuses and potential harm to the remaining twins. However, in these circumstances, we concluded and our patients agreed that selective termination held out more potential benefits than the other two alternatives.

SELECTIVE TERMINATION & ABORTION RIGHTS

Views on the morality of abortion are obviously relevant to choices in multiple pregnancy because both raise the question of whether deliberate killing of a fetus is justified. We argue in the following discussion that abortion *practices* are not sufficient to justify selective termination in multiple pregnancies. However, the structure of an ethical argument concluding that some abortions are morally justified is highly similar to the argument for selective termination in multiple pregnancies.

A typology of responses to selective termination can be constructed by inference from the literature on the morality of abortion. The actual views of particular authors and the variation within religious and philosophical traditions are far richer than the typology presented here.

Position 1: Any human act deliberately taken to destroy human embryonic or fetal life ought to be morally condemned.[12] This position rules out selective termination in any case.

Position 2: An exception to Position 1 is permitted for abortion only to save the life of a pregnant woman,[13] as in cases of uterine cancer or ectopic pregnancy. Whether this position would favor or reject selective termination in multiple pregnancies turns mainly on the empirical questions of the degree of threat to the life of the mother of continuation of pregnancy with premature delivery.

Position 3: Although abortion is a serious moral problem, some abortions are permissible for ethically valid reasons.[14] It follows that some selective terminations in multiple pregnancies are permitted, especially to avoid predictable harms to the pregnant woman, to remaining fetuses, or to survivors. Since this position attempts to draw lines between morally valid and invalid reasons for abortion, it follows that a compatible position on selective termination would search for some moral lines between permissible and impermissible cases.

Position 4: A position for abortion on request for any pregnancy at any stage[15] favors a stance on selective termination that permits termination of any number of fetuses, including twins, to any remainder. The main concern would be the health and well-being of the pregnant woman.

Positions on the morality of abortion mainly rest on three sorts of premises: 1) the moral status of the human embryo and fetus; 2) the relative strengths of countervailing moral claims made in the interests of the pregnant woman, the family, or society; and 3) how much moral weight should be given to whether the pregnancy is wanted or unwanted by the woman. All positions on abortion tend to accept the premise that each pregnancy should be wanted and planned with medical advice, if available.

Position 1 accords moral status of "personhood" to embryos from fertilization and requires that society protect every fetus equally in every pregnancy. This position allows for no countervailing moral claims and accords little moral significance to the unwantedness of a pregnancy.

Position 2 gives the same high moral status to the fetus throughout pregnancy and allows only one higher moral claim to override when continuation of pregnancy actually threatens the woman's life. An important variation of this position extends slightly the range of countervailing moral claims and bends to permit abortions in "tragic" circumstances. These are presumably pregnancies resulting from rape, incest, and for diagnosis of genetic disorders that are totally incompatible with physical or mental life.[16]

Position 3 involves a "graded"[17] approach to the moral status of the fetus that resists indifference at any stage but gradually raises society's protection of the nascent human being with stages of development.[18,19] This view is more likely to recognize countervailing moral claims, especially in the first trimester of pregnancy. It gives an important, but not an absolutely overriding, weight to the wantedness of pregnancy. For example, some unplanned pregnancies that occur after failure of contraception would not result in substantial harm to the woman, family, or society. Abortion under such circumstances, in this view, is morally objectionable because the harm done by abortion is worse than the supposed but empty harm that would be prevented by the abortion. This view is probably dominant in the sense of prevailing in practice and public policy in this society. "Dominance" is used here as a descriptive term and not as a moral judgment.

Position 4 is skeptical of claims for significant moral status or the interests of the fetus until birth, and even them claims to personhood and equal protection might be overridable in certain cases.[20] "Wantedness" of the pregnancy is treated as a matter of moral supremacy in any context.

Do abortion practices justify selective termination in multiple pregnancy? Some might argue, "if society permits abortion of a normal, unwanted fetus, what is so wrong about terminating eight, four or three to two, or two to one in a wanted pregnancy?" It is true that if society proscribed abortions, selective terminations would also be illegal. However, what is legally permitted is not always ethically sound. Using abortion practices as a sole source of justification for selective termination is inadequate, given the premises of the third position above, because some abortions are done for reasons that cannot be justified by ethical principles and that violate respect for fetal life (*e.g.*, abortions for gender choice).[21]

To argue from the premise of what society permits in abortion would also encourage selective termination in cases of normal twins, a direction which would result in the loss of many normal fetuses. To reason from abortion practices and make ethical conclusions is dangerous because many other wrongs could be justified with this approach, such as exploitative experimentation with the embryo and fetus, especially with fetuses to be aborted.

Also, arguments based on abortion practices *per se* could be extrapolated to justify infanticide or euthanasia. For example, if a mother in Africa has eight children and enough food for two, and no help is available or on the way, is she justified in killing six of her children to save two? Two reasons are against it: each child has an equal right to protection, and food, even though scarce, will maintain life. If killing starving children is wrong, and if the moral status of the first trimester fetus is the same as that of such children, then selective termination is *prima facie* wrong. However, if the moral status of starving children were held to be no higher than that of the first trimester fetus, and if contemporary abortion practices were a source of moral guidance, then mercy killing might be more justifiable. If the moral status of the first trimester fetus is such that it is justifiable under some conditions to do an abortion (*e.g.*, maternal health, rape, incest, genetic indications, or social and economic reasons), then moral lines can be more clearly drawn between acceptable and unacceptable cases of abortion, selective termination, and euthanasia. Selective termination can be justified, under some circumstances, whereas killing children in extreme danger from starvation cannot.

An action by a physician that may or will result in fetal harm or death requires a justification in the light of basic ethical principles. Otherwise, physicians are open to moral blame for indifference to many ethical traditions transmitting respect for human life. Along these lines, a basic ethical justification for fetal research, independent of arguments for and against abortion, was developed in the mid 1970s.[22] Also, society's members, including physicians, should help to reduce and prevent the underlying causes of unjustified abortions or casual taking of fetal life.

ETHICAL PRINCIPLES AND MULTIPLE PREGNANCIES

Ethics involves the study and recommendation of bodies of guidance—rules, norms, and principles—that help to resolve difficult problems of moral choice, such as were faced in these cases of selective termination.

In these cases, a conflict exists between two duties. If the pregnancy is wanted, there is a duty to benefit the pregnant woman by preserving her pregnancy, unless unacceptable physical or mental harm to her would ensue. However, there is a second moral duty not to destroy human life, including fetal and embryonic life, without ethically justifiable reasons. Are there ethically justifiable reasons for selective termination?

What are the basic criteria of ethical reasoning? Having the facts, decision makers must then make choices about the best approach to the problem. The facts are not the source of ethics. Human beings choose among various forms of practical guidance to resolve ethical problems. Many physicians claim to approach ethics on a case-by-case basis, as if ethical guidance must be created for each problem. This claim likely rests on unexamined ideas and professional ideology. Systematic studies of what physicians actually do in ethical problems in clinical research and surgery[6] find that they rely on constant sets of ethical beliefs and practices, rather than variable case-by-case choices.

In our view, the selection of ethical guidance involves two interdependent claims. First, ethical guidance ought be judged by the consequences of following it. Second, the consequences should be examined in terms of ethical principles widely respected across cultural, philosophical, and religious lines. A set of principles with wide acceptance in biomedical ethics is outlined below.

Ethical Principles for the Practice of Medicine and Clinical Research

1. *Respect for persons:* The duty to respect the self-determination and choices of autonomous persons, as well as to protect persons with diminished autonomy (e.g., young children, mentally retarded persons, and those with other mental impairments).
2. *Beneficence:* The obligation to secure the well-being of persons by acting positively on their behalf, and moreover, to maximize the benefits that can be attained.
3. *Non-maleficence:* The obligation to minimize harm to persons and, whenever possible, to remove the causes of harm altogether.
4. *Proportionality:* The duty, when taking actions involving risks of harm, to balance risks and benefits so that actions have the greatest chance to result in the least harm and the most benefit to persons directly involved.
5. *Justice:* The obligation to distribute benefits and burdens fairly, to treat equals equally, and to give reasons for differential treatment based on widely accepted criteria for just ways to distribute benefits and burdens.

The consequences of the four positions of ethical guidance outlined previously for cases of multiple pregnancies can be briefly examined in terms of these five principles:

Position 1: Proceeding to delivery in each case of multiple pregnancy because abortion and selective termination are ruled out 1) violates self-determination; 2) rarely results in the benefits of completely healthy children; 3) increases long-term harm and suffering to more persons; 4) effects a disproportionate relationship between the risks of premature delivery and the possible benefits of survival, because more persons will be harmed than benefitted; and 5) is unfair to parents by burdening them with multiple children, some of whom may be severely impaired or suffer a lengthy, costly process of dying in neonatal intensive care.

Position 2: Aborting each multiple pregnancy in hope of starting a new pregnancy: 1) restricts choice of selective termination, if the procedure is available; 2) brings little benefit to infertile couples who may have great difficulty in a new pregnancy; 3) avoids the long-term harms and complications of premature delivery; 4) avoids many risks and harms but with few benefits; and 5) may be unfair to older couples with a long-term history of infertility.

Position 3: Selective termination in any multiple pregnancy, including twins, on request: 1) maximizes self determination; 2) if effective, benefits parents with at least one surviving child; 3) prevents abortion, reduces harms and complications of premature delivery, reduces or prevents stay in neonatal intensive care, increases incidence of selective termination to a larger number of cases (twins), increases incidence of fetal loss, and when ineffective will increase chances of spontaneous abortion, resulting in no child at all; 4) in light of fewer risks of twin pregnancies compared with multiples of three or more, it disproportionately results in more deaths of normal fetuses who would be less apt to suffer serious harm at delivery; and 5) distributes the benefits of selective termination fairly to all parents in all multiple pregnancies.

Position 4: Selective termination in pregnancies of three or more, but to no fewer than twins: 1) restricts self determination only of parents of normal twins; 2) if effective, benefits parents with two surviving children; 3) prevents abortion, provides protection against total loss of pregnancy in case of one fetal demise, reduces harms and complications of premature delivery; reduces length of stay in neonatal intensive care; prevents extension of selective termination to twins; when ineffective, runs risk of spontaneous abortion; 4) proportionately avoids the worst harms of the most dangerous multiple pregnancies with the most benefit to parents and survivors; and 5) distributes benefits and burdens of selective termination fairly to all parents in the most dangerous multiple pregnancies.

SUMMARY

Selective first trimester termination satisfies the criteria of enabling the pregnancies to continue with the least harm and most benefits to all involved. The surviving infants can be saved from certain death (abortion) or higher risks of severe harm and death and of (premature delivery) an extended stay in neonatal intensive care. In the hands of trained operators, selective termination is, in our opinion, the best means to protect the mother's health and well-being, given it is available and approved by the parents. Selective termination avoids the trauma of abortion of a wanted pregnancy, enables the parents to achieve the goal of having their own child, and avoids the dangers of delivery of multiple premature infants.

There is no doubt that any procedure that involves the death of a fetus will be hotly argued despite the potential for greater good.[17] We acknowledge that it will be impossible to convince those who cannot morally accept the taking of any life regardless of the circumstances. We hope, however, that we have shown a place for selective termination in a very limited number of circumstances, and the ethical probability of selective termination as an option in such cases.

REFERENCES

1. Aberg A, Mitelman F, Cantz M: Cardiac puncture of a fetus with Hurler's disease avoiding abortions of unaffected co-twin. Lancet II:990, 1978
2. Antsaklis A, Politis J, Karagiannopoulos C et al: Selective survival of only the healthy fetus following prenatal diagnosis of thalassemia major in binovular twin gestation. Prenat Diag 289:196, 1984
3. Berkowitz RL, Lynch L, Chitkara U, et al: Selective reduction of multifetal pregnancies in the first trimester. New Engl J Med 318:1043, 1988
4. Dumez Y, Oury JF: Method for first trimester selective abortion in multiple pregnancy. Contrib Gynecol Obstet 15:50, 1986
5. Evans MI, Fletcher JC, Zador IE et al: First trimester selective termination in octuplet and quadruplet pregnancy. Obstet Gynecol 71:289, 1988
6. Fletcher JC: Moral problems and ethical guidance in prenatal diagnosis. In Mulunsky A

(ed): Genetic Disorders and the Fetus, 2nd ed pp 819–859. New York, Plenum, 1986
7. Gindoft PR, Yeh MN, Jewelewicz R: The vanishing sac syndrome. J Reprod Med 31:322, 1986
8. Harrison MR, Filly RA, Golbus MS et al: Fetal treatment. N Engl J Med 307:1651, 1982
9. Kanhai HH, Van Rijssel EJC, Meerman RJ, Gravenhorst JB: Selective termination in quintuplet pregnancy during first trimester. Lancet ii:1147, 1986
10. Kerenyi TD, Chitkara U: Selective birth in twin pregnancy with discordancy for Down's Syndrome. N Engl J Med 304:1525, 1981
11. Landy H, Werner S, Conson SL et al: The vanishing twin: Ultrasonic assessment of fetal disappearance in the first trimester. Am J Obstet Gynecol 155:14, 1986
12. Levene MI: Grand multiple pregnancies and demand for neonatal intensive care. Lancet ii:347, 1986
13. MacLennan AH: Multiple gestations. In Creasy RK, Resnick R (eds): Maternal Fetal Medicine: Principles and Practice, pp 527–538. Philadelphia, WB Saunders, 1984
14. McCormick RA: How Brave a New World? Washington DC, Georgetown University Press, 1981
15. National Commission for the Protection of Human Subjects of Biomedical and Behavioral Research. Report and Recommendations. Research on the Fetus. Washington DC, US Government Printing Office, DHEW Pub No (05) 76-127, 1975
16. People Magazine, May 26, 1986
17. Robertson JA: The right to procreate and in utero fetal therapy. J Leg Med, 333, 1982
18. Rodeck C: The twin fetus. Br J Obstet Gynaecol (In press)
19. Rodeck CH, Mibashan RS, Abramowicz T, Campbell S: Selective feticide of the affected twin by fetoscopic air embolism. Prenat Diag 2:189, 1982
20. Schinker JC, Yarkoni S, Granat M: Multiple pregnancies following induction of ovulation. Fertil Steril 35:205, 1981
21. Seibel MM, McArdle CR, Thompson IE et al: The role of ultrasound in ovulation induction: A critical appraisal. Fertil Steril 36:573, 1981
22. Tiefel HO: Human in vitro fertilization: A conservative view. JAMA 247:3235, 1982
23. Varma TR: Ultrasound evidence of early pregnancy failure in patients with multiple conceptions. Br J Obstet Gynaecol 86:290, 1979

SECTION 5: Breech Presentation

Martin L. Gimovsky and Roy H. Petrie

Obstetricians have long recognized the excessive perinatal morbidity and mortality associated with breech presentation. Although only 3% to 4% of all labors are complicated by breech presentation, multiple factors result in a three- to fourfold increase in poor outcome compared to vertex presentation in labor.[5,12,34] The three major factors include congenital malformations, prematurity, and birth trauma.[4] Congenital anomalies occur with breech at a rate three to four times higher than with cephalic presentation.[41] Prematurity complicates up to one in four breech deliveries. Birth trauma with severe sequelae,[11] a common cause of perinatal morbidity and mortality in the past, is an isolated event today; however, it is still more common with breech presentations than with cephalic presentations.[19] Adverse obstetric factors (placenta previa, abruptio placentae, intrauterine growth retardation, abnormalities of amniotic fluid volume, and multiple gestation) also play a role in compromising the overall outcome for the breech fetus.

It is the purpose of this chapter to review the clinical factors associated with breech presentation, present an approach to labor and delivery, and include three basic alternatives in management: cesarean section, a selective trial of labor, and external cephalic version (ECV).

Finally we will review selective protocols that attempt to minimize the need for cesarean section while maintaining a margin of safety for those breech fetuses in whom vaginal delivery may be attempted.[8,23,24,38,44,66] We feel that selected breech-presenting fetuses may safely be allowed a trial of labor under certain circumstances and that the resulting decrease in the use of cesarean section will maximize the benefits and minimize the risks to both mother and infant.[8,24]

HISTORICAL BACKGROUND

Today, the majority of fetuses presenting breech will be delivered by cesarean section,[43] but such was not always the case. In an era before blood banking, antibiotics, and safe anesthestic techniques, routine vaginal delivery was eminently reasonable. Maternal safety was the overwhelming concern of early practitioners. In a sense, since maternal morbidity and mortality associated with cesarean section presented a greater (societal) threat than the adverse neonatal outcome inherent in vaginal delivery, cesarean section was reserved for those cases in which either the life of the mother or her child was clearly in jeopardy.

The liberalization of indications for cesarean section has logically followed the development of increasingly safe operative procedures. As cesarean section become safer, its application in breech delivery increased dramatically. In 1959, Wright[65] went so far as to state that "any patient of more than 35 weeks gestation who enters labor with a living baby in breech presentation should be delivered by cesarean section," provided there was no maternal disease that contraindicated abdominal delivery. Wright based his conclusion on an earlier study by Hall and Kohl.[29] These authors had concluded that cesarean delivery produced the lowest perinatal mortality, but that *this did not imply it should be used in all breech deliveries.* Perhaps their most important contribution was the statement, "In discussing perinatal mortality, breech presentation . . . is not the same as breech delivery."

It should be stressed that such historic data did not usually separate perinatal morbidity and mortality on the basis of etiology or current obstetric and pediatric practice. Thus, without neonatal intensive care facilities, heroic interventions such as cesarean section delivery to save the premature infant were deemed unreasonable. In the past decade, the practice of obstetrics has evolved dramatically. The use of continuous electronic fetal monitoring, the ability to safely perform emergency cesarean section delivery within minutes, and the support of neonatal intensive care units have made childbirth much safer. Obviously, these advances have made an impact in the outcome of breech delivery by whatever route. Cesarean section has been extremely useful in decreasing the risks of birth trauma to the breech-presenting fetus.[10] However, morbidity secondary to congenital anomalies (Table 9-10) may be only minimally altered by route of delivery.[19,41]

Review of data from several retrospective series during the forties and fifties, excluding deaths secondary to prematurity and congenital anomalies, reveals that for infants above 2500 g a direct relationship could be found between the cesarean section rate and perinatal mortality (Figure 9-4).[22] A current rate of 80% to 90% suggests that many of the cesarean sections performed (perhaps a majority) may not be absolutely necessary. This observation has led to the ongoing search

Table 9-10. **Congenital Abnormalities Observed More Frequently in Breech Presentations than in Vertex Presentations**

Central nervous system
  Hydrocephalus
  Anencephaly
  Meningymyelocele
  Familial dysautonomia
Urinary system
  Potter's syndrome
Cardiovascular system
Respiratory and gastrointestinal systems
  Inguinal hernia
Skeletal system
  Myotonic dystrophy
  Dislocation of hips
Multiple abnormalities
  Prader-Willi syndrome
  Trisomy 13 syndrome
  Trisomy 18 syndrome
  Trisomy 21 syndrome
  de Lange's syndrome
  Werdnig-Hoffman syndrome
  Zollinger syndrome
  Smith-Lemli-Opitz syndrome
  Fetal alcohol syndrome

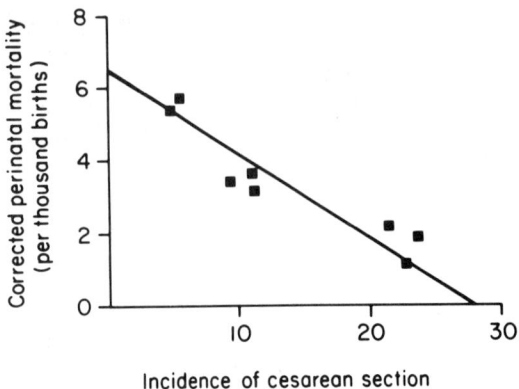

FIGURE 9-4. A direct correlation can be seen between cesarean delivery rates and decreased perinatal mortality in these series of term breech infants from the 1940s and 1950s.

for selective protocols to choose the route of delivery best suited to each individual.[3,8,23,44,62,24]

In the United States in 1984, it was estimated that approximately 9 of 10 breech-presenting infants were delivered by cesarean section. Such a policy was undertaken with an enormous cost emotionally, psychologically, physically, and financially. It is necessary to ask whether there may be reasonable alternatives. This includes methods that allow a trial of labor[8,24] as well as those that convert the breech to a cephalic presentation prior to labor.[51,54,58]

BREECH LABOR AND DELIVERY

Management of breech presentation presents a challenge to the clinician, and experience in the conduct of breech labor and delivery is crucial to outcome. Skilled operators are necessary in order to maximize the safety of allowing labor and vaginal delivery. Many training programs face the problem of insufficient numbers of patients for residents to develop the necessary manual skills to perform a safe vaginal breech delivery. This is also true for delivery by cesarean section.

The total breech extraction required at cesarean section delivery has an intrinsic risk that at times may equal or exceed that of an assisted vaginal breech delivery. Since the maternal risk is also increased with surgery, a balanced approach should be sought. Many breech-presenting fetuses require delivery by cesarean section, and it is our opinion that safe cesarean section delivery demands a clear mechanical understanding of the techniques used in vaginal breech delivery because the breech-presenting fetus may require complex manipulation to effect delivery, regardless of route.

Definitions

Breech Presentation

Breech presentation refers to the longitudinal lie of the fetus with the breech or buttocks as the presenting part. The position of a breech presentation refers to the orientation of the sacrum with respect to the maternal pelvic outlet. Station-in-breech presentation refers to the lowermost portion of the buttocks in relationship to the level of the maternal ischial spine. It is often stated that at a given point in labor the breech is one station higher than its vertex counterpart.

There are several varieties of specific breech presentation (Table 9-11), distinguished by the attitude of the hip and knee joints. In the *frank* breech presentation, there is flexion at both hip joints and extension at both knee joints. This is the most common type of breech presentation at term, comprising over 50% of fetuses during breech labor. Although a pelvic examination is helpful in deciding which type of breech presentation is present, confusion may occur (e.g., between double footling and complete, or between complete and incomplete breeches). In the case of the *incomplete* breech, there may be incomplete flexion at either the hip or knee joint, such as flexion at both hips with flexion at one knee and extension at the other, or flexion at one hip and extension at the other hip, as in a *single footling* breech.

More useful than ultrasound in clarifying the exact type of breech presentation is the

Table 9-11. Varieties of Breech Presentations

Type	Attitude at Hip	Attitude at Knee
Complete	Flexion (both)	Flexion (both)
Incomplete	Flexion (both)	Flexion (one), extension (one)
Double footling	Extension (both)	Flexion or extension
Single footling	Extension (one)	Flexion or extension
Frank	Flexion (one)	

simple abdominal flat x-ray film. The x-ray examination also allows for evaluation of the normalcy of the bony skull, and evaluation of the fetal skull and the attitude between the skull and cervical spine (the degree of flexion or extension).

During the second stage of labor, the breech-presenting infant will deliver by successively larger diameters through the bony pelvis, culminating with the largest diameter, the aftercoming head. By comparison, the vertex presentation may have hours for molding of the head, which allows for adaptation and safe navigation through the pelvis. The aftercoming head in breech presentation will have only minutes to accomplish the same feat. Thus, any significant disproportion between the pelvis and aftercoming head may result in significant fetal injury or even death.[23,49,56] The breech does not fill the birth canal as completely as the head and, because the cord is physically closer to the breech than the head, there is an increased risk of umbilical cord prolapse during the first stage of labor[56] or of compression during the expulsive maneuvers of the second stage and delivery. These are the major factors in the controversy regarding the optimal management of breech presentation.

External Cephalic Version

ECV refers to the conversion of breech presentation to a cephalic presentation, in general, prior to labor.[51] Using tocolytic drugs to relax the uterus and appropriate antepartum surveillance methods, (nonstress testing (NST), ultrasound, and Kliehauer-Betke testing) Van Dorsten and colleagues[58] were able to show the safety and efficacy of ECV at 37 to 39 weeks gestation. In the control group (not chosen for ECV), 17% spontaneously converted from breech to vertex prior to labor. Thus the recognition of breech presentation at term is not necessarily an indication for elective cesarean section prior to the onset of labor. The physician should inform the patient of the potential options: attempted version with breech presentation, cesarean section, or a selected trial of labor. If her fetus remains breech, she must present herself for evaluation at the earliest suggestion of labor or rupture of membranes. At this point, either in early labor or with rupture of membranes, the decision regarding cesarean section, trial of labor, or ECV will be made.

The Mechanism of Labor

Labor in breech presentation is influenced by the mechanical disadvantages presented by the breech. In comparison to the flexion that occurs at the cervical vertebrae in vertex deliveries, flexion in breech presentation must occur at the lumbar vertebrae, with lateral flexion of the trunk for delivery itself. Flexion of the trunk is even more difficult in the frank breech presentation, since the legs tend to splint the body.

During labor, following lateral flexion the anterior hip is forced against and underneath the symphysis. The expulsive phase that follows delivers the anterior and then posterior buttocks; the abdomen follows, and then the chest. As the back rotates anteriorly, the shoulders enter the pelvic inlet transversely. The shoulders rotate 90 degrees and deliver in the anterior/posterior diameter. At this point, the obstetrician is called upon to assist the delivery. As the anterior scapula is recognized at the introitus, the operator sweeps the infant's right humerus across his or her chest. Careful rotation of the body causes the posterior scapula to appear; then the left humerus may be delivered in a similar manner. At this point the aftercoming head enters the pelvic inlet obliquely, and internal rotation and flexion occur. The back of the neck extends against the symphysis and the chin passes over the perineum.

Delivery Procedures

Many manual and operative procedures are available to assist in the delivery of the breech fetus.

Assisted Breech Delivery

As the name implies, assisted breech delivery is one in which the infant is supported and helped to deliver with minimal interference. The infant is allowed to deliver spontaneously to the umbilicus. In the frank breech presentation, this may require slightly greater expulsive efforts to allow the legs to be born.

Several maneuvers may be used in assisted breech delivery. The Lövsett maneuver begins when the lower angle of the posterior scapula becomes visible. Rotation of the shoulder girdle with minimal resultant trauma is the goal of this technique.[13] The fetal back is anterior and the trunk is encircled with both hands so that the thumbs lie against the infant's thighs. The fingers are applied to the baby's posterior pelvis with care to avoid excessive force in the area of the kidneys or adrenal glands. The trunk is guided downward with minimal traction. When the posterior scapula appears, rotation is employed to effect delivery of the upper extremities. The arms appear, followed by the head at the vulva. Manual pressure at this point helps the fetal head to be born.

Another technique commonly employed in assisted breech delivery is the Brandt maneuver. Once the infant has delivered spontaneously to the umbilicus, the obstetrician wraps the fetal body in a warm towel and both hands are then applied to the posterior aspect of the fetal pelvis. One must avoid applying pressure over the fetal kidney and adrenal glands, which are susceptible to significant crush and possibly fatal injuries. Traction is then made in a downward direction. When the lower angle of the anterior scapula becomes visible, a finger is swept over the chest to release the arm. This having been accomplished, gentle rotation is used to bring the other scapula anteriorly. The second arm is released by gentle sweeping across the fetal chest. In performing the rotation at the cervical spine, the operator should remember that the vertebral arteries are susceptible to trauma at this point and that excessive rotation (past 90 degrees) may result in either cervical spine injuries or trauma to the vertebral arteries. The head is next delivered by either manual or operative technique.

During delivery of the abdomen and chest, excessive hast may result in the loss of flexion of the aftercoming head or arms, which is potentially a serious problem. Delivery of nuchal arms may be managed by rotating the trunk. Most authors feel that deflexion of the aftercoming head is the single most difficult situation that may be encountered. Suprapubic pressure should be attempted to regain flexion.

Delivering the Aftercoming Head

As with other aspects of breech delivery, there are varying degrees of invasive techniques available for effecting delivery of the aftercoming head. Maintaining flexion of both the head and arms is the cardinal principle to be followed in effecting safe breech delivery, regardless of route. By placing one hand on the head abdominally, the operator may "follow the head" into the pelvis to aid in maintaining this attitude (Naujoks maneuver).

The Mauriceau-Smellie-Veit (MSV)[40,55,60] maneuver is useful for effecting delivery when the head of the infant is in the occiput anterior position and the back is turned toward the symphysis. The body of the infant, abdomen down, is supported on the operator's left arm while the index finger is inserted into the baby's mouth; two other fingers are applied to the face to maintain flexion. The head is then delivered by downward traction until the back of the neck extends under the pubic arch. The child's face is delivered by gradually extending the neck of the infant under the pubic arch. A modification of the MSV maneuver encourages the maintenance of flexion in the aftercoming head by pressure on the malar eminenses and without placing a finger in the mouth. Another modification of the MSV maneuver is the Wigand-Martin-Winkle maneuver. If the aftercoming head is higher than the operator had previously thought, the first tractive efforts made to accomplish delivery will need to complete flexion and internal rotation. Suprapubic pressure is made with one hand, while the other keeps the head flexed and helps guide it out of the pelvis.[57]

Many times the aftercoming head can be successfully delivered by the use of suprapubic pressure (Kristellar pressure). The principle applied is the same one vital to all methods of effecting delivery of the aftercoming head: the maintenance of flexion. This allows the most optimal diameter of the aftercoming head to present. The loss of flexion will substitute a greater diameter, thus making delivery more difficult.

Occasionally the occiput has turned posteriorly. The technique employed for delivery in this situation (modified Prague maneuver) is with the baby laid with his back on the operator's arm.[37] The index and middle fingers of the hand hook onto either side of the fetal neck from behind. An assistant inserts the index fingers of his hands into the child's mouth (or uses two fingers to maintain flexion on facial bones) and the infant is delivered maintaining flexion. Should the aftercoming head be directed posteriorly and is also complicated by deflexion, delivery may be effected as follows: The back of the baby is laid on the attendant's forearm, the other hand grasping the legs above the ankles. The baby is then raised in a large arc to the mother's abdomen. This results in the occiput passing forward over the sacral concavity and then over the perineum. The fetal larynx serves as a fulcrum in this type of delivery.

Forceps in Breech Delivery

In 1924, Edmond Piper of Philadelphia introduced a special forcep for managing the aftercoming head in breech delivery.[9,48] Its main advantage are long shanks which allow a more suitable pelvic curve. The handles can be at a lower level than the blade of the forcep, making Piper forceps relatively easy to apply to the aftercoming head. Very little traction is necessary.

The aftercoming head must be descended to fill the pelvis and must be in the direct occiput anterior position. Delivery of the fetus using the forceps to rotate the aftercoming head about a point formed by the posterior aspect of the fetal neck where it meets the pubic symphysis allows for delivery with maintenance of flexion.

The Breech Delivery Team

In effecting any vaginal breech delivery, several factors are important. The obstetrician must have a gowned and gloved assistant. When feasible, the delivery room should be set up in advance and include warm towels and Piper forceps in addition to a cesarean section table. One would hope to anticipate and conduct the second stage of all breech deliveries in the delivery room rather than in the labor room. The delivery room should be equipped with a fetal monitor to allow for continuous monitoring of the fetus up to the point of delivery. Ideally, it should be a room equipped for either cesarean section or vaginal delivery.

It cannot be stressed too often that the reliance on expert anesthesia and pediatrics is crucial to the successful outcome of breech delivery whether vaginally or by cesarean section. In about 10% of our vaginal breech deliveries, general anesthesia is employed during the delivery of the aftercoming head. Crawford has shown the efficacy of regional anesthesia in breech delivery.[9] By limiting maternal expulsive efforts, regional anesthesia may be very helpful in special situations associated with breech delivery, primarily premature breech infants and term nonfrank breech presentations. In both instances prolapse of either the umbilical cord or of the fetal body through a partially dilated cervix is a major concern. By keeping the fetal membranes intact as long as is possible and using regional anesthesia, these two difficult groups of breech presentations may be managed safely through the vagina.

The first few minutes after breech delivery are invariably associated with some degree of asphyxia.[15,28,64] This is evidenced by the high incidence of low 1-minute Apgar scores seen at term breech delivery independent of delivery mode.[24,28] Umbilical cord gases frequently evidence some degree of respiratory acisosis (an elevation of P_{CO_2}), probably as a result of partial cord compression as the body passes through the birth canal. Since breech infants are generally subjected to greater degrees of cord occlusion than uncomplicated vertex deliveries, one may generally anticipate that the mild respiratory acidosis will resolve and 5-minute Apgar scores will demonstrate no consistent disadvantage for vaginal delivery in comparison to a cesarean section when a conservative selective protocol has been employed.[19,24,64]

In providing the best possible care of the parturient and her breech fetus, several other areas of concern should be considered:

- Standards of practice (medicolegal issues): Is there one or are there several equally satisfactory standards?
- Informed consent from the patient, after consideration of the risks both to mother and fetus
- The desires and preferences of the patient

X-Ray Evaluation

X-ray pelvimetry appeared in Europe in the late 1800s following Roentgen's discovery of the x-ray. Its history is a long one, punctuated by increasing and decreasing popularity, along with questions regarding its necessity, usefulness, and risk to the fetus and infant.

We have already noted the *importance of excluding a patient with a borderline pelvis from an attempt at vaginal breech delivery* (i.e., lack of time for the moulding process).[49,56] Entrapment of the aftercoming head (by the cervix) is less likely for the term infant than is the danger of difficulty in effecting delivery of the aftercoming head due to bony obstruction offered by a borderline pelvis.[19] The exception is the premature infant for whom entrapment by the cervix is the greater risk.[19,20] The premature infant's head is disproportionately larger than the term infant's. The trauma that may be sustained by either entrapment to the skull or to the cervical spine has lethal potential.

Many different methods of x-ray pelvimetry exist that involve the use of similar triangles to correct for the distance between the patient and the x-ray film. These are relatively cumbersome techniques.[17,59] Pelvimetry by digital radiography provides less exposure to radiation and is currently being assessed in comparison. The decreased exposure required in computed tomography (CT) is desirable because of the oncogenic potential of fetal irradiation. In one study, the maximum radiation required to perform pelvimetry by CT scan was on the order of 20% to 30% that of traditional methods.[16] Fetal gonadal exposure from traditional x-ray pelvimetry has been estimated to be in the order of 800 millirads.[45] By comparison, a single digital radiograph exposes the fetus to only 20 to 30 millirads.

As important as the absolute amount of radiation dosage delivered, however, is the techniques' applicability (the correlation between the traditional measurements and those derived from CT studies). In a prospective study in which traditional methods were compared with CT scanning of the pelvis, the authors noted that CT scanning was at least as accurate as well as technically simpler than conventional methods (Table 9-12).[25] Other factors that require consideration are cost and availability. Evaluation of the fetus and bony pelvis by CT scanning holds exciting poten-

Table 9-12. Comparison of Measurements by Computed Tomography (CT) and Conventional X-Ray Pelvimetry (in cm)

	CT	CONVENTIONAL PELVIMETRY	DIFFERENCE
MINIMAL DIAMETER OF PELVIC INLET >11 cm IN ANTERIOR-POSTERIOR PLANE			
Patient 1	12.1	11.4	0.7
Patient 2	11.2	13.2	2.0
Patient 3	11.7	12.3	0.6
Patient 4	11.3	11.9	0.6
Model	10.5 (10.4)*	10.9	0.4
MINIMAL DIAMETER OF PELVIC INLET >12 cm IN WIDEST TRANSVERSE DIAMETER			
Patient 1	12.1	11.8	0.3
Patient 2	13.5	13.6	0.1
Patient 3	11.7	12.3	0.6
Patient 4	12.0	12.6	0.6
Model	11.7 (11.5)*	12.4	0.7
MINIMAL DIAMETER OF MIDPELVIS >10 cm BETWEEN ISCHIATIC SPINES			
Patient 1	9.8	10.6	0.8
Patient 2	12.1	11.2	0.9
Patient 3	10.5	9.6	0.9
Patient 4	10.1	10.6	0.5
Model	9.6 (9.8)	9.9	0.3

* Figures in parentheses indicate actual measurement in model.[25]

tial because it enhances the safety of delivery in breech presentation. Since many hospitals are equipped with CT scanners it seems likely that this technique, if proven accurate and cost-effective, will gain in popularity in the future.

MANAGEMENT OPTIONS

External Cephalic Version

As mentioned earlier, ECV performed before labor or during early labor is a viable option for the management of the term breech presentation.[51,54,58] In order to perform ECV, it is necessary to ascertain that the breech is not engaged, that uterine activity is minimal, that there is sufficient amniotic fluid to safely attempt rotation, and that placentation is normal. We demand a reactive NST to establish fetal well-being as well as a normal ultrasound prior to attempting ECV. We agree with Saling and Muller-Holve[54] that anesthesia for this procedure is contraindicated, since avoidance of pain or major discomfort during the procedure is a safeguard which limits the amount of force applied. ECV should be performed in proximity to the labor and delivery suite because it is possible, although unlikely, that an emergency situation may arise that demands delivery room care.

A tocolytic agent, generally a betamimetic drug (magnesium sulfate in a diabetic), is given to promote uterine relaxation. The operator places one hand over the breech for elevation and the other over the head and begins to rotate through the shortest arc. Rotation is accomplished slowly, carefully, and without undue force.

This procedure has been successful in 70% to 80% of breech presentations at 37 to 39 weeks gestation. Currently we are evaluating the efficacy of external version for both breech and transverse presentations in early labor when the membranes are intact.

Selective Trial of Labor

The patient with known breech presentation prior to labor is advised to present herself to labor and delivery at the earliest signs of labor or rupture of membranes. It is our opinion that these patients represent a high-risk group and that even on an obstetric service that permits a trial of labor, the majority of women with breech presentations will require cesarean section and its attendant preparations.[19] At Women's Hospital, Los Angeles, the overall use of cesarean section for all breech presentations averages about 70%. This rate ranges upward from 33% for frank breech fetuses in multiparas to 50% to 60% for trial of labor regardless of type of term breech. We have not noted a significant difference between primiparous and multiparous patients in this regard, although our cesarean section rate for primiparous patients is slightly higher than for multiparas.

The protocol for the management of term breech presentation in labor is the same for both frank and nonfrank breech presentations. The protocol outlined in Figure 9-5 has a historic basis (the Sloane Hospital for Women at Columbia University)[23,56] as well as an ongoing clinical experience (Women's Hospital and White Memorial Medical Center, both in Los Angeles).

Ultrasound is our initial tool after considering the diagnosis of breech presentation. The number of diagnosable congenital anomalies, as well as abnormalities of the placenta, dictate the need for this to be the first evaluation of a breech-presenting fetus.

Informed Consent

We begin our approach to these patients with a detailed discussion as to both the fetal and maternal risks and benefits of a trial of labor or an elective cesarean delivery. Our recent experience with several hundred patients within this category provided the background data that we describe to each patient (Figure 9-5). In summary, we feel that the risk to the breech-presenting fetus of a trial of labor and vaginal delivery is not unreasonable in select circumstances. Neonatal morbidity among groups undergoing carefully monitored labor and assisted breech delivery and cesarean section are similar. The risk of neonatal mortality is greater with vaginal delivery, but is distinctly rare, approximately 1 in 300 deliveries.[8,19,23,24,44,62] Maternal morbidity is clearly greater with abdominal delivery.[8,20,44] In our preliminary study, one asphyxiated infant was lost as a result of apparent inadequate resuscitation[24]; subsequently we have not lost another infant due to a trial of labor. Curiously the occurrence of injuries at vaginal delivery and cesarean section has been strikingly similar (1/100–1/500). Thus the fetal/neonatal risk associated with vaginal delivery, which must be weighed against the increased maternal morbidity (>50%) and maternal mortality (1 in 10,000) seen with cesarean delivery provide a clinical equation for decision analysis. The final choice becomes an individual decision that each patient, the family, and physician must consider.

Preparation for Delivery

After informed consent is obtained, the patient is prepared for abdominal delivery. Ce-

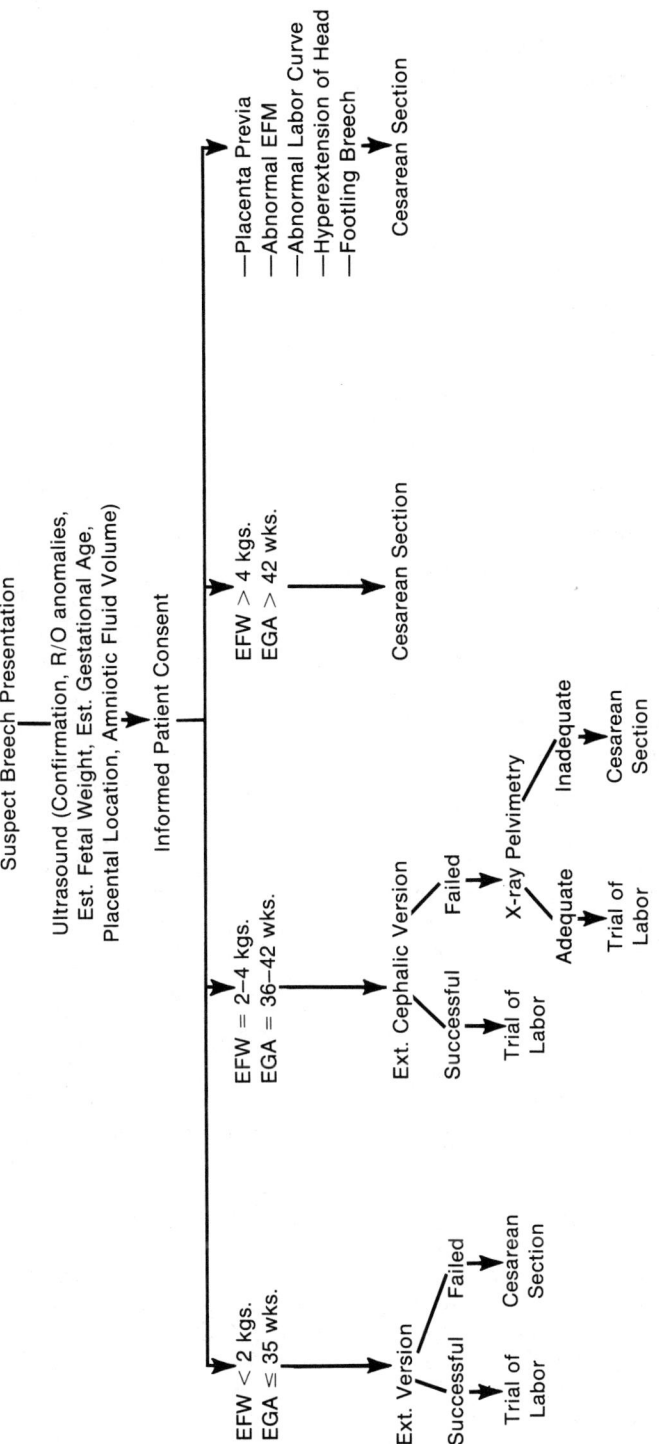

FIGURE 9-5. Overview and flow diagram of the management of breech presentation in early labor.

sarean section, if elected, is performed, using regional anesthesia if appropriate. If cesarean section is not chosen, the patient is next sent for x-ray evaluation. Significant factors in the x-ray evaluation of the fetus and maternal pelvis include the bony pelvis, hyperextension of the head, and the bones of the fetal skull.

Todd and Steer[56] reported on the delivery of over 1000 term breeches at Columbia Presbyterian Medical Center in the 1950s and 1960s. The ultimate safety of vaginal delivery was seen to rely on the adequacy of pelvic measurements obtained at x-ray. When the inlet of the bony pelvis measured 11 cm in the anterior-posterior view and 12 cm in the transverse, the vast majority of infants were delivered vaginally (85%) and safely, perinatal mortality being limited to one case in 200 (0.5%). If either of these measurements was not achieved, the majority of infants required cesarean delivery (60%); of those infants still allowed vaginal delivery, the perinatal mortality was 12 times greater (6.7%). Twenty years later in an update on the same obstetric service, Gimovsky and colleagues[23] added to Todd and Steer's measurements an interspinous diameter of greater than 10 cm. This simple 10,11,12 (cm) rule provides the current basis for excluding the borderline pelvis. In the follow-up study, perinatal morbidity was fivefold greater when x-ray pelvimetry was omitted or when these measurements were not met. However, as Steer and others have shown, clinical pelvimetry alone is not sufficient in this regard.[19]

The x-ray appraisal must also evaluate the relation between the head and cervical spine to exclude hyperextension, which may occur in up to 5% of term breech presentation.[19] The anterior angle between the mandible and cervical spine is used to judge the degree of flexion or extension of the fetal head. Extension is diagnosed when this angle exceeds 105 degrees. Caterini and co-workers showed that extension of the head in breech presentation was associated with spinal cord trauma and traumatic injury at vaginal delivery.[6] Indeed these fetuses may be difficult to deliver even by cesarean section.[2] The etiologic causes of hyperextension include fetal neck masses, nuchal cord,[62] uterine abnormalities such as myomas or septae,[5] pathologic shortening, (torticollis),[6] and neurologic abnormalities of the fetal neck musculature (Table 9-13).[2] When these radiologic criteria are met, the patient returns to the fetal intensive care area for fetal monitoring during labor.

Table 9-13. Etiology of Hyperextension

Fetal
Nuchal cord
Neck mass
Trisomy 21
Torticollis
Hydrocephalus
Anencephalus
Maternal
Uterine
Myoma
Septae
Bicornuate uterus

Augmentation of Labor

Fetal distress is managed similarly to the vertex presentation. However, several authors present data suggesting that the breech fetus may become acidotic during labor more rapidly than his or her cephalic counterpart.[52,58-60] A pelvic examination should be performed upon spontaneous rupture of membranes or with evidence of abnormal fetal heart rate (FHR) patterns to exclude prolapse of the umbilical cord or fetal extremities. Theoretically, fetal blood sampling may be obtained from the fetal buttocks. On the rare occasions that we have used fetal blood sampling, similar criteria in fetal pH or trends of base excess were seen as predictive of fetal distress requiring imminent delivery.[30] In general, serious abnormalities in FHR in the breech will lead to cesarean delivery.

The use of oxytocin in breech labor and delivery is an extremely controversial point. Induction of labor because of toxemia, postdates, or abnormal antepartum testing may be considered if the breech is engaged in the pelvis and the radiologic criteria for adequacy are met. We have seen no increased risk to breech presentations induced for these indications.[8,19,23,24] Macrosomia as well as the potential for fetal compromise on the basis of uteroplacental insufficiency, as seen in severe pregnancy-induced hypertension or postdates, should be considered as a relative contraindication for induction in a breech presentation.

Augmentation of labor, however, may present a significant risk. Brenner and coworkers[5] demonstrated that when rupture of membranes was used to augment breech labor, the fetus was at increased risk over the breech infant with spontaneous labor. Augmentation with oxytocin should offer improved safety.

Friedman has suggested that arrest of active labor in breech presentation is consistent with a large fetus.[18] This fetopelvic disproportion may be a teleologic sign that cesarean section should be used. In our own experience the majority of infants with active phase arrest of labor, or with arrest of descent or protraction disorders, are indeed large infants and thus cesarean section is preferential to oxytocin augmentation of labor.[24]

Conduct of Delivery

The second stage of labor ideally should be managed in the delivery room. With anesthesia and pediatric personnel present, the patient is prepared in the usual fashion for vaginal delivery. Our preference is for anesthesia on standby, with prompt general anesthesia should circumstance mandate.

After bladder catheterization, pudendal anesthesia is given. A general episiotomy (or episioproctotomy) is performed when the buttocks crown. It is essential to allow the fetus to deliver spontaneously as far as is possible. By using continuous electronic fetal monitoring within the delivery room, fetal evaluation is possible virtually to the completion of delivery. The membranes are left intact as long as possible. At this point there is often tremendous anxiety on the part of the inexperienced accoucheur, which must be consciously suppressed. After all, we have preselected an average-size fetus in an average-size pelvis who has not had significant fetal distress (or serious labor abnormality) and may expect a safe delivery. The majority of these infants will deliver spontaneously to the umbilicus without assistance.

At this point, a loop of umbilical cord may be freed. The infant's body should be supported with the left hand by a right-handed obstetrician. The Mauriceau-Smellie-Veit or Wigand-Martin maneuver may then be employed. In delivering the aftercoming head, a common error when Piper forceps are used is to attempt to apply them before the head has fully descended into the pelvis.

The differences in outcome between breech infants delivered by elective cesarean section or by protocol are minimal for infants between 1500 g to 4000 g, whether frank or nonfrank presentations, and among nulliparous or multiparous women. Thus we will consider a patient a candidate for a trial of labor at 36 weeks gestation, or greater than 2000 g. A head-abdomen ratio of less than 1:1 by ultrasound is desirable.

Among all breech fetuses 25% will be premature, and we believe a reasonable application of cesarean section delivery for the breech may be routinely applied between 750 g and 2000 g. Controversy exists as to the efficacy of cesarean section below 1000 g for the breech fetus, but neonatal intensive care unit experience may make a prospective study difficult to perform.

It should be noted that approximately one-half of women entered into protocol evaluation will ultimately require cesarean section, the vast majority of these (60%) because of failure to meet minimal pelvimetry criteria (Table 9-14).[24]

Elective Cesarean Section

Many practitioners have elected to deliver the breech-presenting fetus by cesarean section regardless of other considerations.[43] This decision revolves around a multitude of issues including obstetric, social, and medicolegal

Table 9-14. Failures of Trial of Labor in 39 Patients[24]

Reason	No. of Patients	Trial of Labor Failures (%)	All Trial of Labor Patients (0%)
X-RAY EVALUATION			
Fetal head hyperextended	2	5	3
PELVIMETRY			
1 diameter contracted	18	46	26
2 diameters contracted	5	13	7
LABOR			
Latent phase arrest (with oxytocin)	2	5	3
Active phase arrest (with oxytocin)	2	5	3
Active phase arrest (no oxytocin)	1	3	1
Arrest of descent	1	3	1
PROLAPSE (FIRST STAGE)			
Umbilical cord	3	8	4
Body	2	5	3
EXCLUDED AFTER RANDOMIZATION			
Progressed too rapidly	2	5	3
Elective	1	3	1

factors. The overwhelming concern is to avoid potentially preventable birth injury, umbilical cord prolapse, and the infrequent but potentially disastrous entrapment of the aftercoming head.

Recent experience with breech labor and delivery conducted with the protocol described suggests that performing cesarean section routinely for breech presentation is most beneficial in certain situations:

- Patients delivering in facilities not equipped with full-time support services in both anesthesia and pediatrics
- Women delivering breech fetuses of 34 weeks or less, 42 weeks or more, and/or estimated fetal weights less than 2000 g or more than 4000 g
- Any viable breech in which hyperextension of the head is demonstrated by x-ray (anterior angle >105 degrees)
- Patients who desire cesarean section
- Double footling breech (at highest risk for major labor and delivery problems among breech presentations)

Bony injury and peripheral nerve damage are well known to be increased in breech delivery.[5,12,19,49] Not generally appreciated is that injury occurs to some breech fetuses at cesarean section. Gimovsky and Paul[19] showed that the spectrum of injuries sustained by breech-presenting infants was similar for cesarean section and vaginal delivery using a selective protocol. Erb's palsy, bony fractures, and low 5-minute Apgar scores were equal in both groups. We conclude that adequate incisions of the uterus and the abdominal wall are critical to avoid such trauma at cesarean section for breech presentation. Care should be taken when employing a Pfannenstiel incision to guarantee an adequate opening in the anterior fascia. The uterine incision, when transverse must also be generous. The assistant should maintain pressure on the fundus and follow the fetal head down to maintain flexion.

Care should be taken to perform extraction slowly to prevent deflexion of the head as well as to lessen the incidence of nuchal arms. When a nuchal arm occurs, rotation of the trunk and shoulders is necessary, as at vaginal delivery. The aftercoming head should be delivered by pressure on the fundus to maintain flexion. Excessive lateral pressure to the head should be avoided, since this may result in brachial plexus injury. Additional uterine relaxation with halothane is only rarely necessary to effect delivery and may be associated with hemorrhage.

The uterus should be explored after delivery of any breech presentation for uterine anomalies. Septate uterus as well as myomas and minor uterine anomalies are more frequent with breech-presenting fetuses.[5,19]

THE PRETERM BREECH

We have mentioned the disadvantages that all breech-presenting infants may encounter during labor and delivery. Comparison of the relative differences in the significant fetal diameters (biparietal, bisacromial, and intratrochanteric) reveals that the preterm breech fetus presents an even less optimal shape (a head-abdomen ratio >1) for negotiating the pelvic outlet. Other significant negative factors include an increased incidence of nonfrank presentations with the attendant increased risk of umbilical cord prolapse;[26] the increased incidence of premature rupture of membranes, which results in a further decrease in the dilating wedge[19]; the decreased ability of the premature infant to tolerate the repetitive stress of labor[20,50,61]; and the problem of differentiating the growth-retarded fetus from the truly premature infant.

The partially dilated cervix, and not the bony pelvis, is more likely to entrap the head of the premature infant. In comparing the sequelae suffered at birth by breech-presenting infants of all weights, Gimovsky and Paul found that those infants weighing less than 1500 g were the only breech infants to suffer death or significant depression at birth on the basis of umbilical cord prolapse or head entrapment at delivery.[19] The only deaths that occurred to term breech infants were those infants with lethal congenital anomalies. With entrapment of the aftercoming head, Duhrssen's (cervical) incisions may not allow salvage of the preterm breech infant delivered vaginally. Cesarean section has come to be more common for the delivery of the low birth weight (LBW) breech fetus.[27] Cruikshank and Pitkin[10] asked the pertinent question when they wanted proof of benefit of cesarean section for the premature breech. Even though they could not find prospective data to support this clinical recommendation, they noted that it would be difficult to perform a prospective randomized study.[10,14,20,26,32,33,35]

Management Options

Vaginal Delivery

When choosing to allow a trial of labor in the group of breech infants in the borderline weight range (1500–2000 g), several safeguards are germane. Conduction anesthesia may play a significant role by reducing maternal expulsive efforts during the end of the first stage of labor and delivery, and may decrease the risk of cord prolapse and the potential for delivering the fetus through an incompletely dilated cervix.[9]

Milner showed in a retrospective manner that the application of forceps to the aftercoming head was associated with decreased mortality among breech infants weighing between 1000 g to 2500 g.[42] Wheeler and Greene[65] suggest that fetal monitoring would play a role in avoiding serious asphyxia in labor prior to delivery. The increased vulnerability of the umbilical cord has been associated with an increased tendency to respiratory acidosis during labor.[15,30,64]

Among the subgroups of breech infants in whom cord prolapse would be least expected (i.e., frank and complete breeches), Kaupilla has suggested that a prospective study be performed among fetuses of transitional age.[35] The other groups of preterm breech infants (i.e., footling and incomplete breeches) are probably best managed by cesarean section in view of problems with incomplete dilatation of cervix, the high risk of cord prolapse, and entrapment of the aftercoming head by the cervix and maternal soft tissues.[21]

Cesarean Section

In performing abdominal delivery, the impact of anesthesia and operative technique must be considered paramount. If there has been no or little labor, the uterine incision of choice may be the low vertical incision. Since the indication for cesarean section is the avoidance of trauma, both uterine and abdominal wall incisions must be large enough to permit an atraumatic delivery.

Outcome

Although opinions are many, little prospectively derived data are available on the long-term outcome of preterm breech infants isolating the effect of delivery modes alone.[32] The many other complications of prematurity, as well as iatrogenic complications, have made isolation of the effect of mode of delivery difficult to study.[21] It does seem reasonable to conclude that, as in the vertex presentation, the nonasphyxiated infant born with a minimum of birth trauma will be the highest quality survivor. It is for this reason that cesarean section is recommended and used by most practitioners for the delivery of a LBW breech infant.[8,22,38] Retrospective studies are limited by selection bias, and until a longitudinal prospective randomized study is performed, are likely to remain so.

Of the available studies, two are worth review. Ingemarsson and co-workers[32] followed surviving premature breech infants for 1 to 5 years after birth. Although their study is limited because their vaginal delivery group and cesarean section groups were not controlled or randomized, it is worth noting that the incidence of developmental or neurologic abnormalities was tenfold greater among premature breech infants delivered vaginally. What is even more disconcerting is that the mean birth weight in their study group was greater than 2000 g (gestational age 33–34 weeks). The incidence of cerebrospinal fluid bleeding was two to four times greater among the vaginally delivered infants. One-third of the breech infants in whom significant neurologic sequelae did occur were small for gestational age as well as extremely LBW ($\leq$800 g). A case-controlled retrospective study by Duenhoelter and associates[14] showed a much higher frequency of neonatal death among vaginally delivered breeches. The deaths occurred secondary to asphyxia, hyaline membrane disease, and intracranial hemorrhage. Their cohorts had a mean gestational age of 34 to 35 weeks and a mean birth weight of 1950 g, again a relatively high weight for a premature infant. A dramatic change in outcome has been seen by many authors when the 1500-g mark was obtained at birth (Table 9-15). Although all the data is retrospective, several independent groups did arrive at the same weight range— 1500 g—as the cutoff between LBW breech infants who suffered obvious sequelae as a result of vaginal delivery, and term-size infants, in whom this observation has been controversial.

The following are considerations for the use of cesarean section for the breech fetus who weighs less than 2000 g, is less than 34 weeks gestation, or who is term and suffers from growth retardation (and thus is estimated at less than 2000 g):

- Since the majority of breech-presenting fetuses weighing less than 2000 g will be nonfrank, the risk of umbilical cord prolapse and the attendant compromise is greater than that for the term fetus (Table 9-16).
- Among premature breech infants the head-abdomen circumference will be proportionately greater than at term, leading to an increased potential for head entrapment.
- The ability of the premature infant to toler-

Table 9-15. Outcome of LBW Vaginal Breech Delivery

	1000–1500 g		1500–2000 g	
	Incidence of 5-minute Apgar Score < 7	Corrected Mortality	Incidence of 5-minute Apgar Score < 7	Corrected Mortality
Gimovsky and Petrie (protocol)[20]	50%	50%	33%	8%
Gimovsky and Petrie (nonprotocol)[20]	75%	50%	40%	8%
Goldenberg and Nelson[26]	75%	55%	10%	6%
DeCrespigny and Pepperell[12]		41.2%		10.3%
Mann and Gallant[39]		46%		8.8%
Kauppila et al.[35]		43%		13%

(Modified from Gimovsky ML, Petrie RH: The intrapartum and neonatal performance of the low birth weight vaginal breech delivery. J Reprod Med 27:451, 1982)

ate asphyxia during labor may be severely limited.[50,61]

- Combining the retrospective data available, the breakoff point between the excessive risks of birth trauma associated with premature vaginal breech delivery and relatively safe term breech vaginal delivery appears to be between 1500 g and 2000 g.

On our service we define the preterm breech as either estimated fetal weight of less than 2000 g or gestational age less than 34 weeks. It is our opinion that until more data is available the premature breech, particularly the footling varieties, should be delivered by cesarean section. Premature frank and complete breeches between 32 and 35 weeks may represent another selected group of breeches in which a trial of labor may be considered. Current studies are under way to evaluate the efficacy of an intensively monitored and carefully conducted vaginal delivery in this gestational age/weight group.

Table 9-16. Type of Breech Presentation in Labor by Gestational Age*

	PRESENTATION				
Gestational Age (Weeks)	Frank	Complete	Double Footling	Single Footling	Other
41–42	64	27	52	19	11
39–40	72	41	46	15	4
37–38	80	43	45	11	9
35–36	55	31	38	9	5
33–34	36	22	30	12	2
31–32	20	11	20	14	3
29–30	14	10	19	15	4
27–28	6	2	13	9	8
25–26	6	3	14	12	9

* Diagnosed by x-ray in labor, best clinical estimate gestational age. Data pooled from obstetrical services at LAC/USC Women's Hospital, White Memorial Medical Center, Los Angeles, and Columbia-Presbyterian Medical Center, New York.

THE IMPACT OF SOCIETY AND SOCIAL MORES

Once breech presentation has been diagnosed, the patient and her family rarely will not understand the potential problems to be encountered. The media as well as collective experience has educated the majority of women to the fact that breech presentation presents a risk to the baby. The conclusions drawn by the media profoundly influence the millions of women who will deliver infants in any year. It is the physician's responsibility to explain to patients that under most circumstances cesarean section is a reasonable approach to breech delivery, although certainly not the only one.

In an era of decreasing family size and increasing expectations for a perfect baby and an atraumatic birth, physicians must often choose between the pressure exerted by the patient and the threat of litigation. It is important to allow the patient's participation in the choice of selecting the most appropriate means of management.

Thus the standards of practice applicable to breech management currently include the following:

- Liberal use of cesarean section
- Conversion of the breech fetus at term to a cephalic presentation
- Selective use of a trial of labor in a carefully screened population of term breech-presenting fetuses (36–42 weeks gestation)

It is unreasonable to attempt to equate maternal morbidity (and even perhaps maternal mortality) with fetal risk. It is clearly not possible to do more than explain the actual risks and to use the data available to help the patient understand why in any given situation external cephalic version, a trial of labor, or cesarean section may be reconsidered. If we consider perinatal death as an end point, there is one additional maternal loss with every 10,000 cesarean sections. Our recent data concerning 500 breech deliveries at term conducted by protocol encountered one death attributable to a trial of labor and vaginal delivery. This begets the question, is the risk of one in 10,000 for the mother equal to the risk of one in 500 for her baby?

The risk of morbidity must also be considered for both the mother and the fetus. Again we must ask, is the risk of a transfusion reaction or AIDS for the mother greater or lesser than the risk of Erb's palsy for her baby? Or of hysterectomy versus cerebral palsy?

What role does a cost-benefit analysis play? Although we endeavor to allow a trial of labor after previous cesarean section at our institutions, most women (97%) will not have this option. Thus the cost is not of one cesarean section hospitalization and associated fees, but of repeat procedures also. In a country in which 3,700,000 deliveries occur annually, 120,000 are complicated by breech presentation in labor. If the (breech) cesarean section rate remains at the 90% level, the ultimate cost is measured in hundreds of millions of health care dollars. The cost in terms of psychological effects (cesarean delivery v. vaginal delivery) is an issue that also needs to be raised. These costs also must be viewed together, not just individually.

FUTURE GOALS

One of the earliest protocols described for breech fetuses when home delivery by midwives was the rule is worth remembering. Obstetricians recommended that women with recognized breech presentation be sent to the hospital to be delivered by a senior staff obstetrician.[36] In the 1920s DeLee stated that the delivery of a breech-presenting fetus was "the measure of an obstetrician."[36] In the 1980s, this is no less true. Our increased use of cesarean section has resulted in a dramatic decrease in injury and death during the intrapartum period for breech-presenting fetuses. We should, however, endeavor to minimize its use in order to minimize maternal risk.

We anticipate that the future may hold a decrease in the use of cesarean section for all indications, including the term breech fetus. More and more obstetric units will be able to provide comprehensive services including continuous electronic fetal monitoring, 24-hour availability of anesthesia, and neonatal intensive care.

A potential problem is the current lack of experience among resident physicians, which will produce a generation of obstetricians trained to rely almost exclusively upon cesarean section for breech delivery. The ability of the obstetrician to allow labor and to effect assisted breech delivery will be suspect. Continual reports of birth injuries suffered at cesarean section by breech-presenting infants confirm this belief. Resident physicians should be permitted experience to develop the skill necessary to effect a safe breech delivery by both vaginal and abdominal routes, as well as the maneuvers of version, in order to offer reasonable alternatives to their patients.

We feel that there exist subgroups which provide the lowest risk for a carefully monitored trial of labor and potential vaginal delivery. Studies are under way to consider the breech infants at a transitional age (32–35 weeks) in frank or complete breech presentation as candidates for a trial of labor.

CT scanning of the pelvis for mensuration of the significant pelvic diameters may eventually replace traditional x-ray pelvimetry. The measurements obtained by this technique are likely more accurate and deliver less radiation to the patient.

REFERENCES

1. Axelrod F, Leistner H, Porges R: Breech presentation among infants with familial dysautonomia. J Pediatr 84:107, 1974
2. Ballas S, Toaff R, Jaffa A: Deflexion of fetal head in breech presentation. Obstet Gynecol 52:653, 1978
3. Bird C, McElin T: A six-year prospective study of term breech deliveries utilizing the Zatuchni-Andros prognostic scoring index. Am J Obstet Gynecol 121:551, 1975
4. Braun F, Jones K, Smith DW: Breech presentation as an indicator of fetal abnormality. J Pediatr 86:419, 1975
5. Brenner WE, Bruce RS, Hendricks CH: The characteristics and perils of breech presentation. Am J Obstet Gynecol 118:700, 1974
6. Caterini H, Langer A, Sama JC et al: Fetal risk in hyperextension of the fetal head in breech presentation. Am J Obstet Gynecol 123:632, 1975
7. Chervenak F, Johnson R, Berkowitz RC et al: Is routine cesarean section necessary for vertex-breech and vertex-transverse twin gestations? Am J Obstet Gynecol 148:1, 1984
8. Collea JV, Chein C, Quilligan EJ: The randomized management of frank breech presentation. Am J Obstet Gynecol 137:235, 1980
9. Crawford B: An appraisal of lumbar epidural blockade in patients with singleton fetus presenting by the breech. Br J Obstet Gynaecol 81:867, 1974
10. Cruikshank DP, Pitkin RM: Delivery of the premature breech. Obstet Gynecol 50:367, 1977
11. Daw E: Hyperextension of the head in breech presentation. Am J Obstet Gynecol 119:564, 1974
12. DeCrespigny LJC, Pepperell RJ: Perinatal mortality and morbidity in breech presentation. Obstet Gynecol 53:141, 1979
13. Douglas RG, Stromme WB (eds): Operative Obstetrics, 3rd ed, p 600. New York, Appleton Century Crofts, 1976
14. Duenhoelter J, Wells C, Reisch R: A paired controlled study of vaginal and abdominal delivery of the low birth weight breech fetus. Obstet Gynecol 54:310, 1979
15. Eilen B, Fleischer A, Schulman H: Fetal acidosis and the abnormal FHR tracing: The term breech fetus. Obstet Gynecol 63:233, 1984
16. Federle M, Cohen J, Rosenwein M: Pelvimetry by digital radiography: A low dose examination. Radiology 143:733, 1982
17. Fine E, Brackers NM, Berkowitz RC: An evaluation of the usefulness of x-ray pelvimetry. Am J Obstet Gynecol 137:15, 1980
18. Friedman EA: Clinical Management of Labor, 2nd ed. New York, Appleton Century Crofts, 1978
19. Gimovsky ML, Paul RH: Singleton breech presentation in labor: Experience in 1980. Am J Obstet Gynecol 143:733, 1982
20. Gimovsky ML, Petrie RH: The intrapartum and neonatal performance of the low birth weight vaginal breech delivery. J Reprod Med 27:451, 1982
21. Gimovsky ML, Petrie RH: Optimal method of delivery of the low birth weight breech fetus:

An unresolved issue. J Calif Perinat Assoc 4:34, 1983
22. Gimovsky ML, Petrie RH: Strategy for choosing the best delivery route for the breech baby. Contemp Obstet Gynecol (April) 21:201, 1983
23. Gimovsky ML, Petrie RH, Todd WD: Neonatal performance of the selected term vaginal breech delivery. Obstet Gynecol 56:687, 1980
24. Gimovsky ML, Wallace RL, Schifrin BS, Paul RH: Randomized management of the nonfrank breech presentation at term. Am J Obstet Gynecol 146:34, 1983
25. Gimovsky ML, Willard K, Neglio M, Howard T, Zerne S: X-Ray pelvimetry in a breech protocol: A comparison of digital radiography and conventional methods. Am J Obstet Gynecol 153:887, 1985
26. Goldenberg R, Nelson G: The premature breech. Am J Obstet Gynecol 127:240, 1977
27. Granati B, Rondinelli M, Capot C: The premature breech presentation. Am J Perinat 1:145, 1984
28. Green J, McLean F, Smith L: Has an increased cesarean section rate for term breech delivery reduced the incidence of birth asphyxia, trauma and death? Am J Obstet Gynecol 142:643, 1982
29. Hall J, Kohl S: Breech presentation: A study of 1456 cases. Am J Obstet Gynecol 72:977, 1956
30. Hill J, Eliot B: Intensive care of the fetus in breech labor. Br J Obstet Gynaecol 83:271, 1976
31. Huchcroft S, Wearing M, Buek C: Late results of cesarean and vaginal delivery in cases of breech presentation. Can Med Assoc J 125:726, 1981
32. Ingemarson I, Westgren M, Svenningsen N: Long term follow up of preterm infants in breech presentation delivered by cesarean section. Lancet 2:172, 1978
33. Karp LE, Doney JR, McCarthy T et al: The premature breech: TOL or C/S? Obstet Gynecol 53:88, 1979
34. Kauppila D: The perinatal mortality in breech deliveries and observation of affecting factors. Acta Obstet Gynecol Scand (Suppl) 39:1, 1975
35. Kauppila O, Gionross M, Aro P et al: Management of low birth weight breech delivery: Should cesarean section be routine? Obstet Gynecol 57:289, 1981
36. Kerr M: Breech prevention. In Myciscoyh P, Mori J (eds): Munro Kerr's Operative Obstetrics, 8th ed, p 139. Baltimore, Williams & Wilkins, 1971
37. Kiwisch FH: Beiträge zur Geburtskunde Wurzbury, I Abth, 69, 1846
38. Lyons ER, Papsin FR: Cesarean section in the management of breech presentation. Am J Obstet Gynecol 139:558, 1981
39. Mann LI, Gallant JM: Modern management of the breech delivery. Am J Obstet Gynecol 134:611, 1979
40. Mauriceau F: The method of delivering the woman when the infant presents one or two feet first, p 280. Traite de Maladies des Femmes Grosses, 6 me ed, 1721
41. Mazor M, Hagay Z, Leiberman JR et al: Fetal malformations associated with breech delivery: Implications for management. J Reprod Med 31:717, 1986
42. Milner RDG: Neonatal mortality of breech deliveries with and without forceps to the aftercoming head. Br J Obstet Gynaecol 72:783, 1975
43. NIH consensus development task force statement on cesarean childbirth. Am J Obstet Gynecol 139:902, 1981
44. O'Leary J: Vaginal delivery of the term breech. Obstet Gynecol 53:341, 1979
45. Osborne SB: The implications of the reports of the Committee on Radiological Hazards to Patients. Symposium, British Institute of Radiology, 1962. Br J Radiol 36:230, 1963
46. Phelan J, Bethel M, Devore G et al: Use of ultrasound in breech presentation with hyperextension of the fetal head. A case report. J Ultrasound Med 2:373, 1983
47. Pinard A: On version by external maneuvers. Traite de Palper Abdominal, Paris, 1889
48. Piper EB, Bachman C: The prevention of fetal injuries in breech delivery. JAMA 92:217, 1929
49. Potter MG, Heaton CE, Douglas GW: Intrinsic risk in breech delivery. Obstet Gynecol 15:158, 1960
50. Quirk J, Raker R, Petrie R: The role of glucocorticoids, unstressful labor and atraumatic delivery in the prevention of RDS. Am J Obstet Gynecol 134:768, 1979
51. Ranney B: The gentle art of external cephalic version. Am J Obstet Gynecol 116:239, 1973
52. Robinson G: Birth characteristics of children with congenital dislocation of the hip. Am J Epidemiol 87:275, 1968
53. Rovinsky JJ, Miller JA, Solomon S: Management of breech presentation. Am J Obstet Gynecol 115:497, 1973
54. Saling E, Muller-Holve W: External cephalic version under tocolysis. J Perinat Med 3:115, 1975

55. Smellie W: Smellie's treatise on the theory and practice of midwifery. London, The New Sydenham Society, 1876
56. Todd WD, Steer CM: Term Breech: Review of 1006 term breech deliveries. Obstet Gynecol 22:583, 1963
57. Taylor ED (ed): Becks Obstetrical Practice, 9th ed, p 252. Baltimore, Williams & Wilkins, 1971
58. Van Dorsten P, Schifrin BS, Wallace RL: Randomized control trial of external cephalic version with tocolysis in late pregnancy. Am J Obstet Gynecol 141:417, 1981
59. Varner M, Cruickshank D, Laube D: X-ray pelvimetry in clinical obstetrics. Obstet Gynecol 56:296, 1980
60. Veit G: On version by external manipulation. Hamburgisches Magazin für die Geburtschulfe, 1907
61. Watashsky D, Hockner-Celnikier D, Beller U: Neonatal outcome in cesarean section under general anesthesia related to gestational age, induction-delivery, and uterus-delivery intervals. Isr J Med Sci 19:1059, 1983
62. Watson WJ, Benson WL: Vaginal delivery for the selected frank breech infant at term. Obstet Gynecol 64:683, 1984
63. Wheeler T, Greene K: FHR monitoring during breech labor. Br J Obstet Gynaecol 82:208, 1975
64. White PC, Cibils L: Clinical significance of FHR patterns during labor VII: Breech presentation. J Reprod Med 29:45, 1984
65. Wright RC: Reduction of perinatal mortality and morbidity in breech delivery through routine use of cesarean section. Obstet Gynecol 14:748, 1959
66. Zatuchni A: Prognostic index for vaginal delivery in breech delivery at term. Am J Obstet Gynecol 93:237, 1965

10

Keeping "Dead" Mothers Alive During Pregnancy

SECTION 1: Maternal Brain Death During Pregnancy

David R. Field and Russell K. Laros, Jr.

Brain death, the unequivocal and irreversible loss of total brain function, is a diagnosis that has gained wide acceptance in the medical and legal communities.[4] Because brain death is uniformly followed by cardiovascular collapse in spite of aggressive supportive care, most states have passed brain death statutes which equate that diagnosis with the pronouncement of death. Once such a diagnosis is made, it is generally considered unethical to prolong the family's suffering and to squander costly medical resources by continuing to support vital functions by artificial means. However, short-term support for these brain-dead patients is frequently given in order to provide organs that are optimally perfused for transplantation. Thus, many surgeons involved in transplant programs, as well as a number of neurologists, neurosurgeons, and other physicians practicing critical care medicine, have gained some experience in the short-term maintenance of these "beating heart cadavers."

Since brain death occurs so infrequently during pregnancy, most obstetricians have no experience managing these patients and have not given much thought to the unique fetal considerations raised by such dire maternal circumstances. Maternal brain death during pregnancy might be one instance where the prolonged maintenance of the mother's vital functions is justified for fetal indications. Dillon and co-workers[12] recently reported the first case in which prolonged support of a brain-dead mother resulted in the birth of an infant who survived. Though they suggested guidelines for the management of these patients, the decision of whether or not to continue maximum supportive care in these rare and tragic cases remains a controversial one.[42]

Fundamental to this controversy are unanswered questions concerning the physiologic consequences, to both mother and fetus, of the prolonged support of those organ systems most prone to failure after brain death. We will examine these questions using as a framework for our discussion the case report of a woman who delivered a surviving infant 63 days after the diagnosis of brain death was made. The focus of our discussion will be on the medical and perinatal issues illustrated by the case, rather than the moral, ethical, and economic questions that contribute to much of the controversy.

A CASE REPORT

On January 25, 1983, a previously healthy 27-year-old gravida 1, para 0 Caucasian female presented to her local hospital at 22 weeks gestation with a 5-day history of worsening headaches followed by several hours of vomiting and disorientation. Physical examination was consistent with a 22-week gestation and was otherwise unremarkable with normal vital signs and no focal neurologic deficits noted. A lumbar puncture was normal except for a slightly elevated opening pressure of 20 cm of water and the presence of 4 segmented neutrophils per cubic millimeter of cerebral spinal fluid. Four hours after presentation, the patient had a generalized seizure and a respiratory arrest.

After cardiopulmonary resuscitation, the patient was placed on a ventilator in the intensive care unit (ICU), where examination revealed no response to painful stimuli, fixed and dilated pupils, papilledema, and absent doll's eye movements. Computed tomography (CT) of the head showed marked dilatation of the lateral and third ventricles with a mass obstructing the fourth ventricle. A ventriculostomy was placed and revealed clear cerebrospinal fluid, which had an opening pressure of 50 cm of water. Dexamethasone and mannitol were given, but the electroencephalogram was again isoelectric 2 days later. There was no change in the patient's condition, and a diagnosis of brain death was made at that time using the Harvard criteria.[9]

During this period the fetal heart rate pattern remained normal. In accordance with the strongly expressed wishes of the father, a decision was made to provide maximum cardiorespiratory support to the mother in an attempt to maintain the fetus in utero until a gestational age compatible with fetal viability was reached.

Bilateral patchy pulmonary infiltrates, consistent with adult respiratory distress syndrome (ARDS), soon appeared radiographically. Diabetes insipidus developed, which required injections of vasopressin to control the massive diuresis and hypernatremia. Trimethoprim with sulfamethoxazole was given to treat a *Klebsiella* urinary tract infection. Total parenteral nutrition (TPN) was begun, providing 1500 kcal per day, and the patient was transfused 2 units of packed red blood cells. She was transferred to the University of California at San Francisco (UCSF) Moffitt Hospital on the 14th day of her hospitalization at 24 weeks gestation.

On admission at UCSF, the patient had a temperature of 38.9 °C, and the neurologic examination was consistent with the diagnosis of brain death. The uterine fundus measured 23 cm, and a sonogram revealed a vigorous fetus with anthropometric criteria consistent with 24 weeks gestation. Full ventilatory support was continued and modulated on the basis of frequent arterial blood gas determinations. Maximum effort was directed at treating the severe hypotension, temperature fluctuations, diabetes insipidus, hypothyroidism, and cortisol deficiency that were thought to be the result of loss of the autoregulatory function of the brain. The hypotension responded to plasma expanders and a combination of vasopressors. Heating and cooling blankets stabilized the temperature. A vasopressin infusion alleviated the signs of diabetes insipidus, and both thyroxin and cortisol were administered in normal replacement doses.

A trial of nasogastric feedings failed. Therefore, TPN was restarted and maintained at a rate that supplied 2250 kcal a day. On this regimen, hyperglycemia developed and was treated with a continuous insulin infusion. Nutritional assessments revealed that the patient was in positive nitrogen balance and the serum albumin rose from 2.5 to 3.1 gm/dl during the hospitalization. Fetal heart tones were monitored every shift, and serial obstetric sonograms were performed. After 26 weeks gestation, weekly betamethasone injections (12 mg every 12 hours for 2 doses) were given, and nonstress tests (NST) were performed twice a week.

On the 28th day of hospitalization enterococcal bacteremia developed, which was initially treated with ampicillin and gentamycin. This regimen was changed to piperacillin after the sensitivities were reported, and the bacteremia resolved. However, a *Staphylococcus aureus* bacteremia developed on the 58th day of hospitalization, and was treated with nafcillin. During the course of that treatment, a repeat sonogram showed no evidence of fetal growth over the previous 2 weeks. Because of the suspected intrauterine fetal growth retardation and recurrent septicemia, a decision was made to deliver the fetus by cesarean section on the 63rd hospital day at 31 weeks gestation. A 1440-g male infant with Apgar scores of 8 at 1 and 5 minutes was delivered on March 29, 1983. Maternal ventilatory support was discontinued postoperatively, and cardiac activity ceased shortly thereafter.

The infant was cared for in the neonatal ICU where he developed mild respiratory distress syndrome. However, he generally did well and was transferred to a hospital nearer his home at 3 weeks of age. On follow-up examination at 48 months of age, he was found to be growing and developing normally.

DISCUSSION

Brain death can be diagnosed using several sets of guidelines,[3,4,32] the most frequently used being the Harvard criteria.[9] All of these diagnostic guidelines have in common the documentation of absolute and incontrovertible cessation of total brain function. Brain death is thus clearly delineated from other states of profoundly decreased brain function in which supportive care to preserve vital functions is also required. The most severe of these other conditions, variously called cerebral death,[32] persistent vegetative state,[29] or the apallic syndrome,[26] is characterized by a loss of cerebral and other supratentorial functions with retention of at least some brain-stem function. This residual brain-stem function allows patients, with the proper ventilatory support, to sometimes survive for years. Brain death, in which the entire brain is destroyed as surely as if decapitation had occurred, is distinctly different from cerebral death. The preservation of vital functions, even with the most intensive care, is said to never last for more than 14 days after brain death.[28]

Somatic survival after brain death is not a natural event. It represents the culmination of the impressive advances in medical knowledge, skills, and technology as applied to life-support strategies in critical care medicine. The use of such resources on a person already declared dead, however, has previously been advocated only for relatively short periods of time to preserve viable organs for transplantation.[5,23,41] The longer term sequelae of such support is unknown. Nevertheless, several reviews have examined the fate of patients receiving maximum supportive care who retrospectively fit the criteria of brain death. These surveys conclude that cardiopulmonary respiratory function can, on the average, be maintained for only a few days after brain death.[4,14,27,28,32] In their series of over 1200 brain-dead patients, Jennett and Hessett[28] were unable to find a single case of brain death with cardiac survival beyond 14 days. One case has subsequently appeared in the literature in which a regular heart rate persisted in a 49-year-old man for 68 days after the criteria for brain death were satisfied.[37] To our knowledge this is the only reported instance in which somatic survival was preserved for longer than 2 weeks after the diagnosis of brain death was made. It is possible that this lack of prolonged somatic survival is due as much to the prognostic futility of maintaining cardiorespiratory support in a brain-dead patient as it is to any inherent technical difficulty in maintaining such support.

Brain death complicating pregnancy is one instance in which prolonged maternal cardiorespiratory support might be justified for fetal indications. Ours is the second reported case in which this was undertaken with successful neonatal results and represents, by far, the longest time that a mother has received such support. Dillon and colleagues[12] reported two cases of pregnancy complicated by maternal brain death. In their first case, however, the mother was at 18 weeks gestation, and although the procedures for documenting brain death were not fully carried out, they decided to stop life support. Their second case is more applicable to our discussion since brain death was diagnosed at 25 weeks gestation, and the maternal vital functions were maintained for 7 days until maternal hypotension associated with variable fetal heart rate decelerations prompted the delivery of a surviving 930-g infant.

Dillon and associates[12] suggested a management plan for these patients based on the neonatal survival statistics in their nursery,[11] economic considerations, and lack of evidence that support could prolong somatic life for more than a couple of weeks after brain death. They recommend that when maternal brain death occurs before 24 weeks gestation, no extraordinary measures should be undertaken for either mother or fetus; when it occurs after 28 weeks, delivery by cesarean section should be done as soon as possible; and when brain death occurs between 24 and 27 weeks gestation, life-support measures should be started with immediate delivery reserved for instances of fetal distress or significant maternal deterioration. In contrast to these recommendations, our case demonstrates that stable somatic survival can sometimes be maintained for months, and in these instances the pregnancy might safely be allowed to continue past 28 weeks gestation.

The management of our patient required the cooperative teamwork of health care professionals from a variety of specialties. None of these specialists, however, had experience with similar cases, and there was a paucity of information in the literature regarding the complications to be expected from such prolonged somatic survival. As we faced these problems and attempted to evaluate the impact of our therapeutic regimens on the fetus, we extrapolated information from knowledge gained in the management of isolated organ system failure during pregnancy. That knowledge was incorporated into a coherent plan directed at maintaining an optimum environment for the developing fetus. The following discussion will focus on the fetal ramifications of supporting those systems that fail after maternal brain death. The discussion is not intended to be a comprehensive review of the principles of critical care medicine, but rather a means of addressing the unique implications that supportive care of a brain-dead mother might have on her fetus.

FETAL CARE FOLLOWING MATERNAL BRAIN DEATH

Respiratory Support

The respiratory center, located in the brain stem, has two main parts: the medullary center, which is responsible for the initiation and maintenance of spontaneous respiration, and the pneumotaxic center in the pons, which helps coordinate cyclic respirations. Since both of these areas cease to function with brain death, cessation of spontaneous respirations is a prerequisite for the diagnosis.[28] Thus, brain-dead patients are always maintained on mechanical ventilators. The general principles involved in the ventilator adjustments are the same as for any patient with respiratory failure. During pregnancy, however, there are some differences in the respiratory physiology that affect ventilatory care and deserve mention (Table 10-1).

Pregnancy is associated with a central, hormonally mediated increase in ventilation, leading to a chronic respiratory alkalosis. Maternal hypocarbia establishes a diffusion gra-

Table 10-1. Suggested Measures for Physiologic Support in Pregnancy Complicated by Maternal Brain Death

I. Mechanical ventilation with volume-preset ventilator
  1. Start with a tidal volume of 10 to 15 cc/kg, a respiratory rate of 10 to 12 breaths per minute, and a FIO_2 of 1. Make subsequent ventilator adjustments on the basis of arterial blood gas determinations.
  2. Decrease the FIO_2 to less than 0.6 while maintaining the arterial oxygen saturation at 90%.
  3. Adjust the respiratory rate to maintain the $PaCO_2$ at 28–32 mm Hg.
  4. If the PaO_2 is below 60 mm Hg on an FIO_2 of greater than 0.5, add PEEP by starting at 3–5 cm H_2O and titrating upwards until the oxygenation improves or the cardiac output declines.
II. Vasopressors to treat fluid-resistant hypotension
  1. Start with a continuous intravenous infusion of dopamine (2–5 µg/kg/minute) and titrate upward until a mean arterial pressure (MAP) of 80–110 mm Hg is obtained.
  2. If the desired MAP is not achieved at dopamine infusion rates of 12–15 µg/kg/minute, add dobutamine at continuous infusion rates of 2.5–15 µg/kg/minute.
III. Warming or cooling blankets to treat temperature lability
IV. Nutritional support using enteral tube feedings or TPN
  1. Maintain daily caloric intake of 30–35 kcal/kg ideal body weight
  2. Treat hyperglycemia with insulin
V. Treat endocrine abnormalities with replacement hormones
  1. Vasopressin
  2. Thyroxin
  3. Corticosteroids
VI. Aggressive surveillance for and treatment of infections
VII. Heparin prophylaxis

dient across the placenta that facilitates the elimination of carbon dioxide from the fetus. Because of this, maternal carbon dioxide tensions should be maintained in the normal pregnancy range of 28 to 32 mm Hg, rather than 38 to 45 mm Hg seen in normal nonpregnant patients.[48] The respiratory rate is the major determinant of carbon dioxide levels in the mother, and the rate should be adjusted in the ventilated patient to achieve the desired level. The use of controlled hyperventilation to maintain a degree of hypocarbia has long been advocated as a standard measure of brain-oriented life support of comatose patients because it decreases intracranial pressure, counteracts cerebral acidosis, and improves intracerebral blood flow distribution.[39] However, once brain death has occurred, the brain, by definition, is irretrievably lost, and moderate controlled hyperventilation is only being advocated in this instance to enhance the intrauterine milieu.

Nevertheless, using hyperventilation to decrease the maternal $PaCO_2$ to levels below 30 mm Hg for prolonged periods has been shown in lambs to cause marked reductions in placental perfusion,[33] and this degree of hypocarbia should be avoided. By maintaining a small degree of hypocarbia there will be a compensatory renal bicarbonate loss resulting in a serum level of 18 to 21 mEq/liter (normal 24 to 30 mEq/liter), while *p*H is maintained in the normal range of 7.40 to 7.45. This compensatory respiratory alkalosis approximates that seen in normal pregnancy.

Some patients who suffer brain death on the basis of severe head trauma will quickly develop neurogenic pulmonary edema. This is felt to result from a centrally mediated, massive, sympathetic discharge which produces transient systemic and pulmonary vascular hypertension. The patient is left with abnormal permeability of the pulmonary capillaries, leading to pulmonary edema in the face of normal hemodynamics and cardiac function.[46] In our case report, the patient had a clinical picture consistent with the diagnosis of ARDS. Whether this ARDS was truly neurogenic or secondary to a hypoxia insult occurring during her initial resuscitation becomes a moot point. The use of positive end-expiratory pressure (PEEP), beginning at 5 cm H_2O and titrating upwards until the respiratory parameters improve or until the cardiac output declines, is beneficial in this situation. The ventilator-perfusion relationships improve with PEEP, and the inspired oxygen concentrations required to maintain the arterial saturation above 90% can be reduced.[19] The effect of prolonged high levels of FiO_2 on the fetus are unknown, but evidence suggests that an FiO_2 of 0.5 can be administered indefinitely without adverse effects on the mother or, presumably, the fetus.[49]

Cardiovascular Support

Cardiac activity is usually determined by the dynamic balance between the two components of the autonomic nervous system. The nucleus of the vagus nerve is located in the medulla, and in cases of brain death there is a subsequent complete cessation of vagal activity. On the other hand, the nuclei which operate the sympathetic nervous system are located in the spinal cord, and they survive. Thus, cardiac activity after brain death would seem to be determined by the sympathetic system alone, and the existence of spinal reflex circuits without any cerebral influence has been demonstrated in these patients.[35] However, in brain-dead patients whose electrocardiograms were analyzed, tachycardia was reported in less than half and then only during the initial phase of brain death.[14] Subsequent slowing of the heart rate was noted in all of these patients, suggesting that additional influences, such as hypothermia or subclinical myocardial hypoxia, were counteracting the stimulatory effect of the sympathetic nervous system. It is possibly because of these influences that cardiac arrest generally occurs within a few days of brain death. In spite of maximum support, the conventional wisdom states that cardiac activity never persists for longer than 14 days after brain death.[4,14,27,28,32] Our report, as well as that of Parisi and associates,[37] disproves that dictum and suggests that, with meticulous attention to the maintenance of optimum oxygenation, perfusion, and fluid and electrolyte parameters, a "beating heart cadaver" can be maintained for months.

Experience with cardiac and renal transplant donors has demonstrated that hypotension, requiring treatment with pressor agents, develops in the vast majority of brain-dead patients.[5,23] The problem of hypotension is particularly important in pregnant women because the uterine vasculature is not an autoregulated system, and maternal hypotension will severely decrease uteroplacental blood flow.[22] Therefore, control of maternal hypotension must become a major area of emphasis in these patients. The development of diabetes insipidus, with its attendant intravascular volume contraction, can complicate the differentiation between hypovolemia and loss of central autoregulation as the cause of the hypotension. We therefore recommend the determination of central venous pressures as an important aid in the management of the fluid status. If pulmonary edema develops, we strongly recommend that a Swan-Ganz catheter be used to differentiate cardiogenic pulmonary edema from ARDS and to guide fluid therapy. Once fluid-resistant hypotension is documented, the hypotension should be aggressively treated pharmacologically. The use of vasopressors requires that an arterial line be inserted to continuously monitor blood pressure.

Because of its unique pharmacologic properties, low-dose dopamine was chosen as the initial agent for treating the hypotension. In low doses, dopamine has a weak betamimetic effect on the heart, increasing contractility and heart rate without increasing myocardial oxygen consumption disproportionately. It also stimulates dopaminergic receptors in the renal, mesenteric, and coronary vasculature causing vasodilatation. Unlike pure beta stimulants, dopamine causes vasoconstriction of skeletal muscle, so while its net effect is to elevate blood pressure, the renal and splanchnic blood flows are preserved.[21]

These actions of dopamine are dose-dependent. In doses exceeding 15 to 20 µg/kg/minute, the principle effect is on alpha receptors, resulting in the same generalized vasoconstriction seen with such conventional vasopressors as metaraminol and ephedrine. This effect would be detrimental for the fetus since the uterine vascular bed is also capable of alpha-adrenergic–induced vasoconstriction, which results in decreased placental perfusion.[22] Dopamine, therefore, needs to be administered by continuous intravenous infusion starting at 2 to 5 µg/kg/minute and titrating upward to achieve the desired hemodynamic effect. If that effect is not seen by the time infusion rates approach 12 to 15 µg/kg/minute, we recommend adding dobutamine (see Table 10-1).

Dobutamine is a sympathomimetic amine which has major cardiac beta-1-adrenergic activity with minor beta-2- and alpha-adrenergic activity. Like dopamine it should be given by intravenous infusion, and it also appears to have a biphasic effect on peripheral blood vessels with low doses (5 µg/kg/minute) causing some increase in tone with higher doses (30 µg/kg/minute) induce muscle relaxation.[26] Dobutamine has the ability to improve ventricular contractility without markedly increasing heart rate or dilating resistance vessels, which suggests that in low doses it is a useful adjunctive measure for the control of hypotension in this setting.

The endocrine problems caused by the development of panhypopituitarism contributed to the hypotension in our patient. The most prominent of these was diabetes insipidus, a condition developing in the majority of brain-dead patients who are maintained for more than a few days.[36] In this condition, the massive polyuria and resultant hypernatremia can generally be controlled by giving vasopressin, either intramuscularly or by intravenous infusion, and by using Swan-Ganz monitoring parameters to guide fluid replacement.[5] Hypotension is also associated with secondary adrenocortical insufficiency, which should be anticipated in these patients and treated with replacement doses of corticosteroids if found.

Finally, the mother should always be maintained in a lateral or lateral tilting position to avoid the supine hypotensive effects of the gravid uterus pressing on the great vessels. The importance of this is emphasized by the case report of maternal survival after "postmortem" cesarean section emptied the uterus and allowed effective blood flow to return.[10]

By using fluid resuscitation, invasive hemodynamic monitoring, aggressive pharmacologic support, hormonal replacement therapy, and optimal maternal positioning, hypotension was effectively treated in our patient and the mean arterial pressures were maintained in a range felt to ensure optimal uteroplacental perfusion pressures.

Temperature Lability

Because of the loss of the hypothalamic thermoregulatory mechanism, the normal diurnal fluctuations of body temperature are characteristically absent in brain death. Poikilothermia is the condition in which the body temperature tends to follow that of the environment because there is no thermoregulatory mechanism. In Jorgensen's study,[30] poikilothermia was a constant finding when somatic survival was maintained for more than 24 hours. Although a minority of his patients demonstrated initial hyperthermia, all of these had final asystole within 24 hours. Thus, hypothermia seems to be the predominant manifestation of the loss of thermoregulation in brain-dead patients with prolonged somatic survival, unless specific steps are taken to prevent it. Although a mild degree of hypothermia may be beneficial for preserving organs in a satisfactory condition prior to removal for transplantation, ventricular fibrillation can occur at temperatures below 30° C.[5]

Prolonged maternal hypothermia is not a situation often encountered in clinical practice, and its effect on the fetus is unknown. The fetus normally depends on passive thermoregulation by heat exchange occurring with the mother's blood at the intervillus space. Our knowledge concerning the degree of active thermoregulation present in the fetus is limited. However, Gluckman and co-workers[20] have shown that the fetal lamb responds to cooling with shivering, and that cooling cutaneous thermoreceptors on the fetus can alter fetal electrocortical activity and breathing patterns. This suggests a deleterious state, since fetal energy utilization would be directed away from the primary process of growth and development during hypothermia. We therefore recommend vigilance in maintaining normal maternal temperature by using warming blankets and warm, inspired humidified air.

Though rarely seen during prolonged support after brain death, our patient also had periods of hyperthermia. After an infectious process had been ruled out, we felt that the hyperthermia was a further reflection of poikilothermia in this patient with an internal autonomous heat generator, the metabolically active fetus. In regard to the deleterious effects of prolonged maternal hyperthermia on the fetus suggested by previous studies,[15,44] we also recommend the use of cooling blankets as needed to maintain the maternal core temperature in the normal range.

Nutritional Support

Our patient had been in a state of good nutritional balance prior to her intracranial catastrophe, and she had no intrinsic gastrointestinal pathology. Since her bowel sounds were present on admission to our unit, she was begun on enteral tube feedings with the aim of providing 2400 kcal per day. Sampson and Peterson[40] had previously reported the case of a pregnant patient in a post-traumatic vegetative state who was maintained on nasogastric feedings for 7 months before she delivered an adequately grown infant at 33 weeks gestation. Smith and colleagues[43] also reported that successful experience with the use of long-term enteral hyperalimentation in two pregnant diabetics with hyperemesis gravidarum. In our patient, however, the plan to provide enteral nutrition through a nasogastric tube was thwarted due to the poor motility of her gastrointestinal tract. This poor motility was reflected by large gastric residuals and reflux regurgitation in spite of the feeding tube being passed through the pylorus into the duodenum. Therefore, TPN was initiated through a subclavian vein.

There are a number of reports of TPN being used during pregnancies complicated by a variety of disorders.[8,25,34,38,47] The use of TPN during pregnancy has been shown to be beneficial as judged by the criteria of maintenance of a positive nitrogen balance, maternal weight gain, and normal fetal growth as reflected by sonographic measurements and birth weight.[43] However, there are major risks of TPN, including hyperglycemia, sepsis, and complications resulting from central line placement. Hyperglycemia is a common complication in any patient receiving TPN, but seems especially prone to occur when TPN is given during pregnancy, a condition which is itself inherently diabetogenic. If not controlled, maternal hyperglycemia will stimulate fetal insulin as well as human placental lactogen production and result in increased fetal fat storage. In theory the fetus could then develop a syndrome similar to that seen in infants of diabetic mothers. Therefore, when maternal hyperglycemia appears during TPN, we recommend aggressive treatment with a continuous insulin infusion to maintain euglycemia.

We calculated the patient's daily caloric needs to be 2250 kcal, based on the recommendation of 30 to 35 kcal/kg/day of ideal body weight.[7] These daily calories were given in the form of a fat emulsion (500 kcal), 100 g of protein (400 kcal), and a 20% dextrose solution which supplied the rest of the calculated caloric requirement. Heller,[24] in studying TPN in pregnant rats receiving 50% of their caloric intake as fat, concluded that there is a risk of fatty infiltration of the placenta if parenteral fat emulsions are used during pregnancy. However, this complication has not been seen in the clinical use of commercial fat emulsions supplying up to 20% of daily caloric requirements during pregnancy. We therefore recommend that moderate amounts of fat emulsion be added to the TPN solutions used during pregnancy, not only to prevent maternal essential fatty acid deficiency but also to provide linoleic acid for the fetus. By using this regimen, our patient's nutritional status was judged to be adequate on the basis of positive nitrogen balance tests, a 16-kg weight gain, and a rise in her serum albumin to normal pregnant levels. However, there was sonographic evidence of intrauterine growth retardation after 28 weeks, which was one of the factors that prompted delivery.

Miscellaneous Medical Problems

In addition to diabetes insipidus and secondary adrenal insufficiency, the patient's panhypopituitarism was evidenced by secondary hypothyroidism requiring physiologic replacement doses of 1-thyroxin. By aggressively treating hypotension, perfusion of the kidneys was maintained, and the renal function remained normal throughout the course. Because of the increased risk of thrombosis associated with prolonged bed rest in the absence of any muscle tone, prophylactic heparin was given subcutaneously in doses of 5000 units every 12 hours.

Intensive infection control precautions had to be an integral part of the patient's care. She remained continuously at high risk for septicemia being on a mechanical ventilator, receiving TPN, and having a Swan-Ganz catheter, as well as a urinary catheter and an arterial line, in place. Since she had lost the ability to demonstrate many of the signs of infection, because of her poikilothermy and hypotensive state, infection surveillance consisted of maintaining a constant high suspicion and using frequent blood, urine, and sputum cultures as a screen for pathogenic organisms. Bladder and respiratory colonizations were aggressively treated. Great care was exercised in maintaining strict asepsis in handling the intravenous lines, and these lines were changed regularly. Finally, the importance of expert, dedicated nursing care in the overall management of this case cannot be overstated.

OBSTETRIC STRATEGIES

The premise, when we began, was that by artificially supporting the maternal vital functions we could maintain an intrauterine environment that was at least adequate for allowing the fetus to develop in utero until it had reached a gestational age compatible with a chance of extrauterine survival. A UCSF, 28 weeks gestation is associated with a greater than 80% chance of neonatal survival. The attainment of this gestational age was our initial goal. However, the care of a 28-week neonate in the ICU Nursery is itself a costly and precarious proposition, which becomes less so with each subsequent week of gestation.[31] We, therefore, decided to prolong our maternal support until 34 weeks gestation, as long as there were no indications of maternal or fetal deterioration. (This strategy is at odds with the guidelines proposed by Dillon and colleagues[12].)

The determination of that gestational age at which it becomes reasonable to intervene for fetal indications is always a difficult process for the obstetrician. Usually the fetal benefits, measured in the chance of good quality survival, must be weighed against the risks to the mother during operative delivery. Since a postmortem cesarean section entailed no additional risk to the mother, at 26 weeks gestation we were prepared to intervene for fetal indications if there was any significant deterioration in the mother's physiologic parameters. As recommended by others, the mode of delivery was to be by classical cesarean section to provide the most expeditious and least traumatic birth for the fetus.[1] A surgical kit was kept at the patient's bedside, and standing orders were made to increase the mother's inspired oxygen to 100% at the first sign of acute maternal deterioration. Informed consent was obtained from the father who was in complete agreement with this plan.

Our primary means of providing the most beneficial intrauterine environment for the fetus was to ensure that the various maternal physiologic parameters we were following were as close to normal as possible. However, it would be naive to presume that we could, even with our sophisticated supportive and monitoring techniques, maintain an intrauterine environment as conducive to fetal growth and development as the one present in an otherwise healthy gravida. Because of this, at 27 weeks gestation we instituted the same strategy of aggressive fetal surveillance that we would use in any extremely high-risk pregnancy. Although the usefulness of antepartum fetal heart rate monitoring at that gestational age has been questioned,[6,45] there is evidence of its predictability between 27 and 30 weeks gestation.[2,18] We therefore used a regimen of twice weekly NSTs, with oxytocin challenge tests reserved for use if the NST was suspicious or nonreactive.[16,17] Ultrasound examinations were performed every two weeks to document adequate fetal growth. It was, finally, the lack of fetal growth during the last 2½ weeks of the pregnancy, coupled with recurrent maternal sepsis, which prompted us to deliver the baby.

The economic costs of the total care rendered were considerable. The charges for the maternal care totaled $183,081, and the cost of the neonatal care was $34,703. However, the total cost of $217,784 must be put in the perspective of the spiralling costs of care for other advanced procedures such as heart transplantations. Whether these procedures are justified on an economic basis is something society will have to decide. Rather than proposing rigid guidelines, we feel that when these rare cases appear, the decision of whether or not to proceed with prolonged cardiorespiratory support should be based on the particulars of each individual case. In obtaining informed consent from the family of a brain-dead mother, it is important to be able to prognosticate as much as possible concerning the medical problems and fetal issues such prolonged support entails.

REFERENCES

1. Arthur RK: Postmortem cesarean section. Am J Obstet Gynecol 132:175, 1978
2. Barrett JM, Salyer SL, Boehm FM: The nonstress test: An evaluation of 1000 patients. Am J Obstet Gynecol 141:153, 1981
3. Bernat JL, Culver CM, Gert B: On the definition and criterion of death. Ann Intern Med 94:389, 1981
4. Black PM: Brain death. N Engl J Med 299:338, 393, 1978
5. Cooper DKC, DeVilliers JC, Smith LS et al: Medical, legal, and administrative aspects of cadaveric organ donation in the RSA. S Afr Med J 62;933, 1982
6. Cooper JM, Soffronoff EC, Bolognese RJ: Oxytocin challenge test in monitoring high risk pregnancies. Obstet Gynecol 45:27, 1975
7. Coustan DR, Lewis SB: Clinical approaches to diabetes in pregnancy. Contemp Obstet Gynecol 7:27, 1976
8. Cox K: Home TPN during pregnancy: A case report. J Parenter Enteral Nutr 5:246, 1981
9. A definition of irreversible coma: Report of the Ad Hoc Committee of the Harvard Medical School to examine the definition of brain death. J Am Med Assoc 205:337, 1968
10. DePace NL, Betesh JS, Kotler MN: "Postmortem" cesarean section with recovery of both mother and offspring. J Am Med Assoc 248:971, 1982
11. Dillon WP, Egan EA: Aggressive obstetrical management in late second trimester deliveries. Obstet Gynecol 58:685, 1981
12. Dillon WP, Lee RV, Tronolone MJ et al: Life support and maternal brain death during pregnancy. J Am Med Assoc 248:1089, 1982
13. Dollery CT, Follath F, Lewis GRJ: Cardiovascular effects of dobutamine. Br J Clin Pharmacol 2:182P, 1975
14. Drory Y, Quaknin G, Kosary IZ, Kellerman JJ: Electrocardiographic findings in brain death: Description and presumed mechanism. Chest 67:425, 1975
15. Edwards MJ, Wanner RA: Extremes of temperature. In Wilson JG, Fraser FC (eds): Handbook of Teratology, vol 1, p 421. New York, Plenum Press, 1977
16. Evertson LR, Gauthier RJ, Schifrin BS, Paul RH: Antepartum fetal heart rate testing: 1. Evolution of the nonstress test. Am J Obstet Gynecol 133:29, 1979
17. Freeman RK: The use of the oxytocin challenge test for antepartum clinical evaluation of uteroplacental respiratory function. Am J Obstet Gynecol 121:481, 1975
18. Gabbe SG, Freeman RD, Goebelsman U: Evaluation of the contraction stress test before 33 weeks gestation. Obstet Gynecol 52:649, 1978
19. Gallagher TJ, Civette JM, Kirby RR: Terminol-

ogy update: Optimal PEEP. Crit Care Med 6:323, 1978
20. Gluckman PD, Gunn TR, Johnson BM: The effect of cooling on breathing and shivering in unanesthetized fetal lambs in utero. J Physiol 343:495, 1983
21. Goldberg LI: Dopamine—Clinical uses of an endogenous catecholamine. N Engl J Med 291:707, 1974
22. Greiss F Jr: Concepts of uterine blood flow. Obstet Gynecol Annu 2:55, 1973
23. Griepp RB, Stinson EB, Clark DA et al: The cardiac donor. Surg Gynecol Obstet 133:792, 1971
24. Heller L: Clinical and experimental studies in complete parenteral nutrition. Scand J Gastroenterol (Suppl) 4:4, 1968
25. Hew IR, Dutel M: Total parenteral nutrition in gynecology and obstetrics. Obstet Gynecol 55:464, 1980
26. Ingvar DH, Brun A, Johansson L, Samuelsson SM: Survival after severe cerebral anoxia with destruction of the cerebral cortex: The appallic syndrome. Ann NY Acad Sci 315:184, 1978
27. Jennett B, Gleave J, Wilson P: Brain death in three neurosurgical units. Br Med J 282:533, 1981
28. Jennett B, Hessett C: Brain death in Britain as reflected in renal donors. Br Med J 283:359, 1981
29. Jennett B, Plum F: Persistent vegetative state after brain damage. Lancet (April 1):734, 1972
30. Jorgenson EO: Spinal man after brain death. Acta Neurochir 28:259, 1973
31. Kirkley WH: Fetal survival—What price. Am J Obstet Gynecol 137:873, 1980
32. Korein J: The problem of brain death: Development and history. Ann NY Acad Sci 315:19, 1978
33. Levinson G, Shnider SM, deLorimier AA, Stefanson JL: Effects of maternal hyperventilation on the uterine blood flow and fetal oxygenation and acid base status. Anesthesiology 40:340, 1974
34. Main AH: Intravenous feeding to sustain pregnancy in a patient with Crohn's disease. Br Med J 283:1221, 1981
35. Malliani D, Peterson DF, Bishop VS, Brown AM: Spinal sympathetic cardio-cardiac reflexes. Circ Res 30:158, 1972
36. Outwater KM, Rockoff MA: Diabetes insipidus accompanying brain death in children. Neurology 34:1243, 1984
37. Parisi JE, Kim RC, Collins GH, Hilfinger MF: Brain death with prolonged somatic survival. N Engl J Med 306:14, 1982
38. Rivera-Alsina ME, Saldana LR, Stringer CA: Fetal growth sustained by parenteral nutrition in pregnancy. Obstet Gynecol 64:138, 1984
39. Safar P: Brain resuscitation. In Tinker J, Rapin M (eds): Care of the Critically Ill Patient, p 751. Berlin, Springer-Verlag, 1983
40. Sampson MB, Peterson LP: Post-traumatic coma during pregnancy. Obstet Gynecol 53:2s, 1979
41. The shortage of organs for clinical transplantation: Document for discussion by the British Transplantation Society. Br Med J (Feb 1):251, 1975
42. Siegler M, Wilker D: Editorial: Brain death and live birth. J Am Med Assoc 248:1101, 1982
43. Smith CV, Rufleth P, Phelan JP, Nelson KJ: Long term enteral hyperalimentation in the pregnant woman with insulin-dependent diabetes. Am J Obstet Gynecol 141:180, 1981
44. Smith SW, Clarren SK, Harvey MAS: Hyperthermia as a possible teratogenic agent. J Pediatr 92:878, 1978
45. Sorokin Y, Dierker LJ, Pillay SK et al: The association between fetal heart rate patterns and fetal movement in pregnancies between 20 and 30 weeks gestation. Am J Obstet Gynecol 143:243, 1982
46. Theodore J, Robin ED: Pathogenesis of neurogenic pulmonary edema. Lancet (Oct 18):749, 1975
47. Webb GA: The use of hyperalimentation and chemotherapy in pregnancy: A case report. Am J Obstet Gynecol 137:263, 1980
48. Weinberger SE, Weiss ST, Cohen WR et al: Pregnancy and the lung. Am Rev Respir Dis 121:559, 1980
49. Winter PM, Smith G: The toxicity of oxygen. Anesthesiology 37:210, 1972

SECTION 2: Legal Issues

Philip Reilly

A CASE STUDY

On June 27, 1986, Donna Piazzi was admitted to University Hospital in Augusta, Georgia. The young woman was comatose, apparently due to a drug overdose. Her condition deteriorated, and by mid-July she was brain dead. She was also pregnant.

On July 16, after being informed that his wife was brain dead, Robert Piazzi asked hospital officials to turn off her respirator. But David Hadden, claiming to be the father of the unborn child, asked them to maintain all necessary life-support systems in order to nurture the developing fetus. University Health Services, Incorporated, which operates University Hospital, filed a petition for declaratory relief, asking for resolution of "the rights and relations of the parties and, in particular, an order that life-support systems be maintained to give the unborn child of Donna Piazzi the opportunity to develop and be delivered."[14] The court appointed a guardian ad litem for the fetus and a hearing was held on July 25. In addition to Robert Piazzi, David Hadden, and the guardian ad litem, the Division of Family and Children Services of the Georgia Department of Human Resources was also named as a respondent.

Neither the husband nor the self-declared father testified at the hearing. The court heard testimony from a gynecologist who described the developmental status of the 20-week fetus and stated that it was 4 weeks short of the earliest point at which physicians considered a fetus to be capable of life outside the womb. A neurologist testified that there was no clinical means available to assess the neurologic status of the fetus (presumably, including whether or not the drug overdose and Donna's subsequent clinical course had compromised fetal brain development). The hearing, including the oral arguments, lasted only 45 minutes.[4] On August 4, Superior Court Judge William H. Fleming ordered that "life support systems for Donna Piazzi be maintained."

The Opinion

The court made several findings of fact, of which the crucial ones pertained to the fetus. It found that the fetus had "quickened," that there was a reasonable possibility that "with continued life support Donna Piazzi's *body* (emphasis added) can remain functioning until the point that the fetus would be viable and could be delivered with a reasonable possibility of survival," that "if the fetus is delivered and survives there is a possibility it will suffer from abnormalities such as mental retardation, but it was and is impossible to determine the existence of such abnormalities prior to birth," and that "(t)here also exists a reasonable possibility that the child, if it survives, will be normal."[14]

In framing the legal issues before it, the Court formulated two questions: (1) whether it had "jurisdiction to decide a dispute involving the maintenance of a non-viable fetus," and (2) whether, assuming jurisdiction, it "should order that life support systems be maintained in order to give the fetus the opportunity to develop and be delivered." The Division of Family and Children Services argued that the right to privacy articulated in *Roe v. Wade*[12] precluded judicial action to protect a nonviable fetus. The court, noting that the mother was dead (Georgia has a brain death law), opined that her privacy rights were no longer "a factor". It further noted that *Roe v. Wade* expressly recognized the state's interest in protecting potential life, and took jurisdiction.[14]

Reviewing Georgia common and statutory law, the court found that there was a public policy that favored "protecting life." But, it cited only two Georgia decisions: a decision by the Supreme Court not to stay a lower court order requiring the mother of a viable fetus to undergo a cesarean section (a procedure she opposed on religious grounds),[8] and a decision limiting the right of family members "to terminate life" unless the patient is terminally ill *and* in a chronic vegetative state without hope of recovery.[7] Turning to the statutes, the court noted that when it enacted a "living will" law, the legislature precluded its use by pregnant individuals. It also noted that in Georgia the killing of a quickened fetus was a crime. It concluded that "public policy in Georgia *requires* (emphasis added) the maintenance of life support systems for a brain-dead mother so long as there exists a reasonable possibility that the fetus may develop and survive."[14]

The Outcome

On August 14, 10 days after the court issued its order, physicians performed a cesarean section when the fetal heart rate "dropped to a critical level."[3] Two hours after the delivery of the one-pound, 1½-ounce boy, the life-support systems of the mother were disconnected. The premature infant died the next day.[2]

DISCUSSION

The Georgia Superior Court ruled that "public policy in Georgia *requires* the maintenance of life support systems for a brain-dead mother so long as there exists a reasonable possibility that the fetus may develop and survive." It also dismissed *Roe v. Wade* and its progeny as "inapplicable" because those decisions were based on the mother's right to privacy, which is extinguished at death. *Piazzi* articulates an unusually powerful formulation of the well-recognized and long-established state interest in protecting life. Read literally, it claims that when a pregnant woman is brain dead the fetus has a *right* to be nurtured and delivered regardless of gestational age at the woman's death. Although it does not explicitly so state, *Piazzi* strongly suggests that at the moment when a pregnant woman becomes brain dead the fetus acquires a right to life that has constitutional stature.[14]

The implications of this are far-reaching. I read *Piazzi* to require routine ascertainment of pregnancy in all brain-dead women who may be fertile and, in those women who are pregnant, the maintenance of life-support systems for that period of time needed by the fetus to mature for safe surgical delivery. The stated limitation of this right to those pregnancies in which the fetus has a "reasonable possibility" of survival is not particularly helpful. The only cases that definitely fall outside this limitation are those in which the fetus is determined to be anencephalic or be burdened with some other devastating malformation. *Piazzi* declines to permit the dead woman's husband or the self-declared father of the fetus to decide whether or not to continue the life-support system. In its words, there is "no case law or authority in Georgia which supports the right of *anyone* (emphasis added) other than a mother to terminate a quickened fetus that is not yet viable."[14]

Rights of Father and Family

Unfortunately, in its rush to protect fetal life, the Court failed to consider adequately the parties whose interest in the pregnancy are not extinguished by the death of the mother. I shall focus on the husband (or self-declared father), but other immediate relatives of the dead woman (children, parents, and siblings) also have an important interest. Because it does not even consider the legitimacy of a husband's interest in whether or not to maintain his dead wife's life-support system so that his child may be delivered from her, *Piazzi* is analytically flawed and incomprehensibly cruel. Contrary to what *Piazzi* suggests, there *is* commentary in the case law to assist us in weighing the interest of the husband/father upon the brain death of his pregnant wife.

In *Roe v. Wade* the Supreme Court explicitly declined to discuss the father's rights in the abortion decision. Three years later, however, in evaluating the constitutionality of a Missouri statute that regulated abortion, the high court considered a spousal consent requirement that focused its attention on the husband.[11] Although it decided that a woman's decision to undergo an abortion during her first trimester of pregnancy should not be contingent upon the husband's consent, the Court nevertheless acknowledged that it was "not unaware of the deep and proper concern that a devoted and protective husband has in his wife's pregnancy and in the growth and development of the fetus she is carrying." The Court's discussion of this problem permits one to conclude that it perceived the husband to have the second most important interest in the pregnancy.

Piazzi fails to consider that there exists an important body of case law that extends a zone of privacy around the marital relationship. For example, in a concurring opinion to a decision that forbade the State of Connecticut from preventing access by married couples to birth control devices,[6] Justice White argued that there was a realm of a family life into which the state cannot enter without substantial justification. *Griswold* stands on a corpus of earlier decisions[9,10] that recognize that the family is special and that its intimate decisions are best kept beyond the reach of state regulation. In a recent abortion decision[13] the Court cited this line of cases to argue that a constitutional promise of a certain private sphere of liberty to be kept largely beyond the reach of government "extends to women as well as to men." I would argue that it extends to men as well as to women.

Consider the perspective of the father. *Piazzi* shows no regard for the deep anguish that he might suffer during those months in which his dead wife's body remains unconsecrated. Indeed, maintenance of life-support systems in a pregnant woman after a diagnosis of brain death may violate the religious beliefs and practices of the woman or her husband. Does the court expect that he, his children, and other family members will be able to suspend their grief until a fetus reaches viability? How is he to cope with the legitimate fear that this period of anguish will conclude with the birth of a child burdened with serious neurologic deficits? And who is to bear the economic costs of this extraordinary gestation? Of course, some men would want very much to maintain life-support systems. The decision to nurture the fetus and, hopefully, raise the child surely is a loving statement about their marital relationship. The key issue is not how to decide, but the preservation of the right to choose.

Piazzi gives no indication that it considered the incalculable suffering that a woman's children might feel as they struggle to understand how their mother could be both dead and alive for the months that it took for a fetus to mature. What of elderly parents who must each day confront the image of a dead child? Is the state's interest in protecting previable fetal life really so compelling that it should be permitted to force these experiences on a family? I think not.

There are other problems. *Piazzi* removes a heart, two lungs, two kidneys, and a liver from the reach of persons who are dying from organ failure. It is no overstatement to argue that in ordering that extensive medical resources be used to nurture a previable fetus with a relatively slim chance of survival, the court may have deprived several adult patients of their only hope for survival. Nor should it be forgotten that the decision to tie up an intensive care unit bed, a respirator, and the highly skilled people needed to care for the dead woman is an act of triage. In death Donna Piazzi commandeered an intensive care unit bed for a substantial period of time. This, too, may have prevented the salvage of an unknown number of patients.

The Issue of Viability

Nor does *Piazzi* adequately consider at least one legal dilemma that it creates for physicians. Under *Piazzi* a physician who withdrew life-support systems from a brain-dead woman who was pregnant with a possibly viable fetus without first obtaining the express request to do so from her husband is theoretically liable for a wrongful death action. More than 30 states recognize the rights of patients to sue for the tortious death of a viable fetus. In situations when the pregnant woman is unmarried and the father not easily ascertainable, it is impossible to eliminate this theoretical risk. What is the physician to do?

Roe v. Wade held that it was not until the point of *viability* that the state's interest in protecting fetal life became compelling, and even then it could not proscribe abortions if they were medically indicated to preserve the life or health of the mother. Since then the Supreme Court has been asked to mediate a withering attack on *Roe v. Wade*, and its own membership has changed. In the last few years it has become clear that some Justices see little justification in using viability as a fulcrum upon which to balance competing constitutional interests. For example, Justice Sandra Day O'Connor recently pointed out that because medical advances were reducing the risks inherent in childbirth and increasing the prospects for survival of ever younger fetuses, *Roe v. Wade* was "on a collision course with itself."[1] Her further speculation that fetal viability "in the first trimester may soon be possible" is a thinly disguised hope that advances in neonatology may resolve the abortion controversy.

In a more recent case, Justice White characterized the choice of viability as the point at which the state's interest becomes compelling as "entirely arbitrary."[13] He wrote that the "substantiality of this interest is in no way dependent on the probability that the fetus may be capable of surviving outside the womb at any given point in its development," because that depends on medical factors which are "constitutionally irrelevant." He concluded that the state's interest in the fetus is as compelling before viability as after that point. Justice White apparently would approve the outcome, if not its reasoning, of *Piazzi*.

The Supreme Court has never considered a fact situation like *Piazzi* nor has it overturned *Roe v. Wade*. In a recent Supreme Court decision that rejected several provisions of a Pennsylvania law that chilled the exercise of a woman's right to obtain an abortion, Justice Harold Blackmun, writing for the majority, reminded the states that they "are not free, under the guise of protecting maternal health or *potential life*, to *intimidate women into continuing pregnancies*" (emphasis added).[13] In a sense Donna Piazzi was compelled to continue her pregnancy.

A PROPOSED SOLUTION

For as long as *Roe v. Wade* remains the law of the land, the state interest in protecting fetal life is not compelling until the point of viability. The zone of privacy which shields the intimate choices of family life from government regulation is broad enough to preclude the state from dictating how a husband should decide the issue of whether or not to maintain life-support systems for the previable fetus of his brain-dead wife. Since neither maternal life nor health is at issue in a case like *Piazzi*, the logic of *Roe v. Wade* would permit the State to intervene in favor of maximizing the chance for survival of a fetus that is viable. Given that the husband and other family members are much more affected by this choice than any other citizen, I argue that, in the absence of a statutory resolution of the question, the husband's wishes should control, even if the fetus may be viable. Situations where the fetus is clearly viable are not at issue; in such cases, prompt surgical delivery would be provided.

This resolution would balance the legitimate interests of both State and spouse and remains consistent with the holding in *Roe v. Wade*. It also has the beneficial consequence of temporally limiting the emotional burden that sustaining the dead woman would have on husband, children, and other family members.

Given the trend since *Roe v. Wade*, I imagine the following statute (which does not exhaustively address the issue) would be constitutionally valid:

> Any woman between the ages of 12 and 45 who has been determined to be brain dead must undergo ascertainment of pregnancy prior to pronouncement of death. If a licensed physician determines that she is pregnant with a *viable* fetus, that woman may not be pronounced dead and must be maintained

on appropriate life-support systems until such time as a licensed physician determines that the fetus . . . has a reasonable chance for successful surgical delivery. Immediately after the delivery, a licensed physician may pronounce the woman dead and disconnect her respirator.

If it is determined that the fetus is not viable, the husband shall have the right to decide whether or not to maintain his wife's life-support systems on behalf of the fetus.

Roe v. Wade spoke forcefully on the issue of privacy. It is, I think, not a misreading of *Roe* to suggest that the right to privacy that permits a woman to terminate a pregnancy should logically extend to the husband/father upon the wife's death.

REFERENCES

1. Akron v Akron Center for Reproductive Health, 462 US 416, 1983
2. Baby in court battle dies after one day. New York Times August 16, 1986
3. Baby is weak after birth to brain-dead woman. New York Times August 15, 1986
4. Byrd R: Judge tells hospital to keep brain-dead mother, fetus alive. Associated Press July 26, 1986
5. Eisenstadt v Baird, 405 US 439, 1972
6. Griswold v Connecticut, 381 US 479, 1965
7. In re L.H.R., 321 SE 2d 716, 1984
8. Jefferson v Griffin Spaulding County Hospital Authority, 274 SE 2d 457, 1981
9. Meyer v Nebraska, 262 US 390, 1923
10. Peirce v Society of Sisters, 268 US 510, 1925
11. Planned Parenthood of Missouri v Danforth, 428 US 52, 1976
12. Roe v Wade, 410 US 113, 1973
13. Thornburgh v American College of Obstetricians and Gynecologists, 90 L. Ed. 2d 776, 1986
14. University Health Services v Robert Piazzi et al (Sup Ct Ga No CV86-RCCV-464), 1986

SECTION 3:
Ethical Issues

Thomas A. Shannon

Since 1982 there have been at least three reported cases of pregnant women who were declared brain dead and then maintained on life-support systems until the fetus could be safely delivered. In a 1983 case in San Francisco, the fetus was maintained for 64 days. Such a possibility arises because the maintenance of physiologic functions through advanced life-support systems is not incompatible with the diagnosis of brain dead.

In this article I wish to raise and evaluate several ethical problems associated with this phenomenon. Even though there have been only three reported cases, the problems raised are critical and, if we do not begin thinking about these kinds of situations now, we may find ourselves once again with a practice that has arisen through default rather than conscious choice.

GENERAL ISSUES

For several decades now there has been a substantive discussion about the validity of brain criteria for determining whether or not an individual is dead. These discussions have culminated in the 1981 report of the President's Commission which recommends that death be defined as either an irreversible cessation of respiratory and circulatory functions or an irreversible cessation of the entire brain, including the brain stem. Such a definition is in effect in at least 37 states which have either statutory law or case law which recognizes such a definition. Thus, there is increasing coherence over the use of the concept of brain death as a standard for determining death.

The use of this standard raises several issues. The first is a psychological one, in that the person declared dead is typically on a life-support system, still breathing and with heart still beating. Although he or she is dead by virtue of the lack of brain function, nonetheless the person's bodily functions are maintained by a respirator and may not be *perceived* as totally dead.

The second problem arises from the growing practice of using a life-support system to preserve organs for donation. Having been declared brain dead, the cadaver is maintained so that the organs to be donated will retain the best physiologic quality possible. Typically the cadaver would be maintained for a day or two while the tissue typing and recipient search could be conducted.

Because of the psychological perceptions of brain death and the maintenance of cadavers on life-support systems, it is no wonder that there is some confusion about what brain death means. Many years ago the psychiatrist Willard Gaylin[1] described such an individual as a "neomort" and argued that such a maintained cadaver could be used for a variety of purposes such as research or professional training. We see another purpose being fulfilled now in the maintenance of the cadaver for organ donation.

A third general problem is the treatment of the body or a specific organ of the body as a commodity or object. Once this body was a living individual, and the cadaver still bears a relationship to that presence. Thus we need to evaluate what is appropriate care for a cadaver, especially in the new context of the capacity to maintain a cadaver through a life-support system. In speaking of the specific problem of organ transplantation, William May observed the following.

> The detached organ or member becomes, in a sense, a fit object for ridicule. It has lost its raison d'etre and therefore its centeredness. It has become an eccentricity, an embarrassment, an obscenity. It seems to have committed the indecency of refusing to vanish along with the self, while simultaneously failing effectively to remind us of what has vanished. The severence of death has been crazily compounded by a different order of severence that leaves the community charged with picking up leftovers rather than laying to rest remains. . . .

The development of a system of routine salvaging of organs would tend to fix on the hospital a second association with death—as devourer. In the course of life a breakdown in health is often accompanied by a sense that one has been exhausted and burned out by a world that has consumed all one's resources. The hospital traditionally offered a respite from a devouring world and the possibility of restoration. The healing mission of the hospital is obscured, however, if the hospital itself becomes the arch-symbol of the world that devours. Categorical salvaging of organs suggests that eventually and ultimately the process of consumption that dominates the outer world must now be consumated in the hospital. One's very vitals must be inventoried, extracted and distributed by the state on behalf of the social order. What is left over is utterly unusable husk.

> While the procedure of routine salvaging may come in the short run, furnish more organs for transplants, in the long run its systemic effect on the institutions of medical care would seem to be depressing and corrosive of that trust upon which the arts of healing depend.[2]

While these observations refer primarily to organ transplantation and speak to a proposal to harvest organs routinely, nonetheless they offer interesting insights into the case of a brain-dead pregnant woman maintained on a life-support system. One has to wonder if this may not constitute a reduction of an individual to a specific biologic function. This is where May's point becomes quite relevant. Instead of a detached organ that is the cause of embarrassment, the entire body may be a cause of embarrassment. Although the brain is dead, the body has a new status, albeit a confusing one: a living cadaver. The community may be unsure of how to react to that. Even though one could argue that saving fetal life is an important social function, one also has to recognize that such maintenance is a further extension of functionalism or objectification of the person into the heart of medical practice.

A fourth general issue is the allocation of resources. Assumedly a brain-dead pregnant woman could be maintained on a life-support system only in an intensive or acute care unit. This will require much of the hospital's physical and personnel resources, as well as careful monitoring to maintain the appropriate physiologic conditions essential to the fetus. It is an expensive and substantive use of hospital resources.

One also must raise the issue of who will bear the cost. It is unclear whether third-party payers will be willing to maintain a cadaver on life-support systems. No benefit is being derived by the cadaver, and a third-party payer may be uncomfortable reimbursing a hospital for treatment of a cadaver on behalf of a third party—of questionable social and moral status—for an extended period of time.

Some decisions need to be made at the hospital level with respect to how resources for this purpose can be allocated and on what basis. The insurance company needs to be consulted about whether or not it will pay for such a procedure and on what basis. In addition, some sort of plan needs to be devised by the hospital in the event that a higher priority arises for the use of the equipment maintaining the cadaver. By having a plan that determines when to remove the cadaver's life-support system, the hospital may be better able to save the lives of other individuals.

There are, then, four general problems that surround the discussion of a pregnant brain-dead woman:

- The confusion of perceptions about the status of a cadaver
- The maintenance of bodily functions through life-support systems
- The objectification of the body and the reduction of an individual, including the whole body, to particular biologic functions
- The allocation of resources

These issues, while considered individually, may not resolve the dilemma of brain death and pregnancy. Nonetheless they provide a frame of reference for an ultimate decision about the status of the cadaver and fetus.

THE INTERESTS OF THE MOTHER

Many cultures see childbearing as the primary function of the female and the basis for her value and status within society. It is also argued that the reduction of a woman to a biologic function is degrading and demeaning.

The maintenance of a female cadaver on a life-support system to salvage the fetus is, in effect, a reduction of the woman to her reproductive function. This is an important statement which can be read on different levels. This statement can be symbolic of a society's value of life or it can be a reduction of the female to the status of an incubator.

One of the issues that must be faced and evaluated is what implications does such maintenance of brain-dead pregnant women have for the image and status of women within our society. While it is biologically clear that women bear the child, it is also clear that the reduction of the female to only her reproductive capacity is extremely detrimental. Does a pregnant cadaver maintained on life support enhance the perception of the woman as an incubator?

A second issue is under what conditions a woman would be required to undergo heroic measures to support the life of her fetus. The issue is complicated by the fact that in this particular case the woman is dead. Generally speaking, most ethical commentators argue that no one is required to undergo heroic measures to support one's own life, let alone the life of another, for three reasons. First, extraordinary measures are recognized as transcending any moral duty we have to preserve our own life. Second, a mother is morally permitted to have surgery or take medications that, while benefiting her, directly or indirectly compromise the life of the fetus. Third, the common duty of beneficence sets limits to the duty to prevent harm to third parties (i.e., economic harm to an extant family or denial of a life-support system to a living person).

Use of a life-support system implements the technologic imperative, We can do it; therefore, we ought to do it. It is true that its capacity to maintain a cadaver as well as a fetus provides us with options otherwise unattainable. Nonetheless, this capacity needs to be evaluated in the light of the limits of beneficence and the obligation to use heroic means.

THE INTERESTS OF THE FETUS

If one approaches the fetus from the legal tradition, it is clear that the fetus has no legal rights until it is viable. And one can make a strong argument that there is no basis for requiring that the fetus be maintained until viable.

From a moral point of view, the status of the fetus is debatable, to say the least. On the right-to-life side of the spectrum, one finds a clear argument that the fetus is a human person from the moment of conception and is entitled to any and all rights that other human persons have. Within this context one would be able to make a strong argument for maintaining the cadaver's bodily functions so that the fetus can continue to enjoy its right to life. But on the other hand, even other human beings cannot make the claim that others ought to be maintained for the purpose of supporting their life. Thus, even if one would view the fetus as a full human being, I do not think that the fetus's moral status would require maintaining the cadaver on the life-support system so that it could attain viability. If the fetus's moral status is questionable, the argument for maintaining the cadaver as host is all the more difficult.

If one approaches from the pro-choice side, a range of opinions about the fetus must be considered. Most, if not all, would acknowledge that the fetus is a living member of the human species. At a relatively early point in its development, it has the capacity to experience pain; around the sixth week of its life, the fetus begins to develop measurable brain waves. Because it has a certain genetic and developmental level, many would argue that the fetus is entitled to some rights, though not all that an adult human person would have. Other opinions maintain that because the fetus is in a process of development its moral status is unclear or, in some cases, absent. A case by case evaluation has to be made with no predetermination as to whose rights may achieve priority.

If one looks at the fetus from the point of view of medical practice, one finds a variety of conflicting and perplexing situations. It is clear from developments in both gene therapy and surgery that the fetus is becoming a patient. The growing practice of in vitro fertilization and embryo transfer also recognizes the fetus as a desired entity and as having an important moral status. Based on these practices a strong argument can be made for the fetus as a patient. The next question is whether or not this patient has rights and on what basis. Does the fetus have rights because it is a patient, or does the fetus have rights because it is a person who is also a patient?

The growing accessibility of the fetus—through the externalization of conception and through surgery and other technologies—is going to add a further layer of complication to the abortion debate as well as to the debate about the moral status of the fetus. Once we recognize that the fetus is a patient simply on the basis of providing services for the fetus, we may find it more and more difficult to justify abortions. Out of medical practice we have developed a new vision of the fetus.

Finally, there is the issue of the postnatal status of the fetus. Typically a certain amount of publicity surrounds the birth of a fetus of a brain-dead woman. Even if names of individuals are not used, the possibility remains that such an infant's birth would be well publicized. Although the infant would not be able to learn of this or read about it for quite a period of time, such knowledge has the potential for inflicting harm. The child may at some point question how his or her mother died. Such a process of gestation may constitute a family secret that may or may not cause problems in the rearing of the infant. Nonetheless, I would argue that the history of the Dionne quintuplets, as well as many of the other individuals who have had a very highly publicized birth and infancy, may serve as a helpful reminder that there are significant issues at stake with respect to publicity.

THE INTERESTS OF THE FATHER

Fathers have typically been perceived in a variety of ways ranging from the traditional picture of the absentee parent to that of the totally involved, nurturing primary care giver. According to the legal literature on abortion, the father has no veto rights over an abortion during the first trimester of the pregnancy and assumedly during the second trimester. Since the state has been denied that power, so has any individual other than the mother. Thus, the father has no say whatsoever unless the fetus is viable. On the other hand, one could argue that since the pregnancy has been allowed to continue, the father has a very strong interest in the fetus and would be the one to exercise proxy consent on its behalf if the mother cannot.

Moreover, because the next of kin typically make decisions with respect to the disposition of the cadaver or parts of the cadaver, one would assume that the husband could make decisions with respect to the continuation or withdrawal of a life-support system to maintain the fetus's life. If, however, the father is not also a husband, he does not qualify technically as the next of kin and, therefore, his status as a decision-maker for the disposition of the cadaver is technically unclear.

In any event, the father may have a strong ethical interest in the survival of the fetus. How that interest may be protected is unclear given the legal situation and the uncertain status of the fetus. Having rejected the image of the child as property of the parents, society has not yet articulated or accepted another model that can clarify the father's moral interest in a previable fetus.

ETHICAL PROBLEMS SPECIFIC TO THE MOTHER-FETUS RELATIONSHIP

The first problem is the technologic imperative: If we can do something, we should do it. When this imperative is followed, especially uncritically, we do things simply because we have a technical capacity to do so. We avoid considering whether what we are doing is appropriate or inappropriate. The justification is capacity, not moral obligation.

A second problem, derived from the technologic imperative, is the inappropriate use of the technology. Life-support systems and intensive care units have a clear clinical purpose of aiding patients with massive trauma or who are recovering from major surgery. Various technologies or life-support systems, including the respirator and the interaortic balloon pump, allow the body or specific organs either to rest or operate at a reduced capacity until the body or a specific organ heals and can reassume its appropriate work.

Frequently, though, equipment which was originally appropriately used to help a patient becomes their sole support when there appears to be little or no hope of the patient ever recovering. Is this an appropriate use of a life-support system? How does this relate to the design of the technology as a temporary support system? The question becomes even more critical in our situation of a dead pregnant woman. Are we being guided primarily by the technologic imperative and using technology inappropriately?

A third problem centers on brain criteria for death. Death of the whole brain as a criterion for determining death is gaining acceptance in our country. Maintaining a cadaver declared dead by virtue of brain criteria will confuse this definition in the minds of many people. We will be in a situation of having criteria of death that are not universally applicable. It is one thing to say that the life-support system of a person declared brain dead will not be turned off until an organ recipient can be found; it is another thing to maintain such a cadaver for up to 2 months to ensure the viability of the fetus.

Fourth, in the general tradition of medical ethics there has been a strong common acceptance of the principle that no one is ever required to use extraordinary means to preserve one's own life or the life of another. The basis of this judgment is that no one is bound to the heroic and that the virtue of beneficence has a limit when the individual is put at a disproportionate amount of risk.

Maintaining a cadaver with a life-support system for a period of 2 months is a clear case of extraordinary means as well as an inappropriate use of life-support technology. I think from that point alone one can argue very strongly against maintaining such a cadaver, even for the sake of the fetus. With respect to beneficence, one can argue that since the individual in question is a cadaver, she is not being placed at great risk. On the other hand, a degree of risk comes from the potential for mistreating a cadaver by focusing specifically on only one part of the body and reducing the individual to that particular status. There is also the risk of confusing the appropriateness of the brain death definition, as indicated. Such risks and their impact on the definition of brain death constitute for me a risk sufficient to argue against using life-support systems to maintain a cadaver.

Two very critical issues remain to be discussed. The first is, Did the mother consent? If the mother had the opportunity to discuss the situation with her spouse or the father of the child and the medical team and she consented to being maintained on the life-support system, then the situation would be close enough to the situation of an organ donor that I would not be completely uncomfortable with maintaining her cadaver. I think the consent of the mother is critical because it is her body that will be maintained, and other people will have to deal with the consequences of her decision. Her consent removes or qualifies many of the problems I have raised.

The other issue is, How close to viability is the fetus? If the mother had not consented but the fetus was very close to viability, then the fetus should be allowed to be born. I am conscious that the phrase "very close" is vague, since in fetal development, 2 or 3 weeks can make a huge difference with respect to viability. However, a fetus that is close to viability should be aided by the life-support system so that it can be born.

But absent the last-mentioned two conditions, I strongly argue that there is no obligation to maintain a pregnant cadaver on a life-support system so that the fetus can survive.

REFERENCES

1. Gaylin W: Harvesting the dead. Harper's, September 1974, pp 23–30
2. May WF: Attitudes toward the newly dead. The Hastings Center *Report* 1, p 3ff, 1973

11

Delivery Methods

SECTION 1: Midforceps Deliveries

David A. Richardson, Mark I. Evans and Robert J. Sokol

The controversy over the use of midforceps has continued to heat, if not light, the obstetric literature. In recent reviews, questions as to the effect of midforceps on maternal morbidity, fetal mortality, and perinatal morbidity have been reopened.[8,24] There are those who believe midforceps and even low forceps have become an anachronism and should no longer be used in the modern practice of obstetrics. Others have looked at the same data and have reached either dramatically or marginally different conclusions and feel that the judicious use of instrumental deliveries can be advantageous to both mother and infant.

Fortunately or unfortunately, depending upon one's perspective, the recent work of Emanuel Friedman has been considered something of a landmark, in regard to the evaluation of midforcep deliveries.[6-8] It is probably fair to assert that in the medicolegal arena, these studies have been overinterpreted, the level of inference having been extended very possibly beyond that intended by the original investigators, and certainly beyond a level consonant with the amount of confirmatory evidence available in the literature. Much of the argument, however, has been caught in the medical malpractice quagmire, and many competent obstetricians have given up even the judicious use of midforceps rather than risk litigation.

The purpose of this chapter is to discuss the risks inherent with forceps usage including the contribution of midforceps to brain damage, and to put into perspective the role, albeit a limited one, of midforceps in modern obstetrics.

ASSOCIATED RISK FACTORS

Recent studies have examined various antepartum and intrapartum conditions thought to influence the relationship between the use of midforceps and subsequent neonatal morbidity and intellectual impairment.[5,11,27] Maternal factors affecting perinatal outcome include both younger and older maternal ages, short maternal stature, nulliparity, grand multiparity, and pre- and post-term delivery. Intrapartum associations include relative cephalopelvic disproportion, malposition, a protracted first stage, type of anesthesia, oxytocin augmentation, and secondary arrest of labor. The condition of the fetus at the time of forceps intervention (i.e., meconium staining, abnormal fetal heart tones, or hypoxia), as suggested by abnormal fetal scalp pH, can likewise influence fetal outcome.

Each of these factors influence the demographics of the patient population in which midforcep procedures are performed. Of greater importance is that these factors may *themselves* be associated with adverse outcome jointly with, or independent of, midforceps use. Thus, they may confound any apparent relationship of midforceps use to maternal and infant morbidity. This confounding of the interrelationships may well explain much of the disparity of thought and conflicting conclusions regarding the role of midforceps in modern obstetric practice.

Immediate Outcome

In absolute terms, overall maternal and infant mortality are negligible when compared to the rate of such complications presented in the first detailed studies of midforceps use.[24] Arguments against the use of midforceps now rest mainly on maternal/offspring morbidity attributable to instrumental delivery. Furthermore, since the use of midforceps is now generally limited to very clear indications, comparisons should not be made against normal vaginal deliveries as has been the case in some studies, but against alternative delivery procedures used in identical complicated pregnancies (i.e., cesarean section or vacuum extraction).

It is generally appreciated that maternal morbidity such as cervical lacerations, vaginal trauma, rectal sphincter tears, and blood loss is increased with midforceps compared to normal spontaneous vaginal deliveries.[5,9] The emotional trauma of midforceps delivery also has been reported to discourage patients from wanting further children. On the other hand, the overall morbidity of cesarean section (i.e., increased pain, blood loss, longer hospital stays, and increased risk of infection) is significantly greater than that from midforceps deliveries. Most physicians consider the various aspects of maternal morbidity amenable to therapy and believe that fetal considerations must remain paramount. For example, longer hospital stay or postpartum endometritis is inconsequential when compared to the neonatal morbidity of a permanent brachial palsy or other neurologic deficit.

Over the years, evidence linking the use of midforceps with increases in immediate neonatal morbidity has accumulated. Studies have shown that midforceps usage can have a major impact on birth asphyxia and birth trauma.[4,22,23] Kadar and Romero, in a series of 87 midforceps deliveries and 62 vacuum extractions, found 2 infants with serious traumatic morbidity—skull fractures. The one delivered with Kielland's forceps developed cerebral palsy; the other, a vacuum extraction, contracted seizures. There were 2 cases of shoulder dystocia in the forceps group with one infant developing an Erb's palsy. Two additional cases of facial palsy were reported after Kielland rotations.[12] Levine and co-workers retrospectively studied 13,870 full-term deliveries to assess those factors associated with birth trauma. Logistic regression analysis revealed that midforceps delivery was one of several variables increasing the child's risk for brachial plexus injury, facial nerve injury, or fractured clavicle.[14] This viewpoint is generally strengthened by the clinical experiences of most obstetricians who have been involved with or witnessed obstetric disasters from the overzealous or incorrect use of midforceps instruments. Perhaps the most important result of the work of Friedman has been to impress upon physicians the fact that forceps can be a dangerous weapon.

It should be remembered, however, that most midforceps deliveries especially low midforceps, are uneventful and nontraumatic. Three recent studies of immediate neonatal morbidity have suggested that, with similar indications, infants delivered by cesarean section or midforceps have similar rates of neonatal acidosis.[5,9,15] Babies delivered by midforceps are at an increased risk of low 1-minute Apgar scores, delayed respiratory effort, birth trauma, cephalohematomas, neonatal apathy, or irritability when compared to vaginal deliveries. When midforceps patients were matched to similar groups delivered by cesarean section, however, there was no significant difference in short-term neonatal morbidity. In a large study of 2700 deliveries controlled for parity and indications, Cardozo and colleagues showed that infants delivered by Kielland's forceps did as well as those delivered vaginally. Those infants delivered by cesarean section showed considerably increased rates of morbidity.[3] This work has been criticized because it compared forceps to emergency cesarean sections performed at different stages in labor for varying indications, which may have biased the results in favor of midforceps.[12A]

Traub and associates recently compared the neonatal outcomes of infants delivered by Kielland's forceps (n = 132) to those after cesarean section (n = 101) in the second stage of labor. There were no differences in Apgar score, the need for active resuscitation, increase in neonatal jaundice, or abnormal neurologic behavior. Outcomes after failed Kielland delivery did not appear to appreciably affect neonatal outcome.

In conclusion, the relationship between fetal morbidity and midforceps delivery is dependent on how one asks the question and against which group the comparisons are made. If one looks at midforceps deliveries as a whole, compared to other modes of delivery, they are generally safe and without major complications. If one concentrates the study on traumatic deliveries or adverse outcomes, midforceps have a negative impact on subsequent neonatal morbidity. The issue left unanswered in the current literature is whether we can identify prospectively those midforceps deliveries in which difficulty will arise, and with improved guidelines eliminate the rare but devastating adverse outcomes.

Long-Term Neurobehavioral Outcome

The use of midforceps also raises the issue of subsequent neurobehavioral and intellectual development of the infant. In some older retrospective studies, an increased frequency of midforceps was identified in children with cerebral palsy. However, others have found no association between midforceps and cerebral palsy or mental retardation.[24] McBride and colleagues, in a series of 771 children evaluated at age 5 and controlled for race, pregnancy complications, and low birth weight, found no association between midforceps delivery and abnormal neurobehavioral outcome.[18]

The most comprehensive analysis of the effects of labor and delivery variables on long-term intellectual development was presented by Broman and co-workers in an analysis of the intellectual performance of 26,760 children from the National Collaborative Perinatal Project (NCPP).[2] The intent of the monograph was to identify which prenatal, neonatal, infant, and childhood variables were related to intellectual performance at age 4 and to determine the relative impact attributable to the different factors in accounting for IQ variation. Using a step-wise multiple regression analysis in groups separated by race and sex, they found that in all groups tested, by far the largest proportion of explained variance in IQ was attributable to maternal education and the socioeconomic index. The relative importance of specific variables differed by race and sex. (Table 11-1) Method of delivery was not significant in any group; fetal weight was significant only in black females.

Although forceps were originally hypothesized to have a serious deleterious effect on a child's intellectual performance, Broman's group found an unexpected relationship. Controlling the data for socioeconomic status, race, and fetal sex, forceps usage was associated with significantly higher

Table 11-1. Prenatal and Delivery Variables With an Impact on IQ at Age 4*

WHITE MALES
Mother's education (years)
Socioeconomic index
Number of prenatal visits
Neonatal brain abnormality
Head circumference at birth (cm)
Parity
KUB infection during pregnancy
Mother married
Mother's age at menarche (years)
Mother's age (years)
Mothers prepregnant weight (lb)
Maximum weight gain during pregnancy (lb)
One-minute Apgar score
Anemia during pregnancy

WHITE FEMALES
Mother's education (years)
Socioeconomic index
Number of prenatal visits
Neonatal brain abnormality
Head circumference at birth (cm)
Parity
Mother's age (years)
Duration of pregnancy (weeks)
Lowest hematocrit of mother during pregnancy
Length at birth (cm)
Maximum weight gain during pregnancy (lb)
Mother's prepregnant weight (lb)
One-minute Apgar score

BLACK MALES
Socioeconomic index
Mother's education (years)
Length at birth (cm)
Mother's age (years)
Number of prenatal visits
Neonatal brain abnormality
Mother's age at menarche (years)
Number of hypertensive blood pressures during pregnancy
Lowest hematocrit of mother during pregnancy
Father present in the home
X-ray exposure scale

BLACK FEMALES
Socioeconomic index
Mother's education (years)
Birthweight (kg)
Number of prenatal visits
Mother's age (years)
Mother's age at menarche (years)
Parity
Cigarettes smoked per day during pregnancy
Length at birth (cm)
Convulsions during pregnancy
Lowest hematocrit of mother during pregnancy

* Variables listed in order of relative importance
(Broman SH, Nichols PL, Kennedy WA: Preschool IQ: Prenatal and Early Development Correlates. Hillsdale, NJ, L Erlbaum Associates, 1975)

IQ scores than spontaneous vaginal deliveries (Table 11-2). This relationship disappeared when parity was controlled for simultaneously. The study has been criticized for not controlling for fetal weight.[8] Whether fetal weight would significantly affect the overall relationship demonstrated between IQ and forceps is not known.

Once later study contradicted the general conclusions of the Broman study. Friedman and associates (using NCPP data) demonstrated a relationship between labor patterns, method of delivery, and future intellectual development (IQ at age 4).[7] This is an important paper, strongly recommended for review by the reader. Their data implicate midforceps as an important etiologic agent in diminished neurobehavioral function. However, their results are questionable because of a possible selection bias and failure to use suitable control variables, such as mother's education and socioeconomic status.[24] The nonrandom patient selection criteria probably contributed to a higher number of abnormal, difficult midforceps operation than in the NCPP group as a whole. This is an impor-

Table 11-2. Relationship Between Type of Delivery and IQ at Age 4

	Spontaneous	Low-Forceps	Midforceps Low Mid	Midforceps High Mid
White				
IQ	102.3	106.6	106.7	106.1
(n)	(4561)	(2586)	(2118)	(1420)
Black				
IQ	91.1	91.4	91.7	92.1
(n)	(8696)	(1928)	(1591)	(662)

(Broman SH, Nichols PL, Kennedy WA: Preschool IQ: Prenatal and Early Development Correlates. Hillsdale, NJ, L Erlbaum Associates, 1975)

tant consideration since, with a higher proportion of difficult midforceps operations in the sample, one would expect increased statistical efficiency and ability to detect smaller differences than might otherwise be possible. Although it is certainly reasonable to conclude from this study that midforceps should not be used in situations in which severely aberrant labor patterns are present,[2,7] care must be taken not to draw broad sweeping conclusions.

The NCPP data have recently been analyzed for relationships between midforceps delivery and intellectual and neurologic development at age 7.[8] In this report, Friedman and colleagues stated that the "seven year intelligence quotient data for matched pairs of cases showed significant long-range adverse impact from mid-forceps operations, but not from low-forceps procedures." The study controlled for race, parity, birth weight, institution, type of delivery, and labor pattern. The mean IQ in the midforceps group was 91.5 ± 1.8 (n = 70) compared to match vaginal delivery controls of 97.26 ± 1.68 (n = 70). This difference reached statistical significance.

When determining the validity of any hypothesis, it is important to ascertain the necessary control variables. A matched pair design is an advanced form of statistical analysis, but it is only as strong as the relevant variables for which one can control. The importance of this distinction is presented in Table 11-3, which shows the major impact of socioeconomic status, mother's education, and sex of the child on IQ variance. These variables are uncontrolled in the Friedman study. Without appropriate control variables, it is possible that the conclusions reached in this work may have overstated the case against midforceps.

Friedman's paper engendered a barrage of letters to the editor from many authorities who disagreed with the conclusions.[13] The ensuing dialogue makes fascinating reading and is quite pertinent to the present discussion. It was pointed out that it was unrealistic to compare complicated midforcep deliveries with normal vaginal deliveries and that cesarean sections would have been a more appropriate control group. In rebuttal to this legitimate criticism, Friedman expanded on the materials and methods of his study, and pointed out that the midforceps selected were essentially elective forcep deliveries free of significant antepartum or intrapartum problems. This comparison of normal forceps to normal deliveries significantly enhances the strength and applicability of the study. Hauth and associates felt that since the predelivery state of the neonate (i.e., presence or absence of fetal distress or asphyxia) was not controlled for in the NCPP (the technol-

Table 11-3. Relationship Between Type of Delivery, Socioeconomic Status (SES), and IQ at Age 4

	White Female Child		White Male Child	
	Vaginal	*Midforceps*	*Vaginal*	*Midforceps*
Low SES				
IQ	95.5	95.2	93.4	95.2
(n)	(308)	(62)	(282)	(38)
High SES				
IQ	111.9	112.8	107	109.1
(n)	(748)	(346)	(750)	(410)

	Black Female Child		Black Male Child	
	Vaginal	*Midforceps*	*Vaginal*	*Midforceps*
Low SES				
(IQ)	88.8	89.4	87	89.4
(n)	(1469)	(75)	(1406)	(75)
High SES				
(IQ)	99.0	98.8	96.3	94.3
(n)	(394)	(52)	(357)	(42)

(Broman SH, Nichols PL, Kennedy WA: Preschool IQ: Prenatal and Early Development Correlates. Hillsdale, NJ: L Erlbaum Associates, 1975)

ogy of continuous fetal monitoring and scalp pH was not available at the time), the data base of the collaborative project was the real anachronism and not the use of midforceps.[10]

Long-Term Minimal Brain Dysfunction

The work of Nichols and Chen, an extension of the NCPP, attempted to demonstrate relationships among symptoms of minimal brain dysfunction and more than 300 prenatal and postnatal variables.[19] They could not document any relationship between midforceps and learning disabilities of hyperkinetic-impulsive behavior. A significant association was found on a univariate basis for white males between neurologic "soft signs" and midforceps. To interpret the significance of this relationship, discriminant analysis was performed to determine which of the different pregnancy and labor and delivery variables made the largest, independent contribution to differentiate abnormal from normal children; that is, which variables were no longer significant when other variables were controlled. The variables identified as important discriminators between children with neurologic "soft signs" and children with no minimal brain dysfunction symptoms were number of cigarettes smoked per day during pregnancy, short cord length, low fetal heart rate, diabetes during pregnancy, hospitalization during pregnancy, chorioamnionitis, and low hematocrit during pregnancy. In other words, although midforceps was found to be significant in an initial screening, when other factors were controlled, the differences were no longer significant. Midforceps were, therefore, not implicated.

Long-Term Intellectual Development

Nilsen compared the intelligence scores of 62 males delivered with forceps (32 low, 13 mid, 16 high) at age 18 with all Norwegian military conscripts.[20] Intelligence scores of the entire forceps group was higher than the national average. The midforceps subgroup exhibited no significant difference from the national average. Socioeconomic status was not controlled for in this study and no demographics were presented, showing that the children delivered by instrumental delivery would be, as a group, comparable to the larger population. The small sample size in this study significantly limits its impact, and one would not want to conclude from it that difficult forceps deliveries are beneficial. It would be well to keep clearly in mind not only this study's weaknesses but also those of studies apparently documenting the adverse consequences of forceps delivery.

ASSESSMENT OF STUDIES AND INFERENCES FOR PRACTICE

A randomized clinical trial of midforceps use is almost surely impossible in today's practice of medicine for a number of reasons, including legal and ethical concerns, the rarity of adverse outcomes, and the enormous numbers needed for adequate statistical power. One problem with past experimental studies is that the age and quality of the data make their applicability to today's situation questionable. Additionally, while adverse outcomes with midforceps may in fact be higher than with other modes of deliveries, serious outcomes are still a very rare event.

The statistical manipulations necessary to analyze such huge numbers of appropriate variables, depending upon the particular biases of the person designing the study, can lead to several problems, including both undercontrolling or overcontrolling mediating factors, with consequent inappropriate attribution of risk. Furthermore, many of the studies dealing with neurologic impairments have been retrospective, introducing problems of ascertainment bias. All of the prospective studies described earlier may suffer from attrition bias. In addition, interactions of midforceps with other risks have not been calculated in any of the neurobehavioral studies reviewed here. It might be added that since several studies have come up with different answers for essentially the same question, it is most likely that the affect of midforceps on neurobehavioral outcome, if any, is very small. Finally, it might be argued that even if the relative risk for an adverse outcome is higher with midforceps delivery, the absolute risk may still be very low and, for most pregnancies, negligible.

The prudent clinician might decide to avoid any use of midforceps, particularly if he or she has not been adequately trained in their use. On the other hand, equally prudent clinicians have concluded from the same evidence that a definite, if very limited, role for midforceps remains, since midforceps may lower maternal morbidity without significantly increasing infant morbidity in comparison with the alternative of cesarean birth. This portion of the discussion is from the latter perspective.

It is incumbent on all physicians performing operative deliveries to document a legitimate indication for their use. The arbitrary shortening of the second stage or the use of midforceps for teaching purposes is clearly not justifiable. The procedures can legitimately be employed in cases of fetal distress in the second stage of labor or in instances of maternal exhaustion. The following guidelines should be assessed before midforceps are applied:

- The cervix should be fully dilated.
- Instrumental deliveries should generally be avoided in the face of significant labor abnormalities.
- The vertex should be engaged and forceps should not be applied if there is any significant suggestion of disproportion (caput/molding).
- Membranes should be ruptured.
- Position should be carefully determined with certainty.

- There should be adequate analgesia or anesthesia.
- Extreme caution should be used with forceps rotations for other than right or left occipito-anterior presentations. If the forceps cannot be applied easily and rotation accomplished with light pressure, the procedure should be abandoned.
- Vaginal instrumental delivery of infants over 4000 g should be avoided.
- Multiple instrumentations should be shunned, and prolonged traction should be avoided. Persistence is not a virtue in modern obstetrics.
- The obstetrician must know his or her limitations.

The applicability of midforceps in modern obstetrics continues to be a much debated issue. Even the authors of this section differ among themselves in the role forceps play in the present milieu.

The first author believes that forceps are very seldom necessary in the modern obstetrician's armamentarium. He feels that the difficult forceps rotation and extraction, especially in the face of an arrested labor pattern, have no place in modern obstetrics and that the trauma and serious sequelae of indiscriminant forceps intervention must be eliminated. It is likely over the next decade that this country will experience a continued decrease in the number of forceps deliveries performed. Not only is there an increase in the total number of cesarean sections, but an educated patient population is demanding a more "natural" labor and delivery process. With a dwindling number of forceps deliveries being performed in many institutions, it will likely become impossible to teach aspiring obstetricians the proper skills and techniques needed for safe forceps use. The first author recommends that the Silastic vacuum extractor is the more appropriate instrument, being less traumatic to mother and fetus, easier to use and teach, and designed with built-in safeguards. He uses the vacuum extractor in cases of maternal exhaustion or fetal distress while adhering to the guidelines as outlined above.

The second author believes that midforceps and midforceps rotations (when performed by appropriately trained obstetricians in proper circumstances) are inherently safe and should continue to be performed on obstetric services. Unfortunately, because the true indications for midforceps are few and the fear of litigation so high, the use of midforceps has plummeted. "Modern" obstetrics is rapidly reaching the point of having a generation of obstetricians incompetent to perform rotations. Thus, midforceps use will undoubtedly die out, killed not by the weight of medical evidence but by a few disasters caused by improper use, ill-advised hands, and a litigious society in which a bad outcome associated with forceps use is considered prima facie evidence of malpractice. Both situations are intolerable but are unlikely to be changed.

The third author would take a middle ground. The indications for midforceps use are and should be very limited. An expected rate for an obstetric service might be in the range of 1.5% to 2%. Difficult midforceps, with its inherent risks of maternal and fetal trauma should be avoided by choice of cesarean birth when it becomes clear that vaginal delivery is likely to be difficult. In this context, cesarean is the more conservative approach, one for which the risks to mother and baby are well defined and in which the obstetrician is experienced.

There are some situations which the third author believes are best and most atraumatically handled with operative vaginal delivery. These might best be termed the easy, low midforceps. In these cases, there is no significant disproportion; that is, macrosomia is not suspected and pelvic architecture and size appear normal. The vertex is not impacted but may require slight rotation at a relatively low station (+2 to +3). There may be evidence of significant fetal distress or, perhaps, the patient's bearing down is less than optimal. Abdominal delivery may require too much time or anesthesia to be considered the safest alternative. In such circumstances, the third author believes that a *gentle* midforceps procedure may well represent the best alternative. We shall continue to train obstetricians in this limited use of the obstetric forceps. Surely, midforceps use should not be considered prima facie evidence of obstetric malpractice.

REFERENCES

1. Beverly DW, Chance GW, Coates CF: Intraventricular hemorrhage, timing of occurrence and relationship to perinatal events. Br J Obstet Gynaecol 91:1007, 1984
2. Broman SH, Nichols PL, Kennedy WA: Preschool IQ: Prenatal and Early Development Correlates. Hillsdale, NJ, L Erlbaum Associates, 1975
3. Cardozo LD, Gibb DMF, Studd JWW, Cooper DJ: Should we abandon Kielland's forceps? Br Med J 287:315, 1983
4. Cyr RM, Usher RH, McLean FH: Changing patterns of birth asphyxia and trauma over 20 years. Am J Obstet Gynecol 148:490, 1984
5. Dierker LJ, Rosen MG, Thompson K et al: The mid-forceps maternal and neonatal outcome. Am J Obstet Gynecol 152:176, 1985
6. Friedman EA: Patterns of labor and indicators of risk. Clin Obstet Gynecol 16:172, 1973
7. Friedman EA, Sachtleben MR, Bresky PA: Dysfunctional labor: XII. Long-term effects on infant. Am J Obstet Gynecol 127:779, 1977
8. Friedman EA, Sachtleben-Murray MR, Dahrouge D, Neff RK: Long-term effects of labor and delivery on offspring: A matched-air analysis. Am J Obstet Gynecol 150:941, 1984
9. Gilstrap III LC, Hauth JC, Schiano S, Connor KD: Neonatal acidosis and method of delivery. Obstet Gynecol 63:681, 1984
10. Hauth JC, Gilstrap III LC, Hankins GDV: Letter: Examination of data base in mid-forceps delivery study. Am J Obstet Gynecol 153:814, 1985
11. James DK, Chiswick ML: Kielland's forceps role of antenatal factors in prediction of use. Br Med J 188:769, 1984
12. Kadar N, Romero R: Prognosis for future child bearing after mid-cavity instrumental delivery in primi gravidas. Obstet Gynecol 62:166, 1983
12A. Kielland or Caesar: Letters to the editor. Br Med J 287:609, 1983
13. Letters to the editor: Midforceps. Am J Obstet Gynecol 152:604, 1985; 153:233, 1985
14. Levine MG, Holroyde J, Woods JR et al: Birth trauma incidence and predisposing factors. Obstet Gynecol 63:792, 1984
15. Livnat EJ, Fejgin M, Scommegna A et al: Neonatal acid base balance in spontaneous and instrumental vaginal deliveries. Obstet Gynecol 29:549, 1978
16. Maltau JM, Egg EK, Moe N: Retinal hemorrhages in the preterm neonate: A prospective randomized study comparing the occurrence of hemorrhages after spontaneous vs forcep deliveries. ACTA Obstet Gynecol Scand 63:219, 1984
17. Maryniak GM, Frank JB: Clinical assessment of the Kobayashi vacuum extractor. Obstet Gynecol 64:431, 1984
18. McBride WG, Black BP, Brown CJ et al: Method of delivery and development outcome at 5 years of age. Med J Aust 1:301, 1979
19. Nichols PL, Chen TC: Minimal Brain Dysfunction—A Prospective Study. Hillsdale, NJ, L Erlbaum Associates, 1981
20. Nilsen ST: Boys born by forceps and vacuum extraction examined at 18 years of age. ACTA Obstet Gynecol Scand 63:549, 1984
21. Niswander KR, Gordon M: The women and their pregnancies. DHEW Pub No (NIH) 73-379, 1972
22. O'Driscoll K, Moagher D et al: Traumatic intracranial haemorrhage in firstborn infants and delivery with obstetric forceps. Br J Obstet Gynecol 88:577, 1981
23. Paintin DB: Mid-cavity forcep delivery. Br J Obstet Gynaecol 89:495, 1982
24. Richardson DA, Evans MI, Cibils LA: Midforceps delivery: A critical review. Am J Obstet Gynecol 145:621, 1983
25. Schwartz DB, Miodovnik M, Lavin JP: Neonatal outcome among low birth weight infants delivered spontaneously or by low forceps. Obstet Gynecol 62:283, 1983
26. Traub AI, Marrow RJ, Ritchie JWK, Dorwan KJ: A continuing use for Kielland's forceps. Br J Obstet Gynaecol 91:894, 1984
27. Varner MW: Neuro psychiatric sequelae of mid-forceps deliveries. Clin Perinatol 10:455, 1983

SECTION 2:
Changes in Indications and Incidence of Cesarean Birth

Gregory L. Goyert and Robert A. Welch

Cesarean section should be performed to protect the mother or the fetus.[16]

Against the backdrop of a cesarean birth rate that has more than quadrupled during the last 20 years,[58] today's dedicated obstetrician is left to ponder whether or not he or she is actually effecting protection of mother or fetus. Although the rising rate of cesarean birth does not appear to be related to the simultaneously decreasing rate of perinatal morbidity and mortality,[23] today's threatening medicolegal climate[3,10] is bringing ever-mounting pressure to deliver a "perfect" baby. In addition, while the obstetrician may view the rising cesarean birth rate from the standpoint of physician-scientist and humanitarian, government and insurance industry bureaucrats consider the issue from the perspective of health care financing. Regardless of the obstetric indications, third-party payers are already reducing incentives for clinicians to perform cesarean birth. It will be difficult to overcome these biases and derive clinical significance from future studies assessing the indications and incidence of cesarean birth.

The myriad of social, medical, legal, and economic factors responsible for increasing the cesarean birth rate from approximately 5% in 1965 to more than 25% 20 years later[54] are of small concern to the clinician attempting to answer a seemingly simple question. Is resorting to cesarean birth really the optimal mode of management for obstetric complications, or is it a compromise that may potentially jeopardize the outcome for this patient pair?

This chapter reviews a variety of clinical situations for which cesarean birth is resorted to frequently. Particular attention has been given to the areas of concensus and controversy regarding the use of cesarean delivery.

DYSTOCIA

One of the most prominent diagnoses responsible for the increased rate of cesarean birth is dystocia.[3] Dystocia refers to difficult or abnormal labor and birth and is reported to account for 18.3%[24] to 50.9%[26] of the increased rate of primary cesarean births. Dystocia may be classified as being either relative[3,53] or absolute[3] (rare), and as reiterated by Perkins[53] is a function of the four Ps: pains (efficacy of uterine contractions), passageway (adequacy of pelvis), passenger (fetal size, lie, and position relative to a specific pelvis), and provider (positive or negative influence of the health team's actions). As pointed out by Bottoms and colleagues,[3] absolute cephalopelvic disproportion is a rare event, while absolute dystocia in general[53] (e.g., transverse lie, hydrocephalus, conjoined twins) represents a small fraction of pregnancies terminated by cesarean birth. Thus, relative dystocia (e.g., failure to progress, dysfunctional labor, or uterine inertia) exerts a profound influence on the current rate of cesarean births in the United States. Since it is extremely unlikely that the incidence has more than doubled in 20 years,[3,24,30] the frequency and accuracy of the diagnosis as well as subsequent management are of primary concern.

Unresolved Controversy in Management Approach

The experience at the National Maternity Hospital (NMH) in Dublin with respect to dystocia, its management, and its outcome contrasts sharply with the United States' experience. O'Driscoll and Foley[47] reported a perinatal mortality rate at NMH that declined from 42.1 per 1000 in 1965 to 16.8 per 1000 in 1980 for infants of birth weight 500 g or more, while the cesarean birth rate remained essentially unchanged at 4% to 5%. They attributed their excellent perinatal mortality rate and low cesarean birth rate to their technique in the management of labor. Further, they suggested that the number of cesarean births in the United States might be decreased by more aggressive use of oxytocin in early labor, also known as the "active management of labor."[47-49] The principles of active management include a correct initial diagnosis of labor, frequent reevaluation in early labor, and the liberal use of oxytocin whenever the rate of cervical change is slow in nulliparous women.[48]

In what now appears to be an unresolved controversy, Leveno and associates[39] recently provided "an answer to the House of Horne" in a comparison of obstetric practice and perinatal outcome at Parkland Memorial Hospital (PMH) in Dallas and NMH for 1983. The authors confirmed striking differences in overall rates of cesarean birth (18% at PMH v. 6% at NMH), as well as significant differences in the rate of primary procedures (10.1% at PMH v. 4.4% at NMH). With respect to the indications for primary cesarean births, the PMH experience clearly differed from that of NMH. While dystocia accounted for 50% of the primary abdominal procedures at Parkland, it was the indication for only 27% of the primary cesarean births in Dublin. In contrast, only 15% of the primary cesarean births were performed for fetal distress at NMH versus 21% at PMH.

The Parkland group stressed[39] that the diagnosis of fetal distress justified their cesarean birth rate. They emphasized the sevenfold increase in intrapartum fetal deaths for infants more than 2500 g and the twofold increase in subsequent seizure activity among term infants delivered at NMH. An explanation for the more frequent diagnosis of dystocia at PMH was based on contrasting maternal demographic and obstetric characteristics (e.g., increased frequency of nulliparous patients). Whether active management of labor would benefit maternal-fetal outcome could not be answered based on the previously collected data. More recent data describing uniform application of active management of labor[4,5] and a prospective, randomized trial of active management[8] report conflicting results with respect to the effects on the cesarean birth rate. Although the fetal outcome is apparently uniformly excellent in these trials, differentiating the effects of dystocia from fetal distress confounds attempts at determining optimal management of many of these labors.

Effect on Fetal Outcome

Minkoff and Schwarz[44] in 1980 asked if the rising cesarean birth rate for the diagnosis of dystocia had improved overall fetal outcome and provided an important perspective in a 1980 review. They noted that in a population with stable indications for cesarean delivery (i.e., patients undergoing elective repeat procedures for which the cesarean birth rate remains unchanged at 100%), the perinatal mortality rate at the Downstate Medical Center in 1977 was one-third the rate observed in 1961. Using this perinatal mortality rate as a standard for comparison of other expanding indications for primary cesarean birth (e.g., dystocia), they concluded that the perinatal mortality rate for patients with dystocia decreased at a pace that was unaffected by the mode of delivery (i.e., decreasing rates were similar for patients delivered vaginally and abdominally).

A recent report from Wilford Hall, United States Air Force Medical Center,[17] suggests that the influence of dystocia on the increasing total and primary cesarean birth rate may be curbed without adverse perinatal effects. They examined the indications for cesarean birth during three time frames between 1970 and 1981 and reported a consistent decline in the frequency of dystocia as an operative indication from 1970 to 1973, through 1974 to 1977, and through 1978 to 1981 (39% v. 33% v. 24%). Interestingly, cesarean births performed for dystocia as a percentage of all deliveries increased significantly from 1970 to 1973, through 1974 to 1977 (3.2% v. 5.6%) and then decreased significantly from 1978 to 1981 (5.6% v. 3.6%). The authors attributed the reversal to "informal criteria and policies (that) were established and directed toward assuring an adequate trial of labor . . . (and) assessment (that) included mandatory intrauterine pressure monitoring with oxytocin usage."

Other recent reports have demonstrated identical[23,57] perinatal outcomes between cesarean and vaginal births for dystocia. Porreco[57] prospectively analyzed modification of house officers' attitudes towards cesarean birth in clinic patients at St. Luke's Hospital in Denver. Compared to the control group (private patients), the clinic patients had a lower total cesarean birth rate (5.7% v. 17.6%) and fewer primary procedures for dystocia (36% v. 44%). Porreco's interventions with respect to the diagnosis and management of dystocia were characterized in broad terms and included "an appreciation for the latent phase of labor, usefulness of ambulation in labor, internal fetal monitoring, . . . and judicious use of Pitocin."[57] Corrected perinatal mortality rates and frequency of low 5-minute Apgar scores were essentially identical between the two patient groups.

Haynes de Regt and co-workers[23] reported a review of 65,647 deliveries at four Brooklyn hospitals and found that for both primiparous and multiparous patients, private patients diagnosed with dystocia were significantly more likely to undergo cesarean delivery than clinic patients with the same diagnosis. Of greater importance, they found that private patients were delivered of significantly more infants with low Apgar scores and birth injuries (1:28; $p < 0.001$).

It appears, then, that the increased rate of cesarean delivery for the diagnosis of dystocia has not accounted for the improved perinatal outcome observed over the past 20 years. (Effects of primary cesarean birth versus midforcep delivery for dystocia are addressed in Section 1.) While noting the absence of a survival advantage with cesarean birth for infants weighing more than 2500 g, the National Institutes of Health (NIH) Cesarean Birth Task Force recommended that the issue of dystocia be reevaluated with in-hospital peer review; additional research examining the factors that affect labor progress, including oxytocin stimulation; and examination of the utility of current methods of monitoring the process of labor, with special attention to maternal and fetal morbidity and mortality.[45]

REPEAT CESAREAN SECTION

The management of patients who have experienced a prior cesarean birth is still guided by Dr. Edward Craigen's 1916 pronouncement that "Once a Cesarean, always a Cesarean."[9] In the United States in 1981, more than 98% of patients underwent a repeat procedure following a primary cesarean birth.[45] In 1980, Bottoms and associates[3] reported that repeat cesarean birth accounted for 23% of the increase in the overall cesarean birth rate, while Anderson and Lomas[2] found that the same entity accounted for 68% of the observed increase in the rate of cesarean birth in Ontario, Canada, from 1979 to 1982. In the United States today, repeat procedures constitute approximately one-third of all cesarean births[28] and more than 5% of all deliveries.[44] The absolute number of repeat procedures, as well as its relative contribution to overall rates of cesarean birth, will continue to rise as the rate of primary cesarean births increases.[44,45]

Support for Vaginal Delivery After Cesarean

The issue of elective repeat cesarean birth has received intense scrutiny in the recent literature.[15,16,18,36,43] There is a consensus among current authors that Craigen's proclamation[9] (issued in an era of classical uterine incisions and prior to the advent of sophisticated maternal-fetal monitoring procedures, blood banking capabilities, effective antibiotic therapy, and predictably safe anesthesia) appears to have little role in modern obstetrics. Further, "the uniformity of the reports showing safe and successful results with trial labor suggests that the persistence of elective repeat cesarean birth is based on philosophical rather than scientific reason."[18]

In a cogent 1980 article, Flamm[15] reviewed the literature describing approximately 10,000 vaginal births after previous cesarean birth. A maternal mortality related to a ruptured uterine scar has never been reported. In fact, with a realistic maternal mortality figure of approximately 1 per 5000 elective repeat procedures,[34] it may be argued that these successful trials of labor actually prevented 2 maternal deaths. It is becoming increasingly clear that Meier and Porreco's[43] 1980 assertion that "a trial of labor after previous cesarean delivery constitutes the best and safest form of obstetrical management" is more appropriate in modern obstetrics than Craigen's 1916 dictum.

The fetal outcome associated with trials of vaginal birth after previous cesarean birth has been uniformly excellent.[16,36] In 1982, Lavin and associates[36] reviewed the literature from 1950 to 1980 describing approximately 3200 labor trials after previous cesarean birth with a successful vaginal delivery rate of 67%. Of the 14 fetal mortalities related to uterine scar rupture, 12 occurred due to prior classic uterine incision rupture, and the remaining 2 occurred in unmonitored patients in the early 1960s. Flamm and colleagues[16] reviewed the 1980-1984 literature describing approximately 6200 labor trials with an 86% vaginal delivery rate. Of the 5 fetal deaths related to uterine scar rupture, one involved the rupture of a low vertical incision,[13] one labor was induced with a vaginal prostaglandin pessary, and one fetus weighed 1200 g.[13] Flamm[15] extrapolated that with the exclusion of patients with a known classical or low vertical uterine incision, the corrected perinatal mortality rate is approximately 0.5 per 1000 labor trials. Similarly, Shy and colleagues[64] described the mathematical framework of decision analysis and projected that 37 perinatal deaths would be avoided in a cohort of 10,000 patients undergoing labor trials, compared to 10,000 patients subjected to elective repeat cesarean birth, primarily by elimination of iatrogenic prematurity.

Recent evaluations of more controversial aspects of the practice of labor trials after previous cesarean birth have described excellent fetal outcome in terms of neonatal morbidity as well as mortality[14-16,18,28,43,52,61,65] Flamm and co-workers,[16] Paul and associates,[52] and Silver and group[65] have reported approximately 500 trials of labor in which oxytocin (induction and augmentation) was employed. Similar rates of vaginal delivery were noted (59%-70%) for these patients and no excess perinatal morbidity or mortality attributable to oxytocin use was found. Preliminary reports describing trials of labor after prior cesarean birth, conducted under continuous epidural anesthesia (approximately 700 patients),[15,16,61] have noted excellent maternal and fetal outcomes.

Finally, there are increasing numbers of reports documenting uniform maternal and fetal safety with labor after two or more prior cesarean sections (approximately 120 patients to date).[14,42,52,71] Although controversial and not readily accepted by the majority of obstetricians, these preliminary reports encourage closer scrutiny of the safety of vaginal delivery after more than one low-transverse cesarean birth.

Recommendations Concerning Elective Repeat Cesarean Birth

Elective repeat cesarean birth does not appear to contribute to improved fetal outcome. In fact, in the absence of uniform assurance of fetal pulmonary maturity,[43,63] the opposite may be the case. While all authors stress that importance of appropriate maternal-fetal monitoring techniques during trials of labor after prior cesarean birth, patient and physician enthusiasm for labor is noted to be high.[43] In addition to compelling financial considerations,[15] there is a consensus in the literature that, in properly selected patients, "a trial of labor is associated with lower risks of death and less significant morbidity for both mother and fetus."[43] Although there is a pressing need for further research to elucidate under what "controversial conditions" a trial of labor may be safely conducted (e.g., use of oxytocin, regional anesthesia, and more than one prior cesarean birth),[14,43,45,52] it is clear that there is overwhelming evidence to suggest that "Craigen's old dictum . . . should be abandoned"[11] and that "Once a

Cesarean, always a Cesarean is an outmoded dictum."[34]

FETAL DISTRESS

During the last two decades, the diagnosis of fetal distress has been among the most rapidly increasing indications for cesarean birth.[17,44] While accounting for only 10% to 15% of the overall increase in cesarean birth rates,[3,45] several authors have reported that cesarean births performed for fetal distress increased from five- to eightfold between 1970 and 1980.[17,44] The NIH Cesarean Birth Task Force noted that "although evidence is lacking that the actual incidence of fetal distress has changed, the diagnosis of fetal distress has been made more frequently during the past ten years."[43]

Electronic Fetal Monitoring

A clear relationship has emerged between the introduction of continuous electronic fetal monitoring (EFM) and the increased diagnosis of fetal distress.[45] In contrast, EFM's role in the escalating rate of cesarean birth is somewhat more controversial.[17,21,22,25,31,41,44,51,55,56,60] Undeniably clinicians have demonstrated an increasing willingness to terminate labor by cesarean birth in an attempt to reduce the potential for fetal hypoxic morbidity and mortality.

Petrie[55] has recently offered a comprehensive history of the development of the methodology for intrapartum fetal evaluation. In tracing the evolution of fetal monitoring from Marsac's initial description of the fetal heart rate in 1650 to modern practice, Petrie noted that the "outstanding value of fetal heart rate monitoring during the intrapartum period is the reasonably sensitive ability of this technique to confirm fetal well-being and to permit labor to continue without unnecessary intervention. Unfortunately, this method of surveillance is less able to identify accurately the fetus that is clearly in distress."[54] Similarly, Iams and Reiss[27] outlined the statistical basis for the fundamental difference between EFM employed as a screening test in contrast to its use as a diagnostic test. The authors confirmed the relatively high sensitivity and positive predictive value associated with a reassuring test, but emphasized the low positive predictive value associated with an abnormal EFM result.

Whether routine EFM has improved fetal outcome remains hotly debated. EFM was introduced as a new technology and assimilated into clinical practice before critical analysis of its potential risks and benefits were available.[19] In evaluating the pooled results of nine nonrandomized trials,[1,12,26,29,35,46,50,64] Quirk and Miller[59] concluded that "the use of EFM improves perinatal outcome in both low risk and high risk patients." The authors also noted, however, that "the benefits of EFM in reducing perinatal morbidity have not been tested vigorously."

Results of Early Randomized Trials

Thacker[67] has characterized the randomized controlled trial as "the ideal method to assess the efficacy of clinical interventions in human populations." At the time of this manuscript's preparation, there were eight randomized trials in the literature[21,22,35,40,41,60,74] that assessed the impact of continuous EFM (v. intermittent auscultation) on perinatal outcome. In his critique of the first seven trials, Thacker[67] praised the Dublin trial[41] for design and implementation (a standardized quantitative score of 86%)[6] while noting deficiencies in the initial six trials.[21,22,35,60,74] These deficiencies notwithstanding, however, he analyzed the pooled data from these six initial trials (3928 patients) and found no significant difference in any measure of perinatal outcome (i.e., perinatal death rate, low Apgar score, neonatal seizure activity) between the EFM group and the intermittent auscultation cohort. Further, the combined rates of operative delivery (abdominal and vaginal) were similar in the two groups, but the rate of cesarean birth was significantly higher in the EFM group of patients.[32,41]*

Similar results were reported in a recent prospective trial (alternate-month design), that evaluated selective versus universal continuous EFM at Parkland Memorial Hospital in Dallas.[38] Although this study differed from the eight randomized trials in several fundamental design characteristics, these authors detected no significant difference in perinatal outcome between the two groups. In this large trial of almost 35,000 patients, a small but significant increase in the rate of cesarean birth was found in the universal monitoring group. In contrast, in a recent small (246 patients) randomized trial of EFM versus intermittent auscultation in a preterm population (700–1750 g), Luthy and associates[40] found no significant difference in the frequency of abdominal delivery in the continuously monitored group. As with the other trials, however, perinatal outcome was similar in both groups and the authors concluded that for gestations less than 33 weeks, "continuous electronic [fetal heart rate] FHR monitoring [did] not improve clinical management of premature labor enough to reduce intrapartum acidosis, perinatal morbidity, or perinatal mortality."

The Dublin Trial

The Dublin Trial[41] represents the largest randomized clinical trial designed to evaluate the efficacy of intrapartum EFM in comparison to intermittent auscultation. The 12,964 study patients were enrolled between April 1981 and April 1983, and were randomly allocated to either the intermittent auscultation group, or the continuous EFM group. Analysis of

---

* It is imperative that the reader not equate intermittent auscultation during labor with unmonitored labor. In fact, intermittent auscultation during labor almost universally required nursing care on a one-to-one basis in all eight randomized clinical trials surveyed by Thacker. This fact, in addition to the current medicolegal climate in the United States that demands almost continuous documentation of fetal well-being, may preclude wide acceptance of intermittent auscultation as the primary method of intrapartum fetal evaluation.

this trial found no significant difference between groups in the rate of perinatal mortality, low Apgar scores, requirement for endotracheal intubation, or admission to the special care nursery. The overall operative delivery rate (abdominal and vaginal procedures) was significantly greater in the EFM group (primarily due to indicated procedures for fetal distress), but the rates of cesarean birth were similar.

Most importantly, however, the authors found that EFM was associated with a significantly lower frequency of infants with neonatal seizures (55% reduction) and other "abnormal neonatal neurologic features." Stratified post-hoc analysis revealed that this effect was limited to labors lasting more than 5 hours and appeared unrelated to oxytocin use. The authors suggested that clinicians may opt to be guided by the finding that "the benefits of the more intensive method of fetal monitoring are restricted to relatively long labors." Regardless of indications for its use, EFM has been widely accepted in the United States and it now appears unlikely that a rigorous protocol for intermittent auscultation will ever be possible in most labor and delivery suites.

Fetal Scalp pH Determinations

Regardless of one's interpretation of the retrospective studies, the Parkland trial, and the eight randomized control trials evaluating the efficacy of continuous EFM, it is clear that the primary modality for intrapartum surveillance today is continuous EFM and is likely to remain so for the foreseeable future. As a result, the clinician must decipher whether a given worrisome fetal monitor tracing indicates fetal distress requiring intervention, or if the pattern represents a false-positive result that is often associated with this surveillance modality. The technique of fetal scalp pH determination, originally introduced by Saling[62] in 1961, may significantly reduce the frequency of the false-positive diagnosis of fetal distress.[55] Several reports[23,44,57,75] have demonstrated that in conjunction with more sophisticated analysis of EFM patterns,[17] intermittent fetal scalp pH determination has enabled clinicians to allow the process of labor to continue and has significantly lowered the frequency of cesarean birth performed for fetal distress. A concise diagnostic and therapeutic treatise on this common dilemma is available in a recent essay by Petrie.[55]

The rapid evolution of this technology, with almost equally rapid assimilation into clinical practice, prompted the NIH Cesarean Birth Task Force[45] to call for the further evaluation of "the present accuracy of the diagnosis of fetal distress and to develop new diagnostic techniques." The authors expected that such efforts would "improve fetal outcome and lower cesarean birth rates."

BREECH PRESENTATION

Management of the infant in the breech presentation has undergone dramatic change during the last 15 years.[45] In 1970, fewer than 15% of breech infants were delivered abdominally, compared to more than 60% less than 10 years later.[45] Although the incidence of breech presentation is only 4%, it has accounted for 10% to 15% of the observed increase in the cesarean birth rate.[3,45] Given the controversial literature related to the impact of cesarean delivery on perinatal outcome for these infants, the current medicolegal climate, and the ever-dwindling educational opportunities available for mastering the skill required for safely accomplishing a vaginal breech delivery,[2,23,44] it is unlikely that this trend will soon be reversed.

The issue of the optimal mode of delivery for infants with a breech presentation is explored in greater detail in Chapter 9, Section 5.

THE LOW BIRTH WEIGHT INFANT

The remarkable advances in neonatal care and technology over the past 15 years have resulted in the intact survival of infants that previously were considered previable. Tertiary level neonatal centers have realized survival rates of greater than 90% for infants between 1000 g and 1500 g, 70% to 80% in the 750 g to 1000 g range, and 30% to 40% for infants weighing between 500 g and 750 g.[72] In the mid-1970s, this dramatic improvement in outcome for low birth weight and very low birth weight infants prompted clinicians to reevaluate the impact of the mode of delivery on the perinatal and long-term outcome of these infants.[66]

The decision-making process is handicapped, however, by the absence of randomized controlled trials evaluating the efficacy of cesarean birth for the very tiny baby.[73] Most studies have been unsuccessful at differentiating the effects of fetal trauma (while negotiating the birth canal) from perinatal asphyxia. Contrary to the established practice of many clinicians trying to reduce the incidence of intraventricular hemorrhage, available retrospective studies[32,72,73] do not support cesarean birth for the very low birth weight infant in the vertex presentation. In contrast, most authors advocate cesarean birth for infants less than 1500 g when a breech presentation is detected.[73] (For a comprehensive discussion of the literature related to breech presentation and management of the low birth weight infant, see Chapter 9, Sections 1 and 5.)

THE ANOMALOUS FETUS

Increased reliance on ultrasound has allowed the prenatal diagnosis of a multitude of fetal anomalies previously discovered only at the time of delivery. The clinician is now confronted with the difficult task of determining the best mode of delivery for an anomalous infant while considering maternal well-being. Perkins,[53] commenting upon fetal hydrocephalus, noted that "for many generations . . . management plans were built largely around avoiding unnecessary operative intervention resulting in reproductive handicapping conditions for the mother. Babies . . . were regularly sacrificed." Today, however, certain congenital anomalies are amenable to surgical repair in the immediate neonatal period with resultant encouraging long-term outcomes. Unfortunately, a definitive body of literature detailing the impact of the mode of the delivery on the majority of these abnormalities is not available because of their infrequent occurrence and the still emerging ultrasound technology.

Fetal Anencephaly and Hydrocephalus

Fetal anencephaly is easier to manage than hydrocephalus on both ethical and clinical grounds. It does not require a cesarean birth unless there are maternal indications.[69] In contrast, fetal ventriculomegaly may present a diagnostic and therapeutic challenge to the entire perinatal team. As outlined by Vintzileos and colleagues,[70] management revolves about serial ultrasonography in an attempt to detect associated anomalies, determine the etiology of the fetal hydrocephalus, and monitor the progression of the disease.

In cases of idiopathic isolated congenital hydrocephalus, elective cesarean birth with immediate ventricular shunting has been advocated once fetal pulmonary maturity has been documented by amniocentesis.[69,70] When idiopathic congenital hydrocephalus is associated with spina bifida, the perinatal and long-term outcome are more discouraging. "When the cortical thickness is less than 10 mm, or the spinal defect is very extensive, the prognosis is poor and management should be conservative."[70] Vintzileos and associates have provided a comprehensive overview of the etiology, pathophysiology, diagnosis, and perinatal management of congenital hydrocephalus.[70]

Other Neural Tube Defects

The combination of maternal serum alpha-fetoprotein (AFP) screening and the escalating use of utrasound has allowed for the more frequent antenatal detection of neural tube defects. The differential diagnosis for these lesions includes sacrococcygeal teratoma, hemangioma, lipomyelomeningocele, and myelomeningocele. When detailed ultrasound examination is inconclusive, the determination of amniotic fluid AFP and acetylcholinesterase levels are useful. Diligent ultrasound examination will detect ventriculomegaly in over 80% of fetuses suffering with spina bifida.[70]

The frequent occurrence of dystocia associated with sacrococcygeal teratoma favors cesarean birth as the preferred mode of delivery, while cesarean birth should be reserved for standard obstetric indications only for infants with lipomyelomeningocele.[69] The perinatal management of spina bifida hinges upon the extent of the lesion and the presence or absence of associated anomalies. In instances of isolated spina bifida, cesarean birth has been reported to improve perinatal and long-term outcome by increasing the rate of traumatic rupture of the myelomeningocele sac.[7,69,70] As is the case for infants found to have congenital diaphragmatic hernia,[70] planned cesarean birth in instances of spina bifida would also facilitate preparation of the neonatal resuscitation and surgical teams.

Abdominal Wall Defects

The optimal mode of delivery for fetuses detected antenatally to have either omphalocele or gastroschisis remains controversial[20,33,37] Advocates for cesarean birth of fetuses with these anomalies cite the decreased rate of trauma (omphalocele) and lower rates of bowel contamination and vascular compromise (gastroschisis) associated with planned abdominal delivery.[20,37] Although gastroschisis is not frequently associated with other anomalies,[69] more than 50% of fetuses with omphalocele will have an additional malformation (e.g., genitourinary, cardiovascular, central nervous system).[69] Thus a careful sonographic survey may prove useful when deciding upon the appropriate mode of delivery. Ideally, it would be preferable to reach management decisions on the basis of randomized prospective trials that evaluate alternative methods of delivery.[32,37] The relative infrequency of abdominal wall defects (and other congenital anomalies) will likely preclude the generation of such data in the foreseeable future.

General Guidelines

The list of congenital anomalies for which antenatal diagnosis is possible has expanded with the increased use of ultrasonography. In addition, widening attempts at fetal therapy have increased the complexity of perinatal management of these fetuses. In a recent survey detailing current diagnosis and management of a wide variety of sonographically detected fetal anomalies, Vintzileos and group[69] noted that "the factors crucial for reasonable perinatal management include: an accurate antenatal diagnosis, evaluation of associated anomalies (structural and/or chromosomal) to establish possible etiology and prognosis, and appropriate parental counseling." With respect to general guidelines for determining the most appropriate mode of delivery, Vintzileos's study suggested that "when the fetal abnormality is incompatible with life, or is thought to have a poor prognosis, the management should be conservative, and vaginal delivery is indicated even if fetal distress occurs. If the prognosis for the anomaly is promising, then the perinatal management should consist of frequent antepartum fetal evaluation and cesarean birth, if fetal distress occurs."

REFERENCES

1. Amato JC: Fetal monitoring in a community hospital: A statistical analysis. Obstet Gynecol 50:269, 1977
2. Anderson GM, Lomas J: Determinants of the increasing cesarean birth rate: Ontario data 1979 to 1982. N Engl J Med 311:887, 1984
3. Bottoms SF, Rosen MG, Kelso RJ: The increase in the cesarean birth rate. N Engl J Med 302:559, 1980
4. Boylan PC: Active management of labor. Proceedings Society of Perinatal Obstetricians 131, San Antonio, 1986
5. Boylan PC, Parisi VM: The effect of "active management" on the latent and active phases of labor in the nullipara. Proceedings Society of Perinatal Obstetricians 354, Orlando, 1987
6. Chalmers TC, Smith H Jr, Blackburn B et al: A method for assessing the quality of a randomized control trial. Controlled Clin Trials 2:31, 1981
7. Chervenak FA, Duncan C, Ment LR et al: Perinatal management of meningomyelocele. Obstet Gynecol 63:376, 1984
8. Cohen GC, O'Brien WF, Lewis L, Knuppel RA: A prospective randomized study of the active management of labor. Proceedings Society of Perinatal Obstetricians 214, Orlando, 1987
9. Cragin E: Conservatism in obstetrics. NY State J Med 104:1, 1916
10. Danforth DN: Cesarean section. JAMA 253:811, 1985
11. Demianczuk N, Hunter D, Taylor D: Trial of labor after previous cesarean section: Prognostic indicators of outcome. Am J Obstet Gynecol 142:640, 1982
12. Edington PT, Sibanda J, Beard RW: Influence on clinical practice of routine intrapartum fetal monitoring. Am J Obstet Gynecol 129:917, 1977
13. Eglington G, Phelan J, Yeh S et al: Outcome of a trial of labor after prior cesarean delivery. J Reprod Med 29:3, 1984
14. Farmakides G, Duvivier R, Schulman H et al: Vaginal birth after two or more previous cesarean sections. Am J Obstet Gynecol 156:565, 1987
15. Flamm BL: Vaginal birth after cesarean section: Controversies old and new. Clin Obstet Gynecol 28:735, 1985
16. Flamm B, Dunnett C, Fischerman E, Quilligan E: Vaginal delivery following cesarean section: Use of oxytocin augmentation and epidural anesthesia. Am J Obstet Gynecol 148:759, 1984
17. Gilstrap LC, Hauth JC, Toussaint S: Cesarean section: Changing incidence and indications. Obstet Gynecol 63:205, 1984
18. Graham AR: Trial labor following previous cesarean section. Am J Obstet Gynecol 149:35, 1984
19. Greenland S, Olsen J, Rachootin P, Pedersen GT: Effects of electronic fetal monitoring on rates of early neonatal death, low Apgar scoring and cesarean section. Acta Obstet Gynecol Scand 64:75, 1985
20. Harrison MR, Golbus MS, Filly FA: The management of the fetus with a correctable congenital defect. JAMA 246:744, 1981
21. Haverkamp AD, Orleans M, Langendoerfer S et al: A controlled trial of the differential effects of intrapartum fetal monitoring. Am J Obstet Gynecol 134:399, 1979

22. Haverkamp AD, Thomason HE, McFee JG et al: The evaluation of continuous fetal heart rate monitoring in high risk pregnancy. Am J Obstet Gynecol 125:310, 1976
23. Haynes de Regt R, Minkoff HL, Feldman J, Schwarz RN: Relation of private or clinic care to the cesarean birth rate. N Engl J Med 315:619, 1986
24. Hibbard LT: Changing trends in cesarean section. Am J Obstet Gynecol 125:798, 1976
25. Hobbins JC, Freeman R, Queenan JT: The fetal monitoring debate. Obstet Gynecol 54:103, 1979
26. Huguey MJ, La Pata RE, McElin TW, Lussky R: The effect of fetal monitoring on the incidence of cesarean section. Obstet Gynecol 49:513, 1977
27. Iams JD, Reiss R: When should labor be interrupted by cesarean delivery? Clin Obstet Gynecol 28:745, 1985
28. Jarrell MA, Ashmead GB, Mann LI: Vaginal delivery after cesarean section: A five-year study. Obstet Gynecol 65:628, 1985
29. Johnstone FD, Campbell DM, Hughes GJ: Has continuous intrapartum monitoring made any impact on fetal outcome. Lancet 1:1298, 1978
30. Jones OH: Cesarean section in present day obstetrics. Am J Obstet Gynecol 126:521, 1976
31. Kelso IM, Parsons RJ, Lawrence GF et al: An assessment of continuous fetal heart rate monitoring in labor. Am J Obstet Gynecol 131:526, 1978
32. Keppel N, Verma U, Hameed C, Chayen B: Method and route of delivery in the low birthweight vertex presentation correlated with early periventricular/intraventricular hemorrhage. Obstet Gynecol 69:1, 1987
33. Kirk EP, Wah RH: Obstetric management of the fetus with omphalocele or gastroschisis: A review and report of 112 cases. Am J Obstet Gynecol 146:512, 1983
34. Klein L: Cesarean birth and trial of labor. Female Patient 9:106, 1984
35. Koh KS, Greves D, Yung S, Peddle LJ: Experience with fetal monitoring in a university teaching hospital. Can Med Assoc J 112:455, 1975
36. Lavin J, Stephens R, Miodovnik M, Barden T: Vaginal delivery in patients with a prior cesarean section. Obstet Gynecol 59:135, 1982
37. Lenke RR, Hatch CI: fetal gastroschisis: A preliminary report advocating the use of cesarean section. Obstet Gynecol 67:395, 1986
38. Leveno KJ, Cunningham FG, Nelson S et al: A prospective comparison of selective and universal electronic fetal monitoring in 34,995 pregnancies. N Engl J Med 315:615, 1986
39. Leveno KJ, Cunningham FG, Pritchard JA: Cesarean section: An answer to the house of horne. Am J Obstet Gynecol 153:838, 1985
40. Luthy DA, Shy KK, Van Belle G et al: A randomized trial of electronic fetal monitoring in preterm labor. Obstet Gynecol 69:687, 1987
41. MacDonald D, Grant A, Sheridan-Pereira M et al: The Dublin randomized controlled trial of intrapartum fetal heart rate monitoring. Am J Obstet Gynecol 152:524, 1985
42. Martin J, Harris B, Huddleston J et al: Vaginal delivery following previous cesarean birth. Am J Obstet Gynecol 146:255, 1983
43. Meier P, Porreco R: Trial of labor following cesarean section: A two year experience. Am J Obstet Gynecol 144:671, 1982
44. Minkoff HL, Schwarz RH: The rising cesarean section rate: Can it safely be reversed? Obstet Gynecol 56:135, 1980
45. NIH Consensus Development Statement on Cesarean Childbirth. Obstet Gynecol 57:537, 1981
46. Neutra RR, Fienberg SE, Greenland S, Freidman EA: Effect of fetal monitoring on neonatal death rates. N Engl J Med 299:324, 1978
47. O'Driscoll K, Foley M: Correlation of decrease in perinatal mortality and increase in cesarean section rates. Obstet Gynecol 61:1, 1983
48. O'Driscoll K, Foley M, MacDonald D: Active management of labor as an alternative to cesarean section for dystocia. Obstet Gynecol 63:485, 1984
49. O'Driscoll K, Meagher D: Active Management of Labour. Eastbourne, UK, WB Saunders, 1980
50. Paul RH, Hon EF: Clinical monitoring: V. Effect on perinatal outcome. Am J Obstet Gynecol 118:529, 1974
51. Paul RH, Huey JR, Yeager CF: Clinical fetal monitoring: Its effect on cesarean section rate and perinatal mortality: Five year trends. Postgrad Med 61:160, 1977
52. Paul RH, Phelan JP, Yeh S: Trial of labor in the patient with a prior cesarean birth. Am J Obstet Gynecol 151:297, 1985
53. Perkins RP: Fetal dystocia. Clin Obstet Gynecol 30:56, 1987
54. Petitti D, Olson RO, Williams RL: Cesarean section in California—1960 through 1975. Am J Obstet Gynecol 133:391, 1979
55. Petrie RH: Intrapartum fetal evaluation. In Gabbe SG, Niebyl JR, Simpson JL (Eds): Ob-

56. Placek PJ, Keppel KG, Taffel SM, Liss TL: Electronic fetal monitoring in relation to cesarean section delivery for live births and stillbirths in the U.S., 1980. Public Health Rep 99;173, Mar/Apr 1984
57. Porreco RP: High cesarean section rate: A new prospective. Obstet Gynecol 65:307, 1985
58. Quilligan EJ: Cesarean section: Clin Obstet Gynecol 28:689, 1985
59. Quirk JG, Miller FC: FHR tracing characteristics that jeopardize the diagnosis of fetal well being. Clin Obstet Gynecol 29:12, 1986
60. Renou P, Chang A, Anderson I, Wood C: Controlled trial of fetal intensive care. Am J Obstet Gynecol 126:470, 1976
61. Rudick V, Niu D, Hetman-Peri M et al: Epidural analgesia for planned vaginal delivery following previous cesarean section. Obstet Gynecol 64:621, 1984
62. Saling E: Neues vorgehen zur untersuchung des kindes unter der geburt. Arch Gynakol 197:108, 1961
63. Shenker L, Post RC, Seiler JS: Routine electronic monitoring of fetal heart rate and uterine activity during labor. Obstet Gynecol 46:185, 1975
64. Shy KK, LoGerfo JP, Karp LE: Evaluation of elective repeat cesarean section as a standard of care: An application of decision analysis. Am J Obstet Gynecol 139:123, 1981
65. Silver RK, Gibbs RS: Predictors of vaginal delivery in patients with a previous cesarean section, who require oxytocin. Am J Obstet Gynecol 156:57, 1987
66. Stewart AL, Reynolds EOR: Improved prognosis for infants of very low birthweight. Pediatrics 54:724, 1974
67. Thacker SB: The efficacy of intrapartum electronic fetal monitoring. Am J Obstet Gynecol 156:24, 1987
68. Tutera C, Newman RL: Fetal monitoring: Its effect on the perinatal mortality and cesarean section rates and its complications. Am J Obstet Gynecol 122:750, 1975
69. Vintzileos AM, Campbell WA, Nochimson DJ, Weinbaum RJ: Antenatal evaluation and management of ultrasonically detected fetal anomalies. Obstet Gynecol 69:640, 1987
70. Vintzileos AM, Ingardia CJ, Nochimsen DJ: Congenital hydrocephalus: A review and protocol for perinatal management. Obstet Gynecol 62:539, 1983
71. Wadhawaw S, Norone J: Outcome of labor following previous cesarean section. Int J Gynecol Obstet 21:7, 1983
72. Welch RA, Bottoms SF: Reconsideration of head compression and intraventricular hemorrhage in the vertex very low birthweight fetus. Obstet Gynecol 68:29, 1986
73. Westgren M, Paul RH: Delivery of the low birthweight infant by cesarean section. Clin Obstet Gynecol 28:752, 1985
74. Wood C, Renou P, Oats J et al: A controlled trial of fetal heart rate monitoring in a low-risk obstetric population. Am J Obstet Gynecol 141:527, 1981
75. Zalar RW Jr, Quilligan EJ: The influence of scalp sampling on the cesarean section rate for fetal distress. Am J Obstet Gynecol 135:239, 1979

SECTION 3:
Legal Implications of Delivery Options

Barbara W. Sholl and John S. Sholl

The practice of medicine has often been termed an inexact art. In an attempt to bridge the gap between art, science, and law, this section offers an interdisciplinary approach to obstetrics from a legal perspective. The obstetrician/gynecologist is presented not so much with the factors the medical profession considers in choosing between delivery options, but rather with those the law believes the physician ought to consider in choosing the mode of delivery of any given patient.

Obstetric complications should trigger certain clinical judgments relative to delivery modes. A misunderstanding arises between the physician and the lawyer because they analyse poor outcomes retrospectively in totally different ways. An obstetrician will analyze injury resulting from, for example, shoulder dystocia, by questioning whether the complication was predictable or manageable, whereas an attorney will assume a legal duty which attaches to every physician-patient relationship regardless of known natural calamities, and will examine the total conduct of the obstetrician in order to discover whether any factors in the decision-making process "caused" or "contributed to cause" the injury.

The obstetrician's unique position at the receiving end of what the legal profession terms "the long tail of liability" places the specialist in obstetrics and gynecology at the forefront of the medical malpractice crisis. In Illinois, for example, a minor was considered to be under a "legal disability" until the age of majority. Illinois law "tolled" (i.e., suspended the time within which a minor plaintiff could file a lawsuit) by delaying the start-up time of the running of the statute until the date of the minor's age of majority, 18.[8] Until January 1, 1988, the outside limitations did not exceed 4 years beyond the age of majority in a medical malpractice case, and it was therefore conceivable that a lawsuit against an obstetrician could have languished up to 22 years from a child's birthdate. The Illinois limitations statute, as amended,[9] still provides a minor with an extended time frame, eight years from the date of the alleged injury, in which to file a lawsuit.

In addition to the lengthy time parameters available to minor plaintiffs, verdicts against obstetricians have underscored the trend of stratospheric damages awarded by juries against all doctors. Due to the cost of custodial care over the lifetime of an individual who is totally disabled, verdicts in obstetric and pediatric malpractice cases in excess of one million dollars are not uncommon. Malpractice verdicts in Cook County, Illinois, since 1983 involving children who claimed complete custodial care have ranged from 1.5 to 22 million dollars.

The focus of this chapter will be directed at an assessment of frequently targeted patterns of conduct in obstetric cases, avoidance of these hazardous scenarios, and an examination of ways in which to protect one's legal interests before and after a lawsuit is filed.

LEGAL DEFINITIONS

Analysis of Injury

The concept of an injured party is perhaps the most readily understood and least controversial aspect of any lawsuit involving professional services. The ease with which the public accepts the word injury to describe poor outcome is unfortunate, however, since injury is naturally associated with fault. "Whose fault is it?" is the normal response to news of injury, rather than "Is it anyone's fault?"

Obstetricians have often been accused of hiding behind act of God defenses, yet at the same time patients find it difficult to comprehend the physician's explanation that human reproduction, when viewed from a realistic and historical perspective, has always been measurably inefficient, posing hazards to the life and health of both the mother and fetus.

There is general public acceptance and awareness that pregnancies can end in first trimester miscarriage. Beyond the first trimester, however, the existence of multiple natural disasters is less well known, among them incompetence of the cervix, premature labor, intrauterine death from diabetes, erythroblastosis, or hydrops, preeclampsia, cord accidents, placenta previa, abruptio placentae, placental insufficiency, growth retardation, and uterine rupture. There are also a number of uniquely obstetric calamities which have high maternal or fetal mortality and include eclampsia, acute fatty liver of pregnancy, postpartum cardiomyopathy, amniotic fluid embolism, uterine atony, and hemorrhage.

Given the numerous complications and disease processes, why do the majority of obstetric cases focus not so much on prenatal care, but on the delivery itself? The answer is quite simple. A plaintiff, faced with injuries which may be attributable to known complications of pregnancy, is spared much of the difficult and costly proposition of proving that injury resulted from medical negligence by effectively narrowing the scope of proof the law requires to the time around delivery.

It is not illogical to presume that the public (the jury) finds it easier to conceptualize and criticize the events around the time of delivery than to comprehend the natural failures of gestation and the labor and delivery process.

Standard of Care

The law assumes that a special relationship arises out of any physician-patient interaction, which is commonly referred to as the "legal duty" owed, and which is a necessary element of any medical malpractice lawsuit. Secondly, through evidence, or proof, introduced at time of trial by means of expert testimony, the plaintiff must show that the obstetrician acted in a manner not in keeping with the applicable standard of care. Instructions to the jury may set forth the standard of care as follows:

> In treating or operating upon a patient, a doctor must possess and apply the knowledge and use the skill and care that is ordinarily used by reasonably well qualified doctors in the locality in which he practices or in similar localities in similar cases and circumstances. A failure to do so is a form of negligence that is called malpractice.[7]

Due to the fact that specialty boards are nationally recognized, the trend has been to steer away from the old locality or community standards of practice for specialists. Therefore, an obstetrician's actions will be compared to those of other reasonably well qualified obstetricians. What then, is the standard of care which, in legal parlance, attaches to the delivery of obstetric services provided by family practitioners? Ordinarily, family practitioners will not be held to the same standard as board-certified obstetricians. The question will be dealt with retrospectively in terms of legal analysis. If the general practitioner had knowledge of a medical condition (e.g., preeclampsia) or an obstetric complication (e.g., malposition of the fetus), then the practitioner's judgment will be called into question relative to the need for consultation in a situation calling for a higher level of obstetric skill. That failure to consult in the face of an impending obstetric crisis may be sufficient for a jury to impose liability based upon a deviation from the acceptable standard of care for a nonspecialist. Furthermore, in most circumstances a mistake in professional judgment does not equate with a finding of negligence, but if a family practitioner holds himself or herself out as a qualified practitioner in the field of obstetrics, then that practitioner is required to conform to the standard of care of that specialty. To assume that the law will permit a less rigorous standard for a family practitioner in the performance of a forceps delivery than it will impose upon a board-certified obstetrician constitutes wishful thinking. The diagnostic skills and judgment involved in reading and interpreting fetal monitoring strips and in the decision-making of whether a breech presentation should be delivered vaginally or by means of cesarean section, must also be judged by the standards applicable to the specialist.

Expert Testimony

Whether the care giving rise to the lawsuit was provided by an obstetrician or family practitioner, testimony relative to the standard of care must be supplied by another physician (not necessarily an obstetrician, although the same specialty requirements exist in some states) acting as an expert, or by testimony of the defendant doctor. The expert being offered to support either the plaintiff or defendant doctor must possess knowledge and familiarity with the care under scrutiny. Expert testimony is needed in order to support a claim of malpractice, since jurors are presumably unskilled in the practice of medicine and would find it difficult in the absence of medical evidence to determine any lack of specific scientific skill on the part of the physician.[5,14]

In addition to actual live expert testimony, most trial lawyers will cite publications by physicians, particularly those practicing in specialty areas, to bolster their interpretation of the applicable standard of care. It is important to remember that there are often no specific standards which mandate a particular course of action when several choices are available; they serve as guidelines only. The language of the preface to the *Standards for Obstetric-Gynecologic Services* supports this interpretation as follows:

> It is important, particularly to those agencies or individuals who may consult this manual in preparing codes and regulations governing the delivery of obstetric-gynecologic health care, to recognize that the standards set forth here are presented as recommendations and general guidelines rather than as a body of rigid rules. They are intended to be adapted to many different situations, taking into account the needs and resources particular to the locality, the institution, or type of practice. Variations and innovations that demonstrably improve the quality of patient care are to be encouraged rather than restricted.[12]

As a defendant in an obstetric malpractice case, it does not inure to the physician's best interests to accept any general standard without knowing the specific situation to which that standard will be applied. An obstetrician who is questioned in a legal proceeding as to whether certain professional guidelines and publications are authoritative, should evaluate the source being referred to in its entirety before accepting its tenets as being true and applicable in all situations. When testifying during deposition or trial, an obstetrician named as a defendant in a lawsuit may inadvertently establish the standard of care to be applied in judging his or her own conduct. The consideration of the case at hand before accepting any source as authoritative will prevent the setting of standards which are unrealistic and which may be lethal to the defense of the case.

Proximate Cause

Of the four elements which a plaintiff must prove to a jury—injury, duty, breach of that duty, and proximate cause—that of proximate cause is perhaps the most misinterpreted and most misunderstood. The definition of proximate cause means a cause, which in a natural or probable sequence produced the injury. The legal approach to causation differs markedly from the medical approach to which the obstetrician is accustomed. In reviewing a patient's current medical condition, the obstetrician more or less instinctively searches for the basic cause or causes of the disorder that underlies the problem. The trial judge and attorney, in contrast, seek to determine whether one particular event precipitated, hastened, or aggravated the patient's current condition. In the legal sphere, the causation issue must be resolved on the basis of the best evidence reasonably available, even though that evidence would be unsatisfactory for purposes of determining causation from a medical standpoint. For example, the proximate cause issue would be satisfied in court were the expert physician to answer "Yes, it might have," to the complex question, "Doctor, based upon a reasonable degree of medical and surgical certainty, do you have an opinion as to whether the doctor's failure to perform a timely cesarean section might or could be the cause of the child's cerebral palsy?"

The old adage The straw that broke the camel's back is helpful in illustrating the legal perspective. Consider, for example, a real-life situation involving a plaintiff who is injured when he slips off the edge of a platform and is struck by an oncoming train. He is transported to the emergency room of a nearby hospital in apparently stable condition where he is examined by an emergency room physician and treated for his orthopaedic injuries. His condition progressively deteriorates, and 3 hours later he dies on the operating room table from a ruptured spleen and massive internal injuries. In the opinion of the physician, the patient died due to the fatal injuries he sustained when struck by the train. The plaintiff's attorney, however, seeks to gain legal recognition of the failure to immediately diagnose the patient's condition and operate as a proximate cause of the death, since his case and client stand to benefit from the recognition of the physician's failure to promptly diagnose and treat.

As with all forms of negligence suits, the obstetrician's conduct need not be the *only* possible cause of the claimed injury. The physician will be charged responsible for the outcome if the conduct amounts to one of *several* causes.

The obstetrician may feel naively comfortable in a case involving a difficult forceps delivery, knowing that subarachnoid hemorrhage can occur with spontaneous delivery. The law, however, does not require statistical proofs or irrefutable certainty. A reasonable degree of medical certainty—"Is it more probably true than not true?"—will suffice to prove causation in court. However, even if a plaintiff's expert is of the opinion that the treating obstetrician breached the requisite standard of care, the case is legally deficient and may be subject to dismissal prior to trial if the outcome would not have changed given compliance with the standard.

KEY ISSUES IN OBSTETRIC MALPRACTICE DEFENSE

The obstetrician who is presented with medical complications at time of delivery is faced with the choice of prompt intervention in the form of cesarean section or the use of forceps; management by means of medical therapies (i.e., Pitocin, manual rotation, change of position); or with watchful nonintervention, which may result in vaginal delivery. Situations in which such choices often develop into legal issues are many and include fetal distress, abruptio placentae, premature and prolonged rupture of membranes, cord prolapse, abnormal lies, postmaturity, prolonged labor, preeclampsia, premature labor, and multiple gestation.

A key issue in most obstetric malpractice cases is the diagnosis of fetal distress. Since the most helpful diagnostic tool concerning the presence of fetal distress during labor is the fetal monitoring strip, it is almost always alleged in a complaint that a failure to monitor or failure to interpret the tracing resulted in harm to the baby. If, in fact, approximately 30% to 50% of nonelectronically monitored babies who develop fetal distress or die during delivery show no antecedent signs of impending compromise,[1] electronic fetal monitoring may be extremely useful in assisting the obstetric practitioner in making decisions as to the appropriate mode of delivery. Monitor tracings are closely scrutinized together with the hospital records by plaintiff's attorneys in determining whether a case should be pursued.

Electronic fetal monitoring became available in university medical centers and teaching hospitals in the early 1970s. The acceptance of electronic fetal monitoring in community hospitals came more slowly; by the late seventies it had become more widely available and more frequently used.

The use of this device in a non-high-risk patient is a matter for a physician's judgment; however, hospitals have become cognizant of the benefits of fetal monitoring, and most have implemented written policies and procedures concerning its use. The latest *Standards of the American College of Obstetricians and Gynecologists* recommends continuous monitoring of fetal heart rate and uterine activity for all high-risk patients. Even assuming that there may be a difference of opinion among obstetricians as to the standard of care in this regard, the physician should be aware that failure to use electronic fetal monitoring in a high-risk patient who subsequently delivers an injured child may subject him or her to criticism and probable liability.

The use of electronic fetal monitoring during labor has reached such a point of availability and general acceptance that where previously properly performed auscultation in a non-high-risk patient was considered the norm, today the failure to apply a fetal monitor, when available, to a patient in labor may be the subject of opposing expert testimony as to the standard of care. Experience has demonstrated that even if the mother is not considered a high-risk patient, the plaintiff's case will be prepared so as to find some facet of the woman's medical history or condition which will place her in the high-risk category.

From a review of a number of recent obstetric lawsuits involving the use of fetal monitoring, there are certain observations which may be of benefit to the obstetric practitioner:

- Once the decision is made to continuously monitor a patient, both uterine contractions *and* fetal heart rate should be observed, and the external monitor adjusted to provide an intelligible tracing.
- If a monitor is unavailable, auscultation every 30 minutes during the first stage of labor and every 15 minutes during the second stage of labor is reasonable. When the patient is prepared for delivery, the fetal heart rate should be checked at least every 10 minutes.[12]
- The obstetrician should have expertise in interpreting fetal monitoring strips and should understand the limitations of external monitoring.
- The obstetrician should be able to apply internal monitors and interpret the findings provided.
- It is most helpful to have data, such as a change in the patient's condition, medications, and examinations of the patient, noted on the monitor strip by either the obstetrician or the nursing staff.

If the plaintiff is able to demonstrate by means of expert testimony that there is a causal connection between the physician's failure to use fetal monitoring and the claimed injury, then damages will be awarded. If the plaintiff fails to do so, recovery will be denied. This two-step process is achieved by expert testimony to the effect that (1) lack of fetal monitoring is a deviation from the standard of care under that set of circumstances, and (2) that lack of monitoring itself caused the injury.[5,13] If there is no provable causal link (e.g., an allegation that a failure to employ electronic fetal monitoring resulted in a physical malformation), there cannot be a finding of medical negligence.

Hazards of Choice—Cesarean Section Delivery v. Vaginal Delivery

From a medical standpoint, the vaginal-cesarean delivery determination involves complex issues of fetal benefit versus maternal safety. The medical literature reflects the obstetrician's concern for the welfare of the infant at risk for neurologic disorder, but it often fails to demostrate that cesarean delivery improves perinatal outcome.[11] Although cesarean section is recognized as significantly more hazardous to the mother, injury to the neonate is a far greater concern and legal hazard. Therefore, many of those neonates who may be delivered safely vaginally are delivered instead by cesarean section, to presumably avoid injury in some percentage of births.

A recent study sponsored by the National Institute of Child Health and Human Development (NICHD) and the National institute of Neurological and Communicative Disorders and Stroke (NINCDS) concludes that despite increased delivery by cesarean section and a decrease in the use of forceps, there has not been a decrease in the incidence of neurologic damage. The study concludes that prematurity, low birth weight, and asphyxia put the infant at high risk for brain damage and neonatal death.[11]

Most lawsuits involving allegations of a failure to perform a cesarean section, or a failure to perform a cesarean section in a timely manner, are framed so as to imply that earlier delivery would have prevented perinatal asphyxia. The presence of cord problems, placental insufficiency, intrauterine growth retardation, abruptio placentae, prematurity, breech presentation, and a host of other factors, including possible congenital deficits, are ignored. Criticism is directed at the single issue of whether earlier surgical intervention would have made a difference in outcome. Most frustrating to the defense of "bad baby" cases when asphyxia is alleged to be a causative factor is the inability to conclusively determine the severity and duration of asphyxia in the antenatal period. In many cases the defense attorney and doctor must present other factors, such as prematurity, low birth weight, cord entanglement, or placental insufficiency as more likely causes of the injury. Unless the defendant's expert is able to demonstrate that the child did not experience birth asphyxia, the facts of the case will be decided by a jury. The taking of cord blood gas samples to determine whether or not a depressed neonate was asphyxiated is recommended from a defense standpoint.

The legal reality, in light of the lack of reported case law for injuries sustained during the performance of a cesarean section, or for performance of "unnecessary" cesarean sections, appears to support the conclusion that when there are indications supportive of risk for birth asphyxia, the obstetrician should be aware that a damaged baby is far more costly than a patient with an abdominal scar and possible postoperative complications. From a strictly legal jeopardy perspective, cesarean section delivery may be the only acceptable course of action, in the face of an irrefutable finding of fetal distress. (An exception may arise, however, relative to liability involving cesarean section delivery when an infant of presumed advanced gestational age is delivered by premature cesarean section.)

A secondary legal issue relative to cesarean section addresses the claimed delay in start-up time for the procedure. In response to the Standards of the American College of Obstetrics and Gynecology recommendation that 30 minutes should be the outside parameter between decision and incision time,[12] many hospitals have adopted this guideline as part of their protocols. The obstetric practitioner should pay particular heed to his or her departmental rules and regulations which have an excellent chance of being tendered into evidence during a legal proceeding to support the time frame just discussed and proffered as the standard of care.

Another obstetric issue is that of vaginal breech delivery versus delivery of the infant by cesarean section. Although recent reports suggest that careful selection and management allows safe vaginal birth of term breech infants in about 30% of these babies,[3,15] the risk of injury in breech delivery leads to the inevitable legal conclusion that where careful surveillance and emergency support are not available, cesarean section delivery should be chosen in the best interests of the neonate. From a medical viewpoint, the decision of whether to employ midforceps or cesarean section as a delivery mode has also been troublesome. The use of midforceps does appear to have "a place in modern obstetric care"[3] when "properly indicated and skillfully applied."[15] From a lawyer's viewpoint, the foregoing simply implies that there exist strong differences of opinion, and that the medical practitioner's conduct in cases involving midforceps delivery with a bad outcome will be closely scrutinized.

The Risk Management Concept

A review of lawsuits involving a failure to properly implement delivery options demonstrates that most, if not all, of the cases involve an alleged deficiency of basic obstetric skills. For example, frequently occurring legal accusations involve not only the issue of delivery choices, but nearly always include other issues such as failure to recognize and treat preeclampsia; failure to note the gestational age of the infant, resulting in premature delivery; failure to remove the entire placenta after delivery, resulting in later complications involving infection of the mother; failure to manage the post-date infant; failure to properly interpret fetal distress or electronic fetal monitor strips; failure to diagnose and treat the high-risk patient; and failure to attend the actual delivery. With the knowledge that the foregoing are frequently occurring factual and legal scenarios, the obstetrician/gynecologist should be aware that there is an approach to the delivery of obstetric services which is often overlooked, seldom discussed, and rarely effectively implemented on the physician-patient level.

The approach is referred to as "risk management" and has been defined by Elvoy Raines, Esquire, past director of the Department of Professional Liability of the American College of Obstetricians and Gynecologists, as "that practice style by which the physician minimizes the risk of a lawsuit by practicing in a manner that reduces actual error, assures the greatest chance for obtaining desired results in the care of the patient, and presents the most defensible treatment options." In a nutshell, risk management is quite literally identified as the art of managing identified risk exposures.

Once an accurate diagnosis has been made, the obstetrician is thereafter faced with the choice of therapy and delivery modes. Accurate diagnosis is therefore a basic preventive measure of both harm to a patient and of legal claims.

The second major area of risk to the obstetric practitioner is one of communication with the patient. The public's perception of childbirth is increasingly an idealized vision of delivering a normal, healthy term child "naturally" and has taken on the unrealistic meaning of total lack of intervention by the physician, including avoidance of the use of forceps, Pitocin, analgesia or anesthesia, cesarean section, tocolysis, transfusions, intravenous hydration, and electronic fetal heart rate monitoring. Even if an obstetrician assumes that an uncomplicated delivery will ensue, the prudent physician would be well advised to respond to any request for "natural childbirth" by explaining the attendant risks to the mother, preferably in the presence of the patient's spouse. The discussion should be documented in order to avoid a later claim that informed consent relative to the mode of delivery was not obtained.

Another failure of communication has arisen in which the prenatal course was not communicated to either the hospital staff or obstetrician, who may be seeing the patient upon hospital admission for the first time. In some situations, a practitioner is on staff at a number of hospitals where obstetric privileges have been granted. From a risk management standpoint, protocols on an office level are recommended to ensure that patients with risk factors for obstetric complications are known to the physician who may be called upon to perform the delivery in the primary physician's absence. The patient should be advised at the outset of the possibility that another doctor may deliver her, and where feasible the alternate care-giver should be introduced. A doctor-patient relationship which fosters goodwill, evidences concern for the patient, and provides adequate information to the patient and family fosters a climate in which the patient is less likely to call an attorney in the face of a problem.

One aspect of good communication which should not be overlooked is the quality of being a good listener. Assimilation of information provided by the patient does not serve the limited purpose of good rapport, but may also supply the obstetrician with data critical to delivery options. An example of a failure to listen was the cornerstone of a legal claim involving the prenatal care of a young woman with an assumed singleton gestation. Based on fundal height, the obstetrician chose to assign a date for the woman's last menstrual period some 2 months prior to the date given by the patient. Her pregnancy continued uneventfully, fundal heights always corresponding to the age of the fetus. The onset of labor began presumably at term and she was admitted to the hospital where she was examined by the practitioner's partner. After augmentation of labor with Pitocin she was delivered unexpectedly of 32-week-old twins, who developed respiratory distress syndrome. One of the twins expired shortly after transfer to a neonatal intensive care unit.

The foregoing situation illustrates a communication deficiency which led to a failure to diagnose the presence of a twin gestation. Good risk management strategy demands that partners review upcoming deliveries. Additionally, physicians who practice at a number of hospitals should provide prenatal records of their patients to each hospital, if there is a chance that delivery may occur at an institution other than the one initially designated.

Bearing in mind that the most common sources for proof in a malpractice action are office and hospital records, it is of great importance that charting be as accurate and complete as possible. Missing entries, or changes to the record, particularly after the filing of a lawsuit, are devastating to the physician's position because later explanations are often deemed to be a cover-up of wrongdoing. Legitimate changes should be noted, initialed, and dated. Any change in a record should be irreproachable, since there is nothing that can damage a case as much as accusations of tampering. Even if motivations for the change were innocent, the alteration will be carefully scrutinized by the jury, and in all likelihood the credibility of the medical record will be destroyed.

One of the most effective risk management tools is that of keeping informed of current medical advances in the literature. Plaintiff's counsel is placed at a disadvantage when the defendant physician is well read, thoughtful, and able to back up his or her position with an intelligent justification for the choice of therapy and delivery mode.

A popular misconception has arisen that the medicolegal crisis can best be handled through reactionary practice patterns by physicians, which may include an increase in the number of diagnostic tests which are not medically necessary, but which are ordered to protect oneself from legal action; avoidance of potentially litigious patients; and avoidance of what are perceived to be risky procedures such as forceps maneuvers. The practice of "defensive" medicine should not be equated with a risk management approach. The term defensive medicine does not emphasize good practice habits and demonstrates instead a basic lack of security and faith in one's own skills. Any physician who orders tests because of the fear that the patient care given may be judged substandard is allowing the law to set standards of medical practice, and excludes medical training and judgment from guiding treatment modalities.

The Expert Witness

Much of the ease of proof of obstetric malfeasance is provided by the willingness of physicians in the obstetric area to testify against one another. In comparison with other specialties, where plaintiff's experts are difficult to find and retain, the obstetrician is generally willing to review gray areas of conduct and to assess the situation as black or white. The testimony on either side of the issue is reduced to a battle of the experts at time of trial and part of the problem may be due to those obstetricians and gynecologists who are all too willing to assist the plaintiff's bar in putting its imprimatur of acceptable care on the delivery of obstetric services which are textbook perfect.

In addition, the specialty and subspecialty areas of pediatrics and neonatology, despite very convincing evidence to the contrary, continue to associate only perinatal events with neurologic or other injuries, and assume that asphyxia occurred when little or no proof exists. Plaintiffs' attorneys must necessarily preserve and cultivate their most valuable and credible asset in any obstetric case, the pediatric expert witness. Thus, rarely is the postpartum management of the neonate the subject of a lawsuit. When the obstetrician's policy limits are low, or when the pediatrician equivocates on the cause of injury, it is likely that he or she may be added as a party to the lawsuit. Plaintiffs' attorneys have had little difficulty in finding experts to tie up alleged perinatal asphyxia to the events surrounding labor and delivery when the child has low Apgar scores, seizure activity within the first 24 hours, meconium staining, prolonged resuscitation, or requires transfer to a special care center. The pediatric records will often document the conclusion that a preventable asphyxial injury occurred, and therefore bestows upon the plaintiff's case a presumptively unbiased expert opinion. In deference to their colleagues, subsequent treating physicians should exercise great caution in assigning causes to a depressed neonate's condition, particularly when any uncertainty exists as to the underlying cause of a problem. Since the gestational period is 9 months and delivery occurs in one day, the pediatrician may often be playing diagnostic roulette in trying to establish causation without sufficient proof.

With a significant number of cases alleging microcephaly as a result of a perinatal asphyxia, it is extremely important that head and chest measurements be taken by the pediatrician and recorded in the baby's chart. In addition, careful examination of the infant for congenital defects and of the placenta for any abnormal features may provide the key to refute potential charges of medical negligence.

REFERENCES

1. Chicago Metropolitan Healthcare Council: Tactics, no 45, November 1, 1983
2. Chicago Metropolitan Healthcare Council: Tactics, no 83, November 1, 1985
3. Collea JV, Rabin SC, Weghorst GR, Quilligan EJ: The randomized management of term frank breech presentation: Vaginal v. cesarean delivery. Am J Obstet Gynecol 131:86, 1978
4. Dierker LJ, Roger M, Thompson K, Lynn D: Midforceps deliveries: Long-term outcome of infants. Am J Obstet Gynecol 154:764, 1986
5. First National Bank of Chicago v Porter, 114 Ill App 3d 1, 448 NE 2nd 256, 1983
6. First National Bank of Chicago v Porter, ibid, at 264
7. Illinois Pattern Jury Instructions, 105.01, 1973
8. Illinois Revised Statutes, chap 110, Sec 13-212, 1983
9. Illinois Revised Statutes, chap 110, Sec 13-212(b), 1988
10. Nelson KB, Ellenberg JH: Antecedents of cerebral palsy: Multivariate analysis of risk. N Engl J Med 315:81, 1986
11. Prenatal and perinatal factors associated with brain disorders. NIH Publication no 85-1149, April 1985
12. Standards for Obstetric-Gynecologic Services, 6th ed. 1985
13. Walker v U.S., 600 F Supp 195, DC 1985
14. Walski v Tiesenga, 72 Ill 2d 249, 256, 381 NE 2d 279, 1978
15. Watson WJ, Benson WL: Vaginal delivery for the selected frank breech infant at term. Obstet Gynecol 64:638, 1984

PART V
NEW TREATMENT MODALITIES

12

In Vitro Fertilization

SECTION 1: CLINICAL AND RESEARCH ASPECTS

Joseph D. Schulman and María Bustillo

In vitro fertilization (IVF) is a powerful reproductive technology which in standard or variant forms has permitted many previously infertile couples to have children.[25] While simple in theory, IVF is complex in practice and dramatic in its impact on individual patients and medical science.[2,17] IVF has also attracted much attention from the press, lawmakers, governmental agencies, religious spokesmen, and others who are concerned about its apparent revolutionary significance for human reproduction.[7,26]

IVF is now clinically applicable in many types of infertility situations. An understanding of the fundamental medical and laboratory principles underlying this complex technology is essential for an intelligent analysis of the legal and ethical issues raised by IVF and related reproductive alternatives.[8] This chapter will review those principles largely to prepare the interested reader for the legal and ethical discussions elsewhere in this volume. Also, a number of recent comprehensive volumes on the clinical and laboratory methods of IVF are recommended for additional information.[1,5,6,10,11,13,24]

HISTORY

IVF became a clinical reality largely through the pioneering work of Dr. Robert Edwards, a reproductive physiologist and geneticist at Cambridge University, and his surgical colleague, Mr. Patrick Steptoe, from Manchester. Beginning in the 1960s, Edwards began to utilize techniques of tissue culture and animal embryology in an attempt to identify the appropriate conditions needed to accomplish fertilization of the human oocyte outside the body of the female, and then to permit subsequent early embryonic cleavage. The technique of laparoscopy, which Steptoe had a major role in developing in England, provided a safe method for retrieving the eggs for these investigations. It was decided early that best results were likely to be obtained with oocytes matured in vivo almost to the point of ovulation, rather than by the recovery and prolonged in vitro maturation of immature human eggs. By the early 1970s, appropriate culture conditions were developed which permitted human sperm capacitation, oocyte culture, fertilization, and early embryonic cleavage in an apparently normal manner. Infertile couples from Steptoe's medical practice donated the oocytes used in these investigations and were the recipients of the embryos transferred by transcervical catheters, or occasionally by laparoscopically guided transabdominal needles.

The tenacity of these investigators and their patients over almost a decade of frustration as one embryo transfer after another failed to establish a pregnancy is now legendary, as is their stubborn refusal to abandon their course of research despite severe criticism from some religious leaders, lawmakers, and scientific colleagues.

In 1978, for reasons that even now are not clear, the first successful embryo transfers took place, leading to the widely publicized birth of Louise Brown. Originally, it was thought that the key to success was the use of oocytes recovered from natural cycles, rather than those in which follicular stimulation had been employed. This explanation is no longer accepted, and it seems more likely that the true cause involved some improved quality of manufacturing or handling of reagents used in the laboratory for egg/embryo culture.

Once the first pregnancies were achieved, Edwards and Steptoe developed a large and highly successful private center, Bourn Hall, for the treatment of infertility through IVF. In operation since 1980, this center has produced almost 1000 births—many more than any other IVF center in the world. After 1979, the performance of IVF was rapidly developed in Australia particularly, and in 1981 the first IVF facility in the United States was opened. Australian investigators, especially at Monash University and the Royal Women's Hospital, introduced major innovations of follicle stimulation and the use of donor oocytes and embryo cryopreservation.[18] By 1983, several successful U.S. centers including one supervised by co-author Schulman were in operation and many others were active or being developed worldwide.

As of early 1987, there were over 100 centers in the U.S. alone that identified themselves as performing IVF. Most IVF is done at a much smaller number of large centers; for example, our facility in Fairfax, Virginia, conducts about 800 IVF treatment cycles per year. Fewer than 10 U.S. centers had accomplished at least 50 clinical pregnancies as of June 1988, some other centers are effectively nonfunctional, and the remainder do a moderate volume of IVF (perhaps 50–200 cycles per year).

There can be no doubt that IVF will grow in importance over the next decade as it develops acceptance as an effective form of medical treatment. Various estimates suggest that between 500,000 and 2 million currently infertile couples in the United States will be able to have their own children through the use of IVF or a related type of technology.[7]

CURRENT METHODS OF IVF

The IVF process involves a number of stages as outlined below; highlights of these are provided but, again, the larger references[1,5,6,10,11,13,24] are suggested for additional information.

The IVF Process

Patient Selection

Often overlooked, patient selection is the most critical determinant of the success rate of any competent IVF program. Success rate expressed as an average for the treatment of infertility through IVF has no more validity than would the average success rate of a clinic for the treatment of cancer (since it depends heavily on what type of cancer or infertility is treated, and the age and condition of the patients). Patients who are young, especially in their early twenties, will conceive much more readily through IVF than older patients and will have lower miscarriage rates. The average age of women in IVF programs which do *not* heavily select for younger patients is usually about 34 to 35.

IVF has been effective in treating patients with tubal obstruction, male factor infertility, endometriosis, mixed factor infertility, unexplained infertility, and other types. It is most successful for young patients with simple tubal obstruction, who have previously proven fertility. Patients with major ovulatory difficulties, or couples in whom the male factor is severely abnormal, will in general have a much lower probability of success than tubal patients.

In an IVF program in which patients are not heavily selected, usually fewer than 50% will have isolated tubal disease, and the average age of the female patients will be about 34. Under these circumstances, the *average* success rate for IVF is about 10% per initiated cycle in exceptionally fine IVF programs. This will be higher—better than 20%—in tubal patients under age 30.

It is common for IVF programs to express their success using denominators other than "per initiated cycle," such as "per retrieval" or "per embryo transfer," in order to inflate their results. We feel this practice should not be continued and is fundamentally misleading to patients and referring physicians. Patients should also be made aware that claimed pregnancy rates may include "single positive" biochemical pregnancies and always include clinical pregnancies which miscarry. About 20% to 25% of IVF pregnancies miscarry and this figure is heavily influenced, as in natural pregnancies, by maternal age. Above age 40, the combined effect of an IVF pregnancy loss rate of about 50% and the reduced probability of initiating any pregnancy usually reduces the likelihood of childbirth through IVF to under 5% per initiated cycle.

An additional point is that IVF programs frequently use waiting lists for patient selection. This enhances the ability of the program to pick the best patients to cycle. Some programs keep women waiting many months after a cycle failure before trying IVF again. Both these features tend to magnify the success rate of the program but obviously do not reflect better quality of medical service.

Preliminary Counseling and Evaluation

For patients who appear to be reasonable IVF candidates, precycle evaluation should include a detailed history, pelvic examination, basic hormonal studies, cultures, semen analysis, and other tests as appropriate. Alternative therapies, and the risks and benefits of IVF should be reviewed. Routine use of a screening laparoscopy is not justified, especially if a recent laparoscopy has been performed, and is, of course, not needed if ultrasound-guided oocyte retrieval is used instead of laparoscopic recovery.

Follicle Stimulation and Monitoring

Although the first IVF pregnancies were accomplished in natural cycles as noted above, it is now rare not to employ agents which can stimulate the maturation of several follicles. The usual drugs are clomiphene citrate and human chorionic gonadotropins (hCG) in various doses, with hCG being used to accomplished terminal maturation. Common regimens using human menopausal gonadotropins (HMG) alone involve administration of 2 to 4 ampules of HMG (each being 75 IU follicle-stimulating hormone [FSH] and 75 IU luteinizing hormone [LH]) starting on Day 2, 3, or 4 of the cycle, followed by individualized doses after Day 6 or 7. An example of a combination regimen is 100 mg clomiphene per day for 5 days starting on Day 2, 3, or 4 of the cycle, with HMG, 2 ampules, daily or every other day concurrently, and continued on an individualized basis after Day 7.

Other agents have been used for follicular phase stimulation such as tamoxifen and FSH, but experience with them is more limited and clear indications for their justifiable use, if any, in IVF are being assessed. The less commonly employed or newer agents are typically used in clinical trials on patients who have failed IVF with other agents; inevitably, some of these patients conceive on the new drug. Unless the trial has been designed to include concurrent testing with the drug on which prior cycle failures occurred, poor investigational design may lead to the false conclusion that the new drug is more effective than the standard agent(s) on which the patients had previously failed.

The discussion so far has referred to individualized regimens in which the dosages of HMG are evaluated frequently on the basis of daily estradiol levels and ultrasound measurements of follicle size and number. Progesterone and LH monitoring are also employed in many IVF centers to assist with more accurate timing of hCG administration. Recently, some investigators have proposed a fixed medical regimen with a cycle start time and retrieval time that are predetermined (programmed); it remains to be established if this simplified method of IVF will be as successful as the more classic, individualized treatments for the follicular phase.

Retrieval of Oocytes

Retrieval of oocytes is always performed 30 to 36 hours after HCG administration, or at somewhat shorter intervals after a spontaneous LH surge. Retrieval may be laparoscopic or ultrasound guided.

Laparoscopy. Laparoscopy is the original method of oocyte recovery for IVF, and many pregnancies have resulted from its use. The obvious disadvantage is that a surgical setting, usually in a hospital, is required, and the discomforts and real hazards of general anesthesia are present. Furthermore, laparoscopy may be difficult or impossible for some patients, such as those with pelvic adhesions, prior abdominal surgery, and marked obesity.

Laparoscopy also adds to the high cost of IVF. As IVF attempts must frequently be repeated before success is attained, the disadvantages of laparoscopy are magnified. In Australia, in laparoscopic programs more than half of the patients withdraw from IVF before three attempts are completed[14]; it is felt that the difficulties of repeated general anesthesia and laparoscopy may contribute to this patient withdrawal.

Ultrasound. The use of a needle guided by real-time ultrasound to retrieve oocytes in IVF was initially performed by Lenz and Lauritsen[15] in Denmark using an abdominal sector scanner and transabdominal/transvesical needle insertion. The method was popularized by Austrian workers[9] and is still used under local or epidural anesthesia in Israel and elsewhere.[12,16] The method overcomes many of the disadvantages of laparoscopy, but is quite uncomfortable for patients and has not been widely used in the United States.

Dellenbach and associates[4] in France developed an alternative technique known as transvaginal ultrasound-guided egg retrieval under local anesthesia. An abdominal sector scanner is used to guide a needle inserted through the vaginal fornix directly into the ovary or through the bladder into the ovary. This method is substantially more comfortable than the transabdominal route, and bladder puncture can frequently be avoided. This method was introduced into the United States by co-author Schulman, and the first U.S.–born infants from the transvaginal method were delivered at our Fairfax center.[22,23]

A somewhat different method for egg recovery was introduced by Parsons and associates in England.[20] A needle is inserted through the urethra into the bladder, and then the bladder is punctured under guidance of an abdominal scanner to enter the ovary. This "perurethral" technique is rapid and especially useful when the ovary is high and the bladder is filled. The disadvantage of this method is that bladder puncture, which is uncomfortable, is always needed.

A variant of transvaginal ultrasound-guided retrieval has recently become feasible with the development of small vaginal ultrasound probes with needle guides. These probes usually permit better follicle visualization than even the best abdominal scanners, especially in obese patients or those with ovaries in the cul-de-sac. Another advantage of this method is that scanning can usually be done with an empty or only slightly full bladder, enhancing patient comfort, and bladder puncture is almost never required.

Ultrasound IVF retrieval was initially considered by some to be undesirable, because the number of eggs recovered was thought to be less than with laparoscopy, but well designed clinical trials with experienced groups do not support this contention.[16] The authors have recovered up to 22 eggs from patients using ultrasound retrieval. It is now clear that the major determinants of number of eggs recovered are the type of stimulation regimen, the individual patient's response to these drugs, and the skill of the operator. The hazards of bleeding and infection have proven to be minimal in practice.

We feel strongly that ultrasound retrieval, using the transvaginal route, has already become the standard method for IVF egg recovery, and that laparoscopy need no longer be used for this purpose except in special circumstances.[21]

Gamete Preparation

The sperm to be used for IVF are washed free of the fluid components of the semen, and are usually allowed to "swim up" into a tissue culture fluid supernatant. Capacitation of the sperm occurs during this interval. The motile sperm are then used for insemination of the eggs.

The oocytes are removed from the follicular aspirates and flushes using fine pipettes and are inspected under a dissecting microscope. The oocytes are then allowed to undergo terminal maturation in vitro so that insemination is timed to follow first polar body extrusion.

Fertilization

Each oocyte is placed in an embryo culture dish containing 2 to 3 ml of medium, and usually about 50,000 to 200,000 sperm are added. Several different culture media are commonly used for IVF, such as Ham's F-10, Menozo, T-6, or modified Earle's. Maternal, adult, or fetal cord serum, heat inactivated, is also usually added at 5% to 10% concentrations although some completely artificial media have been tried.

Fertilization is indicated by the extrusion of the second polar body and the appearance of two pronuclei within the cytoplasm of the zygote.

Embryonic Cleavage

After fertilization, embryos are transferred into a culture medium which usually resembles the insemination medium but contains a higher concentration of serum. Embryos are allowed to cleave for 2 to 3 days and have usually attained the 4- to 12-cell stage by the time of transfer. Some embryos may be selected for cryopreservation if a large number of embryos is obtained. A detailed discussion of cryopreservation is beyond the scope of this review; however, this process may be performed using several methods and at various times, from the pronucleate to the blastocyst stage.[3,18] It is intended that cryopreserved embryos will be available for use after thawing for replacement into the uterus in a subsequent, usually natural, cycle.

Embryo Transfer

Embryo transfer is performed using a flexible, fine catheter inserted transcervically, either with or without ultrasound guidance, and in either the knee-chest or dorsal lithotomy positions. Many types of end-hole or side-hole catheters are used. Transfer volume is usually between 30 μl and 100 μl. Trauma to the endometrium is avoided to the maximum extent possible, and uterine tocolytics are advocated in some centers to reduce cramping and expulsion of the fluid containing the embryos.

There is debate about the optimal number of embryos to transfer. Current dogma suggests that three or four embryos should be transferred and cryopreservation used on any extra embryos above this number. The pregnancy rate is higher (but not proportionately higher) when three or four embryos are transferred than when only one or two; the risk of twinning also increases. About 15% of IVF pregnancies are twin gestations; triplets and quadruplets are quite rare.

No matter how many embryos are transferred, the likeliest outcome is that no pregnancy will result; the pregnancy rate per transfer rarely exceeds 30%, even in the most favorable subgroups of patients.

It is common, but not universal practice, to administer progesterone or a progestin to support the luteal phase during and after embryo transfer. Convincing evidence is lacking that this is desirable. Similarly no evidence is available to document that hCG boosters during the luteal phase will enhance pregnancy rates, despite anecdotal reports of possible benefit. The luteal phase is often shorter in stimulated IVF cycles than in natural cycles in the same woman.

Pregnancy Management

Occurrence of pregnancy is documented with early quantitative beta-hCG measurements usually started at 11 to 13 days after embryo transfer. A single positive test should not be regarded as convincing evidence of even a biochemical pregnancy. A clinical pregnancy is associated with serial rising HCG titers, delayed menses, and ultrasound documentation of an intrauterine sac. Once a fetal heartbeat is detected, the pregnancy has over a 90% chance of resulting in a live birth.

About 5% to 10% of IVF conceptions are only biochemical pregnancies. About 3% to 5% will be ectopic pregnancies. The clinical miscarriage rate averages 20% to 25% and is heavily influenced by maternal age; it is not clear if this is higher than the natural, age-adjusted loss rate. Miscarriages may be cytogenetically normal or abnormal.

We suggest that prenatal diagnosis be advocated in IVF pregnancies using criteria similar to that for non-IVF gestations. Either amniocentesis or chorionic villus sampling may be employed.

Once a clinical pregnancy is established, progesterone may or may not be continued for a more prolonged period. Management otherwise should be similar to that for a conventional pregnancy. Perinatal expertise is often needed because of the increased likelihood of advanced maternal age, twinning, and other factors including parental concern.

There have been limited studies of the outcome of IVF pregnancies, but available retrospective surveys suggest that there is no increased frequency of birth defects compared to the age-corrected population of natural pregnancies.

DONOR IVF

Embryos, either fresh or frozen, derived from IVF may be transferred into a recipient who is a woman other than the egg donor. This can be performed when the egg is fertilized either with the sperm of the egg donor's husband or the embryo recipient's husband. The cycles of the egg donor and embryo recipient must be approximately synchronized if fresh embryos are used. Hormonal support in the recipient can make pregnancy possible even if she has no ovaries.[19] Ovarian failure, genetic disorders in the embryo recipient, and other factors may lead to the decision for couples to select this type of reproductive option.

IVF may also use donor sperm, such as when a couple is affected with combined tubal and male factor infertility. This is not an uncommon situation in large IVF programs, and we and others have had successful IVF pregnancies with donor sperm.

REFERENCES

1. Beier HW, Lindner HR (eds): Fertilization of the Human Egg In Vitro. Berlin, Springer-Verlag, 1983
2. Cohen J, Fehilly CB, Edwards RG: Alleviating human infertility. In Austin CR, Short RV (eds): Reproduction in Mammals, 2nd ed, book 5: Manipulating Reproduction. Cambridge, Cambridge University Press, 1986

3. Cohen J, Simons RF, Fehilly CB et al: Pregnancies following the replacement of cryopreserved expanding human blastocysts. J IVF ET 2:59, 1985
4. Dellenbach P, Nisand I, Moreau L et al: Transvaginal sonographically controlled follicle puncture for oocyte retrieval. Fertil Steril 44:656, 1985
5. Edwards RG: Conception in the Human Female. London, Academic Press, 1980
6. Edwards RG, Purdy JM, Steptoe PC (eds): Implantation of the Human Embryo. London, Academic Press, 1985
7. Ethics Advisory Board, Department of Health, Education and Welfare: Report and conclusion: HEW support of research involving in vitro fertilization and embryo transfer. Washington, DC, May 4, 1979
8. Evans MI, Hanft RS, Dixler AO et al: Human in vitro fertilization: Political, legal, and ethical issues. In Speroff L, Simpson JL, Sciarra JJ (eds): Gynecology and Obstetrics, vol 5. Philadelphia, Harper & Row, 1985
9. Feichtinger W, Kemeter P: In vitro fertilization and embryo transfer: An outpatient/office procedure. In Feichtinger W, Kemeter P (eds): Recent Progress in Human In Vitro Fertilization. Palermo, Italy, Cofese, 1984
10. Feichtinger W, Kemeter P (eds): Recent Progress in Human In Vitro Fertilization. Palermo, Italy, Cofese, 1984
11. Fredericks CM, Paulson JD, DeCherney AH (eds): Foundations of In Vitro Fertilization. Washington, DC, Hemisphere Publishing Corporation, 1987
12. Hamberger L, Wikland M: Clinical experience with ultrasound guided follicle aspiration. In Feichtinger W, Kemeter P (eds): Recent Progress in Human In Vitro Fertilization. Palermo, Italy, Cofese, 1984
13. Jones HW, Jones GS, Hodgen GD et al (eds): In Vitro Fertilization, Norfolk. Baltimore, Williams & Wilkins, 1986
14. Kovacs GT, Rogers PAW: The assessment of in vitro fertilization success rates by life table analysis (abstr). Fourth World Congress on In Vitro Fertilization, Melbourne, 1985
15. Lenz S, Lauritsen JG: Ultrasonically guided percutaneous aspiration of human follicles under local anesthesia. Fertil Steril 38:673, 1982
16. Lewin A, Margolioth EJ, Rabinowitz R et al: Comparative study of ultrasonographically guided percutaneous aspiration with local anesthesia and laparoscopic aspiration of follicles for IVF. Am J Obstet Gynecol 151:621, 1985
17. Marrs RP, Schulman JD: Historical and practical aspects of in vitro fertilization. In Speroff L, Simpson JL, Sciarra JJ (eds): Gynecology and Obstetrics, vol 5. Philadelphia, Harper & Row, 1985
18. Mohr LR, Trounson AO, Freeman L: Deep freezing and transfer of human embryos. J IVF ET 2:1, 1985
19. Navot D, Laufer N, Kopolovic J et al: Artificially induced endometrial cycles and establishment of pregnancies in the absence of ovaries. N Engl J Med 314:806, 1986
20. Parsons JH, Riddle A, Booker M et al: Oocyte retrieval for in-vitro fertilization by ultrasonographically guided needle aspiration via the urethra. Lancet i:1076, 1985
21. Schulman JD: Laparoscopy for in vitro fertilization: End of an era. Fertil Steril 44:713, 1985
22. Schulman JD, Dorfmann A, Jones SL et al: Outpatient in vitro fertilization using transvaginal oocyte retrieval and local anesthesia. N Engl J Med 312:1639, 1985
23. Schulman JD, Dorfmann AD, Jones SL et al: Outpatient in vitro fertilization using transvaginal ultrasound-guided oocyte retrieval. Obstet Gynecol 69(4):665,1987
24. Seppala Markku, Edwards RG (eds): In Vitro Fertilization and Embryo Transfer. New York, New York Academy of Sciences, 1985
25. Steptoe PC, Edwards RG, Walters DE: Observations on 767 clinical pregnancies and 500 births after human in-vitro fertilization. Hum Reprod 1:89, 1986
26. Warnock M: Report of the DHSS Committee of Inquiry into Human Fertilization and Embryology. London, Her Majesty's Stationary Office, 1984

SECTION 2: LEGAL ANALYSIS

Alan O. Dixler

In vitro fertilization (IVF) can no longer be viewed as a novel medical procedure. Even so, there is very little law on the subject, and regrettably, the hostility of some elements of organized religion may discourage legislatures from enacting much-needed comprehensive legislation. To add to the confusion, the Department of Human Health Services (DHHS) regulations pertaining to IVF, in contrast to most federal regulations, are specifically subordinate to, and do not supersede, local and state laws and regulations which may apply. Accordingly, a center which contemplates IVF research must consult the law of the jurisdiction in which it is located. In any event, the physician must at all times be well aware that this is an emotionally charged issue, the legal ramifications of which are not always clear. In this regard the advice of counsel can be valuable. Flannery and associates have explored many of the legal issues surrounding government regulation of IVF in an excellent article originally prepared as a memorandum to the Ethics Advisory Board.[13]

There are four major areas of legal concern in regard to human IVF:

1. The rights, if any, of the fertilized human egg before implantation
2. The rights of the would-be parents, and any other partners to the event such as ovum donors or surrogate mothers
3. The rights and liabilities of the physician and hospital
4. The public interest expressed through governmental regulation of IVF

RIGHTS OF THE EMBRYO

A fundamental question is whether the in vitro conceptus is a "person" in the contemplation of the law, or perhaps constitutes property. Most states have no law governing the rights of an in vitro conceptus. However, there is a rich body of law governing the rights of the unborn child *en ventue sa mare* (in utero), both before quickening (first detectable fetal movement) and before viability (capable of survival ex utero).[27] Additionally, the State of Illinois has by statute[20b] vested a duty of care in favor of all conceptuses on any person who intentionally causes the fertilization of a human ovum by a human sperm outside the body of a living female. That person shall be deemed to have the care and custody of a child for purposes of applicable Illinois child abuse law, which prohibits putting a child in danger.[20a]

At early common law, quickening was an important event in fixing certain rights of the unborn child.[33,36] The embryo was not considered to be alive until some movement was detected.[12] Abortion was lawful prior to quickening and could be obtained without the consent of the father.[23,36] Over the years, however, the law developed that the child was a legal entity (if not a person) from the moment of conception.[11,34] Such was the theory of many anti-abortion statutes. The contemporary justification for that position in biologic terms is well expressed by Krimmel and Foley[28]: "A zygote is human because with its total DNA conformation are the DNA which determines, and are common to the human species. It is a specific human being because the total DNA conformation of the individual is constant at all periods in the organism's existence." With a few changes of incumbent justices on the United States Supreme Court, it is possible this view will once again be ascendant.

The unborn of whatever gestational age had rights and protections of property, tort, and criminal law. However, in two decisions in 1973, the United States Supreme Court held that women have a constitutionally guaranteed right to abortion, at least during the first 6 months of pregnancy.[9,44] These decisions do permit the states to regulate second trimester abortions and to ban abortions during the final trimester, roughly corresponding to the viability period of the fetus. The inference is that, under the 14th amendment to the Constitution, a fetus is not a person until it is viable.

It is clear that an unborn child is deemed to be living from the moment of conception for the purpose of taking under a will or trust, provided the child is born alive.[18,48] Additionally, there is considerable authority that tort law protection begins at conception if the child is born alive.[25,50,52] The estate of a stillborn child can recover damages if the fetus was viable when lethal, prenatal injuries took place.[37] Some states by statute (e.g. California Civil Code Ch. 29) explicitly recognize the legal rights of the unborn.[35,43]

The unborn also enjoy certain protections of criminal law. Under common law, an attack upon a pregnant woman for the purpose of killing the fetus was not murder even if the child was stillborn as a result.[24,46] However, California, for example, has made such an attack which succeeds in killing the fetus (except for a lawful abortion) murder.[4,40]

RIGHTS OF THE PARENTS OR DONOR

Similar issues are bound to arise in the context of in vitro conception. For example, a donor father could die before the child is born, before implantation in the mother but after in vitro conception. Inheritance rights could be subject to legal challenge. Indeed, IVF can be performed with sperm which have been stored for some time, thus raising the possibility of in vitro (or in utero) conception after the death of the donor father. The resulting child would not only be a posthumous child, but a posthumously conceived child. Such a situation is more real than might be expected. In France, a young widow persuaded a court that she was entitled to the use of sperm which her late husband had banked during their engagement, and two years prior to his death.[39] Despite her legal victory, the widow was not able to conceive from the husband's sperm. Nevertheless, the court's ruling emphasizes that it is imperative for the physician and hospital to ascertain the identities of the parents beyond question.

For many married couples who are infertile solely because of the male partner, a sperm can be donated anonymously and the wife can be fertilized by artificial insemination or by IVF. It has been estimated that artificial insemination results in approximately 20,000 live births annually in the United States.[31] There are 29 states that have statutes pertaining to artificial insemination by donor: Alabama, Alaska, Arkansas, California, Colorado, Connecticut, Florida, Georgia, Idaho, Illinois, Kansas, Louisiana, Maryland, Massachusetts, Michigan, Minnesota, Montana, Nevada, New Jersey, New York, North Carolina, Oklahoma, Oregon, Tennessee, Texas, Virginia, Washington, Wisconsin, and Wyoming.[45] Almost all of these states require written consent by the husband of the woman who is to be impregnated. Several states explicitly relieve the donor from all parental rights and duties.

In the absence of statutory guidance, the legal status of artificial insemination by donor other than the husband of the impregnated woman is not clear. One line of authority concludes that the product of artificial insemination is illegitimate.[11,17,38] Another line of authority states that the product of artificial insemination is illegitimate even when the husband of the impregnated woman is the donor of the sperm.[29] One court even ruled that the impregnated woman had engaged in adultery (except when the donor was the husband) by virtue of the artificial insemination procedure. However, a leading case has stated that the notion that the impregnated woman is guilty of adultery either with the donor or the physician, is absurd.[41] Other courts have held that the product of artificial insemination by donor other than the husband (when the husband has consented to the procedure) is the legitimate child of the marriage.[21] When the donor was known to the recipient and an active participant in the plan of an unmarried woman to become pregnant by artificial insemination, a New Jersey court conferred the legal status of full fatherhood on the donor.[5]

Accordingly, before becoming involved in an artificial insemination procedure, the physician should be aware of the legal issues. In those jurisdictions where a child conceived through artificial insemination is considered legitimate, it would follow as a matter of logic that a disinterested and anonymous donor who fathered by "artificial insemination" an IVF child should have the same protection as with conventional artificial insemination. Further, it can be argued that when the donor has lost dominion over his semen with the intent to abandon it, the donor no longer has a legal relationship with his sperm, even in the absence of an express provision of law or private contract cutting off the relationship.[15]

Because the unborn do have some legal status, the question arises as to what the physician and hospital should do if the donor mother decided not to have the conceptus implanted in her body. The DHHS regulations require that the fetus be kept alive if possible.[14] With present technology, a preimplantation conceptus could be sustained for only a short period without cryopreservation (which raises further legal issues) or without implantation within another woman. If such became the case, questions could arise as to what the responsibilities and options of an "acceptive" mother would be, including the necessity for adoption proceedings or her request to have a subsequent abortion. Additionally, complex issues as to the legitimacy of the child could arise.[7] An actual situation of this kind developed in Australia. In April 1983, both the husband and wife perished in an airplane crash. At that time there were two developing conceptuses which had not yet been implanted in the wife. The development of the embryos was then arrested by storing them at extremely cold temperatures. They remained in that state for over a year. The legislature of the Australian State of Victoria recommended the destruction of the embryos unless the deceased couple had left instructions to the contrary. There followed a storm of protest and political pressure from the right-to-life movement in Australia. More than 100 women volunteered to become pregnant with the embryos, and eventually legislation was enacted to permit the implantation of the embryos in one of the volunteers.[45]

Twenty-five states have statutes that forbid fetal research: Arizona, Arkansas, California, Florida, Illinois, Indiana, Kentucky, Louisiana, Maine, Massachusetts, Michigan, Minnesota, Missouri, Montana, Nebraska, New Mexico, North Dakota, Ohio, Oklahoma, Pennsylvania, Rhode Island, South Dakota, Tennessee, Utah, and Wyoming.[1] The purpose of these statutes would appear to include the regulation of the experimental use of aborted fetuses. Another purpose is to prevent the development of a market in fetuses for experimentation. While neither IVF nor embryo transplantation were contemplated by the various legislative bodies that enacted such laws, often they are written in broad language and could cause concern. Physicians and hospitals should seek the advice of counsel if IVF is to be performed for the first time in a particular state.

RIGHTS AND LIABILITIES OF PHYSICIAN AND HOSPITAL

Another topic of obvious importance to the physician is the tort exposure involved. At least one commentator has argued that the tort law standard to which the physician performing IVF should be subject is not the normal standard of due care (the negligence standard), but the exacting standard of strict liability (no showing of fault required). This effectively makes the physician the insurer of the IVF process, on the theory that IVF is an abnormally dangerous enterprise.[6] Louisiana has, by statute, specifically negated strict liability in IVF cases.[30,32]

Additionally, a defective infant born of the IVF process could have an action for wrongful life, claiming that there would not have been a birth without the wrongful (negligent or reckless) intervention of the defendant. The theory is that it is better never to have been born than to be born with the particular handicaps in question. Courts were hostile to the wrongful life theory in the past, but the trend has changed.[2,16,19,49,51] In addition, the parents rather than the child could have a cause of action for wrongful birth. The parents may claim they would have terminated the pregnancy or would have attempted to prevent conception if they had been advised properly of the danger of having a defective child. Courts have awarded recoveries on the wrongful birth theory.[3]

Liabilities can arise in other ways also. For example, in an unreported federal case, a would-be mother and father sued a hospital and a physician who destroyed, without the couple's consent, a developing in vitro conceptus in an early IVF attempt.[8] First, the plaintiffs argued that the termination amounted to the deliberate infliction of severe emotional distress, and the jury found for the plaintiffs on this point. Next, they claimed that the defendants *converted* the contents of the test tube (conversion is the wrongful taking of the personal property of another person).[42,47] Under this theory, the plaintiffs argued that the contents of the test tube were property and not a person. The court permitted the jury to consider this theory, but the jury found for the defendants.

Because of the legal complexities involved with the IVF procedure, and because of the lack of legal precedent and statutory regulation, a thorough legal analysis and possibly a written contract are indicated before an IVF procedure is begun. Counsel for the medical center must be consulted prior to setting up an IVF program.

GOVERNMENT REGULATION IN THE PUBLIC INTEREST

Clearly IVF is becoming a means of therapy for female infertility related to tubal pathologic conditions. And although the ethical probity of investigators working in the field may seem self-evident, the public does have an interest in setting guidelines to prevent abuses that could potentially develop. Similarly, the investigators deserve the protection of the law in their responsible attempts to allow infertile couples to have their own children. Therefore, the time for comprehensive legislation has clearly come.

The foregoing discussion should have alerted the physician to the legal complexities surrounding the IVF procedure. In the discussion it has been assumed that the ovum was that of the wife and the infertile couple and that, once fertilized, the conceptus was implanted in the wife. That scenario is not technologically mandated. For example, the ovum could come from a donor, or implantation could be performed on a surrogate. When such is the case, the legal complexities are multiplied further. Advice of counsel should be sought before involvement in such procedures, not only by the physician and institution but also by the other participants.

Whereas many states have statutes concerning artificial insemination and the status of the anonymous donor, there is no law with respect to the donor of an ovum. However, if the ovum were donated by a third party, conception occurred in vitro, and the wife then carried the fetus to term, it is likely that the donor would have no claims to the child and no liabilities. This conclusion is based on the principle that the donor lost dominion over her ovum and had the intent to abandon it. However, such reasoning is no substitute for a statutory scheme defining the various rights of the parties.

A more complex scenario is created if conception is to take place in utero and an embryo is then to be transferred to the wife to carry to term. The donor could refuse to permit removal of the embryo, for example. It is far from clear that this possibility could be avoided through contractual language. A contract to surrender a child for adoption by a surrogate mother may be void in most states. It may also be the case that a contract by a surrogate mother to surrender her rights to the embryo would be void. Further, the questions of visitation and other parental rights in such a situation are open. If a third party serves as the gestational mother, there are even further legal complications. A contract by the gestational mother (whether or not the genetic mother) to surrender the child which she has or will deliver is probably void.

Again, the issues surrounding the legal relationships of the various parties are open.

It should be noted that surrogate motherhood has met with less than a warm reception by the judicial authorities, giving rise to such concerns as baby selling. Surrogate motherhood contracts are voidable under the law of Kentucky.[26] Moreover, a Michigan court upheld the constitutionality of a statute forbidding, inter alia, surrogate motherhood for a fee.[10] Finally, in a widely publicized case, the New Jersey Supreme Court ruled that surrogate motherhood for money contracts is void and possibly criminal.[22] That case, in which a trial court decision upholding the contract was unanimously reversed, is currently the leading case on the subject. The wise physician will proceed with great caution and with legal advice.

REFERENCES

1. Andrews LB: The legal status of the embryo. Loyola Law Rev 32:357, 1986
2. Becker v Schwartz, 46 NY 2d 401, 386 NE 2d 807, 413 NYS 2d 895, 1978
3. Berman v Allen 80 NJ 421, 404 A 2d 8, 1979
4. Cal Penal Code 187
5. CM v CC, 152 NJ Supr 160, 337A 2d 821, 1977
6. Cohen ME: The "brave new baby" and the law: Fashioning remedies for the victims of in vitro fertilization. Am J Law Med 4:319, 1978
7. Cusine DJ: Some legal implications of embryo transfer. New Law J 129:627, 1979
8. Del Zio v Presbyterian Hospital, 74 Civ 3588 (SDNY), 1976
9. Doe v Bolton, 410 US 179, 1973
10. Doe v Kelley, 106 Mich App 169, 307 NW 2d 438, 1981
11. Doornbos v Doornbos, 23 USLW 2308, 1954, App disin'd, 12 Ill App 2d 473, 139 NE 2d 844, 1956
12. Evans v People, 49 NY 86, 1872
13. Flannery DM, Weisman CD, Lipset CR et al: Test tube babies: Legal issues raised in in utero fertilization. Georgetown Law J 67:1295, 1979
14. 45 CFR, part 46, subpart B
15. Frey KL: Comment: New reproductive technologies: The legal problem and a solution. Tenn Law Rev 49:303, 1982
16. Gleitman v Cosgrove, 49 NJ 22, 227 A 2d 689, 1967
17. Gursky v Gursky, 39 Misc 2d 1983, 242 NYS 2d 406, 1963
18. Hall v Hancock, 32 Mass 255, 1834
19. Harleson v Parke-Davis, Inc, 98 Wash 2d 460, 656 P 2d 483, 1983
20. Ill Rev Stat 23:2354 (a); 38:81–26(7) (b)
21. In re Adoption of Anonymous, 74 Misc 2d 99, 345 NYS 2d 430, 1973
22. In re Baby M, 109 NJ 396, 537 A 2d 1227, 1988
23. In re Vince, 2 NJ 443, 67 A 2d 141, 1949
24. Keeler v Superior Court, 2 Cal 3d 619, 87 Rptr 481, 470 p 2 cl 617, 40 ALR 3d 420, 1970
25. Kelly v Gregory, 282 App Div 542, 125 NYS 2d 696, 1953
26. Surrogate Parenting Associates v. Commonwealth ex rel Armstrong, 704 SW 2d 209, 1986 (Ky)
27. King PL: The judicial status of the fetus: A proposal for legal protection of the unborn. Mich Law Rev 77:1647, 1979
28. Krimmel HT, Foley MJ: Abortion: An inspection into the nature of human life and the potential consequences of legalizing its destruction. U Cinn Law Rev 46:725, 1977
29. L v L, 1 All Eng R 141, 1949
30. Lorio KV: In vitro symposium: Introduction. Loyola Law Rev 32:311, 1986
31. Louio KV: In vitro fertilization and embryo transfer: Fertile areas for litigation. Southwest Law J 49:303, 1982
32. Louisiana Rev Stat 9:132
33. Means MA: The law of New York concerning abortion and the status of the fetus: 1664-1968. New York Law Forum 14:411, 1968
34. Miller v Bennett, 190 Va 162, 56 SE 2d 217, 1949
35. Note: The fetus as legal entity. San Diego Law Rev 8:126, 1971
36. Note: The unborn child: Consistency in the law? Suffolk U Law Rev 2:228, 1968
37. O'Neil v Morse, 385 Mich 130, 188 NW 2d 785, 1971
38. Orford v Orford, 58 DLR 251, 490 Ont LR 15, 1921
39. Parpalaix v Cecos, judgment of Aug 1, 1984, Trib gr inst, Fr Gazette due Palais, Sept 18, 1984
40. People v Apodaca, 76 Cal App 3d 479, 142 Cal Rptr 830, 1977
41. People v Sorenson, 68 Cal 2d 280, 437 P 2d 495, 66 Cal Rpt 7, 1968
42. Powell v AK Brown Motor Co, 200 SC 75, 20 SE 2d 636, 1942

43. Prosser W, Keeton WP: On the law of torts, 1984
44. Roe v Wade, 410 US 113, 1973
45. Shapiro ED: New innovations in conception and their effects upon our law and morality. NY Law School Law Rev 31:37, 1986
46. State v Dickinson, 23 Ohio App 2d 259, 263 NE 2d 253, 1970
47. Stickney v Monroe, 44 Me 195, 1857
48. Swain v Bowers, 91 Ind App 307, 158 NE 598, 1930
49. Tichauer L: Proposed legislation to regulate the practice of in vitro fertilization in New Jersey. Rutgers Law Rev 38:403, 1986
50. Torigan v Watertown News Co, 225 NE 2d 926, 1967
51. Turpin v Sortini, 31 Cal 2d 220, 182 Cal Rpt 337, 643 P 2d 954, 1982
52. Zepeda v Zepeda, 41 Ill App 2d 240, 190 NE 2d 849, 1963

SECTION 3: ETHICAL ISSUES IN CLINICAL AND RESEARCH APPLICATIONS

John C. Fletcher

This chapter will describe major ethical positions on clinical in vitro fertilization (IVF) and research involving the human embryo. The sources from which these positions have been assembled, namely, the published considerations of 14 commissions and working parties appointed under national, scientific, or religious auspices, are summarized in Table 12-1. In addition, there is a significant literature by individual scholars on the ethical

The help of LeRoy Walters, Ph.D., is gratefully acknowledged for permission to copy the material in Table 12-1, which he collected and has available at the Kennedy Institute of Ethics, Georgetown University. Also, Howard W. Jones, Jr., M.D., and Gary D. Hodgen, Ph.D., provided information relevant to this chapter.

aspects of IVF, which space does not allow analysis of here.[3,11,14,15,18,21,23,36,41]

As these positions are reviewed, clinical IVF emerges as ethically warranted due to its effectiveness in treating types of involuntary infertility that yield to no other mode of therapy. However, IVF's status as a fully accepted clinical practice remains questionable. Research directed toward the human embryo is ethically far more controversial than clinical IVF and embryo transfer. The arguments in favor of limited, nationally regulated, human embryo experiments are based on the potential benefits as compared to the potential harms to persons, families, and institutions, and are far more convincing than arguments against such experiments.

CLINICAL IN VITRO FERTILIZATION

In socioethical debate about clinical IVF, four major positions have emerged in public testimony and majority/minority statements:

1. Only natural reproduction is morally permissible.
2. Clinical IVF and embryo transfer is acceptable only as therapeutic procedures for married couples.
3. Clinical IVF is permissible even with donated gametes and embryos.
4. Both clinical IVF and laboratory research are morally permissible with donated gametes and embryos.

Only Natural Reproduction Is Morally Permissible

This position excludes any medically assisted conception, including artificial insemination by donor (AID). The argument against IVF can stem from positions that appeal to theologically derived beliefs, biologic observations, rights based on natural law, or other philosophical considerations. Opposition to IVF based on an argument that it is "unnatural" can take several forms, which were reviewed by Singer and Wells[32]:

- If the natural is what occurs in the normal chain of events, untouched by human intervention, then IVF violates the limits of the natural. One consequence of holding this view is that one is resigned to whatever disasters that nature brings, including those that are reversible, like plagues and famines. Also, to hold consistently to this view prevents anything being done for the first time.
- IVF is impermissible because God wills conception to occur only by natural means. This view invalidates ethical discourse apart from the premise of a theologically derived ethics, and it consequently alienates religion and science. Also, the idea that something evil occurs contrary to, but preventable by, divine will leads logically to a position of no confidence in the power, goodness, and omniscience of God, a result hardly intended by those who hold this view. Not surprisingly, this view is usually held by well intentioned lay persons rather than the clergy.
- IVF can be opposed as unnatural based on premises of "natural law." Broadly considered, natural law is composed of ethical imperatives or norms of good and right conduct which are known to all persons in different cultures and eras. One way natural law theorists discover the laws of nature is to attempt to discern the naturally appointed goal or end of an act or entity. If procreation is seen as the natural end of the sexual act, then it follows that any act to disrupt the unity between sexual inter-

Table 12-1. Contrasting Viewpoints on the Ethics of In Vitro Fertilization and Embryo Transfer

	US HEW[35]	(AUSTR) NATL HEALTH[4]	CATHOLIC BISHOPS (AUSTR)	WALLER I (AUSTR)[38]	MED RES COUNCIL (BRIT)[25]	RCOG[29] (BRIT)	CATHOLIC COMMITTEE (UK)[8]	ROYAL SOCIETY (UK)[30]	BRIT MED ASSN
THERAPY									
Acceptability in principle	Yes	Yes	No	Yes	Yes	Yes	Yes	Yes	Yes
Freezing of embryos	---	Yes	No	Yes	No	Yes	Yes	No	Yes
Donations of oocytes	No	Yes	No	NR	---	Yes	No	---	Yes
Donation of embryos (IVF)	No	---	---	No	---	Yes	No	---	Yes
Donation of embryos (IVF)	---	---	---	---	---	---	---	---	---
LABORATORY RESEARCH									
Acceptability in principle	Yes	Yes	No	NR	Yes	Yes	Yes*	Yes	Yes
Donation of embryos for research	Yes	Yes	---	---	Yes	Yes	---	Yes	Yes
Freezing of embryos	---	---	---	---	Yes	Yes	---	Yes	Yes
Interspecies fertilization	No	---	No	---	Yes	---	No	---	---
Division of embryos (cloning)	---	---	---	---	---	Yes	No	Yes	Yes
Nuclear transfer (actual cloning)	No	Yes	---	---	---	---	No	---	Yes
Gene repair	---	---	---	---	---	Yes	---	Yes	Yes
Harvesting of embryonic cells for transplant purposes	---	---	No	---	---	Yes	No	---	---
Production of parthenogenones	---	---	---	---	---	---	No	---	---
Teratogenic studies	---	---	---	---	---	---	---	Yes	---
Interspecies fusion of embryos	No	---	No	---	---	---	---	---	---
DISPOSAL OF EMBRYOS	---	Yes	No	Yes	Yes	No	No	---	Yes
SURROGATE MOTHERHOOD	No	NR	No	No	---	No	No	---	No

(Continued)

Table 12-1. Contrasting Viewpoints on the Ethics of In Vitro Fertilization and Embryo Transfer (*Continued*)

	Waller II (Austr)[39]	European Med Res Councils[13]	American Fertility Society[2]	Warnock (UK)[40]	Waller III (Austr)	Ontario Law Reform[28]
Therapy						
Acceptability in principle	Yes	Yes	Yes	Yes	Yes	Yes
Freezing of embryos	Yes	- - -	Yes	Yes	Yes	Yes
Donation of oocytes	Yes	- - -	Yes	Yes	Yes	Yes
Donation of embryos (IVF)	Yes	- - -	Yes	Yes	Yes	Yes
Donation of embryos (IVF)	- - -	- - -	- - -	No	NR	Yes
Laboratory Research						
Acceptability in principle	NR	Yes†	Yes	Yes#	Yes††	Yes
Donation of embryos for research	- - -	Yes‡	Yes	Yes	Yes	Yes
Freezing of embryos	- - -	Yes	Yes	Yes	Yes	- - -
Interspecies fertilization	- - -	Yes§	- - -	Yes**	- - -	- - -
Division of embryos (cloning)	- - -	- - -	- - -	NR	Yes	- - -
Nuclear transfer (actual cloning)	- - -	- - -	- - -	NR	- - -	- - -
Gene repair	- - -	- - -	- - -	NR	NR	- - -
Harvesting of embryonic cells for transplant purposes	- - -	- - -	- - -	- - -	- - -	- - -
Production of parthenogenones	- - -	- - -	- - -	NR	- - -	- - -
Teratogenic studies	- - -	- - -‖	- - -	NR	- - -	- - -
Interspecies fusion of embryos	- - -	- - -	- - -	- - -	- - -	- - -
Disposal of Embryos	NR	- - -	Yes	Yes	Yes	Yes
Surrogate motherhood	NR	- - -	- - -	No	No	Yes

* If research beneficial to embryo itself; - - -, not discussed; NR, not resolved
† Irish MRC had strong reservations
‡ Norwegian MRC limited to embryos following IVF
§ Norwegian MRC limited to infertility studies
‖ Norwegian MRC disapproved
Majority view
** For fertility testing; developmental limit, 2 cells
†† Majority view;' acceptable only if spare embryos used

course and procreation is contrary to natural law. The Catholic bishops of Victoria, Australia, used natural law theory to argue that by locating sexual union in the IVF laboratory man has separated what God has joined together; it "technologizes" sexuality and thus undermines the very essence of the act of sexual intercourse.[7] Some Catholic moral theologians have opposed contraception and IVF on the same natural law grounds.[27]

Singer and Wells identified a serious contradiction in this argument, namely, that if one understands procreation to be the natural end of sexuality, one will favor and not condemn IVF because it restores the loss of fertility and overcomes the previous harms of disease or accidents.[32]

Clinical IVF and Embryo Transfer Is Acceptable Only if Gametes Are Obtained From Lawfully Married Couples and No Nontherapeutic Research Involving Embryos Is Carried Out

Members of a Catholic bishops' committee in the United kingdom were persuaded that IVF could not be intrinsically wrong if used to restore the gift of human life within the context of marriage.[8] In 1979, a United States Ethics Advisory Board (EAB) chose a similar position, differing on one very crucial point.[35]

The EAB was asked to advise the Secretary of the Department of Health, Education, and Welfare on the use of federal funds to support research on the safety and efficacy of clinical IVF. Their report concluded that research could be carried out under certain conditions, including that gametes be obtained from informed and consenting persons, and if embryo transfer were involved, that gametes be obtained from lawfully married couples. The EAB permitted the fertilization of embryos from gametes of informed and consenting unmarried persons to study the safety and efficacy of clinical IVF, provided that no embryo be sustained longer than 14 days. The Catholic bishops' statement permitted only research intended to benefit the embryo, presumably fertilized from gametes of lawfully married couples.

A position that limits clinical IVF to only the orthodox family is vulnerable to challenges about the unfairness of excluding unmarried but infertile persons who desire a child. Singer and Wells correctly state that no empirical research has proved that married couples provide better homes for children than stable unmarried couples.[32] They also argue that a restrictive IVF policy does not allow careful case-by-case assessments of unmarried persons. To favor only married infertile persons for IVF unfairly discriminates against unmarried persons, who would be responsible parents if able to overcome infertility. Also this restriction prevents single persons with higher genetic risks who desire a child from using clinical IVF combined with AID to prevent transmission of a genetic disorder.

The Catholic bishops' position was doubtless derived theologically, but it results in prejudicial treatment in a pluralistic society. The EAB gave no rationale for its recommendation to restrict embryo transfer to married couples, but it is likely the result of a compromise with theological views of marriage as the normative context for parenthood made in order to achieve a procedural consensus. That the consensus was largely procedural is reflected in a key statement by the board, that the use of human embryos in research on clinical IVF was "ethically defensible but still legitimately controverted," as opposed to being "clearly ethically right." Singer and Wells criticized the United States' statement for conceptual confusion, question begging, and "papering over" serious ethical differences in order to achieve consensus.[32]

Clinical IVF Is Permissible Even When It Involves Donated Gametes And Embryos

Study commissions appointed by governmental bodies in the United Kingdom,[34] Australia,[40] and Canada,[28] as well as three medical and scientific bodies[2,5,29] approved of clinical IVF, including use of donated gametes and embryos. Donated sperm can be used in cases of no sperm or a low-sperm count in the male partner. Donated oocytes can be used to avoid a genetic defect (e.g., when the infertile woman is the carrier of an X-linked disorder) or to help a woman who is physically incapable of ovulation. Donated embryos help when both partners are infertile and physically incapable of producing gametes; they can spare the woman the burdens of more surgery to obtain oocytes.

Objections to donated gametes or embryos may be based on the same theologically based argument used against AID (e.g., separation of sexual intercourse and procreation); perceived harmful consequences of genetic dissimilarity of one or both social parents and the child; and potential legal uncertainties about the status of a child so conceived.

Theologically based objections that begin from a premise of the indissoluble unity of sexual intercourse and procreation fail on a theological level because they raise human biology to a transcendent level, a move that violates injunctions against treating the finite as infinite. Furthermore, the basic thrust of the natural law argument against contraception has been so successfully disproved by historical experiences and refuted by Catholic scholars, among others,[10,37] that no more defense is required of the intentional separation of procreation and sexual union in contraception. The hopelessness of the natural law argument was illustrated by Tiefel, a conservative ethicist, who pointed out the irony for infertile couples to "be overjoyed" if they could but link their sexual union with procreation."[33]

The burden of moral proof is entirely on those who would justify no use of contraceptives in human reproduction. That is, contraception is so well integrated in moral evolution and social history that those who use it to prevent or plan pregnancies are not obligated to justify their reasons in any public sense. They are acting in a praiseworthy manner, even though some of their fellow human beings would judge them to be morally wrong. AID and, by extension, IVF with donated gametes and embryos are in different stages of moral and technical acceptability.

At least 20,000 children are born each year in the United States following AID, indicating its benefits as a solution to male infertility or the avoidance of a dominant genetic disorder transmitted by the male partner. Nevertheless, legal problems remain. Capron states that the law created by judicial decision in this field "over the past 35 years has been a patchwork of rules which are, at best, inconsistent—and which generally do not provide a sensible basis for public safety."[6] Nearly half the states have laws to protect the legitimacy of a child born after AID (assuming that the social father consented to the procedure), which also relieves the donor of any parental responsibility. A number of other problems remain, including the availability of AID to unmarried persons, screening donor sperm for genetic diseases, proper record keeping, and the right of children to know the name or identity of the donor. These are ancillary ethicolegal issues that follow after the basic moral acceptability of the innovation has occurred. An ethical imperative exists to protect those who use reproductive technologies after concluding that benefits far outweigh harms. Those who choose to use technical measures to overcome infertility or genetic disease should be treated fairly, just as those who choose *not* to use such measures should not be punished for their choices.

IVF, with donated gametes and embryos, is in the earliest stage of technologic as well as moral evolution. Experience in the practice of adoption and with AID suggests that genetic unlikeness is neither an obstacle to closeness nor a source of insuperable difficulty in later life for the child who wants to know or meet his genetic parent(s). If donors of gametes or embryos request absolute anonymity, some leeway may be possible in reaching prior agreement to disclose some general characteristics to the future, curious child. Absolute secrecy in matters of biologic identity does not appear to be a wise policy.

States can take legal action to protect the rights of children born consequent to IVF, if necessary, to fill the gaps in the law created by the differences in technologic and natural fertilization.

Clinical IVF Is Permissible, Even With Donated Gametes and Embryos and Also Laboratory Research With Early Human Embryos

Two premises make up the basis for this open policy: (1) to date, clinical IVF has proved safe and relatively efficacious in treatment of infertility, and (2) IVF is a rich source for research into the causes of infertility, genetic disorders, and knowledge about human embryology otherwise unattainable.

Is clinical IVF safe? The earliest objections to clinical IVF were based on fears of harm to offspring, such as congenital abnormalities or mental retardation. As of the Fourth World Conference on IVF/ET in 1985, 1098 babies were reported born after IVF, among whom 8 suffered from birth defects for a rate of 0.007%, a lower than expected rate following natural fertilization.[17]

Abnormalities are not the only risk in pregnancy, however. Pregnancies after IVF that result in ectopic pregnancies (4%–15%) or that are lost to spontaneous abortion (24%–28%) are higher than if following natural fertilization. The higher spontaneous abortion rate may be explained by the fact that women who suffer from infertility have a higher rate of spontaneous abortion. The answer to the higher ectopic pregnancy rate is unknown. Additionally, the incidence of twins (5%–20%) is much higher than following natural fertilization, largely due to the transfer of multiple embryos to increase the chance of pregnancy. Twin pregnancies carry higher risks for the infants and the mother.[22] As to the general health and mental condition of the children, the answer must await the findings of the first follow-up study of 80 children born after IVF in the United States, whose health will be compared to 80 children born after natural conception.[26]

Is IVF effective? In the U.S. program with the most IVF experience (1981–1985), 289 pregnancies were achieved in 1078 total transfers involving 775 different patients for a pregnancy rate of 26.8%.[1] This pregnancy rate was steadily maintained or increased for a variety of conditions causing infertility. Jones commented that the pregnancy rate by transfer is "remarkably similar to the pregnancy rate for a single month of exposure during normal reproduction."[19] Eighty-nine pregnancies of the 289 were lost to spontaneous abortion, a rate of 30.8%, higher than the rate associated with natural reproduction, generally understood to be near 20%.[12] Jones noted the uncertain cause of the higher spontaneous abortion rate and stated that it "may well be associated with the IVF process."[19]

For some patients more than one attempt at transferring an embryo is necessary. For patients who became pregnant the chance of doing so in the first attempt was 20%. IVF is an expensive procedure when estimated in terms of such a modest rate of success. Including preliminary screening, laporoscopy, embryo transfer, and counseling, the costs reported at the Fourth World Conference ranged from $3500 to $5000 per attempt in one cycle. Clearly, there is ample room for improvement in the clinical pregnancy rate and in lowering costs.

Jones discussed three goals in developmental biology required to increase the pregnancy rate:

1. To recruit consistently more mature oocytes
2. To mature in vitro oocytes harvested while immature
3. To identify while in vitro the pregnancy potential of a given embryo[19]

These research goals naturally lead to an additional set of topics and questions.

QUESTIONS RELATED TO EMBRYO RESEARCH AFTER IVF

If More Than an Ideal Number of Healthy Embryos Are Fertilized for Transfer, Is It Ethical to Discard Those That Remain?

Jones points out that "the pregnancy rate by number of . . . embryos transferred shows the importance of transfers up to four but indicates that transfers above three are of doubtful value."[19] In the Norfolk program, on average two and one-half embryos have been transferred per patient. Yet 82% of centers reporting at the World Conference stated that "all embryos" were being transferred, meaning that in some centers as many as five or six embryos are being transferred in one procedure. Not only does this practice increase the chances (and risks) of multiple pregnancy, but it gives a strong appearance of an attempt to counter any possible criticism of deliberately destroying excess embryos.

What is the moral status of the human embryo? The EAB stated that the human embryo "is entitled to profound respect; but this respect does not necessarily encompass the full legal and moral rights attributed to persons."[35] The Warnock report came to a similar conclusion, but altered the EAB's emphasis on depth of "respect" and added a consequentialist framework for consideration: "Though the human embryo is entitled to some added measure of respect beyond that accorded to other animal subjects, that respect cannot be absolute, and may be weighed against the benefits arising from research."[34] None of the governmental bodies appointed to make recommendations about IVF gave extended moral arguments to support their findings. These arguments must be sought out in the religious and scholarly literature on IVF.

Catholic bishops of Australia and the United Kingdom opposed the destruction of any excess embryos on the grounds that each fertilized embryo had the potential of becoming a person and ought to be treated in terms of this potential.[7,8] Singer and Wells[32] accord the embryo no special moral status, because they cannot find a morally relevant difference between destruction of the egg and sperm (which will unite), and destruction of an embryo. For them, everything that could be said about the "potential for personhood" of the embryo can also be said about the sperm and egg that become the embryo. If it is not wrong to destroy the sperm and egg by contraception or masturbation, they argue, then how could it be wrong to destroy embryos?

Dunstan, in an outstanding historical essay on the question of the moral status of the human embryo, showed that the claim to "absolute protection for the human embryo 'from the beginning' is a novelty in the Western, Christian and specifically Roman Catholic moral traditions."[9] He defends a tradition that attempts to "grade the protection accorded to the nascent human being according to its stage of development."

A "graded" or developmental view of the moral status of the embryo, fetus, and infant-to-be is compatible both with the older moral tradition, identified by Dunstan, and with a "common sense" view of the issues, as put forward by a moral philosopher, Lockwood.[24] He distinguished between the concepts of a living human organism, a human being, and a person, appealing throughout the essay to a moral level of justification that is "intuitively" apparent or true on a prima facie level. A living human organism is a biologic, not moral, concept; simply a "[complete] living organism of the species Homo sapiens." In this view, an embryo is simply a living human organism.

Lockwood answers the query as to when a human being begins to exist by the degree of "brain life," especially the higher brain functions, as do many other philosophers and scientists. The concept of a person entails a "conscious being" possessing more than sentience, namely, a capacity for self-consciousness and reflection. Lockwood is open to the idea that some nonhuman primates, such as chimpanzees and dolphins, as well as extraterrestrial beings, may be persons in this sense but not human persons. Persons, for Lockwood, are not identical with living human organisms. The prevailing morality that supports the removal of life supports from terminally ill, brain-dying persons, tends also to make the distinction between persons and living human organisms. For Lockwood, the human embryo is neither a human being with interests to be protected nor a "potential" person (a frequently used argument for equal protection of the embryo and early fetus). He opposes the view that no morally relevant differences exist between killing a human embryo and killing a newborn with grave malformations.

Should the human embryo be accorded more protection by society, which implies more respect, than another animal embryo, such as a mouse, or tadpole, simply because it is a living *human* organism? Singer and Wells attribute this as an error of "speciesism," that species membership as *Homo sapiens* is the source of a claim of special protection or a right to life. They argue that species membership is not a morally relevant category upon which to frame an argument for protection of the right to life, but rather is equivalent to an argument based upon race. Morally relevant characteristics, such as rationality and other attributes of persons, ought to be the criteria for selection. The foregoing discussion of speciesism is an important feature in Singer's moral argument for the protection of animals in research and his critique of the moral beliefs about the superiority of humans, which is traditionally used to justify animal pain and suffering in research.[31]

In effect, three views of the moral status of the human embryo exist and contend for dominance. Each has a notable outcome for the question of discard and research. The first is based on a potential for personhood, grounded in the embryo's genetic composition, and argues for strong protection and even prohibition of certain activities. It was used by three members of the Warnock committee to dissent from the majority.[34] They objected to deliberate destruction of the embryo on any grounds as well as to creation of embryos for research alone. A second group of four dissenters objected to the creating of embryos for research alone, but not to the use of excess embryos for research. They thought this act to be morally wrong because of the deliberate intent involved in creating an organism with human potential and then destroying it. Further, the second group said that a moral line should be drawn between the use of embryos created by chance and by intent in order to prevent other foreseeable dangers of exploitation by eugenic experimentation. A precedent for eugenic experiments exists, in the fertilizing of embryos for the sake of genetic research and the discarding of them.

The second view, as stated by Lockwood, regards human embryos as not "the sorts of things that can have interests at all," and that arguments based upon potential are ineffectual and far-fetched due to the significant biologic differences between the embryo and later stages of human life. It would follow that scientists should be unimpeded by society from destroying excess embryos or doing research if the scientific or clinical merit of the research is worthwhile. In this view, no special protection for the embryo is needed.

A third view, which is my own, begins from the premise that moral indifference to the human embryo, regardless of whether it is considered in the context of normal reproduction, transfer after IVF, or research, is inappropriate. However, no moral blame ought to attach to interventions involving the human embryo that fall within socially legitimate purposes of intentional parenthood and biomedical research. This view is skeptical about claims of intrinsic properties of the human embryo that would prevent its destruction, whether by an abortifacient, following IVF as an excess embryo, or in the context of research. The task is not to create a new set of independent moral rules to govern or prohibit research with the embryo, but to extend the ethical considerations of parenthood and research to include activities involving the embryo. This view is compatible with a developmental view of embryonic and fetal development and a "graded" view of the degree of societal protection owed to the embryo, fetus, and developing human being.

This position does not permit moral indifference at any stage of development, including in the preconceptual period, in which the conditions for optimizing the healthy condition of gametes may be studied and implemented.[20] Further, the wantedness of the pregnancy, when it is intentional, is a morally relevant reason to respect the embryo, the subject of conception. We are confronted with a living human organism intended and wanted by human beings for a purpose that is widely regarded as morally grounded, namely, human reproduction. Every fertilized embryo does not have the capacity to be implanted and develop further towards the possibility of a human being. Indeed, many embryos are incapacitated, as is being discovered in the context of IVF. If it is not morally blameworthy to use an intrauterine device to prevent implantation of the fertilized embryo, why would it be any more blameworthy to discard excess and unwanted embryos following IVF? The respect that is owed to the human embryo depends on the context of parenthood, and largely on whether pregnancy is intended and continued. Consent to pregnancy can occur after an unintended fertilization and implantation.

When embryos are intentionally fertilized externally to overcome infertility, it is no moral wrong to discard the excess embryos, assuming that options to freeze or conduct research are unavailable. The significance of the problem of infertility and the well-being of the woman justify taking the step of avoiding the implantation of excess embryos. However, the more morally acceptable path would be to freeze the excess embryos for later transfer to the woman or as donated embryos to another infertile woman. Then, the embryos would not be wasted. A second strong argument can be made for research

Is It Ethical to Freeze and Store Embryos?

The ethical and public policy issues of this question were reviewed by Grobstein, Flower, and Mendeloff.[16] The objections to freezing arise from overriding moral reasons against the practice of IVF and against freezing as unwarranted experimentation, or as a potential cause of chromosomal or genetic damage to the embryo and future child. The major argument for freezing is based upon the beneficence of sparing the infertile woman further pain, suffering, and expense of surgery. An additional benefit could come through donating embryos to other infertile women who could be spared surgery altogether, or for whom surgery presents excessive risks. The main reservation stems from the lack of certainty, based upon sound clinical trials involving human embryos, about the safety and efficacy of freezing. As of 1985, 12 infants had been born following thawing of embryos, and none of these had birth defects.

Is It Ethical to Fertilize Embryos for the Purpose of Research Alone?

The most controversial question associated with the IVF procedure is that concerning pure research. Given the diverse viewpoints on the moral status of the embryo noted above, it is unlikely that they will be reconciled in some common-ground moral argument that clearly supports such research. Therefore, a procedural resolution to the question has been reached in nations that have permitted embryos to be created, with consent from volunteers who donate gametes, for research into the causes of infertility and chromosomal and genetic disorders.

Out of consideration for the viewpoint that holds the embryo has a significant degree of moral status compared to other animals, the practice has been to limit research to no more than 14 days, a point at which the development of the "primitive streak" begins to occur. The fact that research is permitted at all pays some tribute to the view that no moral blame should be attached to destruction of human embryos, especially when the discovery of significant scientific and medical benefits is possible.

One future benefit may be early selection of embryos produced by families of highest genetic risk. Beyond this goal lies the futuristic concept of introducing fetal genetic therapy following an early prenatal diagnosis of a treatable disorder. Studies with the embryo will enhance the likelihood of embryo selection and fetal therapy. Therefore, embryo research must be pursued if we are to realize such foreseeable but now unreachable benefits as prevention of abortion in intended pregnancies and the earliest possible treatment of genetic diseases.

REFERENCES

1. Acosta AA, Andrews MC, Jones GS et al: The indications for in vitro fertilization. Virginia Med 113:216, 1986
2. American Fertility Society: Ethical statement on in vitro fertilization. Fertil Steril 41:12, 1984
3. Andrews L: New Conceptions. New York, St. Martin's Press, 1984
4. Australia National Health and Medical Research Council, Working Party on Ethics in Medical Research: Ethics in Medical Research. Canberra, Australian Government Publishing Service, 1983
5. British Medical Association, Working Group on In-Vitro Fertilisation: Interim report on human in vitro fertilisation and embryo replacement and transfer. Br Med J 286:1594, 1983
6. Capron AM: The new reproductive possibilities: Seeking a moral basis for concerted action in a pluralistic society. Law Med Health Care, p 196, October 1984
7. Catholic Bishops of Victoria (Australia): Submission to the committee to examine in vitro fertilization (unpublished document) August 6, 1982

8. Catholic Bishops' Joint Committee on Bio-Ethical Issues (Great Britain): In vitro fertilisation: Morality and public policy (unpublished document). March 2, 1983
9. Dunstan GR: The moral status of the human embryo: A tradition recalled. Med Ethnics 1:38, 1984
10. Dupre L: Contraception and Catholics: A New Appraisal. Baltimore, Helicon, 1964
11. Edwards R: Fertilization of human eggs in vitro: Morals, ethics and the law. Q Rev Biology 49:3, 1974
12. Edwards DK, Lindsay KS, Miller JF et al: Early embryonic mortality in women. Fertil Steril 38:447, 1982
13. European Medical Councils, Advisory Subgroup: Human in vitro fertilisation and embryo transfer. Lancet 2:1187, 1983
14. Grobstein C: From Chance to Purpose. Reading, MA, Addison-Wesley, 1981
15. Grobstein C, Flower M, Mendeloff J: External human fertilization: An evaluation of policy. Science 222:127, 1983
16. Grobstein C, Flower M, Mendeloff J: Frozen embryos: Policy issues. N Engl J Med 312:1585, 1985
17. Hodgen GD: Summary data from IV World Conference on IVT/ET, Melbourne, Australia, November 18–22, 1985. Personal communication
18. Jersild PT: On having children: A theological and moral analysis of in vitro fertilization. In Edward D. Schnieder (ed): Questions About the Beginning of Life. Minneapolis, Augsburg, 1985
19. Jones HW Jr: Status of basic external human fertilization. Proc Int Cong Reprod Biology, 1986 (in press)
20. Jongbloet PH: Prepregnancy care: Background biological effects. In Chamberlain G, Lumley J (eds): Prepregnancy Care: A Manual for Practice. New York, John Wiley & Sons, 1986
21. Kass L: "Making babies" revisited. The Public Interest 54:32, 1979
22. Keith L, Hughey MJ: Twin gestation. Gynecol Obstet 2:2, 1986
23. Le Roy Walters: Human in vitro fertilization: A review of the literature. Hastings Center Report 9(4):24, 1979
24. Lockwood M: When does a life begin? In Lockwood M (ed): Moral Dilemmas in Modern Medicine, pp 9–31. Oxford, Oxford University Press, 1985
25. Medical Research Council (Great Britain): Research related to human fertilisation and embryology. Br Med J 285:1480, 1982
26. Mills J: NICHD Norfolk IVF Study. Personal communication.
27. Moraczewski AS: In vitro fertilization and Christian marriage. Linacre Q 46:302, 1979
28. Ontario Law Reform Commission: Report on Human Artificial Reproduction and Related Matters. Toronto, Ministry of the Attorney General, 1984
29. Royal College of Obstetricians and Gynaecologists: Report of the RCOG Ethics Committee on in vitro Fertilization and Embryo Replacement or Transfer. London, Chameleon Press, March 1983
30. Royal Society: Human Fertiliztion and Embryology. London, Royal Society, March 1983
31. Singer P: Animal Liberation. New York, Avon Books, 1977
32. Singer P, Wells D: Making Babies. The New Science and Ethics of Conceptions. New York, Charles Scribner's Sons, 1985
33. Tiefel HO: Human in vitro fertilization: A conservative view. JAMA 247:3235, 1982
34. United Kingdom, Department of Health and Social Security: Report of the Committee of Inquiry into Human Fertilisation and Embryology (Chairman: Mary Warnock). London, Her Majesty's Stationery Office, July 1984
35. United States, Department of Health, Education, and Welfare, Ethics Advisory Board: HEW Support of Research Involving Human In Vitro Fertilization and Embryo Transfer. Washington, DC, US Government Printing Office, 1979
36. United States HEW Support of Research Involving Human In Vitro Fertilization and Embryo Transfer, Appendix, chaps 3–7. Washington, DC, US Government Printing Office, 1979
37. Valsecchi A: Controversy: The Birth Control Debate, 1958–1968, Washington, DC, Corpus, 1968
38. Victoria (Australia) Committee to Consider the Social, Ethical, and Legal Issues Arising from In Vitro Fertilization (Chairman: Louis Waller): Interim report (unpublished document). September 1982
39. Victoria (Australia) Committee to Consider the Social, Ethical and Legal Issues Arising from In Vitro Fertilization (Chairman: Louis Waller): Report on donor gametes in IVF (unpublished document). August 1983

40. Victoria (Australia) Committee to Consider the Social, Ethical and Legal Issues Arising from In Vitro Fertilization: Report on the Disposition of Embryos Produced by In Vitro Fertilization (Chairman: Louis Waller). Melbourne, FD Atkinson Government Printer, August 1984

41. Warnock M: In vitro fertilization: The ethical issues II. Philosophical Q 33:238, 1983

13

Surrogate Motherhood: Legal Issues Raised By the New Reproductive Alternatives*

Alexander Morgan Capron

This chapter examines the rapidly expanding legal issues in human reproduction. The law faces many new challenges because of the remarkable developments taking place in reproductive medicine. For example, so-called surrogate motherhood† may have a biblical precedent,[20] but only in the past few years has it been openly practiced by any appreciable number of people. Moreover, the small number of surrogate mothers pales beside other alternatives to traditional human reproduction, such as artificial insemination by donor (AID), which affect a much larger number of people. Still other, even more technologically complicated alternatives, though not yet in widespread use, are already creating ethical and legal complications. The development of this field has been so rapid that a leading textbook on gynecology and obstetrics published in 1981 contains only one paragraph on in vitro fertilization (IVF) in 1300 pages.[35] (See Chapter 12.)

REPRODUCTIVE POSSIBILITIES

Before discussing some of the problems with which the law must cope in the field of alternative birth technologies, the more feasible reproductive possibilities (Table 13-1) must be considered first, and their underlying goals and values analyzed. Surrogate motherhood, the subject of recent headlines, will also be discussed in detail as a test case for society's legal response.

---

* Adapted from the 1987 Bodenheimer Lecture at the School of Law, University of California, Davis.

† The term surrogate mother is inaccurate. In ordinary parlance a woman who raises another woman's offspring would be called the surrogate mother, but the term has come to general usage to designate a woman who gives up the child she has borne to be raised by another woman and her husband, the child's biological father.

Table 13-1. Reproductive Possibilities

No.	Name of Method	Genetic Source	Fertilization	Gestation	Social Parents
1	Traditional reproduction	X_M & Y_M	Natural	M	M & M
2	Artificial insemination, husband	X_M & Y_M	AI	M	M & M
3	Test tube baby	X_M & Y_M	IVF	M	M & M
4	Artificial insemination, donor	X_M & Y_D	AI	M	M & M
5	Donated egg	X_D & Y_M	IVF	M	M & M
6	Transferred egg	X_D & Y_M	AI with embryo flushing	M	M & M
7	Surrogate motherhood	X_D & Y_M	AI	D	M & M
8	Test tube baby in rented womb	X_M & Y_M	IVF	D	M & M
9	Transfer to rented womb	X_M & Y_M	Natural or AI w/embryo flushing	D	M & M
10	Postnatal adoption	X_D & Y_D	Natural, AI, or IVF	D	M & M
11	Substitute father	X_M & Y_D	IVF	M	M & M
12	Brave new world	X_1 & Y_2	IVF or Natural/AI/ w/embryo flushing	3	4 & 5

Abbreviations: X, female; Y, male; AI, artificial insemination; IVF, in vitro fertilization; D, donor; M, member of married couple.

In any discussion of reproductive possibilities, we must consider several very important variables. First there is the genetic aspect of parenthood: who will be the source of the gametes? Next, how and where does fertilization take place? Is it done with the husband's sperm or with donor sperm? After fertilization, does the embryo stay in the uterus, or is it flushed out? Or are egg and sperm united in the laboratory, through IVF?

Next, where will gestation occur? At the present time, "where?" signifies only "in which woman?", although the future may see the use of extracorporeal gestation, an artificial placenta, or a neonatal intensive care unit for 14-day-old embryos. Finally, who will be the child's social or rearing parents?

In the traditional mode of reproduction between a husband and wife, the wife's egg and husband's sperm unite in her fallopian tubes following intercourse; the fetus comes to term in her uterus, and finally the couple rears the resulting child (Table 13-1, method 1).

Moving beyond tradition, technology begins to enter the picture. Artificial insemination (AI) has been used in selective breeding programs in the field of animal husbandry for decades. Although the first use of the technique in human patients was in the 19th century, it has only been in wide use in the past several decades.[2,13] When used with the gametes of a married couple (method 2), all the factors remain the same as for traditional reproduction except that AI can resolve a male fertility problem (by concentrating the sperm before insertion), or a female fertility problem (when the cervix or tubes pose a barrier to normal insemination). The technique may also be used when a husband anticipates damage to his testicles (e.g., because of workplace hazards) and freezes semen deposits in a sperm bank. Artificial insemination by husband (AIH) need not involve anyone other than the couple, since insemination in its most simplistic form can be accomplished with a turkey baster or a drinking straw. When it is performed for the indications previously mentioned, it typically involves a physician and other medical personnel.

In 1978, a decade of research by Steptoe and Edwards in laboratory fertilization of ova retrieved from women with primary infertility due to impatent fallopian tubes[11] resulted in the birth of the first "test tube baby," Louise Brown.[11] Although dramatic from a technical perspective, IVF (method 3) from genetic, gestational, and social viewpoints is similar to conventional reproduction (method 1). Several thousand babies have been born through this technique, and in vitro clinics are increasing, although a large discrepancy remains among success rates of different clinics.

The present demand for medical services aimed at overcoming infertility is generally acknowledged to be a result of the increase in both absolute numbers and the proportion of women postponing child bearing.[3] The availability of a wider range of contraceptive choices and the general availability from 1973 onwards of elective abortion, combined with the entry of large numbers of women into the mainstream work force, have "liberated" women from the dictates of reproductive biology. The exercise of choice has had a dramatic effect on involuntary infertility. Increased maternal age is accompanied by a decline in fertility. The risk of infertility is also inherent in the use of some contraceptive technologies, such as the pill, IUD, and abortion. Infertility has also increased due to sexually transmitted infectious diseases such as gonorrhea and chlamydia, which can damage the fallopian tubes. At the same time, the major traditional alternative for childless couples—adoption—has constricted due to a decrease in the supply of adoptable babies relative to the demand.[1] For these reasons, a large, eager, even desperate public exists for each new reproductive possibility such as IVF.

Up to this point, the major issues involved in aiding men and women who have had some difficulty in generating children of their own, have been simply the relative safety and efficacy of the procedure: will it harm the prospective parents or child, and is it effective enough to qualify as medical practice rather than research, and thus warrant health insurance coverage? From here on, however, the situation grows more complex.

With artificial insemination by donor (AID) the source of the semen is a third party (method 4). This technique would be more accurately termed *artificial insemination by vendor* (AIV), since the traditional source of semen for artificial insemination has been male medical students who submit their sample in exchange for money.[2] Donor semen is used when the husband has an inadequate sperm count or is a known carrier of a genetic disease (such as Tay Sachs). Theoretically the donor could inseminate the woman through intercourse, but for moral and psychological reasons, insemination is usually performed artificially by a physician. As mentioned previously, the technique is simple, and non-physician-assisted AID certainly occurs. In the opinion of some feminists, the ease of use provides a valuable means for women—especially single women or lesbian couples—to have access to this reproductive alternative without medical approval and control. When used by women themselves, AID often involves a donor who is known by the recipient; when administered by a physician, typically the donor is not known. Fresh semen is still widely used, but fear of acquired immunodeficiency disease (AIDS) has led to more semen banks; improved techniques for freezing semen has led to greater reliance on frozen samples* selected from catalogs that

---

* The risk that AIDS (acquired immunodeficiency syndrome) will be transmitted during artificial insemination has led to greater use of frozen semen. A sample of semen is frozen for 90 days, at which time the donor is retested for AIDS, because several months are sometimes required between infection with the virus and the production of a detectable level of AIDS antibodies.

provide basic information on donor characteristics. The physician may also be able to arrange the use of the same donor for future pregnancies.

When the situation is reversed and the wife either has no viable eggs or wishes to avoid passing on her own genes, the germinal material can be obtained from another woman. This leads to two possible variations of IVF (methods 5 and 6). In method 5, ova harvested from a donor are fertilized with Mr. M's sperm and implanted in Mrs. M's uterus (see Chapter 12, Section 1).[25,26] In a newer technique, method 6, AI of a donor with Mr. M's sperm leads to IVF. Before the fertilized egg can implant in the donor's uterus, however, the embryo is flushed out and transferred to Mrs. M.[2]

Suppose that Mrs. M's problems go beyond having no viable ova-at one extreme, including factors that make it dangerous or impossible for her to bear a child, or at the other extreme, her unwillingness to go through the inconvenience of a pregnancy. If the couple wishes to have a child with the genes of one of them, another woman could be fertilized artificially with Mr. M's semen, bear the child, and then give it to Mr. and Mrs. M to raise. This technique (method 7) has been labeled *surrogate motherhood*.

There are other circumstances in which a couple might want to borrow—or rent—a uterus (remembering that a vendor for pay rather a volunteer donor is most likely to be involved). First, a method parallel to method 5 could be used, in which the eggs are harvested from Mrs. M, fertilized in vitro, and then transferred to the rented gestator (method 8). Alternatively, if a woman has healthy eggs but cannot, or does not wish to, carry the fetus to term, the couple could employ natural intercourse or artificial insemination, followed by embryo flushing and transfer to the donor for gestation (method 9).

To return to the familiar again, method 10 represents what happens with postnatal adoption. Such pregnancies usually follow traditional intercourse, but a baby that results from AI or even from IVF might be put up for adoption (e.g., if the parents were to die). Moreover, the timing of the decision by the male and female donors to give up the child to Mr. and Mrs. M may vary a great deal; usually this is a decision made around the time of birth, and it may or may not involve a male donor, depending upon whether his identity is known and he is claiming paternal rights. But the decision might be made earlier, indeed, even before fertilization.

Many more options could be added to Table 13-1. For example, methods 3 and 4 could be combined: IVF because Mrs. M has blocked fallopian tubes, with AID because Mr. M has sperm problems; this is the *substitute father* method (method 11). The ultimate extension of this process of variation and combination would be the involvement of five different people (in addition to medical personnel): the germinal material coming from two, the fetus gestating in the uterus of a third, and two more being the "parents" who raise the child after birth. In looking at this final possibility, one cannot presume that all the participants were alive at the time. One would probably expect the gestator to be alive, unless she is brain dead and supported by mechanical ventilators and drugs while the fetus reaches viability.[4] Similarly, one might expect the parents to be alive, or how could they raise the child? Yet might the child not still be considered their legal offspring if they acknowledged the child as theirs before its birth but died before the child was born? Most obviously, however, the sperm and ovum donors need not be alive, because about 15% of artificial inseminations use frozen semen and the percentage is rising rapidly. Methods are also being developed to freeze ova; already, births have been reported of embryos that were frozen after fertilization and then later thawed and implanted, as for example, when more eggs are harvested and fertilized than can be implanted in a single cycle.[10] Prior to the new reproductive technologies, when a pregnant widow died in childbirth, her baby was born an orphan. Today a child can be born who is an orphan *at the moment of conception*.

ISSUES, VALUES AND GOALS

The reproductive technologies surveyed here raise complex issues. There are those issues raised by the techniques in which human germinal material is controlled and manipulated outside the body; and there are those issues that arise from the separation of genetic, gestational, and social parenthood. Certain goals and values are needed to guide society in resolving issues of these sorts.

Issues Concerning Extracorporeal Germinal Material

As the review of the techniques showed, there are a number of circumstances in which eggs and sperm are removed, stored, and manipulated outside their human source; moreover, they can be combined to create an embryo, or an embryo can be removed from a woman before it implants in the uterus.

Injury and Safety

The first issues raised by these facts are those of injury and safety. In many ways, these issues are no different from the issues that arise with all new biomedical developments. The novel aspect is that medicine usually intervenes to attempt to correct an existing problem in an existing individual, but in this field, the problem of infertility exists separately from the existence of the child, so that harm might be done in the very act of creating the victim. Such a metaphysical conundrum was cited by the courts in the early "wrongful life" cases, such as *Gleitman v. Cosgrove*,[21] but it is my belief that the whole tangled web of rulings in this corner of tort law will eventually be resolved precisely because judges will be willing to allow recovery for injuries caused by physicians' negligence in treating the unborn, as in prenatal surgery.[12]

Control

The second issue of concern is that of control. This was not an issue as long as the materials that went into making a human being were either in a human body or in the process of being transferred from one body to another during sexual intercourse. Once the egg, sperm, or embryo was outside the body, it became a subject of possession. Can we apply conventional property law and deny the full meaning of such possession? Or should we treat the germinal material merely as quasi-property, like a human body, over which certain people may exercise control, but in which they do not have a full-fledged property interest? Or should we confine this limitation to fertilized embryos and continue to allow semen and ova to be treated like blood and other bodily products that are bought and sold?

To answer questions such as these, we must decide the values that are implicated. Is the primary value possessory? That is, because of the expense, effort, and risk that various individuals have undergone to produce the particular germinal material, should they be entitled to a property right in the product of their work? Or are the claims psychological and emotional, and thus, control should lodge with the source of the germinal material because he or she has a special attachment to it. Alternatively, if the primary value is the protection of human life, then control should be given to the party most likely to ensure the well-being of the genetic material and to treat it with appropriate respect.

The issue of control involves not only values but also process. How ought the issue be resolved? Should arrangements about the "ownership" of germinal material be left to private agreements, or does the public have legitimate interests in restricting people's freedom to do as they please with extracorporeal germinal material? In 1984, Congress adopted the National Organ Transplant Act,[30] Section 301, which makes it "unlawful for any person to knowingly acquire, receive, or otherwise transfer any human organ for valuable consideration for use in human transplantation if the transfer affects interstate commerce." Would a similar prohibition on the sale of embryos be advisable? Or legitimate?

I believe that the special sanctity of human life is a legitimate concern of the state and that preservation of this value would justify regulation to prevent actions that are unnecessarily disrespectful of this special status. The Supreme Court has held that a human being before birth is not a person in the constitutional sense, but the Court also recognized that the unborn have interests that the state may protect.[34] In the present context, those nascent human interests are arrayed not against the interests of a pregnant woman who wishes to rid her body of the unborn embryo, but of a physician or scientist who has possession of the material outside of any body. What is the basis of the control over the embryo that Roe v. Wade gave to pregnant women and their physicians? Is it termination of the woman's pregnancy or termination of the life of the unborn being? And at whose command—only the woman, or others?

I am not taking an absolutist position by recognizing a broader social interest in protecting a fertilized extracorporal embryo from its parents' insistence that it be destroyed. Rather, the sanctity value is violated by actions that are unnecessarily disrespectful. If the use of an embryo (e.g., in a biomedical experiment) is necessary for a particular advance in important medical knowledge, the use of an embryo (obviously, without its consent) as a means to a broader benefit does not necessarily violate a moral principle, because in my view an embryo is not yet a full human being. Yet the fashion in which the research is conducted remains a matter of importance and ought to be subject to very rigorous scrutiny.

The conclusions concerning research reached by the Ethics Advisory Board (EAB) in its report to the Secretary of Health, Education, and Welfare in May 1979 remain pertinent, even though many of the reproductive technologies have been developed since that date.[19] The EAB's recommendations have never been acted upon. There has, in effect, been a moratorium on federal funding for IVF research, so that much of the leading research in IVF has occurred abroad.[23] I am in agreement with the EAB report as a good document prudentially, but do not believe its restriction of research to be first 14 days after fertilization enjoys any special constitutional status.

Of greatest concern is that the technology that raises such issues—and will certainly continue to do so with greater frequency—has progressed as far as it has without the development of any real social consensus or well developed body of law on the moral and legal status of the embryo in the laboratory prior to implantation. Even if one places heavy reliance on "private ordering" to handle such questions, cases will arise that fall outside the arrangements made by the involved parties. For example, several years ago, an Australian couple died leaving several frozen embryos without instructions on what should happen to the embryos in such circumstances.[36,38,45] The Australian state legislature insisted that an attempt be made to defrost the embryos and implant them in a volunteer gestator.[24]

Issues Concerning Parenthood

The second set of issues raised by the alternative birth technologies revolves around the separation of parenthood along genetic, gestational, and social lines. Ironically, one of the reasons for the complexity of these issues is that a larger body of law exists that is arguably relevant to this set of issues. For example, there are state laws on child custody and adoption, and many states now have laws concerning AID.

Most of the debate in this field has been framed in terms of the interests of the adult participants, ignoring what ought to be the strongest value to be served, namely, protecting the interests of the child. Perhaps this emphasis is changing as evidenced by the recent situation in New Jersey, referred to in the media as the Baby M case rather than the Stern-Whitehead case.[28] This terminology may signify a recognition of the primacy of the interests of the child.

The Baby M case is not the first one in which the risks to the well-being of a child of the new technologies became apparent. In 1982, Judy Stiver, a Michigan woman, entered into a surrogate mother contract with the Alexander Malahoffs. Noel Keane, the attorney also involved in the Baby M case, drafted the contract that Mrs. Stiver and Mr. Malahoff signed. When a child was born on January 10, 1983, he suffered from a strep infection and microcephaly. Mr. Malahoff, by this point separated from his wife, allegedly denied physicians permission to treat the infection, pursuant to a clause in the surrogate parenting contract that gave him custody of the child. Hospital officials, questioning his authority, obtained a court order allowing them to treat the boy.[41] Thereupon, Malahoff denied paternity of and responsibility for the baby. Mrs. Stiver and her husband disputed his claims and denied their responsibility. Blood tests were taken and the results revealed to the Stivers and Mr. Malahoff on the Phil Donahue television show.[29] The tests proved that Malahoff could not be the father and that Ray Stiver was the probable father. At this point, Mr. Stiver informed his startled wife on camera that in a previous marriage he had fathered a child whose head had stopped developing in infancy and who then died. With millions of people watching expectantly, Mr. Donahue extracted a promise from the Stivers that they would accept responsibility for the baby.

Nor has the issue of the welfare and interests of the offspring arisen only in the context of surrogate motherhood. In 1973, Dr. Raymond Vande Wiele, Chair of Obstetrics and Gynecology at Columbia University's College of Physicians and Surgeons, interrupted an experiment in which Dr. Landrum Shettles was attempting the IVF of ova and sperm from a Mr. and Mrs. Del Zio. The couple then bought suit for wrongful conversion of personal property and infliction of severe emotional distress, for which they collected $50,000.[15] Whatever the merits of the case, the important point is that the state was not exerting its efforts as parens patriae for the vulnerable party, but was merely providing the means to sort out the competing interests of the adults (patients, physician-investigator, and medical administrators).

Lest it seem that the goal of protecting the vulnerable has become an issue only for a few babies at the outer edges of the reproductive frontier, we should remember what has been true in the area of AID for many years, namely, the absence of accurate information of paternal lineage for most children born by AID. Perhaps in response to the early court cases, which labeled the process adultery and its products bastards,[22] or perhaps out of deference to the sensibilities of the young men whose services were being used for a small fee, or possibly based on a desire to avoid complicating the lives of the couple—for whatever reasons, physicians have generally followed a practice of not recording the identity of semen donors.[2,14] This not only frustrates children who want to know something about their "natural" fathers—a desire that has led some of them to undertake very public national searches—but it may also create health problems for AID children and their own offspring, especially when medical data or test samples from both parental lines are needed for diagnosis or treatment. It is estimated that 20,000 babies are born through AID each year in the United States.[2]

In looking at two sets of issues—those raised by the existence of human germinal material outside the body, and those raised by the separation of aspects of parenthood—I have identified three primary values that may need protection*: the sanctity of human life, personal well-being (sometimes associated with duties of nonmaleficence and of beneficence), and autonomous decision making, which may be described in terms of freedom from interference in medical decisions, and in terms of the expectations of control that are embodied, for example, in property or tort rights.

Each of these values is complex and has numerous possible manifestations in the context of the alternative birth technologies. For example, in the context of state regulation,

---

* See Ref. No. 9, which cites four principles—autonomy, nonmaleficence, beneficence, and justice—that themselves reflect the sanctity of life, and that lead to other derivative rules, such as informed consent, veracity, privacy, and fidelity.

the third value—autonomous decision making—may carry primarily the implication of a *negative* freedom, because under the constitutional doctrine of privacy, the government is limited in the regulations and prohibitions it may place on medical choices, but it is not obliged to make possible the use of particular techniques.[8,27] In a private context, however, autonomous decision making may have broader implications, including creating affirmative duties on the part of physicians to inform their patients of options and even to make those options available.

Two additional values are too important in our society to go unmentioned in the present context; both are aspects of justice, namely the values of equal treatment and of procedural fairness. The first of these arises when technologies to meet reproductive wishes are differentially available to men and women; arguably, it also arises when those who are capable of reproducing without the assistance of third parties are treated differently from those who need such aid. The second aspect, procedural fairness, arises when people lack means to assert their interests, or have these interests asserted by a guardian, in a timely fashion before an appropriate decision maker.

Goals for Public Policy

Clearly, some coherent public policy on alternative birth technologies is urgently needed. Such policies must accommodate the various interests outlined above. Society will be best served by policies that minimize the extent to which the technologies disappear from regulatory oversight and are driven underground. We do not want to see "back alley in vitroists" or "black market surrogates." Too much harm to the child as well as the adult participants would result.

It is vital at the outset to establish the safety of reproductive interventions. Clearly, appropriate biomedical testing must be completed prior to the widespread use of such techniques, which will rely on medical and facilities licensure, tort law, and governmental regulations on research with human subjects. But safety also necessitates appropriate procedures for the *use* of proven techniques, such as AID, to ensure adequate genetic and other medical screening of all sources of germinal material and to ensure confidential record keeping.* Surprisingly most of the legislation in the 30 or so states that have enacted AID statutes makes no provision on either score.† Instead, such legislation (for example, Section 7005 of the Uniform Parentage Act of 1979) seems aimed at protecting the husband from responsibility for a medically induced pregnancy to which he did not consent, and at relieving semen donors of any of the usual obligations of fatherhood.[44]

Beyond these concerns about physical well-being, the second goal of public policy in this field should be to protect the social and financial well-being of the children produced. Explicit rules may be needed concerning the financial and other obligations of those who use the new techniques (especially when the results are not as anticipated). Moreover, I

---

* The problem is illustrated by a Pennsylvania statute that apparently aims to improve the safety of IVF (and to prevent fraudulent clinics from operating) by requiring quarterly reports to be filed with the state Department of Health. 18 Pa. Cons. Stat. Ann. Section 3213 (3) (Purdon Supp. 1985). The statute does not, however, require record keeping or reporting of the names of the donors or recipients of eggs and sperm.

† See Ala. Code Section 26-10-8 (1977); Ariz. Rev. Stat. Ann. Section 8-126(c) (1974); Cal. Penal Code Section 273(a) (West 1970); Colo. Rev. Stat Section 19-4-115 (1974); Del. Code Ann. tit. 13 Section 928 (1981); Fla. Stat. Ann. Section 63.212(1) (b) (West Supp. 1983); Ga. Code Ann. Section 74-418 (Supp. 1984); Idaho Code Section 18-1511 (1979); Ill. Rev. Stat. ch. 40 Sections 1526, 1701, 1702 (1981); Ind. Code Ann. Section 35-46-1-9 (West Supp. 1984–85); Iowa Code Ann. Section 600.9 (West 1981); Ky. Rev. Stat. 199.590(2) (1982); Md. Ann. Code 5-327 (1984); Mass. Ann. Laws ch. 210 Section 11A (Law Coop. 1981); Mich. Comp. Laws. Ann. Section 710.54 (West Supp. 1983–84); Nev. Rev. Stat. Section 127.290 (1983); N.J. Stat. Ann. Section 9:3-54 (West Supp. 1984–85); N.Y. Soc. Serv. Law Section 374(6) (McKinney 1983); N.C. Gen. Stat. Section 48-37 (1984); Ohio Rev. Code Ann. Section 3107.10(A) (Baldwin 1983); S.D. Codified Laws Ann. Section 25-6-4.2 (Supp. 1983); Tenn. Code Ann. Section 36-135 (1984); Utah Code Ann. Section 76-7-203 (1978); and Wis. Stat. Ann. Section 946.716 (West 1982)

would urge restricting the use of frozen germinal material from identified persons to the lifetime (or perhaps even to the period of normal reproduction) of such persons, not only to avoid the difficulties otherwise created for family and estate law but also for psychological reasons, to avoid the intentional creation of orphans.*

Third, for a variety of reasons having to do with individual and collective well-being, a limitation should be placed on the number of offspring from any single donor. A few women are already donating (for a fee) five to ten ova a month (which is possible with superovulation drugs); likewise, some semen donors have been used repeatedly.[1,14] Beyond the increased risks of incest among the offspring of such a "super Mom" or "super Dad," the adverse genetic effects are very disturbing. Furthermore, the *voluntary* use of such a pattern may set the stage for mandated use (perhaps on eugenic grounds) of certain "prime specimens" as super breeders, as is done in animal husbandry.

Finally, the laws should preserve the special status of human life to the extent possible in the face of new technical capabilities. Clearly, some of the mysteries and wonders of life have been altered by scientific discoveries and technologic capabilities in a way that the law cannot, and should not even try to, alter. But limitations on the commercialization of the process and on the manner in which human germinal materials are treated outside the body are desirable and could be formulated in a fashion that did not violate constitutional dictates. Some commentators have argued that the protection given by the Supreme Court to reproductive decisions as fundamental rights means that the state may not restrict what they term "noncoital reproduction."[1] Yet even in the context of conventional reproduction, the Court has held the rights not to be absolute, and the true rights that have been recognized are negative ones, that is, freedom from state interference with natural reproduction and with decisions about contraception and abortion. The courts have not recognized any positive right of state assistance in achieving reproduction artificially or of laws specially modified to one's liking.[34] Regulation to protect the well-being of the defenseless or to preserve order regarding a matter of general interest (such as lineage and genetic fitness), would, I believe, aid the sufficiently compelling state interests to be upheld. Already, several courts have upheld limitations on the new technologies.[16,43] Likewise, a state may restrict its adoption procedures to preclude the selling of babies without violating constitutional rights of privacy or property.

SURROGATE MOTHERHOOD

Although not presently covered by statutory law in any state, surrogacy is on the legislative agendas in more than a dozen states; most are considering bills that would legalize the procedure, although legislation has also been introduced to ban it and invalidate surrogacy contracts.[39]

Present Legal Status

What is the legal status of the procedure in the absence of legislation? First, there appears to be no barrier to the parties entering into the agreement itself, although if the surrogate is married her husband would need to be a party to the contract. The payment of money, beyond certain enumerated ex-

---

* The discussion draft of a statutory proposal, entitled simply "Status of Children of the New Biology," under consideration by the National Conference of Commissioners on Uniform State Laws at its summer 1987 meeting, offers a more permissive alternative on this point. Section 6 eliminates the status of parent for the donor of egg or sperm used after the donor's death or when conception has occurred during the donor's life but the embryo was not implanted for gestation until after the donor's death. Optional language in the section, however, would allow a donor in the latter situation to provide to the contrary by will so long as the embryo is implanted within 21 years after the testator's death. This optional language suggests that the main concern of the section is with certainty in the disposition of estates, not protection of children against the misfortune of being intentionally created as orphans.

penses, is illegal under the adoption laws of about half the states,* and the Michigan Supreme Court has interpreted its "baby selling" statute as banning payment to a surrogate.[16] However, in 1986, the Kentucky Supreme Court reached the opposite conclusion on constitutional grounds.[42]

The forbearance of society in permitting people voluntarily to organize their lives to achieve a surrogate child is not the same as saying the contracts are legal or enforceable. Because a surrogate arrangement amounts to a contract for personal services, attempts to enforce it would not be subject to specific performance as, for example, by an injunction to force the pregnant woman to abort a fetus that the father and his wife no longer wanted to have born (perhaps because of the results of prenatal tests). If the action sought by the couple did not involve such a protected decision, it would be possible to assess damages after the fact, in contract or in tort; for example, if the contract required compliance with specific medical or dietary regime during pregnancy and the surrogate failed to comply, leading to provable damage to the child. This action might void the contract for nonperformance or lead to an assessment of damages to compensate the couple for their added expense in caring for the child.†

Goals of Legislation

Should this gray legal area be clarified by legislating a framework for surrogate contracts? In 1983 the Ethics Committee of the American College of Obstetricians and Gynecologists reviewed this area and opposed legislation. Clarification may lead to an increase in the number of such arrangements. Conversely, the primary interest in protection of the offspring is not well served by the absence of a statutorily established system. At a minimum, I suggest the following:

First, all participants in surrogacy should be medically screened to prevent avoidable illness. This could be achieved by the threat of sanctions on the health professionals actively involved. Failure to offer to screen participants the same as regular couples are could be a basis for liability. The risk of eugenic controls by the state places this aspect of the statute into a difficult balancing act, but the interest in protecting the child is compelling enough to merit a solution just short of state control of reproduction.

Second, surrogacy should be regarded as a form of prenatal adoption of the child of one parent by another parent and provisions for state supervision, including confidential record keeping, should parallel those applicable to postnatal adoption. This raises the question as to whether standards of fitness ought to be applied to the couples; it may be enough to achieve this indirectly through medical supervision. However, there will always be some issues that cannot be well resolved by the law but must be left to the development of social norms. For example, should surrogacy be limited to infertile couples and those with genetic or gestational risks? Rather than trying to legally define in-

---

* See, e.g., Ala. Code Section 26-10-8 (1977); Ariz. Rev. Stat. Ann. Section 8-126(c) (1974) (exempts stepparents); Cal. Penal Code Section 273(a) (West 1970) (exempts stepparents); Colo. Rev. Stat. Section 19-4-115 (1974); Del. Code Ann. tit. 13 Section 928 (1981); Fla. Stat. Ann. Section 63.212(1)(b) (West supp. 1983) (exempts stepparents); Ga. Code Ann. Section 74-418 (Supp. 1984); Idaho Code Section 18-1511 (1979); Ill. Rev. Stat. ch. 40 Sections 1526, 1701, 1702 (1981); Ind. Code Ann. Section 35-46-1-9 (West Supp. 1984–85); Iowa Code Ann. Section 600.9 (West 1981); Ky. Rev. Stat. Section 199.590(2) (1982); Md. Ann. Code Section 5-327 (1984); Mass. Ann. Laws ch. 210 Section 11A (Michie/Law. Coop. 1981); Mich. Comp. Laws Ann. Section 710.54 (West Supp. 1983084); Nev. Rev. Stat. Section 127.290 (1983); N.J. Stat. Ann. Section 9:3-54 (West Supp. 1984–85) (exempts stepparents); N.Y. Soc. Serv. Law Section 374(6) (McKinney 1983); N.C. Gen. Stat. Section 48-37 (1984); Ohio Rev. Code Ann. Section 3107.10(A) (Baldwin 1983); S.D. Codified Laws Ann. Section 25-6-4.2 (Supp. 1983); Tenn. Code Ann. Section 36-135 (1984); Utah Code Ann. Section 76-7-203 (1978); Wis. Stat. Ann. Section 946.716 (West 1982)

† I doubt, however, that the contract would allow the child to seek any damages for its breach. See, e.g., Cal. Civ. Code Section 43.6 (Immunity from Liability; Actions Against Parents in Child-birth Claims) (West 1984)

fertility or medical contraindication, it may be sufficient to leave the question of appropriate candidacy to physicians and potential surrogates.

Third, and perhaps most important, the parties to the contract should each be bound by their normal parental obligations of care and support, regardless of the breach or alleged breach of the contract by any party. The Malahoff case indicates the potential for abandonment of a child if the parties are free to regard the situation as one of a contract for delivery of a product.

All of the suggestions made thus far aim to protect the interest of the child, which I view as the primary aim of public policy in this field. Other provisions in a statute would expand on this goal while also attempting to promote additional values.

Fourth, the law should provide that the child is the legal child of the surrogate mother. This was the position of the Warnock committee in England in 1984.[32] Such a legal rule would reinforce the child's interest in having a legally responsible mother at birth; it would also place the surrogate in the same position as any other woman who decides to allow a child to be adopted, which includes having the right to change her mind within a relatively brief specified postnatal time period. The fact that the man in the adopting couple is the genetic father of the child sets the surrogate situation apart from most ordinary adoptions, though the adoption of an illegitimate child by his or her father is not unknown, and stepparent adoptions are not uncommon. In addition, treating children as the legal offspring of the women who bear them would also deter surrogacy by exposing the biologic father to the risk that he might end up with a financial obligation to the child but without any guarantee of other parental rights (which would lodge instead with the surrogate's husband).

The rule I suggest regarding maternity raises the more difficult issues of the presumption of paternity. Under the law in the 30 or so states with AID statutes, a child born after AID is presumed to be the legal offspring of the husband if he has consented to the insemination.* Applying that rule to surrogacy would make the child the legal offspring of the surrogate's husband if he consents, or would open the physician (and others) to suit if the husband were "non-consenting" and later became dissatisfied with the arrangement. A Michigan decision declined to allow the paternity act to be used to declare the paternal status of a contracting father prenatally; it was revised on appeal.[43] A Kentucky court has declined to allow a "mere affidavit" to rebut the presumption of the paternity of the surrogate's husband.[5]

Another control that a statute might exercise would be to regulate the amount of payment made. Obviously, such agreements are notoriously difficult to supervise. The major risk incurred by an individual going outside the terms permitted in the regulation (namely, holding an unenforceable contract) has not proven a major deterrent thus far. Moreover, besides difficulties of enforcement, the question arises of should regula-

---

* Ala. Code Section 26-17-21 (Supp. 1984); Alaska Stat. Section 25.20.045 (1983); Ark. Stat. Ann. Section 61-141 (1971); Cal. Civ. Code Section 7005 (West 1983); Colo. Rev. Stat. Section 19-6-106 (1978); Conn. Gen. Stat. Sections 45-69f to 69n (West 1983); Fla. Stat. Ann. Section 742.11 (West Supp. 1984); Ga. Code Ann. Section 74-101.1, -9904 (Supp. 1984); Idaho Code Section 39-5401 et seg. (Supp. 1984); Ill. Ann. Stat. ch. 40 Section 1453 (Smith-Hurd Supp. 1983–1984); Kan. Stat. Ann Section 23-128 to -130 (1981); La. Rev. Stat. Ann. Section 188 (West Supp. 1984); Md. Est. & Trusts Code Ann. Section 1-206(b) (1974); and Md. Gen. Prov. Code Section 20-214 (1982); Mich. Comp. Laws Ann. Section 333.2824 (1980) and Section 700.111 (1980); Minn. Stat. Ann. Section 257.56 (West 1982); Mont. Rev. Code Ann. Section 40-6-1-6 (1985); Nev. Rev. Stat. Section 126.061 (1986); N.J. Stat. Ann. Section 9:17-44 (West Supp. 1986); N.M. Stat. Ann. Section 40-11-6 (1986); N.Y. Dom. Rel. Law Section 73 (McKinney 1977); N.C. Gen. Stat. Section 49A-1 (1976); Okla. Stat. Ann. tit. 10, Sections 551–553 (West Supp. 1985); Or. Rev. Stat. Sections 109.239, .243, .247, 677.355, .360, 365, .370 (1985); Tenn. Code Ann. Sections 53–446 (Supp. 1983); Tex. Fam. Code Ann. Section 12.03 (Vernon 1975); Va. Code Section 64.1-7.1 (1980); Wash. Rev. Code Ann. Section 26.26.050 (West Supp. 1986); Wis. Stat. Ann. Section 767.47(9) (West 1985); Section 891.40 (West Supp. 1982–1983); Wyo. Stat. Section 14-2-103 (1978)

tion hold payments to the level of actual out-of-pocket expenses (including life and health insurance premiums), which would lead to surrogacy only by true altruists, or should it push the price up to a level commensurate with the values of the service and the time and effort involved? The latter would doubtless lead to a flood of eager surrogates, but without at least some control, more cases are likely to arise like the recent one in San Diego, in which a Mexican woman sued to retain custody of the child she bore under a surrogate contract for $1500.[37]

The resolution of this issue most protective both of the children involved and of society's interests would be to forbid all commercial surrogacy contracts by refusing to enforce them and by not allowing adoptions in such situations based on the prohibition on "baby selling" that now appears in the adoption laws of many states. That prohibition applies to commissioned adoptions (that is, paying to have a child conceived specifically to allow its subsequent release for adoption) as well as to the transfer of already existing children. As the New Jersey Supreme Court concluded in reviewing the agreement between Mary Beth Whitehead and the Sterns in the Baby M case,[6] the payment made to a surrogate mother is not merely for her services but for the transfer of a child to its paternal family to be reared and for "institut[ing] and cooperat[ing] in proceedings to terminate their respective parental rights in said child," in the words of the Stern-Whitehead agreement. "It strains credulity to claim that these arrangements . . . really amount to something other than a private placement adoption for money."* Such contracts are thus in violation of the statutes that punish the paying or receiving of money in connection with the placement of a child for adoption.

Prohibiting commercial surrogacy safeguards several important values besides protecting women—especially poor, single women—from being exploited. The role of paid breeder is incompatible with a society in which individuals are valued for themselves and their reproductive capabilities remain part of a private, and uniquely personal, sphere rather than becoming items of commerce. Likewise, in arguing against allowing sale of human embryos, Dr. Sherman Elias and professor George Annas observe that "we know intuitively that the human embryo is more valuable than a kidney [which cannot be sold[30]] and of much more symbolic importance regarding human life: that is why we believe embryos should not be the subject of commerce."[7] The same applies, even more forcefully, to payments made for rights in actual babies, with all the implications of a product rather than of a person.

The prohibition on baby-selling serves the value of personhood in another way because a market in reproductive services and babies would have adverse effects on all persons, not simply on those who choose to enter that market: all personal attributes of ourselves as well as our children (sex, eye color, predicted IQ, athletic ability, and so forth) would be given a dollar value by the market, whether or not we wanted to regard ourselves and our progeny in these terms.[31] Moreover, even if a child once incorporated into a family is never again thought of as something that was purchased, the fact remains that during the *process* of the transaction the child was a thing in which people had a transferrable ownership interest, the value of which was set by competition among potential buyers looking for particular, desirable attributes. The trial judge in the Baby M case accepted an ownership view when he found New Jersey's baby-selling prohibitions inapplicable to surrogacy contracts because the father "cannot purchase what is already his,"† but the New Jersey Supreme Court re-

---

* Ref. No. 6 at 1241

† Ref. 7 at 372, 525 A.2d at 1157. Even on property grounds, Judge Sorkow's conclusion makes no sense, since Mr. Stern was not purchasing something he owned but rather was attempting to purchase Mrs. Whitehead's interest in the child (an interest that Judge Sorkow valued very little); he was thus in the position of one joint tenant wishing to purchase the other joint tenant's rights in the property (in this case, in order to transfer them to someone else, namely Mrs. Stern).

versed in part because treating a child as property would allow it to be "sold without regard to whether the purchasers will be suitable parents."*

The British have gone partway toward ending commercial surrogacy by making it illegal to broker surrogate arrangements for a fee or to advertize for surrogates. I believe we should go further, in line with the Baby M decision, and permit only unpaid surrogate mother arrangements and decline to enforce the arrangements as contracts that obligate the mother to relinquish the child after its birth. Plainly, this would render surrogate motherhood an unattractive alternative for most infertile couples. Would it therefore violate the constitutional rights of those infertile couples who might wish to use surrogate motherhood, most particularly those with female infertility? The possible constitutional objections fall into two categories: first, that by discouraging surrogacy, the state is discriminating against one group of infertile couples compared to other infertile couples, and second, that by refusing to treat surrogacy arrangements as enforceable contracts the state has violated the couple's "procreative liberty."[33] However, neither objection is persuasive.

Does the fact that AID is facilitated by laws that make a consenting husband the legal father of the child and remove any parental rights or responsibilities from the semen "donor" mean that surrogate motherhood contracts must also be legally protected, lest couples with male infertility be favored over couples with female infertility? An initial response is that the law does not differentiate the reasons people have for using one form of "assisted reproduction" or another. Indeed, surrogacy itself typically involves AID, except that the source of the semen does not view himself as a donor but as one who is making use of the services of a woman to produce a child whom he will then reclaim. On a formal basis, then, the laws adopted for AID can, and should, be applied to surrogacy: the woman who bears a child (and her mate, if any) are presumed to be the parents of the child, until the presumption is overcome or until they give up their parental rights and responsibilities to the biological father and his mate, if any. Thus, the law on AID is neutral on its face among couples with different types of infertility.

Even assuming that the equal protection clause would require that two procedures affecting somewhat different infertile populations must be treated symmetrically, AID and surrogate motherhood are simply not equivalent. The biological parallel to AID is egg or embryo donation, in which case the woman who gestates the donated egg would be the legal mother of the child to whom she gives birth (see Table 13-3, method 5). Furthermore, the physical risk and labor of surrogacy, to say nothing of the emotional attachment of a surrogate mother to the child she carries and bears, is incomparably greater than the risk, labor, and attachment of a semen donor to the child or children that may be produced by inseminations with his ejaculate.[18] Thus, even if the law continues to permit payments for sperm for AID, it does not follow that it would be a denial of equal protection to prohibit payments to surrogates because the latter poses a much greater risk of commodifying both the mothers and the resulting children.[31] Nevertheless, to the extent that semen partakes of humanness—especially because the semen may be valued deferentially for the genetic traits it is believed to transmit—its sale for amounts more than that which is appropriate payment for the costs of "harvesting," testing, storing, and distributing should be discouraged or perhaps even prohibited. And the same policy should be applied to the female equivalent of AID, namely the obtaining of eggs and embryos from women.

The second constitutional claim—that it is an infringement of liberty if the government denies people the right to make enforceable surrogacy contracts—rests on the doctrine of privacy in reproductive and family matters fashioned by the Supreme Court

---

* Ref. No. 6 at 1241.

of the United States in recent years. But the "procreative liberty" argument rests on a misinterpretation of the rationale and effect of the privacy decisions.

The heart of the privacy doctrine has been to shelter individuals from government intrusion into the choices they make about intimate matters such as abortion and contraception. As the Court stated in Eisenstadt v. Baird:

> If the right of privacy means anything, it is the right of the *individual*, married or single, to be free from unwarranted governmental intrusion into matters so fundamentally affecting a person as the decision whether to bear or beget a child.[17]

The right to be *free from* interference obviously does not generate an obligation on the state to ensure that individuals have the *freedom to* achieve the family they desire in whatever manner they choose.

Furthermore, declining to order specific performance of a surrogacy arrangement seems, in the language of Eisenstadt, less an "unwarranted governmental intrusion" into the couple's reproductive liberty than the intrusion into the surrogate mother's rights that would occur were the state to enforce the arrangement. In the Baby M decision, the New Jersey Supreme Court held that fathering Baby M came within Mr. Stern's constitutionally protected right "to have natural children whether through sexual intercourse or artificial insemination."* But, the court continued, this right does not extend to the father's insisting that the child be turned over to him to raise or that the mother and her husband be forced to fulfill their promise to relinquish their parental rights to the father and his wife because to so hold would violate the surrogate's "recognized fundamental interest" to the compansionship of her child, which is protected by the Constitution," though also subject to state regulation.†

---

* Ref. No. 6 at 1253.
† Ref. No. 6 at 1255.

REFERENCES

1. American Fertility Society, Ethics Committee: Ethical considerations of the new reproductive technologies. Fertility and Sterility (Suppl 1) 46:37S, 1986
2. Andrews L: New Conceptions. New York, St. Martin's Press, 1984
3. Aral S, Cates W Jr: The increasing concern with infertility. JAMA 250:2327, 1983
4. Baby born prematurely to brain-dead woman. N.Y. Times, Aug 15, 1986, 1, at 8, col 6
5. Baby Girl, *In re*, No. 83 AD (Jefferson Circuit Ct., 6th Div., March 8, 1983)
6. Baby M, *In re*, 109 N.J. 396, 537 A.2d 1227 (1988)
7. Baby M, *In re*, 217 N.J. Super 313, 525 A.2d 1128 (1987)
8. Beal v. Doe, 432 U.S. 438 (1977)
9. Beauchamp T, Childress J: Principles of Biomedical Ethics, 2nd ed. New York, Oxford University Press, 1983
10. Berg P: The cutting edge. Wash. Post, May 8, 1985, (Health), at 5, col 1
11. Biggers J: In vitro fertilization and embryo transfer in human beings. N Engl J Med 304:336, 1981
12. Capron A: Wrongful life: Will common sense ever prevail? Bioethics Reporter (Commentary) 1:23, 1985
13. Ciba Foundation Symposium 17: Law and Ethics of A.I.D. and Embryo Transfer. London, Associated Scientific Publishers, 1973
14. Curie-Cohen M, Luttrell L, Shapiro S: Current practice of artificial insemination by donor in the U.S. New Engl J Med 300:585, 588, 1979
15. Del Zio v Presbyterian Hosp., 74 N.Y. Civ. Crt. 3588, S.D.N.Y., Nov 14, 1978 (memorandum decision)
16. Doe v Kelly, 106 Mich. App. 169, 307 N.W. 2d 438 (1981), cert. denied, 459 U.S. 1183 (1983)
17. Eisenstadt v Baird, 405 U.S. 438, 453 (1972)
18. Elias S, Annas G: Social policy considerations in noncoital reproduction. JAMA 255:62, 1986
19. Ethics Advisory Board, U.S. Dept. of Health, Education, and Welfare, Report and Conclusions: HEW Support of Research Involving Human In Vitro Fertilization and Embryo Transfer (1979)
20. Genesis 16:19

21. Gleitman v Cosgrove, 49 N.J. 22, 227 A.2d 689 (1967)
22. Gursky v Gursky, 39 Misc. 2d 1083, 242 N.Y.S. 2d 406 (Sup. Ct. 1963)
23. Health Research Extension Act of 1985, Pub. L. No. 99-158, 99 Stat 820 (1985)
24. Infertility (Medical Procedures Act, No 10163 (Vict., Austl. 1984)
25. Jones H, Acousta A, Andrews M et al: Three years of in vitro fertilization at Norfolk. Fertil Steril 42:826, 1984
26. Lopata A: Concepts in human in vitro fertilization and embryo transfer. Fertil Steril 40:289, 1983
27. Maher v Roe, 432 U.S. 464 (1977)
28. Peterson I: Baby M trial splits ranks of feminists. N.Y. Times, Feb. 24, 1987, 2, at 1, col 5
29. Phil Donahue Show: The Case of Layaway Baby (NBC television broadcast)
30. Pub. L. No. 98-507, 98 Stat. 2339 (1984)
31. Radin M: Market Inalienability. Harv L Rev 100:1849, 1987
32. Report of the Committee of Inquiry into Human Fertilization and Embryology. London, Department of Health and Social Security, July 1984
33. Robertson J: Embryos, families and procreative liberty: The legal structure of the new reproduction. So Cal L Rev 59:939, 1986
34. Roe v Wade, 410 U.S. 113 (1973)
35. Romney S, Gray M, Little A et al: Gynecology and Obstetrics: The Health Care of Women, 2nd ed. New York, McGraw-Hill Book Company, 1981
36. Saltarelli J: Genesis retold: Legal issues raised by the cryopreservation of preimplantation human embryos. Syracuse L Rev 36:1021, 1030, 1985.
37. Scott J: Pair duped her on surrogate mother pact, woman tells court. Los Angeles Times, Feb 20, 1987, Pt. I, at 22, col 1
38. State of Victoria (Australia), Report on the Disposition of Embryos Produced by In Vitro Fertilization, 1984
39. State proposals vary greatly, L.A. Daily J., Apr. 1, 1987, 1 at 23, col. 5
40. Surrogacy Arrangements Act 1985, United Kingdom, ch. 49
41. Surrogate mother's deformed baby rejected. N.Y. Times, Jan 23, 1983, 1, at 19, col 1
42. Surrogate Parenting Assocs. v Kentucky, 704 S.W. 2d 209 (Ky. 1986)
43. Syrkowski v Appleyard, 420 Mich. 367, 362 N.W. 2d 211 (1985) (per curiam), modifying, 122 Mich. App. 506, 333 N.W. 2d 90 (1983)
44. Uniform Parentage Act Section 7005, 9A U.L.A. 587, 592–593 (1979)
45. Wallis C: Quickening debate over life on ice. Time, July 2, 1984, pp 68–69

14

Immunologic Therapy

James H. Beeson

The human fetus has frequently been called nature's perfect allograft. Half of its genetic material is paternal, and it survives in spite of a maternal immune system which is hostile to allografted tissue. In 1953, Medawar listed three reasons that the conceptus is able to survive[24]:

- The anatomic separation of fetus from mother
- The antigenic immaturity of the fetus
- The immunologic inertness of the mother

Probably more than one of these mechanisms is operative, and it may well be that different mechanisms operate at different times in the well orchestrated symphony of reproduction. When reproductive failure occurs, aberrations of the immune system have been invoked when no other known mechanisms are apparent.

INFERTILITY AND HABITUAL ABORTION

To begin a discussion of immune-mediated mechanisms of unexplained infertility and habitual abortion, the term *unexplained* must be defined. In order for infertility and abortion to be unexplained, the following factors must be eliminated:

- Male factor (oligospermia, azospermia, infection)
- Anovulation
- Tubal factors (obstruction)
- Endocrinopathies
- Müllerian Abnormalities (e.g., septate uterus)
- Endometriosis
- Luteal phase inadequacy
- Infection

- Problems of sexual technique
- Genetic factors (e.g., balanced translocation)

When all known factors contributing to infertility and habitual abortion have been eliminated, immunologic factors may be investigated. One must yet differentiate between a failure of fertilization and a failure of implantation and growth.

Failures of fertilization have been attributed to antisperm antibodies occurring in either the male or the female and antizona pellucida antibodies in the female. Therapies for the former have included condom therapy for antibodies in the female and steroids for either partner. Only steroids have been offered as possible therapy for the latter. Although these therapies have been less than satisfactory (remembering that about 30% of untreated patients will conceive), the risks to the patient and the fetus are minimal, and these therapies offer few ethical dilemmas. In addition, as the indications for in vitro fertilization (IVF) have widened, many of these patients have been found to benefit from the procedure.

Failure of implantation and growth characterize a second group of patients, which includes those who have recurrent clinical abortions and those in whom the recurrent abortions are subclinical. That pregnancy loss occurs frequently has been confirmed by careful study of the beta-subunit of human chorionic gonadotropin (HCG-β) in normal women not using contraception. It was found that 57% of the positive test results occurred in women who had no clinical evidence of pregnancy.[9] An early hysterectomy study identified 34 early pregnancies of which about a third were morphologically abnormal.[17] Although I am unaware of similar studies in patients with unexplained infertility, such a study might well prove that many of these patients do conceive but abort before the pregnancy is clinically recognized. Another group which is likely to emerge in this category is patients undergoing IVF in whom blastocyst formation is repetitively observed but no pregnancy results from embryo transfer.

Habitual abortion is most frequently defined as three consecutive miscarriages with no intervening live births. In the absence of any live births, the risk of abortion in the subsequent pregnancy is 46%.[27] Many practitioners know of patients who have had 15 or more spontaneous abortions without a single viable pregnancy.

Current approaches to the treatment of this problem are based on the concept that successful reproduction requires recognition of the pregnancy in such a way that produces a protective (enhancing) immune response. (Fig. 14-1) In other words, it is the correct response rather than the absence of a response that allows the pregnancy to continue uninterrupted. The treatments involve immunization of the mother to foreign antigens to produce this protective response. It is because the regulatory mechanisms are so poorly understood and the long-term effects of such immunizations so totally unknown that ethical dilemmas arise. In the following pages, the rationale for this therapeutic approach, the methods for implementation, and the dangers, both real and theoretical, will be discussed.

Rationale for Immune Therapy

The concept that immune recognition is necessary for reproduction has its roots in nature, in the search for an explanation for the selective advantage of antigenic heterogeneity. In the breeding of laboratory animals, semi-allogeneic conceptuses had a selective advantage over conceptuses that were syngeneic to the mother with regard to the major histocompatibility complex (MHC).[26] Eighty percent of lines being inbred in rodents are lost, and it seems that syngeneic rodent strains which have been so important in research in immunology may represent a reproductive artifact, since the only lines which did emerge were those that somehow satisfied the minimal requirements for successful reproduction.[13]

In allogeneic matings of rodents, the weight of the fetoplacental unit and of the para-aortic lymph nodes is greater than in

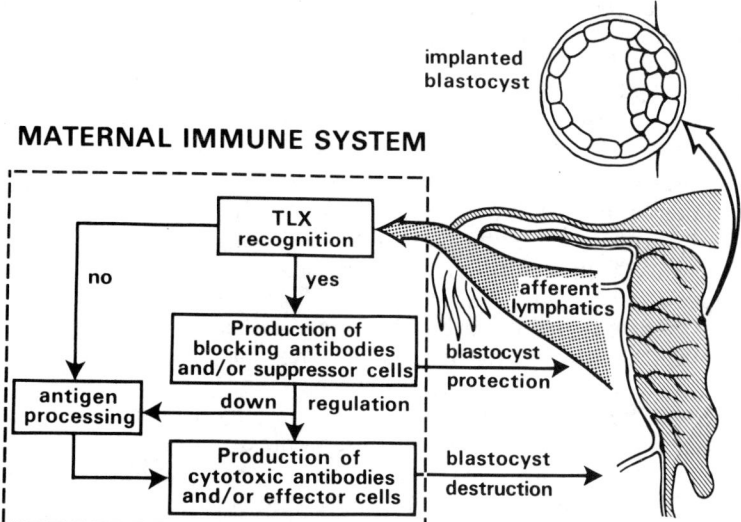

FIGURE 14-1. Schematic representation of the role of trophoblast-specific antigen (TLX) recognition in successful pregnancy.

syngeneic matings. Further, specific immunization of the mother to paternal alloantigens resulted in larger placentas, while excison of the para-aortic nodes resulted in smaller placentas.[2] The importance of the para-aortic nodes in rodent reproduction has been clearly demonstrated by Clark and co-workers who have identified suppressor cells in these nodes which have the ability to inhibit maternal antipaternal immune responses in vitro. Further experiments identified these cells in even greater concentration in the uterine decidua. Of most interest is the fact that these cells were not identified in pregnancies which were being actively resorbed (specifically the mating of a CBA-strain female with a DBA-strain male).[6] It is also worthy of note that the supression did not require cell replication and that it seemed to be mediated by a soluble factor.

Serum-blocking factors have been reported in mice[16] and in the human.[29] In the human experiments, the blocking factor was demonstrated by means of an in vitro lymphocyte migration inhibitory factor assay. The significant finding was that the factor appeared to be an IgG that could be absorbed on lymphocytes but not on platelets, indicating that the antibody was not specific for human leukocyte antigens (HLA). Of more interest is the fact that the serum of women who undergo idiopathic abortions lack this blocking factor.

That mothers recognize and respond to HLA antigens of the MHC is clear. The original source of cytotoxic typing sera for use in the tissue-typing laboratory was multiparous females. Allograft matching for human transplantation is dependent on this fact. Does an HLA mismatch then cause rejection of the fetus? No, in fact, the converse seems to be true.

Gill has summarized the published literature relating HLA compatibility to the incidence of spontaneous abortion.[12] On the whole, the literature supports the contention that couples experiencing idiopathic spontaneous abortion share HLA more frequently than nonaborting couples. In addition, the antigens shared occur more frequently at the HLA-D/DR locus than at the HLA-A or B loci by a factor of two to three. The human HLA-D/DR loci are analogous to the Ia loci of the mouse which function in part as regulatory antigens of immune recognition. Thus, it appears that while the histocompatibility antigens of the HLA loci are not directly involved in immune enhancement necessary for successful viviparous reproduction, there must be an antigen or group of antigens which must be recognized for immunologic enhancement to occur. In addition, these antigens must be coded in the HLA-D/DR region of chromosome 6.

Linked to this hypothesis is the observation that mixed-lymphocyte culture (MLC) hyporesponsiveness occurred more often in women with karyotypically normal abortuses than in normally fertile women and women with karyotypically abnormal abortuses. This depressed reactivity was specific for the one-way culture with the husband as the stimulator. The reactivity was normal for the one-way MLC in which donor lymphocytes were used as the stimulators.[19]

Although the nature of the antigenic determinants necessary for reproduction remain to be rigorously proven, one candidate for this role is the trophoblast-lymphocyte cross-reactive (TLX) antigen system proposed by Faulk and McIntyre.[11,22] Their studies have demonstrated two groups of species-specific cell-surface trophoblast antigens by means of xenogeneic (rabbit) antibodies. These antigen groups were denoted TA1 and TA2. TA1 is specific to the placenta, and TA1 and its specific antiserum have the ability to block human MLC reactivity without blocking interspecies MLC with baboon lymphocytes. TA2 was found to have a wider tissue distribution, and most specifically was present on the membranes of allogeneically stimulated lymphocytes but not mitogen-stimulated lymphocytes. They propose that TA1 modulates cell-mediated immunity and TA2 stimulates maternal recognition in a hapten-carrier model, which taken together is the TLX system. Applying rabbit antisera to ten placentas, they have also presented data suggestive that there are three groups of TLX antigens, and that these sera were not identifying HLA types.[11,22]

The unifying hypothesis then is that TLX recognition is necessary to initiate a protective immune response and allow pregnancy to proceed. Failure of recognition, as manifested by specific one-way MLC hyporesponsiveness, results in a failure of immune supression leading to an absence of blocking factors in maternal serum and a failure of nidation or abortion of the pregnancy. Treatment regimens are then aimed at augmenting TLX recognition.

Before discussing specific treatment modalities, it is worth mentioning that these treatments are experimental, and that humans in this case are the experimental animals. The justification for human experimentation in this case is that no adequate animal model exists—one cannot exist, because the emergence of viviparity in higher vertebrates was the result of parallel evolution rather than conservation of a successful mechanism. For example, there are the anatomic differences in hemochorial placentas such as the hemotrichorial labyrinthine placenta of the mouse versus the hemomonochorial villous architecture of the human. Nevertheless, a mouse model has evolved using the CBA-strain female mated with a DBA-strain male. It has been shown that the high spontaneous resorption rate in these pregnancies can be dramatically reduced by vaccinating the CBA female with BALB/c male spleen cells.[5] This improvement in reproduction correlates with the ability of BALB/c spleen cells to induce MLC suppressor activity in the CBA females.

Therapeutic Approaches

The goal of therapy in cases of idiopathic infertility and habitual abortion caused by failure of TLX recognition is to enhance the recognition process. The nature of this therapy has been compared to improved renal allograft survival after blood transfusion.[23,32]

Two approaches have been taken. Although the human study by Taylor and Faulk appeared before the animal (mouse) model, the approach taken in both is similar. The women involved were repeatedly transfused with leukocyte-enriched plasma from multiple erythrocyte compatible donors.[31] Compatibility was ensured for the ABO, Rhesus, Kell, Duffy, Lewis, Kidd, and MNSs blood groups. Transfusions were done at intervals of about 3 weeks. Of the four patients initially treated, three had normal deliveries at the time of the report, and a fourth, apparently normal, pregnancy was in progress. No complications were noted.

The second approach is that used by Beer and co-workers. Females who are hyporesponsive in the one-way MLC with their spouse are vaccinated intradermally with leukocytes isolated from the peripheral blood of the spouse.[1] At the time of the publication of the study, two of the three patients had established apparently normal pregnancies. A more recent paper presented by the same authors indicated that four of six patients who aborted after this therapy failed to demonstrate humoral MLC blocking activity, while nine similar patients demonstrated the blocking activity and have delivered normal infants.[28]

Related Immune Aberrations

In addition to those cases of infertility and habitual abortion which can be attributed to the TLX recognition framework, there are other immune-related conditions in which abortion or infertility occur. A high rate of fetal wastage has been reported in a number of autoimmune diseases. The best known example is systemic lupus erythematosis (SLE).[33] It has been suggested that the mechanism for spontaneous abortion in SLE involves an aberrant response to trophoblast antigen which produces lymphocytotoxic antibodies rather than blocking antibodies.[4]

Recently, attention has been focused on manifestations of subclinical autoimmune disease in patients experiencing repeated abortion. An incidence of antinuclear antibody (ANA) was noted in aborters which was greater than expected in the general population, and those patients had a poorer prognosis in their next pregnancy than those without a positive ANA.[15] Another study found that ANA plus one other test (antibody to DNA, extractable nuclear antigen, or low complement component 3) was positive in 29% of otherwise normal aborters.[7] Increased frequencies of antibodies to single-stranded DNA have been noted in normal pregnant women (27%) and gestational diabetics (42%).[25] Although the significance of these findings is unclear and no related therapy has been suggested, the fact that this correlation exists should serve as a warning that there may be a relationship between autoimmune disease and normal and abnormal pregnancy.

Related to the incidence of abortion in SLE patients is the lupus anticoagulant. This is an acquired immunoglobulin which prolongs phospholipid-dependent coagulation tests. This immunoglobulin was first described in SLE. Along with anti-Ro, it has been associated with abortion in SLE patients.[18] The lupus anticoagulant has now been reported in women with and without SLE who experienced abortion and mid-trimester fetal death. Treatment of these women with prednisone and aspirin resulted in viable pregnancies and supression of the lupus anticoagulant.[3,20]

Of special interest are women with antisperm antibodies. Although most frequently cited as a cause of infertility, it has been reported that women with these antibodies frequently abort normal pregnancies[30]; subsequently one such patient was vaccinated with paternal leukocytes. The antisperm antibodies disappeared; she conceived, and a normal term fetus was delivered.[14] Although this single case must be considered anecdotal at best, it suggests a strong relationship between this immune aberration and the TLX system.

DANGERS OF MANIPULATION OF THE IMMUNE SYSTEM

The dangers of immune system manipulation are largely unknown. One has only to survey the literature of immunology to grasp the limit of knowledge in this area. At best, leukocyte immunization for the treatment of habitual abortion and infertility represents the application of an immune recognition theory (the TLX system) for which the only real evidence at the moment is the success of the reported experiments in human subjects. Since the total number of patients reported in the literature is less than 20, and only historical controls were employed, the hypothesis itself must be considered unproven. While no complications have been reported, it may well take decades of follow-up to reveal important complications of this type of therapy.

In the preceding pages, an effort has been made to demonstrate that there is an extremely complex and poorly understood relationship between immune enhancement and a variety of diseases. Since the relationships are not understood, they cannot be controlled. Leukocyte immunization could actually reverse these disease processes, but it might also trigger them.

The relationship of pregnancy to carcinogenesis has long been a subject of investigation. The ability of the tumor to escape "immune surveillance" has often been referred to as fetal behavior. Epidemiologic data on breast cancer indicates that early pregnancy is protective against breast cancer, and this has been interpreted to mean that women sensitized to pregnancy antigens manage to destroy developing tumors. Conversely, it has been suggested that late pregnancy may produce blocking immunity that enhances the emergence of these tumors.[8,10]

Another more realistic risk is the identification of another group of aborters, which have been characterized as having normal pregnancies prior to their series of abortions. These aborters demonstrated excessive antipaternal immunity. The immunity did not appear to be directed at paternal HLA allotypes and might well be directed to fetal extraembryonic antigens (perhaps TLX).[21] If this observation is true, then leukocyte immunization carries the risk of converting a habitual aborter of the first type to a habitual aborter of the second type. When the pooled donor leukocyte protocol is used, a small risk exists for the transmission of Acquired Immunodeficiency Syndrome (AIDS). Although human immunodeficiency virus (HIV) antibody testing minimizes the risk, the risk is not zero.

RECOMMENDATIONS

It is not the things that we do not know that cause trouble; it is those things that we know that are wrong.

Ray Robertson, MD
Author's family physician
ca. 1950

The risks which have been cited—cancer and autoimmune disease—are dramatic but primarily hypothetical. Nevertheless, these risks, no matter how small, must be considered in the context of what is being treated. If the disease being treated were life-threatening, these risks would certainly be justified in the minds of all. The health threat of the disease under consideration, however, is primarily psychological. Reproduction is considered by many to be a basic human right, and the failure to reproduce may produce feelings of inadequacy in the victims. While this is unfortunate, it is not life-threatening.

A second factor to be considered in the risk-benefit ratio is the fact that the treatment is not proven. Without adequate controls, inadvertent patient selection or special care might result in dramatic results in a small number of published patients. The methodology is simple and could be applied by any practitioner with the help of a competent blood bank. Thus, many may be tempted to apply these methods to any patient with unexplained infertility or habitual abortion. This type of widespread experimentation is to be deplored. Any patients considered for this therapy must be rigorously evaluated, and true informed consent must be obtained to the extent that it is possible. Both the study protocol and the consent must be approved by a valid institutional review board. Furthermore, when the investigator embarks on such an experiment, he obligates himself to follow the patient for an extended period of time (years) in order to identify and report possible long-term complications.

Finally, it must be reiterated that these are human experiments. The underlying theory is inadequate, and there is no background of animal research. Leukocyte immunization is not a proven therapeutic modality and should not be treated as such.

REFERENCES

1. Beer AE, Quebbeman JF, Ayers JWT, Haines RF: Major histocompatibility complex antigens, maternal and paternal immune responses, and chronic habitual abortions in humans. Am J Obstet Gynecol 141:987, 1981
2. Beer AE, Scott JR, Billingham RE: Histoincompatibility and maternal immunological status as determinants of fetoplacental weight and litter size in rodents. J Exp Med 142:180, 1975
3. Branch DW, Kochenour NK, Herschgold EJ et al: The lupus anticoagulant—A recently discovered and treatable cause of recurrent abortion and fetal death. Am J Reprod Immunol 5:100, 1984
4. Bresnihan B, Grigor RR, Oliver M et al: Immunological mechanism for spontaneous abortion in systemic lupus erythematosus. Lancet 2:1206, 1977
5. Chaouat G, Kiger N, Wegmann TG: Vaccination against spontaneous abortion in mice. J Reprod Immunol 5:389, 1983
6. Clark DA, McDermott MR, Szewchuk MR: Impairment of host versus graft reaction in pregnant mice. II. Selective suppression of cytotoxic T-cell generation correlates with soluble suppressor activity and with successful allogeneic pregnancy. Cell Immunol 52:106, 1980
7. Cowchock S, Dehoratius RD, Wapner RJ, Jackson LG: Subclinical autoimmune disease and unexplained abortion. Am J Obstet Gynecol 150:367, 1984
8. Doll R: The epidemiology of cancers of the breast and reproductive system. Scot J Med 20:305, 1975
9. Edmonds DK, Lindsay KS, Miller JF et al: Early embryonic mortality in women. Fertil Steril 38:447, 1982
10. Faulk WP, McIntyre JA: Immunological aspects of the materno-fetal relationship in human pregnancy. Role of the placenta. Acta Paediatr Belg 33:77, 1980
11. Faulk WP, McIntyre JA: Immunological studies of human trophoblast: Markers, subsets and functions. Immunol Rev 75:139, 1983
12. Gill TJ III: Immunogenetics of spontaneous abortion in humans. Transplantation 35:1, 1983
13. Gill TJ III, Repetti CF: Immunological and genetic factors influencing reproduction. Am J Pathol 95:463, 1979
14. Haas GG, Kubota K, Quebbeman JF et al: Antisperm antibodies and subsequent reproductive performance in females with recurrent abortion (abstr). Soc Gynecologic Investigation, March 1984
15. Harger JH, Archer DF, Marchese SG et al: Etiology of recurrent pregnancy losses and outcome of subsequent pregnancies. Obstet Gynecol 62:574, 1983
16. Hellstrom KE, Hellstrom I, Brawn J: Abrogation of cellular immunity to antigenically foreign mouse embryonic cells by a serum factor. Nature 224:914, 1969
17. Hertig AT: The implantation of the human embryo. Histogenesis of some aspects of spontaneous abortion. In Behrman J, Kistner R (Eds): Progress in Infertility, 2nd ed, p 411. Boston, Little Brown, 1975
18. Hull RG, Harker EN, Morgan SH, Hughes GRV: Anti-Ro antibodies and abortions in women with SLE. Lancet 2:1138, 1983
19. Lauritson JG, Kristensen T, Grunnet N: Depressed mixed lymphocyte culture reactivity in mothers with recurrent spontaneous abortion. Am J Obstet Gynecol 125:35, 1976
20. Lubbe WF, Butler WS, Palmer SJ, Liggins GC: Fetal survival after prednisone suppression of maternal lupus anticoagulant. Lancet 1:1361, 1983
21. McConnachie PR, McIntyre JA: Maternal antipaternal immunity in couples predisposed to repeated pregnancy losses. Am J Reprod Immunol 5:145, 1984
22. McIntyre JA, Faulk WP, Verhulst SJ, Colliver JA: Human trophoblast-lymphocyte cross-reactive (TLX) antigens define a new alloantigen system. Science 222:1135, 1983
23. MacLeod AM, Power DA, Mason RJ et al: Possible mechanism of action of transfusion effect in renal transplantation. Lancet 2:468, 1982
24. Medawar PB: Some immunological and endocrinological problems raised by the evolution of viviparity in vertebrates. Soc Exp Biol Symp 7:320, 1953
25. Melez KA, Halfoun V, Doberson MJ et al: Autoantibodies in pregnancy. Lancet 1:354, 1983

26. Michie D, Anderson NF: A strong selective effect associated with a histocompatibility gene in the rat. Ann NY Acad Sci 129:88, 1966
27. Poland BJ, Miller JR, Jones DC, Trimble BK: Reproductive counseling in patients who have had a spontaneous abortion. Am J Obstet Gynecol 127:685, 1977
28. Quebbeman JF, Hamazaki Y, Jijon A, Broka J: The dynamics of humoral mixed lymphocyte culture blocking factors in women with recurrent abortion prior to, during and following a successful pregnancy (abstr). Soc Gynecologic Investigation, March 1984
29. Rocklin RE, Kitzmiller JL, Carpenter CB et al: Maternal-fetal relation: Absence of an immunologic blocking factor from the serum of women with chronic abortion. N Engl J Med 295:1209, 1976
30. Scott JS, Jones WR: Immunology of Human Reproduction. New York, Grune & Stratton, 1976
31. Taylor C, Faulk WP: Prevention of recurrent abortion with leucocyte transfusions. Lancet 2:68, 1981
32. Williams KA, French ME, Ting A et al: Preoperative blood transfusions improve cadaveric renal-allograft survival in non-transfused recipients. Lancet 1:1104, 1980
33. Zurier RB: SLE and pregnancy. In Schur PA (ed): The Clinical Management of Systemic Lupus Erythematosis. New York, Grune & Stratton, 1983

15

Fetal Therapy

SECTION 1: SURGICAL MANAGEMENT OF FETAL MALFORMATIONS

W. Allen Hogge and Mitchell S. Golbus

Although there have been remarkable advances in the prenatal detection of congenital abnormalities over the last decade, the ultimate goal of the reproductive geneticist is to develop techniques for fetal therapy to complement the ability to diagnose these disorders. With the advent of active fetal intervention[2,5,10,16] has come the consideration of the fetus as a patient, and the first attempts to outline appropriate courses of action for the fetus with a correctable congenital defect.[6,11,15]

CONSIDERATIONS PRIOR TO THERAPY

Fetal Selection Criteria

The most difficult task in prenatal management is the selection of the fetus most likely to benefit from active intervention. As with any disease in medicine, it is essential that the pathophysiology and natural history of the disorder be understood before any attempt at therapy is undertaken. Likewise, the clinical spectrum of the disease must be known, including the normal variation, in order to clearly differentiate the abnormal from the normal state.

Directly correlated with the differentiation of abnormality is an accurate diagnosis of the fetal condition. Once an accurate diagnosis has been established, a careful assessment must be done to determine if intervention is justified. This decision must be based on a consideration of both fetal and maternal risks and benefits. There are certain general criteria that have been suggested as guidelines in considering a particular case for treatment:

- The fetus should be a singleton with no associated anomalies based on an evaluation by a level II ultrasound and amniocentesis for karyotype, alpha-fetoprotein level, and viral cultures.
- The family must be fully informed about the risks and benefits of the treatment proposed, and should agree to all aspects

of that therapy including long-term follow-up.
- A multidisciplinary team, to include (at least) an obstetrician experienced in fetal diagnosis and intrauterine treatment, an ultrasonographer experienced in the diagnosis of fetal anomalies, and a pediatric surgeon and neonatologist who are experienced in the management of the high-risk neonate, should concur on the plan for innovative treatment and should obtain the approval of an institutional review board
- There should be access to a level III high-risk obstetrical unit and intensive care nursery, and availability of appropriate bioethical and psychosocial consultation.[14]

As will be discussed later, there are two other major criteria to be met which relate to the spectrum and time of onset of the disease in question.

- First, prenatal intervention for disease of any severity is not warranted once the fetus can be safely delivered for more definitive postnatal treatment.
- Some fetuses are so severely affected that they cannot be salvaged even by intervention at an early stage of pregnancy.

It is absolutely essential, therefore, that a thorough diagnostic evaluation be carried out prior to an attempt at therapeutic intervention. Without strict adherence to guidelines similar to those outlined, the true efficacy and benefits of fetal therapy will remain unknown.

Treatment Modality Selection

The availability of treatment modalities for the fetus has given rise to a new set of decisions to be made when a fetal malformation is detected. Previously the only question to be answered was whether to abort the fetus or await delivery. Now it is essential that a carefully considered plan of management be outlined for a fetus with a surgically correctable lesion. Because experience in fetal management is limited, any management protocols should be considered tentative and readily altered or discarded as new information becomes available. Certain basic considerations become more critical regarding any fetal condition as our surgical techniques become more sophisticated.

Pregnancy termination. When serious malformations incompatible with postnatal life are diagnosed, the family should have the option of terminating the pregnancy. Those with malformations recognized after the time period for safe abortion is past should be counseled and appropriate postnatal management arranged. Examples of such conditions are anencephaly, bilateral renal agenesis, and lethal bone dysplasias (e.g., thanatophoric dwarfism).

Defects best corrected after term delivery. Most correctable malformations that can be diagnosed in utero are best managed after delivery at term. The mode of delivery should be based on obstetric indications in most instances, although certain situations should be managed by cesarean delivery. A malformation that would cause dystocia is one situation that would require elective cesarean section. The advantage of prenatal detection for disorders correctable at term is that it allows preparation for appropriate prenatal and postnatal care, and insures that appropriate personnel are available at the time of delivery. It should always be kept in mind that the term infant is a better anesthetic and surgical risk than the preterm infant.

Defects that may alter the timing of delivery. Certain fetal anomalies should be corrected as soon as possible after diagnosis. However, in every instance the risk of premature delivery must be weighed against the risk of further damage if the pregnancy is continued. Because of the recent advances in perinatal medicine, including the stimulation of fetal lung surfactant production with corticosteroids, and better techniques of ventilatory management, the time at which delivery can be safely performed has become progressively earlier. Decisions to take this option of early delivery must, however, be made on a clear understanding of the natural history of the disorder or definite evidence of progression of the disease. Surgical conditions that may fall into this category are gastroschisis, ruptured omphalocele, and certain cases of obstructive hydronephrosis and obstructive hydrocephalus.

Anatomic malformations that may require in utero intervention. Considerations of in utero surgical intervention should be based on the rationale that the malformation in question will interfere with fetal organ development and that, if alleviated, would allow normal fetal development. The three anatomic malformations that meet this condition at present are bilateral urinary tract obstruction, obstructive hydrocephalus, and congenital diaphragmatic hernia. Treatment of other more complicated lesions will occur in the future when their pathophysiology is elucidated and techniques for fetal intervention improve.

FETAL STRUCTURAL MALFORMATIONS POTENTIALLY AMENABLE TO SURGICAL THERAPY

Urinary Tract Obstruction

Evaluation

Fetal hydronephrosis is a commonly recognized fetal abnormality because fluid-filled masses are easily detected by ultrasound and because the associated oligohydramnios results in a size-dates discrepancy, prompting sonographic evaluation. If the sonographic findings suggest fetal urinary tract obstruction, an accurate delineation of the abnormality and a thorough evaluation to rule out associated anomalies are absolutely essential. This work-up should include obtaining fetal cells, either from amniotic fluid or fetal urine, for karyotyping because chromosomal abnormalities have been reported to be associated with urinary tract abnormalities.[8,24]

The second criterion to be met is that serial sonographic observation should be done to document that the obstruction is not transient and that the quantity of amniotic fluid is decreased or decreasing. Adequate amounts of amniotic fluid usually signify reasonable fetal renal function and should be a major factor in deciding when intervention is necessary.

Finally, as was discussed previously, a fetus at 32 weeks gestation or longer is better managed by delivery and treatment by conventional approaches. Based on these criteria, an approach to the management of the fetus with urinary tract obstruction can be developed (Fig. 15-1).

Management Options

For the fetus with unilateral obstruction and normal amniotic fluid volume, intervention does not appear warranted. Harrison and colleagues have reported on the expectant management of eight fetuses with these findings[17]: all were followed and delivered near term with no neonatal complications; Subsequently six have had successful pyeloplasties and two have required unilateral nephrectomy. The prenatal diagnosis of these conditions is, however, of significant benefit in view of the fact that in three of the neonates the flank mass was not noted until specifically sought on the basis of the prenatal sonogram.

In the case of bilateral urinary tract obstruction with normal amniotic fluid volume, a similar approach of expectant management is recommended. These pregnancies are followed with serial sonograms to determine whether the process will resolve or progress before intervention is considered. Although it appears that this group does well without intervention, the number of pregnancies followed to date is too limited to provide a clear indication of the natural history of this form of fetal uropathy.

The approach of invasive assessment and therapy for urinary tract obstruction should be reserved for cases that demonstrate isolated bilateral hydronephrosis secondary to obstruction in association with oligohydramnios. However, prior to any surgical intervention, a thorough evaluation of

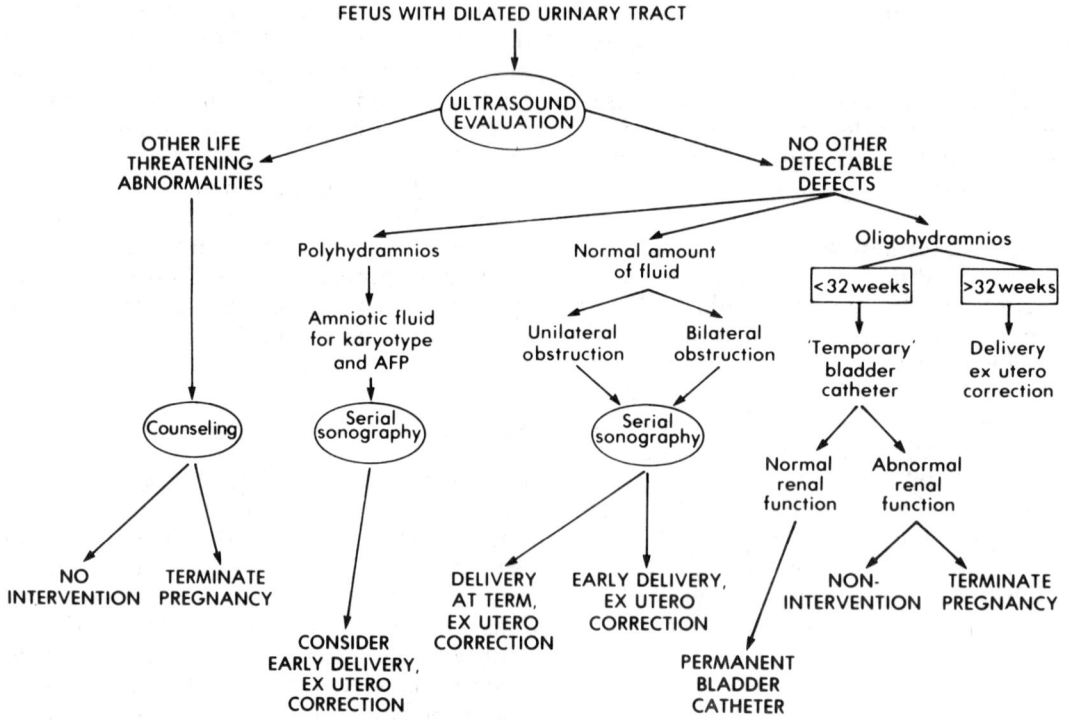

FIGURE 15.1. Approach to the management of a fetus with urinary tract dilatation detected by sonography.

fetal renal function must be done. Sonography by an experienced ultrasonographer can provide some preliminary information on which to make clinical judgments.[22] The presence of increased echogenicity of the fetal kidneys associated with renal cortical cysts indicates severe renal dysplasia, and these fetuses will not benefit from drainage procedures. Unfortunately, the absence of these sonographic findings does not preclude severe dysplasia, and other methods of functional assessment are required. To evaluate renal function, the fetal bladder or renal pelvis is aspirated. The findings of normal urine sodium (<100 mEq/ml), chloride (<90 mEq/ml), and osmolality (<210 mosm) are evidence of relatively normal renal function; severe damage to the fetal kidney appears to be characterized by a salt-losing state. The necessity of aspirating the renal pelvis, rather than the bladder, is emphasized by a recent report by Nicolini et al[25] in which electrolytes from bladder urine were abnormal, but one kidney had normal findings. The favorable outcome in this case strongly suggests that the mixed bladder sample may give misleading information in some instances. Although urine electrolytes appear to be a relatively sensitive indicator of fetal renal function, they must be used in combination with other clinical information. Even with careful evaluation there may be cases in which electrolytes may not be an accurate predictor of neonatal renal function.[26] Thus it is open to debate whether there really are "absolute" criteria for believing that renal function in early pregnancy can be declared irreparable.

In those cases in which renal function appears intact and the gestational age is less than 32 weeks, an attempt to bypass the obstruction is indicated. The technique most

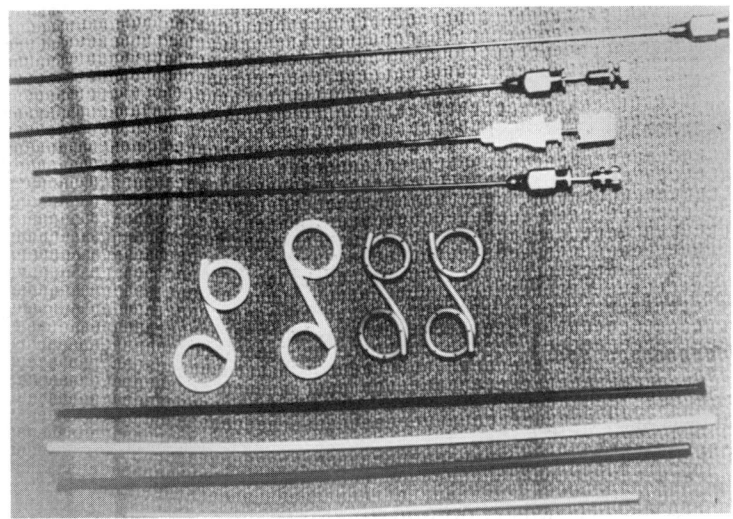

FIGURE 15-2. Harrison bladder catheters with equipment developed for placement of catheter shunts under sonographic control. Catheters are straightened over trochar needles for puncture.

commonly employed is placement of a Harrison double-pigtailed fetal bladder catheter (Fig. 15-2) from the fetal bladder to the amniotic cavity. Bypassing the obstruction should prevent further renal damage, restore normal amniotic fluid volume, and prevent pulmonary hypoplasia. One of the major difficulties with this approach has been the need for multiple catheter placements because of the high incidence of the catheter becoming dislodged after relatively short periods of time (approximately 2–3 weeks). For this reason alternative approaches to the management of a fetus diagnosed in the second trimester are being considered.

With the availability of tocolytic agents, an "open" procedure may offer greater benefit in the long-term management; that is, direct exposure of the fetal abdomen through a hysterotomy incision would allow marsupialization of the bladder and continuous drainage that bypasses the obstruction of the posterior urethral valve syndrome. A similar approach in which bilateral fetal ureterostomies were done has been reported.[16] Although the outcome in this case was not a successful one, it did offer evidence that direct access to the fetus was possible without precipitating preterm labor. Despite the potential this approach has for management of the fetus, both fetal and maternal risks are high. Before undertaking such innovative therapy the techniques must be thoroughly tested in the laboratory in the nonhuman primate, and extreme care is necessary in selection of potential candidates for this management.

For those patients with a fetus having severely compromised to absent renal function and severe oligohydramnios, the outcome has been universally dismal with no survivors.[17] The options for this group are limited to early termination of the pregnancy, or nonintervention awaiting the onset of spontaneous labor.

The multifaceted approach necessary for the evaluation and management of congenital urinary tract obstruction illustrates the necessary prerequisites to be met before undertaking active intervention. It is important that fetal treatment programs be actively engaged in continuing research programs to better understand the mechanism and pathophysiology of the disease process in question. There are many unanswered questions regarding the efficacy and long-term effects of these intervention techniques. At this early stage in its development, fetal intervention should be pursued only in a center committed to research and development in appropriate animal models prior to responsible clinical application.

Congenital Hydrocephalus

Evaluation

In no other fetal structural disorder amenable to potential in utero intervention is the need for proper and thorough evaluation more clearly demonstrated than in fetal ventriculomegaly. The marked technical advances in ultrasonography have made possible the diagnosis of ventricular enlargement at early stages of gestation and have stimulated interest in the field of in utero surgical management of this common malformation.

In theory, this condition should be ideally managed by placement of a ventricular shunt analogous to the methods used for postnatal therapy. However, since the first reports of in utero decompression of fetal hydrocephalus,[2] and the placement of ventriculo-amniotic shunts,[5] much has been learned about the etiologic heterogeneity and natural history of fetal ventriculomegaly detected by ultrasound.[3,9,27] In the study by Glick and colleagues, there were 24 cases of ventriculomegaly as defined previously by Fiske and Filly.[7] The method is based on measurement of the choroid plexus size relative to the transverse diameter of the ventricular body. Careful sonographic evaluation of these 24 fetuses revealed isolated ventriculomegaly in only 11 cases. These 11 cases were followed with serial sonography and, in 10 instances, ventriculomegaly remained stable without significant change in enlargement of the ventricles or the biparietal diameter with advancing gestation. Cerebral cortex thickness measured between 10 mm and 17 mm initially and remained unchanged or increased in size as pregnancy progressed. Postnatally 4 infants required shunting within the first 5 months of life, and 5 have not required shunting. One neonate died shortly after birth from cardiac abnormalities not detected prenatally. Of note is that in one of these cases the ventriculomegaly was seen to resolve spontaneously.

In only 1 of these 11 fetuses with suspected isolated ventriculomegaly did there appear to be progression. Although early serial ultrasounds revealed stable ventriculomegaly, there was mild progressive ventricular enlargement and cortical mantle thinning noted between 33 and 37 menstrual weeks. A recommendation was made for early delivery; however, the patient had the spontaneous onset of labor at 37 weeks and vaginally delivered a normal male infant without signs of increased intracranial pressure. At 2 months of age a ventriculoperitoneal shunt was placed, and subsequent developmental milestones have been normal.

Of significant concern, however, is that 3 of the 11 fetuses thought to have isolated obstructive hydrocephalus had other associated midline central nervous system malformations which were not detected by ultrasound prenatally or on retrospective review of the films postnatally. Each infant had agenesis of the corpus callosum; two additionally had absence of the septum pellucidum, and one had septo-optic dysplasia and was blind. Similar findings have been noted in several fetuses who have undergone in utero intervention.[2,4] The concern regarding precise diagnosis is emphasized by the reports to the Fetal Treatment Registry.[23] Of the 41 cases reported to the Registry, only three fourths had a diagnosis of aqueductal stenosis. Even more significant is that of the 28 survivors following in utero therapy only 40% of the infants were clinically normal on follow-up examination. However, in more recent data following the outcome in 200 untreated fetuses with ventriculomegaly, the outcomes have generally been extremely poor.[6A]

Management

Based on this experience it becomes clear that a thorough and continuing evaluation is necessary when ventriculomegaly is detected sonographically. Amniocentesis should be performed for karyotype, alpha-fetoprotein determination, and cytomegalovirus culture. A careful, detailed sonogram done by an ultrasonographer experienced in the detection of fetal anomalies is essential. In those cases with apparently isolated ventriculomegaly weekly sonograms should be done. If no change in ventricular size or cortical thickness occurs, no intervention should be undertaken. Progression after 32 menstrual weeks is best managed by early delivery and ex utero shunting, if indicated.

On the basis of this management protocol there would appear to be a group of patients with isolated progressive hydrocephalus prior to 32 weeks gestation that might benefit from in utero shunting. However, in our experience with more than 30 patients, there has not been a single patient who met these guidelines. Even in retrospective analyses of cases of hydrocephalus diagnosed prenatally, the number of cases that potentially would have met these criteria is quite low.[27] There are many unanswered questions regarding the management of congenital hydrocephalus, and for the present most investigators have agreed to a moratorium on in utero procedures until further knowledge can be gained on the natural history and pathophysiology of this heterogenous group of disorders. With the identification of a small group of patients who have isolated, progressive ventriculomegaly, it may be appropriate to begin to offer such patients a randomized trial of shunting of ventriculomegaly.[6A]

Congenital Diaphragmatic Hernia

Evaluation

The incidence of congenital diaphragmatic hernia (CDH) is approximately 1 per 2600 births, with most neonates being severely affected and having a mortality that approaches 80%.[13] As with the other disorders just discussed, the advent of real-time sonography has made this a prenatally diagnosed condition rather than a neonatally diagnosed one. The ultrasound findings include herniated abdominal viscera, abnormal upper abdominal anatomy, and a mediastinal shift away from the side of the herniation. Polyhydramnios is a common finding, seen in 76% of the cases reported by Adzick and colleagues.[1] Despite this ability to detect CDH prior to birth and to plan sophisticated postnatal therapy, the mortality rate is no different from that reported for cases diagnosed after birth (80%). The majority of these deaths are secondary to severe pulmonary hypoplasia, a developmental consequence of compression by the herniated viscera. In Adzick's series, 16% of the cases also had other associated lethal anomalies.

Management

Because the prognosis for CDH is so dismal despite optimal neonatal care, the possibility of in utero surgical correction has been raised.[13] Harrison and colleagues have demonstrated in an animal model that CDH is surgically correctable in utero, and that correction can lead to adequate lung development and to neonatal survival.[12,18,20] Before these techniques are extended to the human fetus, the details of this technically difficult procedure must be mastered in the laboratory, and a high degree of success achieved experimentally. Prior to any attempt at intervention, however, an accurate diagnosis must be made, and any associated anomalies ruled out by a careful diagnostic evaluation including detailed sonography and amniocentesis for chromosome analysis. The preliminary experience with this technique is promising. Four cases have been performed with one successful repair in utero. It would appear that in carefully selected cases, surgical repair prior to birth may offer hope for the fetus with congenital diaphragmatic hernia.

THE NEED FOR FURTHER RESEARCH

Our ability to detect and define congenital malformations will continue to improve. Likewise, our ability to intervene and correct the anatomic changes will improve. However, there are certain lessons to be learned from our experience to date. First, to be able to select for treatment only those fetuses which will truly benefit from intervention, we need better techniques to measure fetal organ function. Basing clinical management on morphologic criteria alone has proven to be unsatisfactory. Second, there is considerable potential for doing harm to both mother and fetus with innovative fetal treatments. The techniques must be fully tested in the laboratory before clinical application is undertaken. Most of the important questions about pathophysiology, efficacy of correction, and feasibility and safety of intervention must be answered in animal models, and these models must be carefully established. Although the pathophysiology may be defined by investigation of nonprimate models, the feasibility and safety of a technique must be addressed in the nonhuman primate. By following this logical progression of models a reasonable approximation of the success or failure of clinical application can be made.

An example of this type of approach was discussed previously relative to congenital diaphragmatic hernia, and similar models have been developed for obstructive hydronephrosis.[19,21] Excellent animal models for the study of the pathophysiology of both these conditions were developed in the fetal lamb. Likewise, these models provided information on the benefits of early intervention. However, the uterus of sheep is quite insensitive to surgical manipulation and hysterotomy will rarely induce preterm labor. It is not a good model for evaluating the feasibility and safety of fetal intervention in the human in whom preterm labor is likely to result from surgical manipulation of the uterus. For this type of study the nonhuman primate provides an excellent model. The gravid monkey uterus is very susceptible to preterm labor and provides an extremely rigorous model for the testing of intervention techniques. Surgical intervention for the human fetus with a malformation should not be attempted until success is achieved and competence is demonstrated in this most demanding and critical model.

Fetal treatment has been embraced with enthusiasm, but this enthusiasm must be tempered with caution. Innovative fetal intervention must be fully tested in the laboratory, carefully and continually evaluated in light of current knowledge of the disorder in question, and honestly presented to the patient before it is undertaken. In utero fetal therapy is an experimental form of fetal medicine, and, thus should be applied only in those centers where ongoing research is being done. Surgical therapy must be a logical extension of knowledge gained from thoughtful research in genetics and developmental biology.

REFERENCES

1. Adzick NS, Harrison MR, Glick PL et al: Diaphragmatic hernia in the fetus: Prenatal diagnosis and outcome in 94 cases. J Pediatr Surg 20:357, 1985
2. Birnholz JC, Firgoletto FD: Antenatal treatment of hydrocephalus. N Engl J Med 304:1021, 1982
3. Chervenak FA, Ment LR, McClure M et al: Outcome of fetal ventriculomegaly. Lancet 2:179, 1984
4. Clewell WH: Personal communication, 1984
5. Clewell WH, Johnson ML, Meier PR et al: A surgical approach to the treatment of hydrocephalus. N Engl J Med 306:1320, 1982
6. Diament MJ, Fine RN, Ehrlich R, Kangarloo H: Fetal hydronephrosis: Problems in diagnosis and management. J Pediatr 103:435, 1983
6A. Drugan A, Krause B, Canady A, et al: The natural history of prenatally diagnosed ventriculomegaly. JAMA (in press)
7. Fiske CE, Filly RA: Ultrasound of the normal and abnormal fetal neural axis. Radiol Clin North Am 20:285, 1982
8. Frydman M, Magenis RE, Mohandas TK, Kaback MM: Chromosome abnormalities in infants with prune belly anomaly: Association with trisomy 18. Am J Med Genet 15:145, 1983
9. Glick PL, Nakayama DK, Harrison MR et al: Management of the fetus with ventriculomegaly. J Pediatr 105:97, 1984
10. Golbus MS, Harrison MR, Filly RA: In utero treatment of urinary tract obstruction. Am J Obstet Gynecol 142:383, 1982
11. Golbus MS, Harrison MR, Filly RA: Prenatal diagnosis and treatment of fetal hydronephrosis. Semin Perinatol 7:102, 1983
12. Harrison MR, Bressack MC, Chung AM, deLorimier AA: Correction of congenital dia-

phragmatic hernia in utero. II. Simulated correction permits fetal lung growth with survival at birth. Surgery 88:260, 1980
13. Harrison MR, deLorimier AA: Congenital diaphragmatic hernia. Surg Clin North Am 61:1023, 1981
14. Harrison MR, Filly RA, Golbus MS: Fetal treatment 1982. N Engl J Med 307:1651, 1982
15. Harrison MR, Golbus MS, Filly RA: Management of the fetus with a correctable congenital defect. J Am Med Assoc 246:774, 1981
16. Harrison MR, Golbus MS, Filly RA et al: Fetal surgery for congenital hydronephrosis. N Engl J Med 306:591, 1982
17. Harrison MR, Golbus MS, Filly RA et al: Management of the fetus with congenital hydronephrosis. J Pediatr Surg 17:728, 1982
18. Harrison MR, Jester JA, Ross NA: Correction of congenital diaphragmatic hernia in utero. I. The model: Intrathoracic balloon produces fatal pulmonary hypoplasia. Surgery 88:174, 1980
19. Harrison MR, Nakayama DK, Noall R et al: Correction of congenital hydronephrosis in utero. II. Decompression reverses the effects of obstruction on the fetal lung and urinary tract. J Pediatr Surg 17:965, 1982
20. Harrison MR, Ross NA, deLorimier AA: Correction of congenital diaphragmatic hernia in utero. III. Development of a successful surgical technique using abdominoplasty to avoid compromise of umbilical blood flow. J Pediatr Surg 16:934, 1981
21. Harrison MR, Ross NA, Noall R et al: Correction of congenital hydronephrosis in utero. I. The model: Fetal urethral obstruction produces hydronephrosis and pulmonary hypoplasia in fetal lambs. J Pediatr Surg 18:247, 1983
22. Mahoney BS, Filly RA, Callen PW et al: Fetal renal dysplasia: Sonographic evaluation. Radiology 152:143, 1984
23. Manning FA, Harrison MR, Rodeck CH: Catheter shunts for fetal hydronephrosis and hydrocephalus: Report of the International Fetal Surgery Registry. N Engl J Med 315:336, 1986
24. Nevin NC, Nevin J, Dunlop JM, Gray M: Antenatal detection of grossly distended bladder owing to absence of the urethra in a fetus with trisomy 18. J Med Genet 20:132, 1983
25. Nicolini U, Rodeck CH, Fisk NM: Shunt treatment for fetal obstructive uropathy. Lancet 2:1338, 1987
26. Wilkins IA, Chitkara U, Lynch L, et al: The nonpredictive value of fetal urinary electrolytes: Preliminary report of outcomes and correlations with pathologic diagnosis. Am J Obstet Gynecol 157:694, 1987
27. Williamson RA, Schauberger CW, Varner MW, Aschenbrener CA: Heterogeneity of prenatal onset hydrocephalus: Management and counseling implications. Am J Med Genet 17:497, 1984

SECTION 2: MEDICAL FETAL THERAPY

Mark I. Evans and Joseph D. Schulman

Waves of enthusiasm surrounded the earliest fetal surgical interventions. However, with increasing experiences there has been a considerable sobering of expectations for such surgical procedures.[11] Conversely, medical and pharmacologic alterations in the hormonal milieu of the fetus now appear to be much more promising and ultimately will likely be the mainstay of fetal therapy.[9]

Successes in medical fetal therapy have been clearly demonstrated in two main areas: the prevention of external genital masculinization in female fetuses affected with 21-hydroxylase deficiency congenital adrenal hyperplasia, and the correction of fetal cardiac dysrrhythmias that can lead to nonimmune fetal hydrops and fetal death.[5,29] (Cardiac therapy will be discussed in Section 3.) In some other areas, it has been demonstrated that the pharmacology of the fetus can be altered, although questions as to the usefulness of such alterations remain to be proven.

The potential effects of drugs or maternal metabolites on the fetus are well known. In many cases, as with known teratogens, the effects are adverse and may be in part genetically determined.[25,26] Furthermore, some maternal metabolic diseases may have profound fetal effects, as perhaps best demonstrated by the extensive fetal damage seen secondary to maternal phenylketonuria and resultant fetal hyperphenylalaninemia.[14,23,24]

For decades drugs and other agents have been administered to pregnant women for treatment of fetal disorders not usually classified as metabolic, in the hope of improving the capacity for postnatal adaptation. Well-known examples include exchange transfusions in Rh disease, the administration of corticosteroids for the prevention of respiratory distress syndrome in premature infants, and the administration of phenobarbital prior to birth in the hope of inducing liver enzymes for postnatal reduction of serum bilirubin concentration. However, there are only a very few examples of attempted prenatal treatment for genetically determined metabolic defects.

The Rh-isoimmunization model provides a successful illustration of medical intervention in the developing fetus.[3] Up until the introduction of RhoGAM in the early 1970s, thousands of infants died in utero or in the early neonatal period with acute hemolytic disease secondary to Rh-isoimmunization. Many of the surviving affected infants suffered from mental retardation, incapacitating neurologic disability, or deafness. The first prenatal exchange transfusion was performed by Lilley in the early 1960s and was complemented by the development of postnatal transfusions. Finally, complete prevention of hydrops by passive maternal isoimmunization was made possible by RhoGAM. Unlike other surgical and medical fetal interventions which are still technically experimental, exchange transfusions have clearly moved into the realm of standard practice for Rh-isoimmunization.

MEDICAL MANAGEMENT OF GENETICALLY DETERMINED METABOLIC DEFECTS

Congenital Adrenal Hyperplasia

Evans and colleagues have demonstrated that the fetal adrenal gland can be pharmacologically suppressed by maternal replacement doses of dexamethasone.[7] Their first case involved a woman who sought genetic counseling because she had mild 21-hydroxylase deficiency. The couple had a previous female child with classic congenital adrenal hyperplasia (CAH) and external genital masculinization. She and her husband wished to know if prenatal diagnosis of CAH were possible. They indicated that they would terminate the pregnancy if the fetus were affected. In consultation they were told of an untested technique whereby the fetal adrenal gland might be suppressed and the masculinization prevented. After thorough counseling, they agreed to the attempt at suppression.

Dexamethasone, 25 mg, was administered orally q.i.d., beginning the 10th week of gestation. Maternal estriol and cortisol values indicated rapid and sustained fetal and maternal adrenal gland suppression. Without therapy, the diagnosis of CAH is possible from the elevated levels of cortisol precursors in amniotic fluid, most notably 17-OH progesterone. Amniocentesis was performed at 17 weeks gestation. The karyotype was 46,XX. Analyses of adrenal hormones in the amniotic fluid were found to be in the low normal range, confirming adrenal suppression (Table 15-1). Human leukocyte antigen (HLA) haplotypes were assayed but were not informative. Therefore, the dexamethasone was continued throughout the pregnancy. The patient was followed very closely and had multiple reactive nonstress tests throughout the third trimester. Fetal growth appeared adequate.

At 39 weeks gestation, the patient was spontaneously delivered of a female neonate with normal external genitalia, demonstrating that prolonged dexamethasone suppression of the fetal adrenal gland could be accomplished without making the mother cushingoid and without apparent adverse affects on the fetus. The infant was immediately started on replacement therapy with dexamethasone and Fluorinef. Adrenocorticotropic hormone (ACTH) challenge tests revealed that she did not have the classic disease. Subsequent analysis of the neonatal

Table 15-1. Amniotic Fluid Steroid Hormone Concentrations in the Second Trimester

Hormone	Patient Treated with Dexamethasone	Patient Treated with Prednisone*	Control Range	Specimens Assayed
Cortisol, µg/dl	0.7	2.5	1.5–6.4	111
17-hydroxyprogesterone, ng/dl	21†	129	48–299	111
Progesterone, ng/ml	23	31	14–106	111
17-hydroxypregnenolone, ng/dl	125	136	85–164	9
Pregnenolone succinate, ng/dl	150	168	53–251	9
Estriol$_3$, pg/ml	396	2,580	982–3640	111
Estriol$_2$, pg/ml	15.9	. . .	12–122	109
Esteriol$_1$, pg/ml	92	258	111–895	111
Dehydroepiandrosterone, ng/dl	28.1	66	39–104	9
Δ^4-Androstenediol, ng/dl	60	37	41–152	7
Δ^5-Androstenediol, ng/dl	64.2	50	38–66	9
Dexamethasone	1.12†	< 0.5‡	< 0.5‡	7

* Pregnant woman with Crohn's disease receiving prednisone, 10 mg twice daily, measured two hours after last dose
† Maternal plasma concentration, 5.8 ng/ml
‡ Assay detection limit

HLA haplotypes revealed a crossing over between HLA B and D loci and suggested carrier status.

Following the initial observation of the Evans study, Forrest and David used the same protocol and demonstrated that fetuses known to be clinically affected with the severe form of 21-hydroxylase deficiency CAH were prevented from external congenital masculinization.[10] To date, several infants with classic CAH, who clearly would have been masculinized, have been born with normal genitalia. We believe that these events represent the first prevention of a birth defect and may serve as a model for other attempts at pharmacologic fetal therapy. One interesting element to this first case was the fact that therapy had to begin long before a diagnosis was possible. With the autosomal recessive genetics of CAH, only one of eight pregnancies would be expected to benefit (females with CAH). Now with the availability of a probe for the gene,[20] a nearly definitive diagnosis would be possible by DNA analysis of chorionic villi before therapy would need to be initiated.

The fundamental principles addressed in such attempted prevention of masculinization are logically extended to other medical fetal therapies. The concepts of a thorough informed consent procedure, thorough documentation of progress, and high-risk obstetric management have been followed by investigators in these fields.

Multiple Carboxylase Deficiency

Biotin-responsive multiple carboxylase deficiency is an inborn error of metabolism in which the mitochondrial biotin-dependent enzymes, pyruvate carboxylase, propionyl-coenzyme A carboxylase, and B-methylcrotonyl-coenzyme A carboxylase have diminished activity. Affected patients present as newborns or in the early childhood period with dermatitis, severe metabolic acidosis, and a characteristic pattern of organic acid excretion. Metabolism in patients or in their cultured cells can be restored toward normal levels by biotin supplementation. There have been two reports of prenatal administration of biotin to fetuses affected with this disorder.

Roth and co-workers treated a fetus

without the benefit of prenatal diagnosis in a case in which two siblings of the fetus had died of multiple carboxylase deficiency.[22] The first sibling had died within 3 days of birth, and in the second the diagnosis of biotin responsive carboxylase deficiency was made posthumously.

The patient was first seen at 34 weeks gestation. Prenatal diagnosis was not attempted because of the late stage of pregnancy. The maternal urinary organic acid profile was normal throughout the final 4 weeks of pregnancy. Because of severe neonatal manifestations in the previous siblings and the probable harmlessness of biotin, oral administration of this compound to the mother was begun at a dose of 10 mg/day. There were no apparent untoward effects; maternal urinary biotin excretion increased approximately one hundredfold during biotin administration.

Nonidentical twins were subsequently delivered at term. Cord blood and urinary organic acid profiles, and cord blood biotin concentrations were four to seven times greater than normal. The neonatal course for both twins was unremarkable. Subsequent study of the cultured fibroblasts of both twins compared under biotin-rich and biotin-depleted growth conditions indicated that in biotin-depleted medium, the cells of twin B (but not of twin A) had virtually complete deficiency of all three carboxylase activities. Genetic complementation studies confirmed that despite the normal clinical presentation during the newborn period, twin B was homozygous for mutations of both biotins.

Packman and colleagues have also reported prenatal diagnosis and treatment of biotin-responsive multiple carboxylase deficiency for a mother who had previously given birth to a male with the neonatal-onset form of this disease.[19] In the next pregnancy, maternal urine organic acid profiles were normal. The three carboxylase activities were assayed in cultured amniotic fluid cells obtained by amniocentesis at 17 menstrual weeks. In biotin-restricted medium, the amniotic cells demonstrated the characteristic severe reduction in carboxylase activities.

At 23½ menstrual weeks, the mother started receiving 10 mg/day of oral biotin. After birth, the term female exhibited no clinical or gross chemical abnormalities. Postnatal biotin administration was begun postnatally on Day 4. The diagnosis of multiple carboxylase deficiency was confirmed employing fibroblasts derived from the neonate. Postnatal development of the infant was normal.

The above two cases provide compelling evidence that biotin administration effectively prevents neonatal complications in certain patients with biotin-responsive multiple carboxylase deficiency. No toxicity from treatment was observed. In such patients who also have methylmalonic aciduria (to be discussed next), the traditional approach would be treatment immediately after birth. At this time, it is not possible to definitively assess the relative advantages or disadvantages of prenatal treatment, although such therapy appears both effective and logical.

Methylmalonic Acidemia

Methylmalonic acidemia is related to a functional vitamin B_{12} deficiency. Coenzymatically active B_{12} is required for the conversion of methylmalonyl-coenzyme A to succinyl-coenzyme A. Several genetically determined etiologies for methylmalonic acidemia include defects in methylmalonyl-coenzyme A mutase or in the metabolism of vitamin B_{12} to the coenzymatically active form, 5'-dioxyadenosylcobalamin in the converting enzyme. Some patients may respond to administration of large doses of B_{12}, which can enhance the amount of active holoenzyme (mutase apoenzyme plus 5'-deoxyadenosylcobalamin).

Ampola and associates were the first to attempt prenatal diagnosis and treatment of a B_{12}-responsive variant of methylmalonic acidemia.[1] They followed the pregnancy of a patient who had previously suffered the loss of a child to severe acidosis and dehydration at the age of 3 months. The diagnosis of methylmalonic aciduria was only made posthumously by chemical analysis of blood and urine. In the pregnancy they followed, an amniocentesis was performed at 19 weeks gestation. An elevated methylmalonic acid content was documented in the cell-free amniotic fluid. Cultured amniotic fluid cells had defective propionate oxidation, succinate oxidation, undetectable levels of 5'-deoxyadenosylcobalamin and normal succinate oxidation and methylmalonyl-coenzyme A mutase activity in the presence of added 5'-deoxyadenosylcobalamin. These studies established by approximately 23 weeks gestation that the fetus suffered from methylmalonic acidemia seemingly due to deficient synthesis of 5'deoxyadenosylcobalamin.

It was already known that fetal methylmalonic acidemia is associated with increased methylmalonic acid excretion in maternal urine.[16] Ampola and colleagues documented increased methylmalonic acidemia in a maternal urine sample first collected at 23 weeks gestation; the methylmalonic acid excretion/mg creatinine was approximately twice the upper normal limit and demonstrated a further rise by 25 weeks. Urinary methylmalonate excretion is not abnormal in heterozygous females carrying a normal fetus, as shown subsequently by these same investigators.[1]

At 32 weeks gestation, cyanocobalamin (10 mg/day) was administered orally to the mother in divided doses. The treatment only marginally altered the maternal serum B_{12} level; however, there was a slight reduction of urinary methylmalonic acid excretion which remained severalfold above normal. At approximately 34 weeks gestation, 5 mg of cyanocobalamin/day intravenously was begun. The maternal serum B_{12} level then rose gradually to more than sixfold normal and was accompanied by a progressive decrease in urinary methylmalonic acid excretion. Maternal urinary methylmalonate was only slightly above the normal range when delivery occurred at 41 menstrual weeks. Amniotic fluid methylmalonic acid concentrations were three times the normal mean at 19 menstrual weeks and four times the normal mean at term, despite prenatal treatment.

Postnatally, the diagnosis of methylmalonic acidemia was confirmed. The infant suffered no acute neonatal complications and had an extremely high serum B_{12} level. Long-term postnatal management involved protein restriction; however no continuous cyanocobalamin treatment was required.

In this instance prenatal treatment certainly improved the fetal and, secondarily, the maternal biochemistry. Whether there was any significant *clinical* benefit to the fetus by in utero treatment cannot be adequately assessed. It seems likely that reducing the fetal burden of methylmalonic acid should have some beneficial effect on fetal development and possibly reduce the risks in the neonatal period. Such, however, is only speculation.

Nyhan has suggested that there may be an increased frequency of minor anomalies associated with untreated fetal methylmalonic acidemia.[17] Thus, very early or perhaps even prophylactic treatment with B_{12} prior to prenatal diagnosis in at-risk cases might be indicated for optimal therapy of B_{12}-responsive methylmalonic acidemia.

The report by Ampola and co-workers was the first example of treatment of a vitamin-responsive inborn error of metabolism in utero.[1] A subsequent report of prenatal treatment of methylmalonic acidemia revealed similar results, and other pregnancies have been monitored by the authors.[21] However, a number of important questions raised by the study are still unresolved and may ultimately require many years to treat enough patients to establish the risk-benefits ratio of this approach.

Abnormalities of Mineral Metabolism

Specific prenatal mineral supplementation has yet to be reported for prevention of human fetal disease. However, such additives have been used in animals with genetic deficiencies. Animal studies are of considerable interest and suggest the possibility of analogous human treatment.

Manganese

The effects of prenatal manganese supplementation on the prevention of otolith defects in mice affected with the pallid mutation have been investigated.[6,12] Pallid mice have defective pigmentation, including an absence of pigment from the membranous labyrinth. This pigmentary characteristic is fully penetrant in the pallid homozygous recessive; whereas another manifestation, impaired otolith formation, is variably expressed. Lyon observed a significant correlation of litter size and the expression of the otolith abnormalities in the offspring and hypothesized that the otolith defect may be influenced by competition in utero for an unidentified substance.[15]

Hurley and co-workers reported that development of the inner ear in normal rats and mice was affected by decreased manganese. In mice, experimental manganese deprivation in utero induced a defect of the inner ear which was morphologically and behaviorally indistinguishable from pallid, although manganese deficiency did not mimic the effect of the mutant gene on pigmentation. Subsequently these investigators observed that manganese supplementation of pallid mice throughout gestation with a diet containing from 45 to 2000 parts/million of manganese yielded a dose-dependent decrease in the percentage of abnormal otoliths.[12]

These data have been extended to a genetic basis for susceptibility. In several studies on prenatal manganese restriction, the percentage of otolith abnormalities was influenced by the strain of mice studied. Thus, interactions of manganese intake and genetic predisposition influence otolith development in several strains.[12] These observations suggest that at low or borderline levels of dietary intake of many nutrients, the genotype of the fetus can substantially alter fetal responses.

There are a number of genetic defects in animals with associated pigmentary and inner ear abnormalities. Some data suggest that manganese may play a role in modifying defects expression. Hurley and colleagues have suggested that a sex-linked form of ocular albinism in humans, associated with labyrinthine dysfunction, may be analogous to some of these animal models. We are unaware of any studies of manganese metabolism in human ocular albinism, nor of attempts to administer manganese prenatally in the hope of ameliorating expression of any associated labyrinthine defects.

Copper

Hurley and co-workers have investigated possible deleterious effects of prenatal copper administration on mice with the recessive mutant "crinkled" gene.[13] These investigators have suggested that the "crinkled" gene produces many phenotypic characteristics common to patients with Menkes' kinky-hair syndrome. Dietary supplementation of pregnant mice with copper sulfate partially ameliorated the effects of the crinkled gene in the offspring. Different prenatal copper regimens have resulted in varying degrees of success. Copper nitrilotracete appeared to be superior to copper sulfate in increasing postnatal survival and body copper content of the mutant offspring of heterozygous dams. Postnatal supplementation with copper did not increase survival of the mutants.

These studies may possibly lead to insights relevant to prenatal treatment of Menkes' syndrome, a sex-linked disorder characterized by progressive degeneration of neurologic function in infants. Alterations suggestive of functional copper deficiency are present in affected infants. Fibroblasts from patients with Menkes' disease accumulate excess copper probably present in an abnormally bound form. Howell feels that Menkes' syndrome can be reliably diagnosed in utero by demonstrating abnormally increased copper uptake in Menkes cultured amniotic fluid cells incubated in a high-copper medium. Menkes' disease has been refractory to postnatal therapy with copper; and it is conceivable that by analogy to the crinkled mutation, prenatal treatment might be of greater benefit.[13]

Despite apparent responses to prenatal mineral administration of pallid and crinkled mutations, the relationships of these mutants, if any, to ocular albinism and Menkes' disease, respectively, remain speculative. While animal studies have proven encouraging, they have not yet led to trials of prenatal mineral supplementation in genetically defective human beings.

Galactosemia

Galactosemia is an inborn error of metabolism caused by diminished activity of the enzyme galactose-1-phosphate uridyl transferase. It is inherited in an autosomal recessive manner and results in cataracts, growth deficiency, and ovarian failure. Galactosemia can be diagnosed prenatally by study of cultured amniocytes and chorionic villi. Clinical symptoms appear in the neonatal period and can be largely ameliorated by elimination of galactose from the diet. However, irreversible damage to oocytes has already been done long before birth. Cellular damage in galactosemia is thought to be mediated by accumulation of galactose-1-phosphate intracellularly and of galactitol in the lens.

There are suggestions that even the early postnatal treatment of galactosemic individuals with a low galactose diet may not be sufficient to ensure normal development. There has been speculation that prenatal damage to galactosemic fetuses could contribute to subsequent abnormal neurologic development and to lens cataract formation.[25,28] Furthermore, it has been recently recognized that female galactosemics, even when treated from birth with galactose deprivation, have a high frequency of primary or secondary amenorrhea due to ovarian failure. There also may be some subtle abnormalities of male gonadal function.[27]

Exposure to a high galactose diet has been considered to represent an animal model for human galactosemia. Chen and associates have observed a reduction in the oocyte content of rat ovaries after prenatal exposure to a 50% galactose diet.[4] No analogous alterations in the testes were observed in prenatally treated males. Experiments in rats suggest that toxicity to the female gonads from galactose or its metabolites is most obvious during the premeiotic stages of ovarian development.

These observations in animals and human beings have led to speculation that galactose restriction during pregnancy may be desirable if the fetus is affected with galactosemia. In the human female, ovarian meiosis begins at 12 and is complete by 28 menstrual weeks. Thus ovarian damage, and perhaps neurologic or lens abnormalities, might occur prior to the usual time when prenatal diagnosis by amniocentesis can be accomplished. Thus anticipatory treatment in pregnancies at risk for having a galactosemic fetus might best be initiated very early in gestation or even preconceptually.

Despite these experiments and speculations, we are unaware of studies which adequately assess the impact of prenatal administration of a low galactose diet to galactosemic infants. For obvious reasons such data, especially controlled, will be difficult to obtain. Nevertheless, prenatal galactose restriction is probably desirable in galactosemia and should be harmless. There is little reason to suppose that galactose restriction would have adverse consequences, since galactosemic and normal fetuses are both capable of some endogenous galactose synthesis.

FUTURE DEVELOPMENTS

Only the most preliminary steps have been taken toward the therapy of genetic metabolic disorders in the fetus. Certain categories of diseases may be particular candidates for future attempts at treatment, especially if some newer approaches are developed.

Vitamins

Prenatal therapy has been reported for two vitamin-responsive genetic errors of metabolism. A significant number of other vitamin-responsive defects are known and have responded to postnatal treatment.[18] Antenatal treatment of some of these may be anticipated, especially for those with neonatal manifestations.

We also speculate that in addition to the usual vitamin-responsive errors, there may be genetic defects for which prenatal vitamin

E administration may be justifiable. Postnatally, vitamin E administration prevents abnormalities of leukocyte function and improves the shortened red cell survival in glutathione synthetase deficiency.[23] Because grossly lowered intracellular glutathione levels in this mutant state seem to predispose to oxidant-mediated cellular damage, it might be desirable to consider prenatal antioxidant therapy with vitamin E. Most patients with glutathione synthetase deficiency have neurologic impairment which can be progressive. Functioning as an antioxidant, vitamin E might inhibit the development of neurologic abnormalities. Such speculations can only be confirmed or denied by future clinical studies.

In abetalipoproteinemia, which is associated with very low serum vitamin E levels, progressive and fatal neurologic impairment gradually develops.[23] It is now known that high-dose vitamin E supplementation can retard or prevent neurologic damage.[23] Although patients with abetalipoproteinemia, like glutathione synthase–deficient patients, appear not to manifest gross neurologic abnormalities at birth, prenatal damage could be occurring. Antenatal treatment with vitamin E might be justifiable on an experimental basis.

Pharmacological and Nutritional Approaches

It might be appropriate to consider suppressing excessive cholesterol production prenatally in severe hypercholesterolemia if a safe and effective agent for accomplishing this were available (although there is no clear evidence for hypercholesterolemic prenatal damage). If cysteamine or related agents were to prove an effective treatment for lethal variants of cystinosis, prenatal therapy might be considered, because excessive and possibly harmful cystine accumulation is evident in cystinotic fetuses.

Cysteine levels have been detected in chorionic villi, and significant elevations even at 10 weeks gestation have been hypothesized.[8] Inhibitors of gammaglutamyl transpeptidase, if safe, would elevate intracellular glutathione levels and inhibit oxoproline production in glutathione synthase deficiency, thereby averting the characteristic neonatal acidosis.

In theory, it would be desirable to minimize copper accumulation in Wilson disease as early as possible. If and when reliable prenatal diagnosis of Wilson disease is possible, cautious administration of penicillamine prenatally might be considered. Such would be a double-edged sword, however, as the teratogenic and lathyritic potential of penicillin would demand careful evaluation. Recently, Batshaw and associates have treated certain urea-cycle defects by the administration of arginine and benzoate.[2] Since hyperammonemia in some of these entities develops very acutely after birth, it might be desirable to consider pretreating the fetus with these compounds just prior to or during labor to minimize postnatal hyperammonemia.

Conversely, it may be desirable to consider drug avoidance as an approach to fetal treatment. For example, fetuses with glucose-6-phosphate dehydrogenase deficiency are sensitive to a variety of drugs which can induce hemolysis. It would probably be appropriate to avoid administering such agents to women carrying or known to be at risk for carrying fetuses deficient in glucose-6-phosphate dehydrogenase.

Choronic villus sampling or umbilical cord catheterization under ultrasound guidance may lead to the development of other types of fetal treatment which at present may seem rather futuristic. Systems such as gene replacement are being developed for certain lysosomal storage disorders (see Section 3). Progress is being made in postnatal experimental models on administration of thymic cells for certain immune deficiency states, bone marrow transplantation for a variety of genetic disorders, and gene transfer. The development of better and earlier techniques for prenatal treatment will be complex, especially with regard to gene transfer; but progress will be made, and access to the fetal vasculature may be required for these methods to have a chance for success.

Bone marrow transplantation or thymic cell infusion is actually only a specialized example of organ transplantation. In the future, fetal organ transplantation may become possible and may open many prospects for surgical treatment of certain biochemical genetic disorders.

One can also speculate about therapeutic possibilities involving compounds administered directly into the amniotic fluid or into the fetal intestinal tract. It might be possible, for example, to administer thyroid hormone in this fashion or to prevent meconium ileus in cystic fibrosis by instilling yet to be hypothesized enzymes into the fetal intestinal tract.

REFERENCES

1. Ampola MG, Mahoney MJ, Nakamura E et al: Prenatal therapy of a patient with vitamin B responsive methylmalonic acidemia. N Engl J Med 293:313, 1975
2. Batshaw M, Brusilow S, Waber L et al: Treatment of inborn errors of urea synthesis: Activation of alternative pathways of waste nitrogen synthesis and excretion. N Engl J Med 306:1387, 1982
3. Bowman JM: The management of Rh-isoimmunization. Obstet Gynecol 52:1, 1978
4. Chen YT, Mattison DR, Feigenbaum L et al: Reduction in oocyte number following prenatal exposure to a high galactose diet. Science 214:1145, 1981
5. DeVore G, Donnerstein RL, Kleinman CS et al: Real time-directed M-mode echocardiography: A new technique for accurate and rapid quantitation of the fetal preejection period and ventricular ejection time of the right and left ventricles. Am J Obstet Gynecol 141:470, 1981
6. Erway LC, Fraser AS, Hurley LS: Prevention of congenital otolith defects in pallid mutant mice by manganese supplementation. Genetics 67:97, 1971
7. Evans MI, Chrousos GP, Mann DL et al: Pharmacologic suppression of the fetal adrenal gland: Attempted prevention of 21 hydroxylase sufficiency congenital adrenal hyperplasia in utero. JAMA 253:1015, 1985
8. Evans MI, Gahl WA, Karson EM et al: Normal chorionic villus cystine levels are similar to fibroblast values: Possible basis for first trimester diagnosis of cystinosis. Am J Hum Genetics, Toronto, Canada, 1984
9. Evans MI, Schulman JD: Biochemical fetal therapy. Clin Obstet Gynecol 29:523, 1986
10. Forrest M, David M: Prenatal treatment of congenital adrenal hyperplasia due to 21 hydroxylase deficiency. 7th International Congress of Endocrinology, Abstr #911, Quebec, Canada, 1984
11. Harrison MR, Filly R, Golbus MS: The Unborn Patient. New York, Grune & Stratton, 1984
12. Hurley LS, Bell LT: Genetic influence on response to dietary manganese deficiency in mice. J Nutr 104:133, 1974
13. Keen CL, Saltman P, Hurley LS: Copper nitrilotriacetate: A potent therapeutic agent in the treatment of a genetic sort of copper metabolism. Am J Nutr 33:1789, 1980
14. Levy ML, Lenke RR, Crocker AC: Maternal PKU. DHHS Publication No. (HSA) 81–5299. Washington, DC, US Government Printing Office, 1981
15. Lyon MG: Stage of action of litter size effect on absence of otoliths in mice. J Z Ind Abst Verebl 86:289, 1954
16. Morrow G III, Schwartz RH, Halloc JA et al: Prenatal detection of methylmalonic aciduria. J Peds 77:120, 1970
17. Nyhan WL: Prenatal treatment of methylmalonic aciduria. N Engl J Med 293:353, 1975
18. Packman S: Approach to inherited metabolic disorders presenting in the newborn period. In Rudolph AM, Hoffman JCE (eds): Pediatric, 17th ed, pp 256–258. Norwalk, CT, Appleton-Century-Crofts, 1982
19. Packman S, Cowan MJ, Golbus MS et al: Prenatal treatment of biotin responsive multiple carboxylase deficiency. Lancet 1:1435, 1982
20. Phillips JA III, Burr IM, Orlando P et al: DNA analysis of human steroid 21-hydroxylase genes on congenital hyperplasia. Am J Hum Genet 37:A171, 1985
21. Rosenblatt DS, Cooper BA, Schmutz SM et al: Prenatal vitamin B12 therapy of a fetus with methylcobalamin deficiency. Lancet 1:1127, 1985
22. Roth KS, Yang W, Allen L et al: Prenatal administration of biotin: Biotin responsive multiple carboxylase deficiency. Ped Res 16:126, 1982
23. Schulman JD, Mudd SH, Schneider JA et al: Inborn errors of glutathione and sulfur amino acid metabolism. Ann Int Med 93:330, 1980

24. Schulman JD, Simpson JL (eds): Genetic Diseases in Pregnancy. New York, Academic Press, 1981
25. Segal SS: Disorders of galactose metabolism. In Stanbury JB, Wyngarden JB, Frederickson DS (eds): The Metabolic Basis of Inherited Disease, 5th ed, p 167. New York, McGraw-Hill, 1983
26. Spielberg SP: Pharmacogenetics in the fetus. N Engl J Med 307:115, 1982
27. Steinmann B, Gitzelmann R, Zachmann M: Galactosemia: Hypergonadatropic hypogonadism found already in prepubertal girls but only in adult males. European J Peds 135:337, 1981
28. Vannas A, Hogan MJ, Golbus MS et al: Lens changes in galactosemic fetus. Am J Opthalmol 80:726, 1975
29. Wladimiroff JW, McGhie JS: M-mode ultrasonic assessment of fetal cardiovascular dynamics Br J Obstet Gynecol 88:1241, 1981

SECTION 3: DIAGNOSIS AND MANAGEMENT OF FETAL HEART DISEASE

Joshua A. Copel and Charles S. Kleinman

The field of fetal diagnosis has undergone revolutionary changes over the last 15 years, based in large part on advances in ultrasound imaging techniques. Detailed evaluation of both normal and abnormal anatomy is now possible with high resolution real-time imaging. A wide variety of diagnoses have been reliably established in virtually every system of the body. In addition, fetal behavior has been assessed, and the "biophysical profile" is now an integral part of the assessment of fetal well-being.

The first generation of fetal ultrasound consisted of A-mode imaging, which provided limited information about the fetus and could not be used to diagnose fetal structural anomalies. Static scanning, the next step, provided still pictures. Although high-quality images of the fetus could be obtained, information concerning moving structures was still beyond the limits of the technology. Cardiologists used ultrasound for dynamic cardiac imaging with M-mode echocardiography, but variations in position and the absence of concurrent information concerning fetal movement limited the application of M-mode echocardiography to the fetus. Nevertheless, the first description of fetal echocardiography was based entirely on M-mode ultrasound.[43]

More recently, the availability of high quality two-dimensional real-time ultrasound has permitted detailed examination of the fetal heart. Both normal and abnormal anatomic findings have been described by a number of centers with fetal echocardiography laboratories.[2-4,18,24,26,39,45] The equipment used has included two-dimensional real-time sector scanners with simultaneous or duplex M-mode capability and, recently, pulsed Doppler ultrasound which has been applied to the evaluation of the human fetal heart.

PRINCIPLES OF FETAL ECHOCARDIOGRAPHY

Fetal cardiac structural diagnosis is based on interpretation of the same tomographic sections that are relied upon in pediatric and adult echocardiography (Table 15-2). The sec-

Table 15-2. Standard Views Used in Fetal Echocardiography

Four Chamber
Long Axis Left Ventricle
Short Axis Ventricles
Short Axis Great Vessels
Aortic Arch
Pulmonary Artery/Ductus Arteriosus

tional anatomy of the normal fetal heart has been clarified by a number of studies.[4,18,26] It is important to bear in mind several important factors about the fetal heart prior to undertaking fetal cardiac studies.

Fetal Physiology

The cardiovascular system of the fetus differs from that found postnatally in several significant ways. Although most of our understanding of the fetal circulation is based on the fetal lamb model,[35] similar patterns probably occur in the human. The human brain is larger than that of the lamb relative to carcass mass, which may increase the relative contribution of the left ventricle to the combined ventricular output. Preliminary human studies using Doppler ultrasound appear to confirm the principles initially derived from ovine models.

The ventricles of the fetal heart work in parallel, as opposed to working in series postnatally. Blood returning to the fetus from the placenta crosses the ductus venosus, is briefly carried through the inferior vena cava, and is preferentially shunted across the foramen ovale into the left atrium. Thus, the more oxygenated blood is distributed to the ascending aorta and perfuses the coronary and cerebral beds. The majority of right ventricular output enters the ductus arteriosus and is thereby carried to the descending aorta. This less oxygenated blood is then transported to the placenta, and re-oxygenated. The right ventricle, therefore, is the ventricle responsible for perfusing the organ of respiration prenatally as well as postnatally.

Thus, there are two communications between the right and left sides of the normal fetal heart. These shunts, the foramen ovale and the ductus arteriosus, are not normally visualized postnatally. Failure to demonstrate their presence may indicate pathology in the fetus.

Another consequence of the parallel circulation of the fetus is that pressures in the two ventricles are very similar. Additionally, the fetal ventricles normally appear equal to each other in size.

Finally, it is essential to remember that the fetus is constantly moving, and that orientation must be established at the outset of the study by locating the fetal head, spine, and stomach to ensure normal situs and to permit the sonologist to identify chambers and great vessels.

Technique

Fetal echocardiography requires demonstration of the same standard tomographic planes as used in pediatric and adult echocardiography (see Table 15-2). We rely primarily on two-dimensional imaging, reserving M-mode for analysis of dysrhythmias and measurement of septal thickness in diabetic pregnancies. Other authors have suggested that M-mode-based measurement of cardiac chambers and structures should take a greater role in the diagnosis of fetal structural cardiac anomalies.[12]

While the examination can be conducted with either sector- or linear-array scanning equipment, we find that sector scanners provide greater flexibility in approaching the fetal heart from the necessary angles. We currently use an electronic phased-array scanner with a 5 MHz transducer for virtually all examinations (Hewlett-Packard 77020A Ultrasound Imaging System, Hewlett-Packard, Andover, MA). In selected patients we use a variety of other techniques, including linear-array (GE RT 3600, General Electric, Milwaukee, WI) or mechanical sector scanners (ATL UltraMark 4, Advanced Technology Laboratories, Bellevue, WA).

The simplest and easiest view to obtain is the four-chamber view, which includes both atria and ventricles, along with the atrioventricular valves. It can usually be found by starting from the image of the abdomen used for calculation of the abdominal circumference and angling the transducer cephalad on

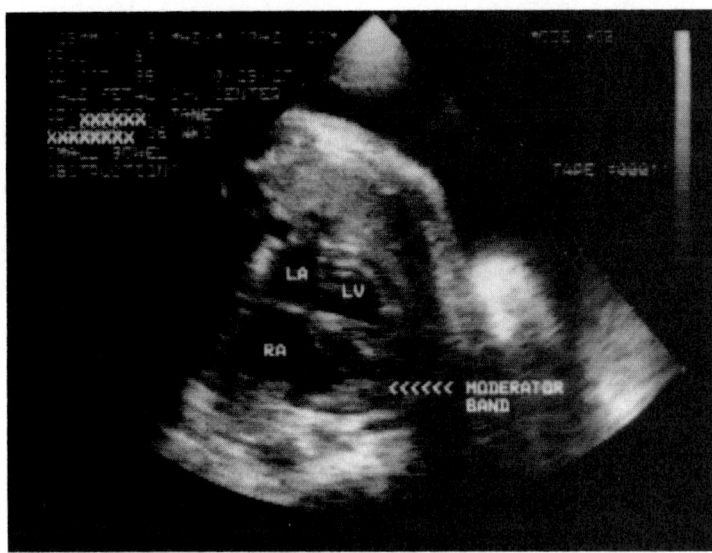

FIGURE 15-3. Normal four-chambered view of the heart at 36 weeks' gestation. The ventricles are approximately equal to each other in size, as are the atria. The moderator band is visible near the apex of the right ventricle.

the fetus. This view is especially useful for assessment of the relative sizes of the cardiac chambers, the anatomy of the atrioventricular valves, and the presence or absence of pericardial fluid (Figure 15-3).

The four-chamber view must be seen in relationship to the fetal stomach, spine, liver, and vena cavae in order to ascertain situs. We find that by maintaining our maternal anatomic orientation (i.e., looking from right to left, or feet toward head on the mother), regardless of the orientation of the heart on the screen, it is easier to adjust the transducer position on the mother's abdomen when necessary.

Further experience will permit the sonologist to adjust the transducer to optimize other necessary views. We include a long axis view of the left ventricle, short axis views of the ventricles and great vessels, and an aortic arch view in each examination. The maneuvers needed to produce each of these will vary with fetal position.

As in postnatal echocardiography, each tomographic section provides information about a specific portion of cardiac anatomy. The four-chamber view can demonstrate lesions of the atrioventricular valves and poste-

rior atrioventricular septum, and allows assessment of ventricular cavity enlargement or hypoplasia (Figure 15-4). As will be discussed, we have found the four-chamber view helpful as an initial screen for fetal heart disease. The long axis view of the left ventricle is most important in the fetus for evaluation of septal-aortic continuity, and failure to establish this relationship suggests override of the aorta. Should such a finding be suspected, serial evaluation of cardiac anatomy is essential, since the lesion may evolve in utero. We have seen several fetuses develop subpulmonic stenosis after aortic override was first appreciated, which progressed to tetralogy of Fallot.

The evaluation of the great vessels, through the short axis, pulmonary artery/ductus arteriosus, and aortic arch views, is important to ensure that the ventriculoarterial connections are correctly aligned. Differentiation of the aorta and pulmonary artery can be difficult in utero, because the ductus arteriosus is quite large and in continuity with the descending aorta. The complete scan must include demonstration of a bifurcating vessel leaving the anterior ventricle and entering the descending aorta (pulmo-

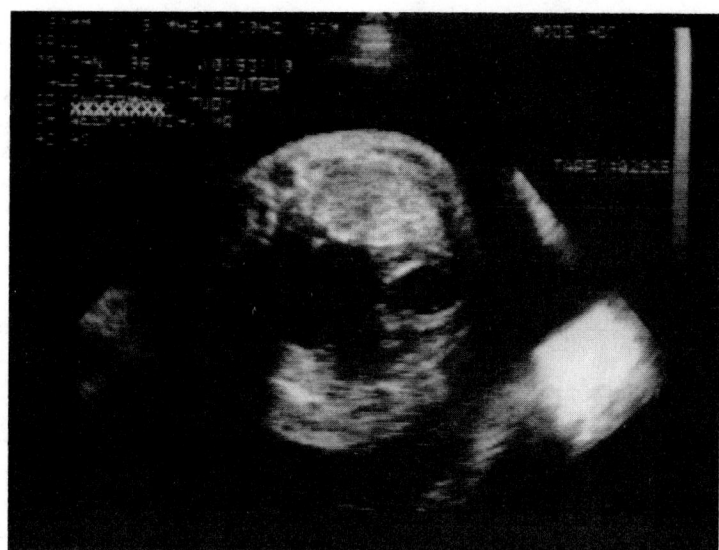

FIGURE 15-4. Four-chambered view of the heart from a fetus at 34 weeks' gestation with severe aortic stenosis. The left atrium is greatly enlarged. The left ventricle is dilated and its wall is echogenic. On real time examination, left ventricular contractility was diminished. Note increased amniotic fluid.

nary artery), as well as the brachiocephalic, left carotid, and left subclavian arteries branching from the aortic arch.

In each view the physician must keep in mind that right and left ventricular outputs are not equal in utero (the right ventricular output appears to be slightly greater than the left,[32,36] and that the right ventricular dimension should be greater in size in utero than postnatally. A similar relationship holds for pulmonary versus aortic root size. Any *major* asymmetry suggests the presence of pathology.

Dectection of Dysrhythmias

Throughout the anatomic examination, the sonologist should pay attention to the cardiac rate and rhythm. The normal fetal heart rate is between 120 and 170 and regular. Sinus bradycardia may cause the fetal heart rate to be 100 to 120, but if the rate is below 90 or if any discrepancy is found between the atrial and ventricular rates, careful evaluation of the rhythm is warranted. Often in such cases co-existent anatomic abnormalities are present.[11] If either second- or third-degree heart block is suspected based on M-mode or pulsed Doppler study, cardiac structures should be examined. Also, an assay for maternal connective tissue autoantibodies, such as anti-Ro, is useful, since these markers for systemic lupus are often present.[6,13,29,38,41]

The most common dysrhythmia seen in our laboratory has been premature atrial extrasystoles.[8] These may be identified with either M-mode or pulsed Doppler visualization of the premature atrial beat, which may or may not be conducted. While these are for the most part benign, they may precipitate supraventricular tachycardia in susceptible fetuses. When these are diagnosed we recommend weekly auscultation of the fetal heart to rule out runs of tachycardia, until they resolve. Isolated extrasystoles almost always resolve spontaneously before or just after birth, so no treatment is recommended. Possible cardiac stimulants, such as caffeine, sympathomimetics (including over-the-counter nasal decongestants as well as beta-adrenergic tocolytics), and illicit drugs such as cocaine should all be avoided, since these may worsen the dysrhythmia.

When supraventricular tachycardia is detected the appropriate management depends on the etiology and the gestational age. If fetal maturity is present, based on well established dates or amniocentesis, delivery may be prudent. For the preterm fetus, determination of the type of tachycardia is important in choosing the therapy. Fetal paroxysmal atrial tachycardia has responded well to digitalis as a first line of therapy in our experience. Fetal atrial flutter and fibrillation have been more difficult to control.[22] Treatment should be undertaken in a hospital, at a center with experience in the management of these patients.

Pulsed Doppler ultrasound has recently been successfully applied to the evaluation of fetal cardiac dysrhythmias. The sample volume can be placed below the atrioventricular valves to examine diastolic flow into the ventricles. In contrast to the postnatal pattern of predominant passive flow, in the fetus most flow into the ventricles occurs with atrial systole. This greater volume and greater velocity results in the a wave being higher than the e wave of atrial flow. In premature atrial extrasystoles, the early a wave can be identified.[25] Similar studies can be carried out in the fetus suspected of supraventricular tachycardia.[19]

INDICATIONS FOR FETAL ECHOCARDIOGRAPHY

Fetal echocardiography is a much more complex procedure than routine obstetric sonography. Although most congenital heart disease (CHD) occurs in children without identifiable risk factors, certain situations can be targeted as placing fetuses at particular risk of CHD. The current indications for fetal echocardiography are shown in Table 15-3. We group these risk factors according to their etiology: fetal, maternal, or familial.

The risk of CHD is increased significantly if a couple has had a previous child with CHD, or if the mother herself has CHD. In the general population, the risk for CHD is approximately 0.8%. If there has been a previous child with CHD it rises to about 2% to 3%, and if the mother herself has CHD, to about 5% to 10%.[31] If the etiology in these cases is assumed to be polygenic inheritance, the risk may be elevated slightly over that of the general population when the CHD occurs

Table 15-3. Proposed Indications for Fetal Echocardiography

Fetal Risk Factors
  Extracardiac anomalies
    Chromosomal
    Anatomic
  Fetal Cardiac Dysrhythmia
    Irregular rhythm
    Tachycardia (>200 bpm)
    Bradycardia (Nonperiodic)
  Nonimmune Hydrops Fetalis
  Suspected cardiac anomaly on Level I Scan
Maternal Risk Factors
  Congenital heart disease
  Cardiac teratogen exposure
  Maternal metabolic disorders
    Diabetes mellitus
    Phenylketonuria
  Polyhydramnios
  Maternal infections
    Rubella
    Toxoplasmosis
    Coxsackie virus
    Cytomegalovirus
    Mumps
Familial Risk Factors
  Congenital heart disease
    Previous sibling
    Paternal
  Syndrome
    Noonan
    Tuberous sclerosis

in more distantly related individuals (e.g., offspring of the patient's siblings), although the precise degree of incremental risk is not currently known.

Maternal exposure to potential teratogens constitutes an area of great concern to pregnant women.[47] Lithium carbonate has been associated with Ebstein's anomaly of the tricuspid valve. Synthetic progestins have also been implicated in some studies as potential teratogens, although this association is now known to be false.[42] We recommend fetal echocardiography for any patient who has taken any of the drugs in Table 15-4, although, to alleviate patient anxiety, women

Table 15-4. Drugs Suspected of Cardiac Teratogenicity

Lithium carbonate
Alcohol
Phenytoin
Valproic acid
Trimethadione
Isotretinoin
Amphetamines
Thalidomide

---

who have taken other medications are often scanned as well.

Insulin-dependent diabetic women (White, class B and above) have a fourfold higher incidence of CHD in their offspring than the general population.[34] There are two distinct fetal cardiac effects of maternal hyperglycemia: first-trimester exposure predisposing to structural CHD, and later exposure causing hypertrophic cardiomyopathy. All women with class B or greater diabetes are therefore offered fetal echocardiography at the same time as a general anatomic survey for other anomalies, at approximately 20 to 22 weeks' gestation. We perform an additional scan between 30 and 32 weeks' gestation to confirm the normal anatomy and to detect hypertrophic cardiomyopathy.

Women with phenylketonuria who were successfully treated with dietary restrictions in childhood are now entering their own childbearing years. These women have often relaxed their diets, and have relatively high phenylalanine levels, which can result in cardiac and other anomalies.[27,28] As in diabetes, these patients should receive preconceptual counseling regarding the need for stricter dietary control in the first trimester, and careful scanning in the second trimester to attempt diagnosis of any anomalies which may be present.[10]

Most of these "historical" risk factors result in slightly higher risks of CHD than are found in the general population. On the other hand, we find that fetuses with either an extracardiac anomaly detected on ultrasound, or with a suspected cardiac anomaly at the time of a general scan, have a much greater risk of CHD. Any fetus found to have an anomaly strongly associated with CHD should have a careful examination of the heart (unless the anomaly is itself invariably fatal), because the presence of CHD may influence the neonatal management and timing of any needed surgical procedures. These anomalies have been recently reviewed[10] (Table 15-5). We offer fetal echocardiography to all patients with an extracardiac anomaly, even if the particular anomaly is from a low-risk group. We scan these patients because the known risks are derived from pediatric data, and fatal associations may be removed from such series due to intrauterine or early neonatal deaths.

Nonimmune hydrops represents congestive heart failure in the fetus.[23] It has further been found that the combination of structural heart disease, atrioventricular valve insufficiency, and nonimmune hydrops carries with it an extremely poor prognosis.[40] The true fre-

Table 15-5. Extracardiac Anomalies Frequently Associated with Congenital Heart Disease

Abnormalities of cardiac position
Hydrocephalus*
Microcephaly*
Agenesis of corpus callosum
Encephalocele (Meckel-Gruber syndrome)
Ectopia Cordis
Esophageal atresia/Tracheo-esophageal fistula
Duodenal atresia
Situs abnormality (Asplenia/Polysplenia)
Omphalocele
Diaphragmatic hernia
Bilateral renal agenesis†
Conjoined twins

* Heterogeneous etiology, some causes associated with congenital heart disease, others not

† Uniformly fatal regardless of presence or absence of congenital heart disease

From Copel JA, Pilu G, Kleinman CS: Congenital heart disease and extracardiac anomalies: Associations and indications for fetal echocardiography. Am J Obstet Gynecol 154:1121–1132, 1985

quency with which structural heart disease and dysrhythmias cause nonimmune hydrops will vary somewhat with the population surveyed. We have found that about one-third of fetuses with nonimmune hydrops have a cardiac etiology, although other centers have reported varying figures.[1,5,15,17,20,33] In many cases this will be difficult to assess, since intermittent supraventricular tachycardia may cause hydrops and fetal death, leaving no signs at autopsy.

We have found CHD in a high percentage of fetuses referred because the heart "looked funny" during a routine scan.[8] In review of 74 fetuses with heart disease, we further found that 92% had abnormalities of the four-chamber view, suggesting that it may be useful as a screen for CHD.[9] Preliminary results of a study testing the value of the four-chamber view as a screen for congenital heart disease have been encouraging.[14] Although a screening ultrasound to detect fetal anomalies is not yet an accepted routine for all prenatal patients in the United States, a high enough percentage of patients are scanned at least once in the course of pregnancy that careful attention to the heart's appearance might be expected to increase the number of lesions identified prenatally.

Review of pediatric studies suggests that chromosomal abnormalities are found in 5% to 10% of cases of CHD. We have found that a much higher number of cases of fetal heart disease have chromosomal abnormalities. In a series of 34 fetal diagnoses of heart disease, 11 (32%) had chromosomal abnormalities.[7] This incidence is similar to the findings of Wladimiroff and co-workers in a smaller series.[44]

There is a clear need to perform fetal echocardiography in the fetus with an extracardiac anomaly, or in the abnormal-appearing heart. We also feel it is important to reverse the same equation. Any fetus at risk of CHD may also be considered to be at risk for extracardiac structural anomalies. We, therefore, perform full anatomic screens and growth measurements on all fetuses referred for echocardiography.

PRESENT AND FUTURE DIRECTIONS

Widening Options in Neonatal Care

Despite the potential future value of screening for fetal heart disease with the four-chamber view, there will still be a need for detailed fetal echocardiography in selected patients. Those with specific risk factors for fetal heart disease will probably continue to require such studies, which should be performed in centers with extensive experience because of the time and expertise required. Since the greatest number of abnormalities will occur in the absence of clear risk factors, many abnormalities will continue to be identified during obstetric scanning for other purposes. The total impact of these diagnoses is complex to measure.

Some anomalies will be incompatible with postnatal survival; for example, the combintion of severe CHD and nonimmune hydrops fetalis. If this is found early in gestation, the parents may choose to terminate the pregnancy. If it is not identified until beyond the period in which termination is an option, or if the parents are opposed to such a course, there are still important benefits to be gained from the information obtained.

Many fetal cardiac diagnoses are made later in pregnancy, usually because of suspicious-appearing hearts during obstetric sonograms. In such cases, accurate prenatal diagnosis permits honest counseling for the parents and adequate medical planning for delivery and neonatal care (e.g., ensuring that prostaglandin E_1 is mixed and ready in the nursery for the delivery of a fetus with a ductus-dependent lesion). Delivery of such fetuses in an institution equipped to provide comprehensive neonatal and cardiac care can be expected to improve outcome for many infants. While our survival statistics for the first 150 fetuses with CHD diagnosed at Yale University Fetal Cardiovascular Center were not, by themselves, impressive (28 out of 150 survivors, 19%), it is striking to note that 21 of the survivors had ductus-dependent lesions (75%). For this group, delivery at an institution with comprehensive neonatal cardiac care capabilities would be expected to improve outcome.

Recently, the options for neonates with lesions previously considered inoperable have been widened. Both neonatal cardiac transplantation and the Norwood procedure have been offered for neonates with hypoplastic left heart syndrome. The complexities of supporting such critically ill newborns make transport to a center offering surgery difficult, so delivery would be best accomplished at an institution capable of providing comprehensive maternal and neonatal care. We also feel it important to allow the parents to consider their options. Informed consent for surgery is difficult in the best of circumstances, but with an unstable neonate at issue, it may be an impossibility. We feel that education of the parents at one or more prenatal visits is essential for their active participation in deciding on expectant management versus cardiac transplantation or the Norwood procedure for their infants.

We offer all patients with fetal heart disease information about the risks of chromosomal abnormalities, and the option of karyotyping. If there is sufficient time prior to term, amniocentesis may be appropriate. In other situations fetal blood sampling, or placentocentesis (transabdominal chorionic villus biopsy) offers the possibility of karyotype results in just a few days. Waiting for delivery to assess facial morphology and other external factors, or for blood cells to karyotype may be fruitless, as many such infants will be stillborn and important information regarding the likelihood of recurrence may be lost.

Future Avenues of Research

Fetal echocardiography can diagnose structural heart disease with a high degree of accuracy. It can similarly evaluate cardiac function, at least in terms of cardiac rhythm. Evaluation of cardiac pump performance remains an important area of investigation. Preliminary studies have attempted to define such parameters as fractional shortening and ratios of ventricular dimensions.[12] Others have considered ventricular function through estimations of cardiac output based on planimetry measurements,[37,46] although such studies are confounded by two factors. The first is the parallel, rather than series, arrangement of ventricular function in utero. The second factor is the difficulty in defining the geometric shape of the fetal ventricles needed for estimations of volume, based on two-dimensional images.

Another technique of great potential value is the use of pulsed Doppler ultrasound, which allows the sampling of a flow-velocity waveform from selected portions of the cardiovascular system. Mathematic manipulation of the waveform shape, including correction for factors such as the incident angle to the direction of blood flow, permits estimation of velocity and volume of blood flow. In order to reduce the random errors that are introduced by each further step in these calculations, various methods of relating velocities during various phases of the cardiac cycle have been proposed for study of flow in the umbilical cord and fetal descending aorta.[16] Similar angle-independent indices of flow during various parts of the cardiac cycle may prove useful in evaluating intracardiac blood flow.

Doppler has already proven useful in the investigation of fetal dysrhythmias and in determining the presence of valvular regurgitation.[30,40] It may be possible to use pulsed Doppler ultrasound to measure the cardiac output in the fetus,[21,32] although the technical difficulty of doing so and the large errors which may be randomly introduced continue to limit the applicability of using it in the research setting. It remains one of the most exciting areas of fetal research.

REFERENCES

1. Allan LD, Chapman DC, Sheridan R, Chapman MG: Aetiology of non-immune hydrops: The value of echocardiography. Br J Obstet Gynecol 93:223–225, 1986

2. Allan LD, Crawford DC, Anderson RH, Tynan MJ: Echocardiographic and anatomical correlations in congenital heart disease. Br Heart J 52:542–548, 1984
3. Allan LD, Tynan MJ, Campbell S, Anderson RH: Identification of congenital cardiac malformations by echocardiography in the midtrimester fetus. Br Heart J 46:358–362, 1981
4. Allan LD, Tynan MJ, Campbell S et al: Echocardiographic and anatomical correlates in the fetus. Br Heart J 44:444–451, 1980
5. Beischer NA, Fortune DW, Macafee J: Nonimmunologic hydrops fetalis and congenital abnormalities. Obstet Gynecol 38:86–95, 1971
6. Chameides L, Truex RC, Vetter V et al: Association of maternal systemic lupus erythematosus with congenital complete heart block. N Engl J Med 297:1204–1207, 1977
7. Copel JA, Cullen M, Green J et al: Congenital heart disease diagnosed by fetal echocardiography and chromosomal abnormalities. Am J Obstet Gynecol (in press)
8. Copel JA, Kleinman CS: The impact of fetal echocardiography on perinatal outcome. Ultrasound Med Biol 12:327–335, 1986
9. Copel JA, Pilu G, Green J et al: Fetal echocardiographic screening for congenital heart disease: The importance of the four chamber view. Am J Obstet Gynecol 157:648–655, 1987
10. Copel JA, Pilu G, Kleinman CS: Congenital heart disease and extracardiac anomalies: Associations and indications for fetal echocardiography. Am J Obstet Gynecol 154:1121–1132, 1985
11. Crawford D, Chapman M, Allan L: The assessment of persistent bradycardia in prenatal life. Br J Obstet Gynecol 92:941–944, 1985
12. DeVore GR: The prenatal diagnosis of congenital heart disease: A practical approach for the fetal sonographer. J Clin Ultrasound 13:229–245, 1985
13. Esscher E, Scott JS: Congenital heart block and maternal systemic lupus erythematosus. Br Med J 1:1235–1238, 1979
14. Fermont L, deGeeter B, Aubry MC et al: A close collaboration between obstetricians and pediatric cardiologists allows antenatal detection of severe cardiac malformations by two-dimensional echocardiography. In Doyle EF, Engle MA, Gersony WM et al (eds): Pediatric Cardiology: Proceedings of the Second World Congress, p 34. New York, Springer-Verlag, 1986
15. Gough JD, Keeling JW, Castle B, Iliff PJ: The obstetric management of non-immunological hydrops. Br J Obstet Gynecol 93:226–234, 1986
16. Griffin D, Cohen-Overbeek T, Campbell S: Fetal and utero-placental blood flow. Clinic Obstet Gynecol 10:565–602, 1983
17. Holzgreve W, Curry CJR, Golbus MS et al: Investigation of nonimmune hydrops fetalis. Am J Obstet Gynecol 150:805–812, 1984
18. Huhta JC, Hagler DJ, Hill LM: Two-dimensional echocardiographic assessment of normal fetal cardiac anatomy. J Reprod Med 29:162–167, 1984
19. Huhta JC, Strasburger JF, Carpenter RJ et al: Pulsed Doppler fetal echocardiography. J Clin Ultrasound 13:247–254, 1985
20. Hutchinson AA, Drew JH, Yu VYH et al: Nonimmunologic hydrops fetalis: A review of 61 cases. Obstet Gynecol 59:347–352, 1982
21. Kenny JF, Plappert T, Doubilet P et al: Changes in intracardiac blood flow velocities and right and left ventricular stroke volumes with gestational age in the normal human fetus: A prospective Doppler echocardiographic study. Circulation 74:1208–1216, 1986
22. Kleinman CS, Copel JA, Weinstein EM et al: In utero diagnosis and treatment of fetal supraventricular tachycardia. Semin Perinatol 9:113–129, 1985
23. Kleinman CS, Donnerstein RL, DeVore GR et al: Fetal echocardiography for evaluation of in utero congestive heart failure: A technique for the study of non-immune hydrops fetalis. N Engl J Med 306:568–575, 1982
24. Kleinman CS, Hobbins JC, Jaffe CC et al: Echocardiographic studies of the human fetus: Prenatal diagnosis of congenital heart disease and cardiac dysrhythmias. Pediatrics 65:1059–1067, 1980
25. Kleinman CS, Weinstein EM, Copel JA: Pulsed Doppler analysis of human fetal blood flow. Clin Diag Ultrasound 17:173–185, 1986
26. Lange LW, Sahn DJ, Allen HD et al: Qualitative real-time cross-sectional echocardiographic imaging of the human fetus in the second half of pregnancy. Circulation 62:799–806, 1980
27. Lenke RL, Levy HL: Maternal phenylketonuria and hyperphenylalaninemia. N Engl J Med 303:1202–1208, 1980
28. Levy HL, Waisbren SE: Effects of untreated maternal phenylketonuria and hyperphenylalaninemia on the fetus. N Engl J Med 309:1269–1274, 1983
29. Litsey SE, Noonan JA, O'Connor WN et al:

Maternal connective tissue disease and congenital heart block. N Engl J Med 312:98–100, 1985
30. Maulik D, Nanda NC, Moodley S et al: Application of Doppler echocardiography in the assessment of fetal cardiac disease. Am J Obstet Gynecol 151:951–957, 1985
31. Nora JJ, Nora AH: The genetic contribution to congenital heart diseases. In Nora JJ, Takao A (eds): Congenital Heart Diseases: Causes and Processes, Mount Kisco, Futura, 1984, pp 3–13
32. Reed KL, Meijboom EJ, Sahn DJ et al: Cardiac Doppler flow velocities in the human fetus. Circulation 73:41–46, 1986
33. Romero R, Copel JA, Jeanty PJ, Hobbins JC: Causes, diagnosis and management of nonimmune hydrops fetalis. Clin Perinatol 19:31–52, 1986
34. Rowland TW, Hubbell JP, Nadas AS: Congenital heart disease in infants of diabetic mothers. J Pediatr 83:815–820, 1973
35. Rudolph AM: Congenital Diseases of the Heart. Chicago, Year Book Medical Publishers, 1974
36. Rudolph AM, Heymann MA: Circulatory changes during growth in the fetal lamb. Circulation Res 26:289–299, 1970
37. Sahn DJ, Lange LW, Allen HD et al: Quantitative real-time cross-sectional echocardiography in the developing normal human fetus and newborn. Circulation 62:588–597, 1980
38. Scott JS, Maddison PJ, Taylor PV et al: Connective-tissue disease, antibodies to ribonucleoprotein, and congenital heart block. N Engl J Med 309:209–212, 1983
39. Silverman NH, Golbus MS: Echocardiographic techniques for assessment of normal and abnormal fetal cardiac anatomy. J Am Coll Cardiol 5:20S–29S, 1985
40. Silverman NH, Kleinman CS, Rudolph AM et al: Fetal atrioventricular valve insufficiency associated with nonimmune hydrops: A two-dimensional echocardiographic and pulsed Doppler study. Circulation 72:825–832, 1985
41. Taylor PV, Scott JS, Gerlis LM et al: Maternal antibodies against fetal cardiac antigens in congenital complete heart block. N Engl J Med 315:667–672, 1986
42. Wilson JG, Brent RL: Are female sex hormones teratogenic? Am J Obstet Gynecol 141:567–580, 1981
43. Winsberg F: Echocardiography of the fetal and newborn heart. Investig Radiol 7:152–158, 1972
44. Wladimiroff JW, Stewart PA, Sachs ES, Niermeijer MF: Prenatal diagnosis and management of congenital heart defect: Significance of associated fetal anomalies and prenatal chromosome studies. Am J Med Genetics 21:285–290, 1985
45. Wladimiroff JW, Stewart PA, Tonge HM: The role of diagnostic ultrasound in the study of fetal cardiac abnormalities. Ultrasound Med Biol 10:457–463, 1984
46. Wladimiroff JW, Vosters R, McGhie JS: Normal cardiac ventricular geometry and function during the last trimester of pregnancy and early neonatal period. Br J Obstet Gynecol 89:839–844, 1982
47. Zierler S: Maternal drugs and congenital heart disease. Obstet Gynecol 65:155–165, 1985

SECTION 4: GENE THERAPY

W. French Anderson

Rapid progress has been made in recent years toward developing the technology for human gene therapy in the pediatric patient.[1] In April 1987, our group submitted a Human Gene Therapy Preclinical Data Document to the Recombinant DNA Advisory Committee (RAC) at the National Institutes of Health (NIH) as a first step toward obtaining approval to treat adenosine deaminase (ADA) deficiency with our bone marrow transplantation/retroviral gene transfer protocol.

The ethical justification for somatic cell gene therapy in patients suffering from severe genetic diseases has been discussed by a number of authors.[2,9,16] There are, however, a number of serious genetic diseases that already produce irreversible damage by the time of birth.

This section outlines our present studies

aimed at testing the possibility for in utero gene therapy and considers the ethical implications involved.

SOMATIC CELL GENE THERAPY IN THE PEDIATRIC PATIENT

Somatic cell gene therapy is designed to correct a genetic disorder in the somatic cells of a patient by inserting a normal copy of the mutated gene. There are many examples of genes which, when defective, produce serious or lethal disease in a patient. Gene therapy should be beneficial primarily for the replacement of a defective or missing enzyme or protein that must function inside the cell that makes it, or of a defective or missing enzyme whose absence leads to a build-up of a toxic level of a normal metabolite (e.g., as in phenylketonuria [PKU]) or of a deficient circulating protein whose level does not need to be exactly regulated (e.g., blood clotting factor VIII which is deficient in hemophilia).

Disease Candidates for Clinical Trials

The initial candidates for gene therapy would need to satisfy these requirements:

- Because this is a new unproven therapy with, therefore, uncertain risks, the initial diseases would need to be severe genetic disorders leading to severe crippling or early death. Thus the benefit-risk ratio would potentially be much higher than for mild disorders.
- The disease should be correctable by treatment of the bone marrow cells, because only the bone marrow can be removed from a patient, treated ex vivo, and then returned to the patient.
- The defect should be an enzyme with simple regulation, not a protein like hemoglobin in which relatively complex regulation is involved.
- The normal gene would need to have been cloned.

The most likely gene to be used in the first experiments attempting human gene therapy is ADA, the absence of which results in severe combined immunodeficiency disease, in which children have a greatly weakened resistance to infection and cannot survive the usual childhood diseases. In ADA deficiency, the clinical syndrome is profoundly debilitating. No, or minimal, detectable enzyme is found in the bone marrow cells of patients who have no copies of the normal gene. In these patients, the production of a small percentage of the normal enzyme level should be beneficial, and a mild overproduction of the enzyme should not be harmful. In addition, the normal gene has been cloned and is available.

Because severe combined immunodeficiency due to a defect in the ADA gene can be corrected by infusion of normal bone marrow cells from a histocompatible donor, selective replication of the normal marrow cells appears to take place. This observation offers hope that defective bone marrow can be removed from a patient, the normal ADA gene inserted into a number of cells through gene therapy, and the treated marrow reimplanted into the patient where it may have a selective growth advantage. If selective growth occurs, elimination of the patient's own marrow would not be necessary. If, however, corrected marrow cells have no growth advantage over endogenous (i.e., the patient's own untreated) cells, then partial or complete marrow destruction (either by irradiation or by other means) may be required in order to allow the corrected marrow cells an environment favorable for expansion. The latter situation would require much greater confidence that the gene therapy procedure would work before a clinical trial should be undertaken.

Previously, clinical investigators thought that the human genetic diseases most likely to be the initial ones successfully treated by gene therapy would be the hemoglobin abnormalities (specifically, beta-thalassemia), because these disorders are the most obvious ones carried by blood cells, and bone marrow is the easiest tissue to manipulate outside the body. Regulation of globin synthesis, however, is unusually complicated. Not only are the embryonic, fetal, and adult globin chains carefully regulated during development, but also the subunits of the hemoglobin molecule are coded by genes on two different chromosomes. To understand the regulatory signals that control such a complicated system and to develop means for obtaining controlled expression of an exogenous (i.e., inserted by gene therapy) beta-globin gene will take considerably more research effort.

Criteria for Successful Treatment Protocols

What criteria should be satisfied prior to the time that somatic cell gene therapy is tested in a clinical trial? Three general requirements (to be proven in animal studies) were first presented in 1980[3]:

1. The new gene can be put into the correct target cells and will remain there long enough to be effective
2. The new gene will be expressed in the cells at an approprrate level
3. The new gene will not harm the cell or, by extension, the animal.

These three requisites, summarized as *delivery*, *expression*, and *safety*, will each be examined in turn.

These criteria are very similar to those required prior to the use of any new drug, therapeutic procedure, or surgical operation. The requirements simply state that the new treatment should get to the area of disease, correct it, and do more good than harm. The exact definitions of what is "long enough to be effective," what level is "an appropriate level," and how much harm is acceptable are questions for ongoing discussion as more is learned about gene therapy. Ultimately, local Institutional Review Boards and the RAC-NIH, with its Human Gene Therapy Subcommittee, must decide if a given protocol is ready for human application. Once the criteria are satisfied, that is, when the probable benefits for the patient are expected to exceed the possible risks, then attempts to cure human genetic disease by treatment with somatic cell gene therapy would be ethical.[2,9,16] The goal of biomedical research is, and has always been, to alleviate human suffering, and gene therapy is a proper and logical part of that effort.

Delivery

At present, the only human tissue that can be used effectively for gene transfer is bone marrow. No other cells can currently be extracted from the body, grown in culture to allow insertion of exogenous genes, and then successfully reimplanted into the patient. In the future, as more is learned about how to package the DNA and to make it tissue-specific, the intravenous route would be the simplest and most desirable. However, attempting to give a foreign gene by injection directly into the bloodstream is not advisable with our present state of knowledge, since the procedure would be enormously inefficient and there would be little control over the fate of the DNA.

Bone marrow consists of a heterogeneous population of cells, most of which are committed to differentiate into red blood cells, white blood cells, platelets, and so on. Only a small proportion (0.1–0.5%) of nucleated bone marrow cells are stem cells (blood-forming cells that have not yet differentiated into specific cell types and which divide as needed to maintain the marrow population). In gene therapy, it would be these rare, unrecognizable stem cells that would be the primary target. Consequently, a delivery system for gene therapy must be efficient.

Several techniques for transferring cloned genes into cells have been developed.[1] Each procedure is valuable for certain types of experiments, but none can yet be used to insert a gene into a specific chromosomal site in a target cell. At present the most promising approach for gene transfer into humans employs retrovirus-based vectors carrying exogenous genes.

Vectors derived from retroviruses possess several advantages as a gene delivery system:

- Up to 100% of cells can be infected and can express the integrated viral (and exogenous) genes.
- As many cells as desired can be infected simultaneously; 10^6 to 10^7 is a convenient number for a simple protocol.
- Under appropriate conditions, the DNA can integrate as a single copy at a single, albeit random, site.
- The infection and long-term harboring of a retroviral vector usually does not harm cells.

Several retroviral vector systems have been developed; those projected for human use at the present time are constructed from the Moloney murine (mouse) leukemia virus. Evidence obtained from studies with experimental animals and in tissue culture indicates that retroviruses can be used as a reasonably efficient delivery system.[5,7,8,10,12,13,15,17]

An ideal delivery system would be tissue-specific. When a genetic disorder is in the blood cells, the isolated bone marrow can be treated. But no other tissue can be removed, treated, and replaced at present. Since many viruses are known to infect only specific tissues (i.e., to bind to receptors that are present only on certain cell types), a retroviral particle containing a coat that recognizes only human blood-forming cells would permit the retroviral vector to be given intravenously with little danger that cells other than those in the marrow would be infected. In the future, such specificity could permit the liver and brain, for example, to be treated individually. In addition, the danger of inadvertently infecting germ cells could be eliminated. One problem, however, is that cell replication appears to be necessary for retrovirus integration. It would not be possible to infect nondividing brain cells, for example, so far as we now know.

The optimal system would not only deliver the vector specifically into the cell type of choice, but also direct the vector to a predetermined chromosomal site. Specific insertion into a selected site on a chromosome can be achieved in lower organisms but has not yet been possible in mammals.

Expression

In order for gene therapy to be successful, there must be appropriate expression of the new gene in the target cells. Even when a delivery system can transport an exogenous gene into the DNA of the correct cells of an organism, it has been a major problem to get the integrated DNA to function. A vast array of cloned genes have been introduced into a wide range of cells by several gene transfer techniques, but "normal" expression of exogenous genes is the exception rather than the rule.[1]

Expression of exogenous genes carried by retroviral vectors into intact animals by treated bone marrow cells has now been reported by a number of laboratories. Most studies have demonstrated the expression of an antibiotic resistance gene in mice,[7,8,13] but the human enzymes hypoxanthine phosphoribosyltransferase (HPRT)[15] and ADA[5] have also been detected in the blood-forming tissues of mice. Our group has demonstrated expression of the human ADA gene in the blood cells of irradiated monkeys that were reinfused with their own bone marrow cells after the cells had been treated in vitro with an ADA retroviral vector.[12] These several reports provide hope that vectors can be built with all the regulatory signals necessary to produce correctly controlled expression of exogenous genes in target cells in vivo.

Safety

Finally, a human gene therapy protocol must be safe. Although retroviruses have many advantages for gene transfer, they also have disadvantages. One problem is that they can rearrange their own structure, as well as exchange sequences with other retroviruses. In the future it might be possible to modify noninfectious retroviral vectors in such a way that they remain stable. At present, however, there is the possibility that a retroviral vector might recombine with an endogenous viral sequence to produce an infectious recombinant virus. What properties such a recombinant would have are unknown, but there is a potential homology between retroviral vectors and human T-cell leukemia viruses so that the formation of a recombinant that could produce a malignancy is possible. There is, however, a built-in safety feature with the mouse retroviral vectors now in use. These murine structures have a very different sequence from known human retroviruses, and there appears to be little or no homology between the two. Therefore, it should be possible with continuing research to build a safe retroviral vector.

Initial safety studies with our ADA-containing retroviral vector (called SAX) suggests that its use might be associated with fairly minimal risk. Four monkeys that underwent the gene transfer protocol have been followed for over 18 months. These animals have shown no sign of viremia, marrow dysfunction, hematopoietic malignancies, solid tumors, or other signs of pathology. In order to produce the worst case scenario, we injected large quantities of SAX-containing viral particles together with wild-type helper virus directly intravenously into three additional monkeys. All three cleared the viruses within 12 minutes, never developed a fever or other indications of viremia, and never demonstrated virus in their bloodstreams (after the first 12 minutes) based on an assay sufficiently sensitive that a single infectious viral particle in a milliliter of blood could have been detected. All these animals will continue to be followed, but at this point the gene therapy protocol with the SAX vector appears to be relatively low risk.

Expectations for Human Trials

It now appears that effective delivery-expression systems are becoming available that will allow reasonable attempts at somatic cell gene therapy in the pediatric patient. The initial protocols will be based on treatment of bone marrow cells with retroviral vectors carrying a normal gene. The efficiency and safety of the procedures are the remaining issues. Patients severely debilitated by having no normal copies of the gene that produces the enzyme ADA are the most likely first candidates for gene therapy.

It is unrealistic to expect a complete cure from the initial attempts at gene therapy. Many patients who suffer from severe genetic diseases, as well as their families, are eager to participate in early clinical trials even if the likelihood is low that the original experiments will alleviate symptoms. However, for the protection of the patients (particularly since those with the most severe diseases, and therefore the most ethically justifiable first candidates, are children), gene therapy trials should not be attempted until there are good animal data to suggest that some amelioration of the biochemical defect is likely. Then it would be necessary to weigh the potential risks to the patient, including the possibility of producing a pathologic virus or a malignancy, against the anticipated benefits to be gained from the functional gene. This risk-benefit determination, a standard procedure for all clinical research protocols, would need to be carried out for each patient.

In summary, Institutional Review Boards and the NIH should carefully evaluate therapeutic protocols to ensure that the delivery system is effective, that sufficient expression can be obtained in bone marrow cultures and in laboratory animals to predict probable benefit, even if small, for the patient, and that safety protocols have demonstrated that the probability is low for the production of either a malignant cell or a harmful infectious retrovirus. Once these criteria are met, it would be unethical to delay human trials. Patients with serious genetic diseases have little other hope at present for alleviation of their medical problems. Arguments that genetic engineering might someday be misused do not justify the needless perpetuation of human suffering that would result from an unnecessary delay in the clinical application of this potentially powerful therapeutic procedure.

POTENTIAL USES FOR IN-UTERO SOMATIC CELL GENE THERAPY

Is there a place for initiating gene therapy in the fetus rather than waiting for the child to be born? There are a number of diseases, particularly involving the central nervous system, in which irreversible damage may already have occurred by the time of birth. Initial studies in fetal sheep suggest that in utero gene therapy is possible. If a vector could be developed that could safely be inserted into the central nervous system directly, or which could bypass the blood-brain-barrier following its introduction into the fetal circulation, then it might be possible to salvage these fetuses who are now doomed to irreversible damage before birth. It is important, as an initial step towards this goal, to determine if in utero bone marrow transplantation from a compatible donor would be beneficial to a defective fetus (e.g., one with Lesch-Nyhan disease).

Fetal Bone Marrow Transplantation/Retroviral Gene Transfer

To test the feasibility of fetal bone marrow transplantation/retroviral gene transfer, an in-utero sheep gene transfer protocol was established.[4] The protocol for infection of cells is shown in Figures 15-5 and 15-6. After the head and neck of a 96-day-old fetal lamb was externalized through a small incision in the uterus, the fetal carotid artery was cannulated with a small-diameter catheter. The fetus was exchange-transfused with maternal blood. After supernatant infection with a retroviral vector (called N2), the blood cells were reinjected into the fetus. The catheter was removed and the animal was allowed to develop to term 55 days later. One week after birth, bone marrow cells from the lamb were evaluated in blood cell colony assays in the presence or absence of a selective agent, G418. As expected, no colony growth was obtained in an age-matched uninfected lamb in the presence of G418. However, G418-resistant colonies were obtained in the infected animal, representing successful gene transfer and expression of the vector gene 62 days after transplantation. Assays over the first 8 weeks of life continued to demonstrate G418-resistant colonies. These results indicate that a functional gene can be efficiently transferred into fetal hematopoietic cells in utero without cytoablation and that the gene will continue to be expressed months later in the young animal.

The fetal sheep experiment demonstrates that fetal lamb stem cells can be infected efficiently. It appears that this high level is due to an inherent quality of fetal cells and is not simply due to species differences. Furthermore, in the absence of cytoablation prior to transplantation, the infected, reinfused cells seemed to have a growth advantage over those remaining in the fetus, as evidenced by a high percentage of G418-resistant colonies. We believe that this finding may be related to the continuing expansion of the hematopoietic system in the mammalian fetus, especially during the last one-third of the gestation period; a naturally occurring change in the primary hematopoietic site from liver and spleen to bone marrow around the time of the transplant; and the relatively large numbers of hematopoietic progenitors (infected and uninfected) made available to the fetus by the bolus reinfusion of these cells right at a time when physiologic space was open in the expanding bone marrow. These findings suggest that in-utero bone marrow transplantation/retroviral gene transfer may provide a viable adjunct to postnatal gene transfer or even an alternative when the diag-

IN-UTERO GENE TRANSFER PROTOCOL

CIRCULATING HEMATOPOIETIC CELLS
FROM 100 DAY-OLD FETAL SHEEP
↓
INFECTED WITH NEO[R] or ADA CONTAINING
RETROVIRUS VECTOR
↓
TRANSPLANTED INTO DONOR FETUS
↓
BONE MARROW CELLS CULTURED IN PRESENCE OR
ABSENCE OF G418 AFTER BIRTH

FIGURE 15-5. Sheep in-utero gene transfer protocol. NEO[R], the gene providing resistance to neomycin; ADA, the gene for human adenosine deaminase.

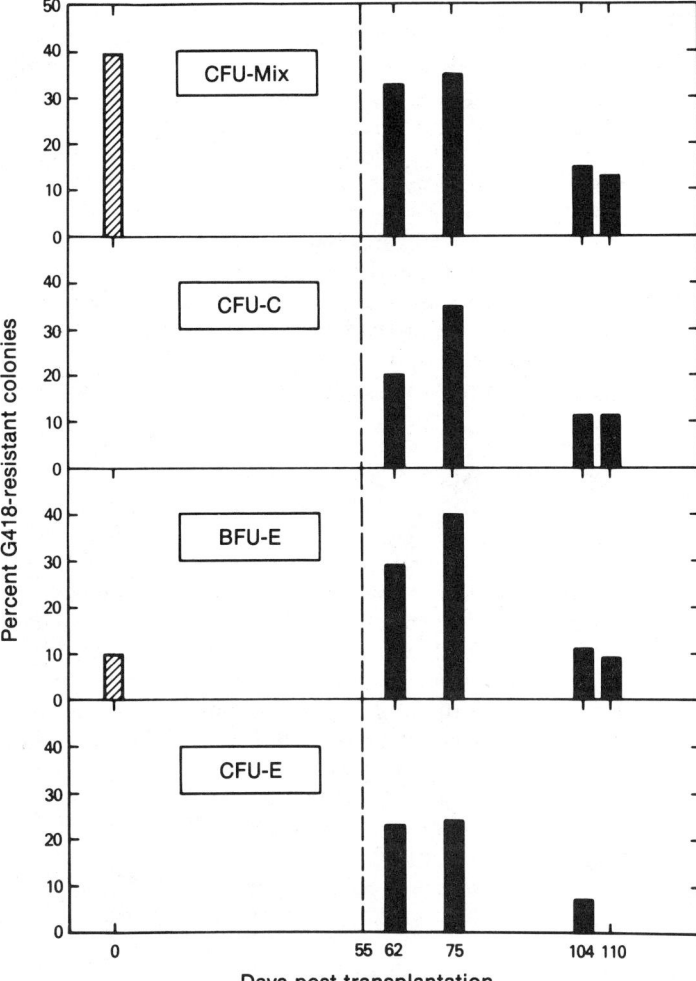

FIGURE 15-6. Percentages of G418-resistant colonies derived from the treated lamb over time. Circulating hematopoietic cells derived from the 96-day-old fetus after infection (*hatched bars*) and bone marrow cells from the lamb 62, 75, 104, and 110 days after gene treatment (*solid bars*) were assayed for G418-resistant progenitor cells. Data from in vitro–infected hematopoietic cells were plotted [(total no. of colonies + G418/total no. colonies − G418) × 100] for both progenitor cells. The dashed line at 55 days represents the day of birth of the animal.

Data for newborn lambs were plotted [(total no. of G418-resistant colonies/total no. of colonies) × 100] for assays performed at 62, 75, 104, and 110 days after transplantation were done similarily. In all situations, results [(total no. of G418-resistant colonies/total no. of colonies) × 100] for the uninfected, age-matched control lamb were less than 1%. See reference 4.

nosis of a severe genetic disease is made in utero.

What additional ethical considerations arise when the fetus is the patient? Much of this volume discusses this issue with regard to other modes of therapy, and the same arguments apply to gene therapy. If the risk-benefit ratio for the fetal patient is acceptable, if all other criteria for somatic cell gene therapy are satisfied, and if there is no additional potential for accidental germ-line gene therapy, then carrying out the procedure in utero should present no additional ethical concerns.

Germ-Line Gene Therapy

Gene therapy of germ-line cells would require a major advance in our present state of knowledge. It would require that we learn how to insert a gene not only into the appropriate cells of the patient's body, but also how to introduce it into the germ line of the patient in such a way that it would be transmitted to offspring and would be functional in the correct way in the correct cells in the offspring. Based on the small amount of information now available from animal studies, the step from correction of a disorder in somatic cells to correction of the germ line would be difficult.

Germ-line transmission and expression of inserted genes in mice has been done successfully by a large number of laboratories but with a technique that is not acceptable for use in human patients, namely, the physical microinjection of fertilized eggs. Microinjection into tissue culture cells has been used for a number of years and has the advantage of high efficiency (up to one tissue culture cell in five injected can be permanently transfected). However, the distinct disadvantage is that only one cell at a time can be injected. The transfection of a large number (e.g., 10^6) of blood-forming stem cells is not feasible.

To obtain a transgenic mouse, DNA can be microinjected into one of the two pronuclei of a recently fertilized egg. This egg can then be placed into the oviduct of a pseudopregnant female, where it can develop into a normal mouse carrying the exogenous DNA in every cell of its body including its germ cells. Consequently, the injected DNA can be transmitted to offspring in a normal mendelian manner. The first success using this technique for correcting a genetic disorder in an animal was to partially correct a mouse with a defect in its growth hormone production.[11] By attaching a rat growth hormone gene to an active regulatory sequence (specifically, the promoter that normally directs the synthesis of metallothionein messenger RNA in mice), researchers obtained a recombinant DNA construct that actively produced growth hormone in the genetically defective mouse and in a number of its offspring. Although the level of growth hormone production was inappropriately controlled (i.e., influenced by signals that normally regulate metallothionein synthesis), these experiments did show that microinjection could be used as a delivery system to put a gene into every cell of an animal's body, that a genetic disorder could, as a result, be corrected, and that the correction could be passed on to the next generation of animals.

Why is the technique of microinjecting a fertilized egg not acceptable for use in human gene therapy at the present time? First, the procedure has a high failure rate; second, it can produce a deleterious result; and third, it would have limited usefulness.

Microinjection has a high failure rate because the majority of eggs are so damaged by the microinjection and transfer procedures that they do not develop into live offspring. In one typical experiment[6] involving microinjection of an immunoglobulin gene into mouse eggs, 300 eggs were injected, 192 (64%) were judged sufficiently healthy to be transferred to surrogate mothers, only 11 (3.7%) proceeded to live birth, and just 6 (2%) carried the gene. These results are from a highly experienced laboratory in which thousands of identical eggs from the same hybrid cross of inbred mice have been injected over several years. The mice were chosen precisely because they gave the best results for gene transfer by microinjection. Attempts to microinject functional growth hormone genes into livestock eggs met with several major biologic and technical problems before being accomplished. Successful gene transfer by microinjection of human eggs, without a long period of trial and error experimentation, is extremely unlikely.

Second, microinjection of eggs can produce deleterious results because there is no control over where the injected DNA will integrate in the genome. For example, the integration of an exogenous rabbit beta-globin gene in transgenic mice can sometimes occur at a chromosomal location, resulting in expression of the beta-globin gene in an inappropriate tissue, such as muscle or testis.[14] There have also been a considerable number of cases reported in which integration of microinjected DNA has resulted in a pathologic condition. Although there is no control over where exogenous DNA will integrate in any gene transfer procedure, the damaging effect caused by a harmful insertion site could be great when it occurs in the egg, but may be negligible when it occurs in one or a few of a large number of bone marrow cells.

The third objection to microinjection of eggs is limited usefulness. Not only is it ethically questionable to experiment on human eggs because of the expected losses, but even if success were obtained, it would be applicable primarily when both patients are homozygous for the defect. When the parents are both carriers of a recessive trait, only one fertilized egg out of four would result in an affected child. Since a homozygous defect cannot yet be recognized in early embryos, and since the procedure itself carries such a high risk, it would be improper to attempt any manipulation in this situation. Furthermore, most of the very serious genetic disorders result in infertility (or death before reproductive age) in homozygous patients. Consequently, there would be little use for the procedure even if it were feasible.

Even when the technical capability becomes available to attempt germ-line gene therapy in humans, there are major medical and ethical concerns to consider. The medical issues center primarily around the question, Will the transmitted gene itself, or any side-effects caused by its presence, adversely affect the immediate offspring or their descendants? Since in this case one must study several generations of progeny to obtain answers, it will clearly take longer to gain knowledge from animal studies on the long-term safety of germ-line gene therapy than on somatic cell gene therapy. Germline therapy deserves careful ethical consideration well in advance of the time when the technical capability for carrying it out arrives.[2]

Enhancement Genetic Enginering

Enhancement genetic engineering is considerably different in principle from the two uses of gene transfer described above. This is no longer therapy of a genetic disorder; it is the insertion of an additional normal gene (or a gene modified in a specific way) to produce a wanted change in some characteristic. Enhancement would involve the insertion of a single gene or a small number of genes that code for a product (or products) to produce the desired effect; for example, greater size through the insertion of an additional growth hormone gene into the cells of an infant or fetus. Enhancement genetic engineering presents a major additional scientific hurdle, as well as serious new ethical issues.

The scientific hurdle to be overcome is a formidable one. Until now, we have considered the correction of a defect—of a "broken part." Fix the broken part and the human machine should operate correctly again. Replacing a faulty part is different from trying to add something new to a normally functioning system. To insert a gene in the hope of improving or selectively altering a characteristic might endanger the overall metabolic balance of the individual cells as well as of the entire body. Medicine is a very inexact science. Every year new hormones, new regulators, and new pathways are discovered. There are clearly many more to be discovered. Most impressive is the enormously intricate way that each cell coordinates within itself all of its thousands of pathways. Likewise, the body as a whole carefully monitors and balances a multitude of physiologic systems. Much additional research will be required to elucidate the effects of altering one or more major pathways in a cell. To correct a faulty gene is probably not going to be dangerous, but to intentionally insert a gene to make more of one product might adversely affect numerous other biochemical pathways.

We possess insufficient information at present to understand the effects of attempts to alter the genetic machinery of a human. Is it wise, safe, or ethical for parents to give, for example, growth hormone (now that it is readily available) to their normal sons in order to produce very large football or basketball players? Unfortunately, this practice is reported to now take place in this country. But worse is insertion of a growth hormone gene into a normal child, since once it is in, there is no way to get it back out. The child's reflexes, coordination, and balance might all be grossly affected. In addition, even more serious questions can be asked, such as, Might one alter the regulatory pathways of cells, inadvertently affecting cell division or other properties? In short, we know too little about the human body to chance inserting a gene designed for "improvement" into a normal healthy person.

Eugenic Genetic Engineering

Eugenic genetic engineering has received considerable attention in the popular press, with the result that at times unjustified fears have been produced because of claims that scientists might soon be able to re-make human beings. In fact, however, such traits as personality, character, formation of body organs, fertility, intelligence, and physical, mental, and emotional characteristics are enormously complex. Dozens, perhaps hundreds, of unknown genes that interact in totally unknown ways probably contribute to each of them. Environmental influences also interact with these genetic backgrounds in poorly understood ways. With time, as more is learned about each of these complex traits, individual genes will be discovered that play specific roles. Undoubtedly, disorders will be recognized that are caused by defects in these genes. Then, somatic cell gene therapy could be employed to correct the defect.

Even so, we should be concerned about the possible misuse of genetic engineering in the future. The best insurance against possible abuse is a well informed public. Gene therapy has the potential for producing tremendous good by reducing the suffering and death caused by genetic diseases. We can look forward to the day when, with proper safeguards imposed by society, this powerful new therapeutic procedure will be available.

REFERENCES

1. Anderson WF: Prospects for human gene therapy. Science 226:401, 1984
2. Anderson WF: Human gene therapy: Scientific and ethical considerations. J Med and Phil 10:275, 1985.
3. Anderson WF, Fletcher JC: Gene therapy in human beings: When is it ethical to begin? N Engl J Med 303:1293, 1980
4. Anderson WF, Kantoff P, Eglitis M et al: Gene transfer and expression in nonhuman primates using retroviral vectors. Cold Spring Harbor Symposia LI:1073, 1986
5. Belmont JW, Henkel-Tigges J, Chang SMW et al: Expression of human adenosine deaminase in murine haematopoietic progenitor cells following retroviral transfer. Nature 322:385, 1986
6. Brinster RL, Ritchie KA, Hammer RE et al: Expression of a microinjected immunoglobulin gene in the spleen of transgenic mice. Nature 306:332, 1983
7. Dick JE, Magli MC, Huszar D et al: Introduction of a selectable gene into primitive stem cells capable of long-term reconstitution of the hemopoietic system of W/W^v mice. Cell 42:71, 1985
8. Eglitis MA, Kantoff P, Gilboa E, Anderson WF: Gene expression in mice following high efficiency retroviral-mediated gene transfer. Science 230:1395, 1985
9. Fletcher JC: Ethical issues in and beyond prospective clinical trials of human gene therapy. J Med Philos 10:293, 1985
10. Gruber HE, Finley KD, Hershberg RM et al: Retroviral vector-mediated gene transfer into human hematopoietic progenitor cells. Science 230:1057, 1985
11. Hammer RE, Palmiter RD, Brinster RL: Partial correction of murine hereditary growth disorder by germ-line incorporation of a new gene. Nature 311:65, 1984
12. Kantoff PW, Gillio AP, McLachlin JR et al: Expression of human adenosine deaminase in nonhuman primates after retrovirus-mediated gene transfer. J Exp Med 166:219, 1987
13. Keller G, Paige C, Gilboa E, Wagner EF: Expression of a foreign gene in myeloid and lymphoid cells derived from multipotent haematopoietic precursors. Nature 318:149, 1985
14. Lacy E, Roberts S, Evans EP et al: A foreign β-globin gene in transgenic mice: Integration at abnormal chromosomal positions and expression in inappropriate tissues. Cell 34:343, 1983
15. Miller AD, Eckner RJ, Jolly DJ et al: Expression of a retrovirus encoding human HPRT in mice. Science 225:630, 1984
16. Walters LR: The ethics of human gene therapy. Nature 320:225, 1986
17. Williams DA, Lemischka IR, Nathan DG, Mulligan RC: Introduction of new genetic material into pluripotent haematopoietic stem cells of the mouse. Nature 310:476, 1984

SECTION 5: LEGAL ISSUES IN FETAL THERAPY

John A. Robertson

Prenatal diagnosis of a fetal malformation ordinarily presents the mother with the stark choice of undergoing an abortion or delivering a handicapped child. Recently, medical and surgical treatments of the fetus in utero have become available, treatments that are of various degrees of safety and efficacy in the journey from investigational to established therapy. The future is likely to hold even greater potential for treatment of the preterm child, as even now the technical possibility of genetic therapy on preimplantation embryos is being discussed.

The availability of prenatal therapy focuses attention on potential conflicts in a clinical relationship that previously received little scrutiny. What are the rights and duties of the mother and physician to a developing fetus after its conception or continuing gestation has been chosen? What are the prenatal rights of the child?

The ethical situation is complex. It contains the traditional pediatric ethical dilemma of whether the mother may provide or refuse a treatment that may injure but also benefit the child with two additional considerations. First, the fetus has uncertain and controversial legal and moral status. Since the right to an abortion was recognized legally in *Roe v. Wade*,[11] the rights of the fetus are deemed secondary to the wishes of the mother up to the point of viability. Yet the possibility of in utero treatment seems to make the fetus a patient with independent rights and interests. Second, therapies to help the fetus must necessarily invade the body of the mother, thus raising the possibility of conflict with the mother's right to bodily integrity.

With a few exceptions, the problems involved are no different from those that arise in pediatric practice. Doctors and mothers acting in good faith may use experimental prenatal fetal therapies when the child would be at great risk without them, but they are not legally or morally obligated to do so. When the therapy is established, a mother's refusal of the intervention in principle may be penalized or overridden by the courts. Of course, the circumstances in which refusal of an established therapy should be punished or lead to direct intervention will be controversial and probably rare. If limits are placed on a woman's freedom, however, they will be limits on her right of bodily integrity, rather than her right not to procreate. Once a woman decides not to abort, she has an obligation to take reasonable steps to ensure the birth of a healthy child.

THE PRENATAL RIGHTS OF CHILDREN

The legal rights and duties of mothers and physicians in using fetal therapy derive from a body of law that imposes prenatal obligations of reasonable care toward fetuses which will be born alive. Fetuses have no right to be conceived nor, once conceived, to be carried to term unless they have reached the point of viability (estimated at 24 to 26 weeks of pregnancy).[3] However, if they are going to be carried to term, they do have rights against the mother, the doctor, or third parties not to be injured or subjected to unreasonable risk of injury.

Since the fetus's right to be born as healthy as is reasonably possible cannot ordinarily be asserted until after birth, it is clearer to speak of prenatal obligations of mothers and physicians to the unborn child. These obligations are contingent on the live birth of the child and ordinarily cannot be asserted before birth. If mother or physician violate these prenatal obligations by intentionally injuring the viable fetus or negligently failing to avert injury, then criminal or civil legal action is possible. State law might permit a variety of criminal charges to be brought. If the child is stillborn or dies in utero after the point of viability, the mother and/or physicians could be prosecuted under abortion or feticide laws. If the child is born alive but then dies as a result of prenatal derelictions, charges of homicide or child abuse could be brought.[4] If the child is born damaged but lives, a charge of child abuse could be lodged against the mother or doctor for prenatal actions.

Civil actions for damages also could be brought. All American jurisdictions recognize a cause of action for reasonably foreseeable and avoidable prenatal and, in some cases, preconception actions that cause death or injury to a child born alive.[2] The reasoning of the cases imposing liability for prenatal injuries applies to negligent conduct on the mother's part as well. A recent case in Michigan shows that previous barriers to such suits, such as doctrines of intrafamilial tort immunity, may no longer apply. In the pathbreaking case of *Grodin v. Grodin*,[10] a suit by a child against his mother for discolored teeth caused by her negligently taking tetracycline during pregnancy was held legally cognizable. Removal of the financial incentives to file such suits by changes in personal liability insurance coverage (in *Grodin*, a broadly stated clause in a homeowner's insurance policy was the incentive for the suit), and the other impracticalities of mounting such suits will prevent most children injured by negligent maternal behavior from suing their mothers. However, recognition that the law would sanction such conduct does set an important principle.

These legal doctrines clearly limit a woman's freedom over her body during pregnancy, but they do not limit her reproductive freedom—her constitutional right not to procreate—since they arise after she has waived that right by choosing not to abort. Recognition of the voluntary nature of pregnancy thus works to strengthen duties to the fetus that a woman chooses to carry to term. Having decided to use her body to procreate, a woman loses some bodily freedom during pregnancy in order to ensure the health of a child that she has chosen to birth. It is against this background of prenatal duties to children that the rights and duties of mothers and physicians regarding fetal therapy emerge.

PRENATAL RIGHTS AND DUTIES OF PARENTS AND PHYSICIANS

Experimental Prenatal Therapies

Because the experimental or established status of a therapy affects the legal rights and duties of parents and physicians, we must at the outset distinguish between the legal and ethical issues that arise when prenatal fetal therapies are innovative and experimental, and those that arise when they become established and accepted therapy.

Duty to Employ Procedures

Few fetal therapies have been established as safe and effective. As of late June 1988, fewer than 500 fetuses have been treated surgically, and few full-scale reviews of these cases or clinical trials have been published. When in utero surgery is experimental and innovative, it offers a possible benefit to the fetus by providing an alternative to abortion. However, parents or physicians are not obliged to try this alternative. Under the Supreme Court decision in *Roe v. Wade*, a mother is free to abort through the end of the second trimester and even beyond, if the state has not prohibited abortion after viability. Since this right exists even if the fetus is normal and would be born healthy, the possibility of correcting a congenital defect in utero with an experimental therapy would not prevent the mother from choosing abortion.

If the mother decides against abortion, she still has no legal or moral duty to have an experimental procedure done. Because reasonable people could differ over whether the benefits of an experimental therapy outweigh the risks, it is clearly the mother's prerogative to decide about the use of an experimental therapy. The mother would have no greater duty to employ an experimental therapy with a fetus than she would with a child. Parents, for example, are free to refuse *experimental* chemotherapy for treatment of their child's leukemia, but they could not refuse an *established* therapy nor treat with an unproven drug, such as laetrile, instead.

The experimental status of fetal therapy also affects the legal duties of the obstetrician. The physician may offer to try an experimental in utero technique but must defer to the mother. If the mother refuses, the physician would have no obligation to take steps to override her decision, as he might if the therapy was established as safe and effective.

Discretion to Employ Procedures

Although mothers and physicians are not obligated to use prenatal surgery to correct a congenital anomaly, the more crucial questions at this stage of development are whether they may choose to do so and what procedures must be followed if they do. These questions are important because experimental in utero therapy could risk harming the fetus and mother to a greater degree than doing nothing. Intervention could induce premature labor and death, whereas the fetus might have survived if nothing had been done, or it could cause greater damage than if no intervention occurred, as would result if the doctors were mistaken in their diagnosis and prognosis. Finally, the intervention might allow the fetus with a lethal lesion to survive in a severely handicapped state. Since one of the patients (the unborn child) is incapable of consent, can the mother decide to subject the fetus to these risks? May the physician concur?

There is little doubt that a mother may legally allow experimental procedures to be performed in utero. As long as the mother is competent and has been fully informed of the unproven status of the surgery, the risks to her and the fetus, and the risks and benefits of the alternatives, she is legally free to undergo some medical risk in order to bring a healthy baby into the world. Although the procedure poses risks to the fetus, doing nothing may impose even higher risks of death or disability. In such circumstances, consent to an experimental procedure may be a reasonable course of action. Even if the therapy leads to the child being more damaged than if the surgery had been postponed until delivery, or if the surgery prevents death but leads to the child surviving in a damaged state when it would not otherwise have been born at all, use of the experimental therapy still may have been a reasonable course of action. A poor outcome that resulted from a series of clinical judgments that were reasonable at the time would not justify legal sanctions.

The legal duties of the physician mirror those of the mother, with some important differences. Since in utero therapy involves specialized knowledge and skills, obstetricians contemplating such procedures must have the requisite training and experience to perform competently. They may then legally use experimental techniques to benefit the unborn child, provided the mother has been fully informed and freely consents. Attempting an unvalidated procedure with maternal consent for the purpose of benefiting a fetus that would otherwise die or be severely disabled would not constitute actionable negligence, provided there are grounds for thinking the procedure would be of benefit. However, the physician must be careful not to overemphasize the benefits of what may still be a speculative and risky procedure.

The physician employing in utero surgical techniques may have additional duties, based on whether the procedure is seen as research or as an innovative, unproven therapy. If the physician is conducting research with the fetus and mother as subjects, then approval of an Institutional Review Board (IRB) may be required, whatever the source of the funding. An IRB reviewing experimental in utero therapy in accordance with Department of Health and Human Services regulations for research on fetuses may approve such research. The regulations permit research on fetuses and pregnant women when "the purpose of the activity is to meet the health needs of the mother or the particular fetus."[8] If the physician has no research intent and perceives the unproven procedure to be innovative therapy, there may be no legal obligation to obtain IRB review, though it is an advisable course of action.

Established Procedures

The rights and duties of mothers and physicians change significantly when prenatal therapies are established as safe and effective for their intended purpose.

Termination of Pregnancy

The mere fact that a congenital defect is treatable prenatally does not alter the mother's right under *Roe v. Wade* to terminate the pregnancy. The right to abort depends on the wishes of the mother and the stage of pregnancy, not on the health or prospects of the fetus. Just as a normal fetus may be aborted, so may a defective though treatable one. In the 25 states that have not prohibited abortion after viability, termination and death in utero is lawful at any point in the pregnancy.

If the state has prohibited postviability abortions, then abortion of a viable fetus with a congenital defect may be prohibited. In that case, a mother might by required to undergo prenatal fetal therapy or be subject to criminal and civil penalties for not taking reasonable steps to protect the child that she has chosen to bring into the world.

Duty to Employ Established Procedures

When prenatal fetal therapies are still experimental, the mother and physician have no duty to use them. When a medical procedure is established as safe and effective by reasonable practitioners and the pregnancy is going to term, it is appropriate medical practice and proper parental behavior to employ that procedure. In such a case, the benefit to the unborn child from the intervention clearly outweighs the risks of the intervention and thus may appropriately be done with maternal consent and without IRB review.

The key legal issue that arises when prenatal fetal therapies are medically established is whether the mother can refuse them. If prenatal therapies are medically acceptable or indicated in a clinical situation, a physician who fails to employ them or to inform the parents of the need for them and their availability elsewhere could be liable under traditional malpractice standards for wrongful death or to the parents and child, if the child is born in a damaged condition, for the costs of care and the pain and suffering involved.

The most difficult question concerns the scope of the mother's duty to the unborn child. If the mother elects not to abort, she may be legally obligated to employ available medical procedures that will prevent the child from being born damaged or in an avoidable unhealthy state. If the child is likely to be born alive, she takes on a legal duty to take all reasonable measures, including employing established in utero therapies, to minimize damage to the child. The parents' duty to children to provide necessary medical care includes the duty to provide essential prenatal therapy when a live birth is expected. Depending on the jurisdiction, refusal of an established therapy could be prosecuted under feticide, homicide, or child abuse/neglect statutes if the viable fetus died in utero or after birth, or was born in an avoidably damaged or handicapped state. With the demise of intrafamilial tort immunity, a child could also sue the parents for failing to employ low-risk in utero therapy that would have prevented the child from being born injured. Practically speaking such suits are rare, but they could arise if the parents have personal liability coverage or if they divorce.

The possibility of criminal or civil action against the mother for prenatal negligence that harms the child carried to term also raises the question of the obstetrician's duty under child abuse reporting laws to report maternal neglect to child welfare authorities. If the mother has prenatal obligations to prevent harm to unborn children, then presumably physicians, nurses, and other persons covered by child abuse reporting laws are also thus obligated. Although no case or action against a physician on this basis has occurred, the logic of the situation would allow the imposition of such a duty on the physician, illustrating once again how prenatal therapies clarify (and complicate) a relationship that previously escaped close scrutiny.

Direct Seizures and Coerced Treatment

The most troubling ethical and legal issue in fetal therapy is whether prenatal therapy may be directly imposed on the mother against her wishes. May child welfare authorities, informed that a mother's prenatal conduct is likely to harm the offspring, obtain a court order compelling the mother to undergo in utero treatment? In the typical pediatric situation, an established treatment could clearly be ordered over the parents' wishes, since parental autonomy ordinarily cannot override the child's interest in life or health. When the child is still unborn, however, treatment of the child over the mother's wishes necessarily invades her body. With fetal therapy, the issue is whether the mother's interest in bodily integrity is great enough to override the unborn child's well-being.

The state probably has the authority to enact legislation that would empower judges to order prenatal treatment in certain cases. (Whether it should use this power is another issue.) Bodily intrusions without the consent of the individual for the sake of another individual are highly disfavored, but not unknown to the law.[5] The state may force persons to have blood drawn or even undergo surgery to produce evidence of crimes. Compulsory vaccination and military service are well-established traditions. Prisoners may be forcibly fed or treated for the sake of prison discipline. Courts have sometimes ordered Jehovah's Witness parents with young children to receive blood transfusions.

Given the precedent for violating bodily integrity when a very important interest is at stake, it is likely that legislation authorizing courts to order parents to undergo a simple blood test, donate a point of blood, or even give bone marrow if it was necessary to preserve the child's life would be found constitutional. As the degree of harm and intrusion to the parent increases, as in the case of a forced kidney donation, the state's power to override bodily integrity weakens and it is less likely that courts would order bodily intrusion for the child's sake. While the loss of a kidney is not itself life-threatening, the burden of forced nephrectomy is considerably greater than the burden of forced blood or marrow donations. But the factor that makes forced nephrectomy hard to justify is the degree of harm and not the fact of coerced bodily intrusion. When the harm is less substantial, bodily intrusions essential to the child's health could be constitutionally ordered.

Although the courts have not yet addressed the constitutional authority of the state to force tissue or blood donation from a parent to a child, there are two cases that uphold coerced medical treatments on the mother for the sake of an unborn child. In a 1964 New Jersey case, *Raleigh-Fitkin-Paul Morgan Memorial Hospital v. Anderson,*[7] a hospital unsuccessfully petitioned a trial court to order blood transfusions on a Jehovah's Witness, age 23, who was 8 months pregnant and in danger of severe hemorrhaging. The New Jersey Supreme Court, reversing the trial court, held that "the unborn child is entitled to the law's protection" and ordered blood transfusions to the mother if the physicians determined that they were necessary.

Then, in 1981, the Georgia Supreme Court ordered a cesarean section to be performed on a woman to save her unborn child. The case, *Jefferson v. Griffin Spalding County Hospital Authority,*[9] involved a woman in the 39th week of pregnancy who had a complete placenta previa. The doctors claimed that neither she nor the child could survive if a vaginal delivery occurred. When the mother refused the surgery on religious grounds, the state child welfare agency petitioned the juvenile court for temporary custody of the unborn child and for an order requiring the mother to submit to the cesarean section. The Georgia Supreme Court affirmed the juvenile court order that the mother submit to a cesarean section if "considered necessary by the attending physician to sustain the life of this child," on the ground that "the intrusion involved into the life of [the mother] is outweighed by the duty of the State to protect a living, unborn human being from meeting his or her death before being given the opportunity to live."

If resolution of the fetal-maternal conflict in *Raleigh-Fitkin* and *Jefferson* in favor of the near-term fetus over the mother's interest in bodily integrity is correct, then the state may have a far-reaching power to intrude on the mother's body and freedom of action for the benefit of the unborn child. In addition to the results seen in the court cases just discussed, this reasoning would support state policies compelling many different kinds of maternal behavior. A woman might be prohibited from using alcohol or other substances harmful to the fetus during pregnancy or be kept from her workplace because of toxic effects on the fetus. She might be ordered to take drugs such as insulin for diabetes, medications for fetal deficiencies, or intrauterine blood transfusions for fetal Rh-isoimmunization. Prenatal screening and diagnostic procedures, from amniocentesis to sonography or even fetoscopy, could be made mandatory. If established as safe and effective, in utero fetal surgery (e.g., to shunt cerebroventricular fluids from the brain to relieve hydrocephalus or to relieve the urethral obstruction causing bilateral hydronephrosis) also could be ordered. Indeed, even extrauterine fetal surgery, if it becomes an established procedure, could be ordered if the risks to the mother were small and if it was a last resort to save the life of or prevent severe disability in a viable fetus.[6]

An important limit on coercing treatment or other behaviors for the sake of the child is the risk presented to the mother. Society's preference for the viable fetus and unborn child over the mother's bodily autonomy is authorized by *Roe v. Wade* only where protection of the fetus does not threaten "the life or health of the mother."[12] The boundaries of this limit, however, are vague, for health interests can range from relatively minor emotional harm to major, permanent physical injuries, and the Supreme Court has not indicated how substantial the threat to health must be. It is likely that minimal or nonsubstantial health risks posed by an intervention to save the fetus will be insufficient to give the mother priority over the viable fetus.

Many types of in utero fetal therapy, such as forced medications or intrauterine transfusions, for example, may carry very small health risks and thus be required of the unwilling woman. Invasive prenatal diagnostic techniques, such as amniocentesis or even fetoscopy, also involve relatively minor risks to the mother. Even in utero surgery performed through fetoscopy may not be so risky as to outweigh a societal interest in preserving the life or health of a viable fetus. Of course, the mother may still be free to undergo medical procedures necessary for her health (e.g., radiation for cervical cancer), even if they risked harm to an expected child.

The hardest case for imposing treatment against a mother's wishes will arise with procedures involving general anesthesia and major surgery, such as extrauterine fetal surgery and, more commonly, cesarean section. The court in *Jefferson* was able to avoid this issue, since the mother's health was also threatened. The risks to the mother of the surgery must be weighed and balanced against the benefit to the unborn child. The decision will depend on the medical condition and risks to the mother in each case. A Colorado trial court, for example, has found that the health risks to the mother of a cesarean section under general anesthesia are not so great as to prevent the state from preferring the interests of the fetus and ordering the surgery.[11]

To put the above discussion in proper perspective, let us recall that the issue being analyzed is the constitutional authority of the state to order treatment of unwilling pregnant women, and does not constitute a recommendation that direct seizures should be ordered. Whether the constitutional muscle of the state should be exercised involves policy considerations that are beyond the scope of this discussion. In any event, the unavailability or undesirability of prebirth seizures to protect unborn children does not mean that the postbirth civil and criminal sanctions discussed above, which seek more indirectly to achieve offspring well-being, must also be rejected.

Resolving Conflicts Over Refusal of Established Prenatal Therapy

Compelling prenatal medical interventions on a woman to protect a viable fetus represent a drastic step that should be taken only after the need for it is clearly established. Indeed, the dilemma is not likely to arise often, for most mothers will want their child to survive in the healthiest state possible. When conflicts do arise and the mother refuses an established procedure, the physician will face a dilemma. If the physician accedes to the mother's refusal and the fetus dies or the child is born defective, the physician could be criminally liable for feticide or child abuse, or could be civilly liable to the child for failing to fulfill obligations to a fetus likely to be born alive. On the other hand, if out of fear of legal liability or concern for the unborn child, the physician insists on the surgery, he or she may face civil or criminal charges for assault and battery on the mother.

CONCLUSION

In describing legal considerations in fetal treatment, legal analysis must distinguish between avoidable and unavoidable harm to offspring, and recall that prenatal duties to offspring arise only afer a woman has decided to continue a pregnancy that she is free to terminate. Analysis must also distinguish postbirth civil and criminal sanctions from forcible seizures prior to birth. The legal status and desirability of each policy differs enormously. Objections to forcible seizures do not necessarily mean that there is no role for postbirth sanctions for egregiously harmful prenatal conduct. In the final analysis, education, services, and voluntary compliance remain the most desirable policies to pursue.

The physician plays an important role in minimizing avoidably handicapped births. He or she must explain to pregnant women options for treating fetuses or avoiding conduct harmful to them, and persuade them to act for the good of the child. There may also be a legal duty to report refusals or risks to child welfare authorities. At that point physicians have done all that may reasonably be asked to fulfill their legal duty to the unborn child whose care they have assumed during pregnancy.

REFERENCES

1. Bowes WA Jr, Selgestad B: Fetal versus maternal rights: Medical and legal perspectives. Obstet Gynecol 58:209, 1981. The outcome in this case could still occur even if the result in Lee v. Winston, 717 F. 2d 888 (4th Cir 1983), refusing the state the power to compel an armed robbery defendant to undergo general anesthesia to remove a bullet relevant to the charges against him, is upheld by the United States Supreme Court. The state's interest in compelling the surgery in Lee is arguably much less than it would be were a full-term fetus' life at stake, because of the mother's refusal of a cesarean section.
2. Id. at 1404–1413
3. Robertson J: The right to procreate and in utero fetal therapy. 3 J Legal Med 333–341, 1982
4. Robertson J: Toward rational boundaries of tort liability for injury to the unborn: Prenatal injuries, preconception injuries and wrongful life. Duke LJ 1401, 1405, 1978
5. Robertson, *supra* note 1, at 353–354
6. Robertson, *supra* note 2, at 357–359
7. Raleigh-Fitkin-Paul Morgan Memorial Hospital v. Anderson, 42 N.J. 421, 201 A. 2d 537 (1964)
8. 45 C.F.R. 46, 206(a) (2)
9. Jefferson v. Griffin Spalding County Hospital Authority, 247 Ga. 86, 274 S.E. 2d 457 (1981)
10. Grodin v. Grodin, 301 N.W. 2d 869 (Mich App. 1981)
11. Roe v. Wade, 410 U.S. 113 (1973)
12. Roe v. Wade, 410 U.S. 113, 165 (1973)

SECTION 6:
ETHICS IN EXPERIMENTAL FETAL THERAPY: IS THERE AN EARLY CONSENSUS?

John C. Fletcher

Modern fetal surgery, as prophetically reviewed by Adamsons,[1] began with Liley's[31] successful blood transfusion by needle into the peritoneal cavity of the fetus affected with erythroblastosis fetalis. Contemporary fetal therapy, still a very new field of medicine with a small number of cases, is mainly comprised of experimental treatments by surgery, drugs, and vitamins. The number of defects and conditions correctable before birth is slowly increasing, but the great majority of treatments are still deferred until after birth.[21,33] The near future will likely see attempts to correct genetic disorders prenatally.[26,41]

Experimental fetal therapy is the occasion for several significant ethical problems. The problems are listed here in terms of their actual appearance in the history of fetal therapy or in the literature, and not by order of the ethical significance of the questions involved:

- Do the risks and benefits of experimental fetal therapy require ethical consideration by prior group review?
- How should cases for experimental fetal therapy be selected?
- What is the optimal consent process for fetal therapy?
- Should experimental fetal surgery be attempted in multiple pregnancies?
- In cases of maternal refusal to allow proven fetal therapy, should the refusal be respected or overridden?

Other ethical issues are sometimes associated with the field of fetal therapy, for example, the ethics of using fetal tissues or organs after elective abortion as a source of therapy for others who will worsen or die without them,[19] or the ethics of fertilizing human embryos for research with the eventual clinical aim of diagnosis, embryo selection, or gene replacement therapy.[7] These issues are intrinsically interesting but do not arise in the field of fetal therapy itself. The fetus as a source of therapy after abortion is a different issue from that concerning the fetus as a fitting recipient of therapy. The issue of embryo research and eventual clinical applications is important but does not yet face practitioners and parents today.

This chapter addresses the immediate question of whether there is an early consensus among practitioners of experimental fetal therapy on their approach to the five problems previously listed. This discussion will be based upon four of the six meetings of the organizers of the International Society of Fetal Surgery and Medicine and the literature on ethical problems in fetal therapy. If experimental fetal therapy indeed leads to proven treatments at levels of acceptable risk to the pregnant woman and the fetus, it will be vital to recall the origins of the ethical standards which were adopted by its founders.

This chapter also addresses the long-term goal of a coherent approach to ethical problems in the three interdependent fields of fetal research, fetal diagnosis, and fetal therapy. The relations between these fields in the United States are now marred by inconsistent ethical premises and public policies that work against one another. The goal of this chapter is to lay groundwork for a long-term study of the evolution of ethics in the field of fetal therapy that will also be constructively related to fetal research and fetal diagnosis.

EVOLUTION OF A DOMINANT APPROACH

In the earliest stage of a new field in science or medicine, technical and ethical issues are intertwined and must be separated for analysis. Practitioners in the new field *can* perform new technical feats, but the question of whether they *ought* to do so must be answered from ethical, rather than technical, premises. The pattern in creating a new field is that clinical investigators take incremental steps by consensus-building in meetings as data and mistakes are analyzed and goals and limits are set, which can be altered on the basis of experience. This process is all contrary to the conventional view that in science and medicine "what can be done will be done." This popular view ignores the search for ethical principles and limits that has increasingly marked the biomedical sciences in the United States and other nations since the mid-1960s. However, deviation from the self-imposed limits defined by clinical investigators is a possibility and occurs.[27]

Beyond the earliest and most experimental stage of a new field lie the first clinical trials and the more familiar territory of research ethics.[3] No true clinical trials have yet been conducted in fetal therapy.

Even though successful technical approaches to medical problems can be proven, ethical objections still arise from a variety of cultural and religious standpoints. Gradually, as the new medical technology becomes accepted, a "dominant approach" to the ethical problems associated with it develops. The dominant approach, like the concept of consensus, is a descriptive rather than evaluative concept. *Dominance* describes the approach as it actually prevails in practice, not its ethical validity. The *dominant approach* is that set of moral beliefs, given the alternatives, that actually prevails in practice in a society. It is far too early, of course, for a dominant approach to the ethical problems of fetal therapy to have developed.

Adequate studies of practitioners and patients are required to describe the actual shape of ethical conflicts, the available options, and the prevailing morality. For example, careful studies[8,32] of the evolution of morality and public policy about abortion show a long-term trend in many societies to permit the pregnant woman's health and interests to transcend claims of a fetal right to life and equal treatment. To be sure, strong ethical objections have been made to the dominant approach to abortion choices,[23] and some of the ethical arguments that are widely used to support abortion are logically flawed and weak.[12] However, a prevailing morality about abortion can be clearly described in many societies. Also, the degree of consensus and variation in approaches to major ethical problems faced by medical geneticists in several nations has been studied.[18]

After clearly defining the ethical problems in a field, the first step in practical ethics is to answer the question, What is the dominant approach to the problems in practice today? The answer ought to be based on careful studies. A dominant approach truly may not exist, owing to the degree of controversy or the novelty of a particular problem. For example, in this country no dominant approach exists regarding surrogate motherhood, although in the United Kingdom it is dominantly held as ethically objectionable.[42] If significant practices have grown up around moral beliefs and distinct approaches to specific ethical problems have evolved, the outlines of a dominant approach may become quite clear. Then the analysis ought to proceed to the harder questions: Is this the best approach, ethically considered? Where will it lead in the long run?

EXPERIMENTAL FETAL THERAPY: AN EARLY CONSENSUS

The first national conference on fetal treatment met in July 1982 at Santa Ynez Valley, California. Discussion mainly focused on scientific and medical analyses of surgical treatment (by shunting) of congenital hydronephrosis and hydrocephalus. However, three of the five ethical problems I listed earlier were debated in the first meeting. A conference report was published[20] with tentative guidelines about these issues. In the 1983 meeting at Aspen, Colorado, the issue of prospective maternal refusal of proven fetal therapy was discussed and, with the exception of informed consent, each issue has been the subject of some discussion at each successive meeting. The discussion that follows will take up each problem in order.

Do the risks and benefits of experimental fetal therapy require ethical consideration by prior group review?

It is common to distinguish between innovative treatment and research.[30] *Innovative treatment* involves a previously untried maneuver done in the reasonable but unproven expectation that it may provide medical benefit, usually in a desperate situation. *Research* consists of techniques designed to gather and analyze information about a procedure, which may or may not be intended to benefit the subject, from which generalizable conclusions can be drawn.

Activities defined as research, if sponsored and supported by the federal government, are required to be reviewed by an Institutional Review Board (IRB) and to conform to all relevant federal regulations. Innovative treatment does not require IRB approval, but falls instead under the modes of surveillance and sanctions usually found in medical practice, such as peer review and malpractice.

Although the fetal therapy that has been carried out in the United States, Canada, the United Kingdom, and in Western Europe falls under the definition of innovative treatment, physicians have nonetheless taken the precaution to submit their plans in writing to an IRB or its equivalent for prior group review. Except for intrauterine transfusion for Rh-hemolytic disease, no other form of fetal therapy could be said to be proven. No true contemporary clinical trials have been conducted. For example, it is not known in a scientifically valid sense if fetal surgery for congenital hydronephrosis is actually better than postnatal treatment. Any study of this question would clearly be research and would require prior group review. However, physicians involved in fetal therapy have preferred, largely because of the risks involved, to review their plans for innovative treatment with an IRB (or its equivalent in other nations).

How should cases for experimental fetal therapy be selected?

Without the benefit of knowledge gained in controlled clinical trials, selection of cases for treatment has been, and remains, the most prevalent and difficult ethical problem in experimental fetal therapy. Which cases will benefit the most from prenatal treatment? The worst consequence of poor selection of cases is a surviving prenatally treated child who might have been better off dead, who lingers due to treatment in a half-way state between life and death.

Given the uncertainty of the earliest stage of fetal surgery, Duckett[9] opposed fetal intervention for *any* urologic anomaly. Hecht and Grix[22] pleaded for clarification of the indications for fetal shunting for hydrocephalus, pointing to its variable causes and poor outcome in one case due to X-linked aqueductal stenosis. From 1982 to 1987, the criteria for selection of cases for experimental surgery have been clarified but never completely agreed upon. As discussed in Chapter 15, Section 1, obstructive hydrocephalus and uropathies have been shunted and four attempts at in utero repair of diaphragmatic hernias have been attempted. While there have been scientific disagreements about the selection of particular cases, there has been little disagreement in the field about the ethical probity of attempts to correct these serious disorders.

What is the optimal consent process for fetal therapy?

Informed consent was discussed briefly at the first conference, but an optimal process was not described in the conference statement. The ethical problem of obtaining a valid informed consent in fetal therapy has been developed in other contexts.[15,17] Due to the possibility that some pregnant women may be prone to disregard their own well-being for the sake of the fetus, special precautions for the consent process were recommended:

- An impartial physician, uninvolved in the fetal medicine team, to "speak for" the fetus
- The mother's own physician, available at least by telephone, to help her reflect on the risks to her
- Involvement of other family members, especially the father, in the various stages of decision making
- Ethics consultation, on request, by physicians or parents
- Psychiatric consultation, on request of the physician, if marital problems or other emotional issues complicate the decision making

Should experimental fetal surgery be attempted in multiple pregnancies?

A controversial ethical question at the first conference was whether experimental surgery should be done in one affected twin when the other twin was presumed healthy. A discussion of the possible consequences ensued. In the absence of enough cases to assess the risks and benefits for even singleton pregnancies, it was deemed excessively risky to incur an added risk to a healthy twin.

The assembly failed to find any sound ethical grounds to answer hypothetical questions about why such risks were justified. Restraint from any experimental surgery in multiple pregnancy was to be the rule until experience proved that added risk was justified by added benefits.

Except for one case of surgery on an affected twin with hydrocephalus in Baltimore in 1986, physicians have exercised restraint in twin cases. Because of the better outcome in fetal surgery for congenital hydronephrosis, the 1985 meeting (Jasper, Canada) made an exception to include surgery on one twin for this condition.

In cases of maternal refusal to allow proven fetal therapy, should the refusal be respected or overridden?

At the 1983 Aspen fetal therapy conference, the major ethical and legal question addressed was what physicians ought to do in the event of a refusal of fetal therapy by the mother. Robertson, the first legal scholar to deal with this question, was a major speaker. Refusals of proven fetal therapy (e.g., for intrauterine transfusion for Rh-hemolytic

Table 15-6. Guidelines for Ethical Problems in Innovative Fetal Therapy (1982–1989)

A. Although many fetal abnormalities can be detected, most defects are best treated after birth.
B. The most difficult medical-ethical problem is to select only fetuses that can benefit from treatment. Intervention can be ethically justified only if there is a reasonable probability of benefit.
C. Criteria for selection of cases for treatment:
　1. Singleton fetus (except congenital hydronephrosis)
　2. No concomitant anomalies using level-II sonography and amniocentesis for karyotype, alpha-fetoprotein levels, and viral cultures
　3. Family fully counseled about risks and benefits
　4. Consent to treatment and long-term follow-up
　5. A multidisciplinary team—perinatal obstetrician, ultrasonographer, pediatric surgeon, and neonatologist—should concur on the plan for treatment approved by a duly constituted institutional review board (IRB)
　6. Access to a level-III high-risk obstetrical unit and neonatal ICU
　7. Access to bioethical and psychosocial consultation

disease) had not been reported but the possibility could not be discounted. Also, court-ordered interventions over refusals of cesarean section in two cases with diagnoses of placenta previa were widely viewed as possible precedents for similar actions in the context of fetal therapy.[5,24]

Drawing upon precedents of court-ordered cesarean sections and maternal blood transfusions to benefit the fetus, Robertson suggested that if these court-ordered actions are correct, then "the state may have a far reaching power to intrude on the mother's body and freedom of action for the benefit of the unborn child."[36] He did not take the position that intrusion is correct, or that it could ever be correct in any circumstances other than perhaps proven fetal therapy at very minimal risk to the woman.[34,35] But a question remains: Is it ethically correct to override a woman's refusal of fetal therapy? Is there any consensus on this question at present?

Since 1983, fetal-maternal conflicts and prospective maternal refusal of fetal therapy have been widely discussed in ethical and legal literature. There are three dimensions to the ethical issue of fetal-maternal conflicts:

1. The effect of technology on moral beliefs about fetal status
2. The justification for fetal therapy despite the refusal of the pregnant woman
3. The public policies needed to regulate what will likely be a small number of refusals

Will Technology Enhance Fetal Status?

Increased reporting of experimental fetal therapy leads me[13,14] to predict that the ability to treat the previable fetus with a correctable disorder will enhance the much-debated moral status of the fetus at that stage of gestation, because of the benefits to the fetus that could be brought about through treatment. With the improvement in fetal status brought about by technology, a much stronger ethical argument could be made for a duty to perform therapy.

Ruddick and Wilcox[39] have objected to what they believe to be the premise of this argument. They hold that because the fetus is not a person in the moral sense, the status of patient cannot be assigned except in the most provisional sense, and even this provision is contingent upon the woman's decision to do anything to help the fetus. Bosk[4] has analysed their objections in detail, noting that fetal therapy is not likely to change people's views on abortion. My original argument was less about the issue of personhood of the fetus than the effect that actual visualization and treatment of the fetus would have on its moral status. I predicted that the ethics of abortion and the ethics of fetal therapy would collide. Shinn[40] has pointed to my argument's speculative character, but has agreed that revisions of ethical perceptions could also occur in the case of the treatable fetus.

Premarternal Duty to Avoid Harm

Englehardt[11] and Callahan[6] each view technical developments in fetal therapy in the context of a more complex future, in which the moral status of the fetus cannot be set aside even while granting a wide sway for legally protected abortion decisions. Englehardt, as well as Robertson, has noted that "the very availability of abortion, perhaps paradoxically for some, has increased the plausibility of maternal duties to fetuses in that a woman's continuing with a pregnancy is more of an expression of free choice than was the case in the past." Robertson suggests that continuation of pregnancy, if abortion were widely available, implies that the woman has waived her right to an abortion.[36] Under such circumstances, if prenatal diagnosis reveals a disorder that is treatable by a proven technique with little risk to the woman, maternal refusal would involve a preventable harm, which could lead to sanctions either at the time or after birth. Robertson and Schulman[38] make a case for legal sanctions after birth for premartial failure to avoid harm (e.g., using a prescribed diet prior to and during pregnancy to avoid the harms of maternal phenylketonuria). Although they question the worth of a public policy option of incarceration and forced treatment of pregnant women who "are unlikely or unwilling to avoid the behavior that is damaging to offspring," they nonetheless show that such actions are within the power of the state and, given sufficient state interests, "there may be rare situations in which prenatal protection of offspring satisfies it, because the benefits to offspring clearly outweigh the burdens of the intrusion."[38]

On the other side of the question, Elias and Annas[10] argue that pregnant women have the legal and moral right to refuse all obstetric interventions involving any risk whatsoever, including fetal therapy, except those involving a slight risk (e.g., a drug that is 100% effective with no adverse maternal or fetal effects). Also, they hold that coerced treatments, even of a safe and effective drug, ought to occur only if the woman is mentally incompetent. Their ethical arguments are based primarily upon protecting the bodily integrity of the woman from unjustified intrusions. Their legal argument is that the concept advanced by Robertson of a waiver of abortion is unacceptable, since abortion may be legally exercised up to the time of birth, if needed to protect the life and health of the woman. Further, about half of the state legislatures have no restriction on abortion in the third trimester. Their constitutional argument is that court-ordered intrusions are a "state-erected penalty on her exercise of her right to bear a child." In a similar but even stronger vein, Johnson[25] argues that the autonomy of pregnant women is the absolute and final measure of any maternal-fetal conflict. She grants that a "general proposition that a pregnant woman has a moral obligation to her future child" exists; however, she denies that it follows that "we should, or even that we can, determine in any particular case that a woman has somehow violated that obligation." She opposes any legal sanctions or legal approaches to resolving maternal-fetal conflicts.

An ethical position that protects the woman's autonomy at all costs must face its responsibility for any harm that results. Is allowing such harm the necessary price to pay to protect the prevailing morality of reproductive liberty? After taking this position[16] and reflecting on its strengths and weaknesses, I now find that it runs too great a risk of moral absolutism by ruling out higher moral claims, especially the claim to avoid harm to a future child at small risk to the pregnant woman. The prevailing morality of virtually absolute parental autonomy must be reshaped whenever it results in avoidable harm to a child whose future life has been irrevocably chosen by its mother.[37] The primary ethical imperative of medicine is to do no harm and to prevent harm if at all possible. The harm caused to a future child by refusal of proven fetal therapy that carries a risk to the mother (but which is acceptable to a "reasonable pregnant woman" in good health) cannot be morally absolved, in my view, by appeal to the doctrine of informed consent. There is a moral duty of the pregnant woman and those who are her care providers to take reasonable actions to protect the health and future well-being of the child, assuming that she has chosen to continue the pregnancy. Clearly, women whose lives or health are threatened by continued pregnancies are ethically justified in ending the pregnancy at any point by abortion. However, the typical case of refused fetal therapy will be by women whose lives are not in danger from the pregnancy, but who disagree with the medical advice they have received and who desire to continue the pregnancy.

Englehardt[11] offers some useful criteria for selection of cases of justified intervention, as well as for societal compensation for intervention:

1. A duty to care for the fetus on the part of the woman must be established. This duty can be shown if
   – abortions are readily available,
   – the woman understands the circumstances, and
   – the woman decides to continue the pregnancy
2. The state must bear the cost of the intervention as well as the upbringing of a

defective child saved through such procedures.
3. There should be a high certainty of success from the procedure and a high probability of injury to the fetus in the absence of intervention.

To these criteria should be added that the risk of harm from the intervention to the pregnant woman should be no greater, considering probability and magnitude, than that incurred in routine obstetric care of pregnant women in good health. This criterion would permit an invasive procedure with minimal maternal risks, comparable to routine amniocentesis, and the administration of drugs, vitamins, or special diets with minimal or small risk to the mother and fetus. Infusion and transfusion of the fetus would also be permitted under this criterion. However, surgical procedures equivalent to hysterotomy under general anesthetic to permit fetal surgery, even if proven, are beyond the level of risk intended to be allowed by the term *routine*. General surgery, including cesarean section in the perinatal period, is not routine obstetric care. Maternal refusal of surgery, including cesarean section, should be respected out of concern to avoid serious bodily and psychological harm to the woman, even though harm to the future child cannot be avoided. Sharp limitations to the risk of bodily intrusions, if these are to be permitted over maternal refusals, should be set by society in the context of pregnancy.

Public Policy and Maternal Refusal of Fetal Therapy

Any public policy steps designed specifically to deal with maternal refusals of fetal therapy are ethically justified only if they rest on a deeper social commitment to deal with far greater injustices that cause far more harm to vastly greater numbers of children. Such commitment includes providing access to good prenatal care to all pregnant women, regardless of their ability to pay or insurability; expanded programs for prevention of low birthweight; expanded educational programs for young persons about reproduction, pregnancy, and childbirth; and expanded genetic services to families known to be at high genetic risk who cannot afford the services. To move independently towards public policies to deal with a relatively few maternal refusals of fetal therapy while ignoring these greater injustices is hypocritical. The results, as noted by Lantos,[29] are the same as those produced by the "Baby Doe" regulations.

The Ethics Committee of the American College of Obstetrics and Gynecology has recommended that physicians should rarely, if ever, resort to court actions for forced obstetric interventions.[2] Instead, in case of refusal, the physician should obtain consultation for the pregnant woman to help her reconsider the merits of the medical advice she has received. Every effort should be made to resolve the conflict by using medical, mental health, and bioethical consultation. In rare cases, the courts could be relied upon for help, but only after all attempts at conciliation have failed.

A recent study[28] shows that obstetricians in the United States do not generally exercise the recommended level of restraint and care in dealing with maternal refusals of obstetric interventions. The study received answers to a survey from 61 of 75 heads of fellowship programs in maternal-fetal medicine (80%) and 14 of 14 directors of divisions of maternal-fetal medicine, for a net response of 83%. Answers were received from 45 states and the District of Columbia. This important study showed that of 21 court orders sought for cesarean section (15), hospital detention (3), and intrauterine transfusion (3), a total of 18 had been successfully obtained. The survey also showed that 80% of the patients involved were minority and single women; 4 used English as a second language. Additionally, 46% of the respondents believed that women who refused beneficial treatments for the fetus should be forcibly detained in the hospital.

The women in this study who have been forced to receive treatment designed to benefit the fetus largely represent groups of women who, along with their children, already suffer harms from injustices presently tolerated by the United States health care system. Furthermore, if one compares actual practice to the ideas expressed by the professional society, the difference illustrates the lack of consensus among obstetricians about this important issue.

Any public policy steps or legislative sanctions about prematernal liability for avoidable harms ought to be taken in tandem with remedies for deeper wrongs. Meanwhile, the best policy for obstetricians to follow is to apply the recommendations of their own professional group fairly to all patients, regardless of their ability to pay for care, their marital status, race, or ethnic background.

REFERENCES

1. Adamsons K: Fetal surgery. N Engl J Med 275:204–205, 1966
2. American College of Obstetricians and Gynecologists: Press release: Court ordered treatment rarely justified for obstetrical care, August 11, 1987
3. Berg K, Tranøy KE: Research Ethics. New York, Alan R. Liss, 1983
4. Bosk CL: Sociomedical and ethical dilemmas in fetal medicine. In Milunksy A, GJ Annas: Genetics and the Law III, pp 381–382. New York, Plenum Press, 1985
5. Bowes WA, Selgestad B: Fetal versus maternal rights. Medical and legal perspectives. Obstet Gynecol 58:209–214, 1987
6. Callahan D: How technology is reframing the abortion debate. Hastings Cent Rep 16:33–42, Feb 1986
7. Ciba Foundation: Embryo Research. Yes or No. London, 1987
8. David HP, Friedman HL, van der Tak J, Sevilla MJ: Abortion in Psychosocial Perspective. Trends in Transnational Research. New York, Springer, 1978
9. Duckett JW: Fetal intervention for obstructive uropathy. Dialogues Pediatr Urol 5:8, 1982
10. Elias S, Annas GJ: Reproductive Genetics and the Law. Chicago, Year Book Medical Publishers, 1987
11. Englehardt HT: Current controversies in obstetrics: Wrongful life and forced fetal surgical procedures. Am J Obstet Gynecol 151:313–318, 1985
12. Fleming L: The moral status of the fetus: A reappraisal. Bioethics 1:15–34, 1987
13. Fletcher JC: The fetus as patient: Ethical issues. JAMA 246:772–773, 1981
14. Fletcher JC: Ethics and trends in applied human genetics. Birth Defects 19:143–158, 1983
15. Fletcher JC: Ethical considerations in and beyond experimental fetal therapy. Semin Perinatol 9:130–135, 1985
16. Fletcher JC: Drawing moral lines in fetal therapy. Clin Obstet Gynecol 29:595–602, 1986
17. Fletcher JC, Jonsen AR: Ethical considerations of fetal surgery. In Harrison MR, Golbus MS, Filly RA (eds): Unborn Patient, pp 159–170. Orlando, FL, Grune & Stratton, 1984
18. Fletcher JC, Wertz DC, Sorenson JR, Berg K: Ethics and human genetics. A cross-cultural study in 17 nations. In Vogel F, Sperling K: Human Genetics. Heidelberg, Springer-Verlag (in press)
19. Harrison MR: Organ procurement for children: The anencephalic fetus as donor. Lancet 2:1383–1386, Dec 1986
20. Harrison MR, Filly RA, Golbus MS et al: Fetal treatment. N Engl J Med 307:1651–1652, 1982
21. Harrison MR, Golbus MS, Filly RA (eds): Unborn Patient, 2nd ed. Orlando, FL, Grune & Stratton (in press)
22. Hecht F, Grix A: Treatment of fetal hydrocephalus. N Engl J Med 307:1211, 1982
23. Hilgers TW, Horan DJ, Mall D: New Perspectives on Human Abortion. Frederick, MD, University Publications of America, 1981
24. Jefferson v. Griffin Spaulding County Hospital Authority et al.: West's Reporter 274 SE 2nd 457 (1982)
25. Johnson D: A new threat to pregnant women's autonomy. Hastings Cent Rep 17:33–40, 1987
26. Kantoff PW, Flake AW, Eglitis MA et al: In utero gene transfer and expression: A sheep transplantation model. Nature (in press)
27. Kolata GB, Wade N: Human gene treatment stirs new debate. Science 210:407–408, 1980
28. Kolder VEB, Gallagher J, Parsons MT: Court-ordered obstetrical interventions. N Engl J Med 316:1192–1197, 1987
29. Lantos J: Baby Doe five years later. Implications for child health. N Engl J Med 317:444–447, 1987
30. Levine RJ: Ethics and Regulation of Clinical Research, 2nd ed. Baltimore, Urban and Schwarzenberg, 1986
31. Liley AW: Intrauterine transfusion of foetus

in haemolytic disease. Br Med J 2:1107–1109, 1963
32. Luker K: The Politics of Motherhood. Berkeley, University of California, 1984
33. Pringle KC: In utero surgery. Adv Surg 19:101–138, 1986
34. Robertson JA: The right to procreate and in utero fetal therapy. J Legal Med 3:333–341, 1982
35. Robertson JA: Procreative liberty, and the control of conception, pregnancy, and childbirth. Va Law Rev 441–457, 1983
36. Robertson JA: Legal issues in fetal therapy. Semin Perinatol 9:140–145, 1985
37. Robertson JA: Personal communication, October 7, 1986
38. Robertson JA, Schulman JD: Pregnancy and prenatal harm to offspring: The case of mothers with PKU. Hastings Cent Rep 17:23–32, 1987
39. Ruddick W, Wilcox W: Operating on the fetus. Hastings Cent Rep 12:10–14, 1982
40. Shinn RL: The fetus as patient. A philosophical and ethical perspective. In Milunsky A, Annas GJ: Genetics and the Law III, pp 317–324. New York, Plenum Press, 1985
41. Simpson TJ, Golbus MS: In utero fetal hematopoietic stem cell transplantation. Semin Perinatol 9:68–74, 1985
42. United Kingdom, Department of Health and Social Security: Report of the Committee of Inquiry into Human Fertility and Embryology (Chairman, Mary Warnock). London, Her Majesty's Stationery Office, July 1984

PART VI
FATE OF FETUSES

16

Federal Regulations for Fetal Research: A Case for Reform

John C. Fletcher and

Kenneth J. Ryan

Human fetal research is controversial for at least five reasons. Paramount are fears of harm to the fetus, especially if the research is nontherapeutic, that is, intended to increase biomedical knowledge but not to benefit the fetus involved. Second, when the research is performed in anticipation of, or at the time of, an induced abortion, societal conflicts over the abortion itself add to the controversy. There is conflict over whether a fertilized egg (a pre-implantation embryo), the embryo, or the fetus in advanced stages of development ought to have the same or a different moral status. Even the selection of terms to describe the fetus at its various stages may be used as metaphors to sway emotions on the issue. Third, it is not always apparent to the public why research is needed or desirable. Fourth, research directly involves the prospective mother and perhaps the prospective father. Fifth, the risks of fetal research are difficult to ascertain. Because the fetus is susceptible to environmental factors during development and natural loss is often due to genetic and teratogenic factors, it is difficult to sort out the added risk of research intervention.

In 1974 the National Commission for the Protection of Human Subjects of Biomedical and Behavioral Research considered many aspects of fetal research. The commission received some detailed ethical, legal, and scientific analyses, invited public testimony, and recommended guidance for biomedical research involving the human fetus.[1] One of the authors (KJR) chaired the commission. Many of its recommendations became federal regulations on fetal research issued in 1975 and bear on research "conducted by the Department of Health and Human Services (DHHS) or funded in whole or in part by a Department grant, contract, cooperative agreement or fellowship."[2]

Baron's[3] legal review observed that fetal

research not funded by DHHS is not subject to these regulations. But he rightly noted that the regulations affect federally funded institutions regardless of the source of funds for fetal research. These institutions must obtain an assurance approved by DHHS that includes "a statement of principles governing the institution in discharge of its responsibilities for protecting the rights and welfare of human subjects of research conducted at or sponsored by the institution, regardless of the source of funding."[4] Institutional statements follow the requirements of federal regulations on fetal research. If alleged violations in fetal research supported by private funds occurred in a DHHS-funded institution, the issues would doubtless be examined within the scope of the federal regulations.

These regulations have been in effect for more than a decade. Little if any federally supported nontherapeutic research has occurred, although the regulations permit it within careful limits. However, during this period practical access to the fetus sharply increased. Ultrasonography, early prenatal diagnosis, and in vitro fertilization (IVF) were as yet undeveloped in the early 1970s. Proposals to use technology in new ways involving the fetus include developments in fetal diagnosis and treatment, therapeutic uses of donated fetal tissues and organs, and the prospect of studies involving the pre-implantation human embryo. These advances call for a review of the regulations. The concepts of *minimal risk* and *no discernible risk*, which played such an important part in the commission's recommendations, also need to be examined in the light of recent knowledge gained about the fetus and pregnant woman. Any system of ethical guidance ought to be evaluated in the light of changes in medical science and the evolution of public attitudes about the issues.

This chapter concentrates mainly on research that seeks new biological knowledge or that is done in observational and investigative stages prior to a trial of a new mode of diagnosis or therapy for the fetus or pregnant woman. The regulations define the fetus as "the product of conception from the time of implantation (through any of the presumptive signs of pregnancy, such as missed menses, or by a medically acceptable pregnancy test), until expulsion or extraction of the fetus."[5] By this definition, the pre-implantation embryo is not considered a fetus. However, scientific and ethical concepts of fetal research must not be artificially separated from research in embryology, human reproduction, or perinatal medicine. Society's goal should be a set of public policies, ethically and procedurally coherent, that allow federal support of needed research and also protect from undue risks, from fertilization to birth, the fetal-maternal dyad, (i.e., the human embryo before and after implantation, the pregnant woman, the developing fetus in or out of the uterus, and the infant in the perinatal period). An excellent forum for study, debate, and recommendations on these necessarily related policies is the Congressional Biomedical Ethics Board and its Biomedical Ethics Advisory Committee, established by the Health Research Extension Act of 1985. One of the board's mandates is to "conduct a study of the nature, advisability, and biomedical and ethical implications of exercising any waiver of the risk standard published in section 46.102 (g) of such part 46 (or any successor) to such regulations."[6]

The first half of this chapter reviews ethical concerns leading to the regulations, describes the main features of the regulations, and summarizes the activities of the Ethics Advisory Board. The second half discusses four needed changes. Two are changes needed to develop new, workable regulations to allow appropriate research as originally intended; two are changes needed in the existing regulations. The regulations, which include a ban on federal funding of research involving IVF, need the following:

- Restoration of an Ethics Advisory Board to advise the DHHS Secretary on applications of scientific and social merit that raise significant ethical questions, and the lifting of the ban on IVF research
- Implementation as originally intended to balance two complex ethical obligations: (1) protection of the fetus, whatever its life chances, from exploitation in research; and

- (2) promotion of socially desirable research
- Amending to permit an increment of higher risk in nontherapeutic research involving first-trimester fetuses
- Amending to clarify the definition of *minimal risk,* which now lacks a frame of reference by which it may be applied to the fetal-maternal dyad

WHY FEDERAL REGULATIONS FOR FETAL RESEARCH?

Before federal regulations were adopted, a major ethical concern was to protect the fetus from harm. However, the change in abortion laws made abortion itself an issue. Fetal research was attacked for the perceived role that it might play in fostering abortion by creating a demand for research material. There was a strong moral perception that fetal research was wrong until proven right by the researchers who desired to do it.

Some objectionable fetal research did exist. The clearest examples involved studies of nonviable but still living fetuses obtained after hysterotomy abortions. A study in the United States in 1963 attempted to learn if oxygen could be provided through the skin to fifteen fetuses while each was immersed in salt solution.[7] One fetus survived for 22 hours. The experiment yielded knowledge relevant to artificial life support for premature infants. Later, researchers in Finland perfused (separated) the heads of eight fetuses after hysterotomy abortions to learn if the fetal brain could metabolize ketone bodies.[8] This study confirmed findings in animal research obtainable from the human fetus by no other method. Also controversial were pharmacologic experiments done before elective abortion to study drug effects in fetal tissues examined in the abortus. Such experiments knowingly inflict harm to fetuses to gain biomedical knowledge that does, in fact, improve treatment for intrauterine infection.

Ramsey,[9] Maynard-Moody,[10] and others[11] chronicled events before 1973 that propelled public and congressional debate about fetal research. Between 1970 and 1972, advisory groups within the National Institute of Child Health and Human Development (NICHD) debated and shaped policy to review and fund fetal research by the National Institutes of Health (NIH). The NIH discussions were reported concurrently with stories of abuses by Scandinavian researchers on live, postabortion fetuses.[12]

On January 22, 1973, the U.S. Supreme Court struck down all state laws prohibiting abortion in the first two trimesters.[13] Public and congressional concern arose in the wake of the decision that fetuses to be aborted would be exploited for research purposes and that abortions would be opportunistically encouraged for research. Following a public demonstration at the NIH in April 1973, officials declared a moratorium on any research with the living fetus before or after abortion.[14]

In 1974 Congress created the National Commission for the Protection of Human Subjects of Biomedical and Behavioral Research. The first of the commission's several mandates was to recommend guidelines for fetal research. The law authorizing the commission[15] continued a ban of fetal research, except to assure the survival of a fetus, until the commission made its recommendations. President Nixon signed this bill on July 12, 1974, and Secretary of Health, Education, and Welfare Weinberger administered the oath to the 11-member group on December 3. Congress gave the commission a deadline of *four months* for recommendations on fetal research. This short timetable reflected the emotionally polarized state of the issue. The commission responded with recommendations,[1] and many were included in federal regulations adopted on July 29, 1975.

The commission commenced with studies of reports by other groups on the problem of protecting the fetus in research regardless of the method of its delivery. In 1972 the British government had authorized an Advisory Group on the Use of Fetuses and Fetal Material for Research, which published its report in May 1972.[16] It recommended that nontherapeutic research be permitted on fetuses to be aborted that weighed less than 300 g, conditional on prior group review and the separation of researchers from medical attendants at abortion. The report cited the study of transfer of substances across the placenta, the reaction of the immature fetus to drugs, and endocrinologic and placental development as examples of important research. The report condemned as "unethical" experiments based on the "deliberate intent" of administering drugs prior to abortion to learn whether the drugs are harmful to the fetus.

Commissioners also examined an NIH proposal to protect vulnerable human subjects, including the human fetus.[17] This document strongly defended equal protection of the fetus to be aborted and explained the health benefits for pregnant women and children derived from continued research with the nonviable human fetus. The commission also received several legal, scientific, and ethical analyses of fetal research that were of outstanding quality. Some of these reports are cited below.[18]

SUBSTANTIVE AND PROCEDURAL ETHICAL ISSUES

Five substantive and procedural ethical issues were debated at length by the commission. The first, third, and fifth issues are most germane to this discussion:

1. What is the soundest ethical reasoning from which to approach fetal research?
2. Does the human fetus in research deserve equal protection with children and other human subjects?
3. Do human fetuses to be aborted deserve as much protection in research as fetuses to be delivered?
4. Who can give a morally valid consent to fetal research?
5. In a society with widely divergent views on the moral status of the fetus, what kind of decision-making process is best to consider specific projects with experimental risks to fetuses to be aborted?

The commission explored alternative approaches to the first question, reconstructed here with the aid of analogies recently coined by Albert Jonsen, a member of the commission.[19]

Basic ethical reasoning about fetal research usually takes one of three general forms. First, one can appeal to benefits to be sought for society, for other fetuses at risk, and for pregnant women. One can argue that if abortion is to occur, which results in death irrespective of the research, then research in the fetus can be morally justified if it does not add to pain or suffering of the fetus. An additional reason is the psychological benefit to the woman of some additional gain to society in the context of the abortion event. Writers such as Lappe, Gaylin, and Joseph Fletcher took this position at the time.[20] Their view of fetal research was the most permissive. The most relevant analogy for this view would be that fetal research is like an autopsy given with permission of the family. No moral guilt should be felt about an autopsy, since its purpose is entirely to promote medical knowledge. Autopsies can be performed with attention to the sensitivities of the family.

A second view, the most restrictive, is based on the belief that most abortions in our society are morally objectionable. This view holds that no one, especially not she who makes a decision to destroy the fetus, can ethically give proxy consent for a fetus to nontherapeutic research. In this view, fetal research, except to save the life of the distressed fetus, cooperates in the immorality of abortion and violates the consent rules of human experimentation. The analogy used in this view is that fetal research is like experiments on condemned prisoners, which may involve coerciveness, cruelty, and injury. Fetal research is morally worse, however, because prisoners deserve punishment but fetuses are innocent victims of research. Ramsey and Louisell, among others, took this position.[21]

Many commission members adopted a third position: fetal research (in association with induced abortion) was morally problematic as was experimental chemotherapy in cancer patients, especially in those who were near death. Phase I trials with desperately ill or dying cancer patients can involve pressure bordering on coercion, great risks, and even death caused by research. Above all, such patients must not be exploited in research. In the ethos of that period, the commission members approached fetal research with two goals in mind. Both goals amounted to negative duties and were very difficult to reconcile. The recommendations are framed between a duty not to exploit the fetus unfairly in research and a duty not to unfairly restrict research. The consensus achieved by the commission did not relinquish either side of this issue and emphasized the procedures to maintain this balance.

The commission found help to support both sides of this view in writings by McCormick and Walters.[22] McCormick stressed that conventional moral reasoning that balanced social benefits against the risks to the fetus could not avoid a "utilitarian" premise that subjugated the individual to the collective. He recommended that the commission ground its reasoning in reflection on proxy consent. McCormick modified and broadened a natural law position, previously taken against Ramsey, explaining why it is ethically acceptable for others (including parents) to give proxy consent for children (and by extension for fetuses in some morally acceptable abortions) to nontherapeutic research—namely, because human beings can be observed to want to save others' lives and to participate in efforts to do so within the limits of "no discernible risk or undue discomfort."[23] Reasoning from this premise, McCormick found it acceptable for parents to give proxy consent for children and for fetuses for research that the subjects *ought* to want to do for others simply "because we are members of the human community."[24]

McCormick opposed linking the research enterprise in "cooperation" with most abortions as presently permitted by society. But he argued that in principle the ethics of therapeutic and nontherapeutic research could be extended from children to fetuses. If one is not pressed to accept the natural law premises in his argument, McCormick's thought based limited fetal research in societal benefits and relieved much of the moral onus that fetal research had been construed to carry.

Walters[25] stressed the equality principle for moral reasoning about fetal research. With McCormick, he saw the ethics of fetal research to be properly an extension of the ethics of research with children. The fulcrum of Walters' position, however, was that the moral line for permissible research ought to be drawn on the side of what one would do or would not do with wanted fetuses to be delivered, since the quality of proxy consent to nontherapeutic research is suspect in the context of a decision to abort. Walters advised the commission that it was possible to "skirt these difficult problems" and "to be ethically consistent" [p. 8–8] by adopting a rule to carry out only research procedures on the fetus to be aborted that one would do with the fetus to be carried to term. He noted that any policy based on the equality principle would be "formal and therefore flexible; it does not prohibit any particular research procedure but establishes a general test which all proposed procedures would be required to meet" [p. 8–10]. Practically, researchers were to act as if the woman's decision to abort the fetus did not alter its moral status in research. In the context of the cancer analogy used above, Walters' position was that the imminent death of a cancer patient is not a morally justifiable reason for taking excessive risks in nontherapeutic research. One ought to treat cancer patients in a similar manner in research despite their proximity to or distance from death. Similarly, the abortion decision was not a pretext to allow higher risks than one would take if the fetus were wanted and expected to live to delivery.

The social basis of McCormick's position and the equality principle as argued by Walters helped the commission take a position favoring fetal research that was formally independent from reasoning about abortion. The commission was clear about its intent to protect the fetus in research on the same level as any other human subject, including the fetus to be aborted. However, the application of the equality principle was a source of discussion. The commission's most controverted issue was the meaning of equal protection in nontherapeutic research with fetuses to be aborted. Most members favored a policy in which, if the research carried some risk but was acceptable to offer to fetuses to be carried to term, initial studies could be offered selectively to fetuses scheduled for abortion. But not all commissioners agreed. For example, if the research involved learning a new procedure in prenatal diagnosis that carries a risk of fetal loss, should one *begin* to learn equally with both classes of fetuses or only with those to be aborted? The commission's report[1] admitted this moral dilemma and left it unresolved with the further potential of national review. The report stated:

> There is basic agreement among commission members as to the validity of the equality principle. There is disagreement as to its application to individual fetuses and classes of fetuses. Anticipating that differences of interpretation will arise over the application of the basic principles of equality and the determination of "minimal risk," the commission recommends review at the national level . . . the appropriate forum for determination of the scientific and public merit of such research. In addition, such review would facilitate public discussion of the sensitive issues surrounding the use of vulnerable nonconsenting subjects in research. [p. 67]

Commissioners knew that conflicts would arise between the obligation to benefit individuals and society by fetal research and the difficulty of practical application of equality to all fetuses. They framed a system of institutional controls with interaction between local and national levels to resolve such conflicts in specific proposals. An already intact system of independent, local institutional review boards (IRBs) was expected to interact with a national Ethics Advisory Board as *necessary* to maintain the complex moral tension in public policy on fetal research.

RECOMMENDATIONS AND RESTRICTIONS

The commission, with one notable dissent by David Louisell on categories 4 and 5, encouraged federal support of six categories of fetal research, conditional on IRB approval, informed consent of the mother, and the lack of objection from the father. The following illustrates the types of research permitted by the regulations:

1. *Therapeutic research directed toward the fetus,* within appropriate medical standards.
2. *Therapeutic research directed toward the pregnant woman,* provided the research imposes minimal risk or no risk to the fetus; altered in the regulations to "fetus will be placed at risk only to the minimum extent necessary to meet" the health needs of the mother [46.207 (a) (1)].
3. *Nontherapeutic research directed toward the pregnant woman,* if the risk to the fetus is minimal.
4. *Nontherapeutic research directed toward the fetus in utero* either: (a) not anticipating abortion, if risk to the fetus is minimal and the knowledge is unobtainable by other means; or (b) anticipating abortion, if risk to the fetus is minimal. Approval of a national ethical review body was required if such research presents "special problems related to the interpretation or application of these guidelines."
5. *Nontherapeutic research directed toward the fetus during the abortion procedure and nontherapeutic research directed toward the nonviable fetus ex utero,* provided that the fetus is less than 20 weeks gestational age, no significant changes in the interest of research alone are introduced into the abortion procedure, and no attempt is made to alter the duration of the life of the fetus. As in category 4, if problems arise about the interpretation of *minimal* or *added risk,* the proposal requires the approval of a national ethical review body.
6. *Research directed toward the possibly viable fetus,* provided that no additional risk to the infant will be imposed by the research and that knowledge is unobtainable by other means.

Federal regulations do not prevent any research conducted with the dead fetus but specify that such research shall be conducted in accordance with state or local laws pertaining to such activities [46.210].

Except for the removal of the 20-weeks gestational age provision in category 5 and minor rewordings, existing federal regulations still embody these key elements, except that the terms *therapeutic* and *nontherapeutic* are not used. Instead, they describe activities to "meet the health of the particular fetus" or "the development of biomedical knowledge which cannot be obtained by other means."

Neither the commission's recommendations nor the regulations defined *minimal risk* specifically for fetal research. A specific definition of *minimal risk* in children's research was developed by the commission in 1975:

> "Minimal risk" means that the risks of harm anticipated in the proposed research are not greater, considering probability and magnitude, than those ordinarily encountered in daily life or during the performance of routine medical or psychological examinations or tests, of healthy children.

In the fetal regulations, the frame of reference phrase, "of healthy children," was omitted, and "physical" substituted for "medical" tests [45 CFR 46. 102 (g)].

THE ETHICS ADVISORY BOARD

The 1975 regulations also required that proposals for IVF be reviewed by an Ethics Advisory Board (EAB), which, among other duties, would advise the Secretary of the Department of Health, Education, and Welfare (DHEW) on their acceptability. An EAB was not chartered until 1977 and not convened until 1978. Thus, a de facto moratorium on federal support continued for nontherapeutic fetal research and on IVF.

In 1977, the NIH received an application for support of IVF research, which was approved by a study section. In May 1978, the EAB agreed to review the proposal. The EAB published its recommendations[26] and forwarded them to the DHEW Secretary in May 1979. The EAB recommended support of research on IVF and embryo transfer to study the safety and efficacy of the technique when used for the treatment of infertility. Conditions included IRB approval, informed consent, a 14-day cutoff to study embryos in vitro, provided that gametes be obtained only from lawfully married couples. These recommendations have yet to be approved by a subsequent DHHS Secretary, and no federal support of IVF research has yet been permitted.

The EAB reviewed only one proposal for fetal research. In 1978, investigators from the Charles R. Drew Postgraduate Medical School proposed to assess the safety of fetoscopy for prenatal diagnosis of hemoglobinopathies in pregnancies of women who had elected abortions for reasons unrelated to the research. Working with data obtained from the earliest use of fetoscopy in the United States, the EAB evaluated a proposal in which the risk of fetal loss was estimated to be at least 5% but was essentially unknown. The EAB did not insist on a rigorous application of the equality principle in this case. Because of the importance of the biomedical information, unobtainable by any other method, the EAB recommended a waiver of provisions of the regulations involving minimal risk.[27] The EAB also stipulated that the timing of the planned abortions was not to be altered by the research. DHEW Secretary Califano granted a waiver for this single research project in September 1979, shortly before his resignation, but took no action on an EAB recommendation of a generic waiver for fetoscopy studies.

CONSEQUENCES OF NO ETHICS ADVISORY BOARD

DHHS Secretary Harris allowed the EAB to lapse when its charter and funding expired on September 30, 1980. Many unfortunate consequences followed. First, applications to DHHS for support of fetal research were discouraged. Aware that no EAB existed, researchers did not apply, preferring to rely on institutional funds or patient fees to support fetal studies.

A review of NICHD grants in 1984–1985 confirmed that U.S. researchers essentially stopped requesting federal support for any fetal research that raised questions about risk. NICHD is the primary source of federal support for fetal research. A review of 183 research projects on high-risk pregnancies and fetal pathophysiology supported by NICHD showed that other than two studies employing ultrasound and one study with antibiotic therapy, no studies even approached the threshold of minimal risk.[28] One study evaluated ultrasound as a predictive test for respiratory distress syndrome following delivery; a second used ultrasound to study fetal heart, lung, and other functions to determine effects of smoking in pregnancy. The antibiotic study was to answer the question of whether infections in the genitourinary tract cause premature labor. Pregnant women with any of three bacterial organisms (but no other symptoms) were given either an antibiotic or a placebo until the 38th week of pregnancy or delivery, whichever occurred first. The effect of treatment on prematurity and the infant's health would be determined.

The second serious consequence of the lapsing of the EAB is that no national process exists to maintain the complex moral tension desired by the commission. Only local review of fetal research now occurs. IRBs are not by design or law the forum to deliberate on the long-range ethical implications of research. No continuing body maintains continuity with the work of the commission or evaluates the ethical cogency of the regulations to contemporary fetal research. Nationally, fetal research is bereft of rigorous ethical and scientific consideration and subjected mainly to continuing congressional scrutiny and political assessment. Consequently, the public, broadly considered, is excluded form participation in ongoing evaluation of an area of research in which there has been much public interest.

Third, funding for fetal research and IVF has been bifurcated. Research with some risk to the fetus or mother is supported in the private realm, but it may not receive optimal scientific or ethical peer review. A small amount of very safe fetal research is federally supported. This double standard of support and review does not exist in any other area of biomedical research. Who loses the most in this situation? Families at higher genetic risk, fetuses at higher risk, pregnant women, and infertile persons are being deprived of the potential benefits of research on problems that affect their life chances. Federal funds for research that would be permitted by regulations and recommendations of an EAB are now blocked by the lack of a means to consider new proposals. We give examples in the next section.

Fourth, because of the social distance between local and national levels created by the lack of an EAB, many researchers mistakenly believe that the regulations prohibit most fetal research. An example is given below.

RESEARCH IN FETAL DIAGNOSIS AND TREATMENT

A balance has not been maintained between the moral tensions desired by the commission. In federally funded research, except for one fetoscopy project, the fetus to be aborted has been shielded from research risks. But little research of significance has occurred prior to introduction into clinical practice of new techniques in fetal diagnosis and treatment. The same situation prevails in the treatment of infertility by IVF and embryo transfer. Alternative approaches to infertility are not rigorously evaluated in scientifically controlled trials. Thus, patients are being placed at higher risk, and physicians are unable to inform them adequately about such risks. Here are some examples of research conducted without federal support:

Prenatal Diagnosis

The most significant advance since amniocentesis is chorionic villus sampling (CVS). CVS is a first-trimester procedure to obtain fetal cells for study and diagnosis. The procedure may be done transcervically or transabdominally. In 1982–1983, with the approval of local IRBs, physicians in the United States brought CVS through an early research stage into the first phase of clinical practice without any federal support. Questions needed to be answered about whether the cells obtained were genetically identical to those of the fetus and what the complications of CVS were for the pregnant woman and the fetus. A few investigators in states with laws banning any nontherapeutic research on the fetus to be aborted used cases of blighted ovum in the earliest studies. However, most initial feasibility studies obtained villi for diagnosis in the context of elective abortions. Women who had decided on first-trimester abortions were asked to participate in the research only after the abortion procedure had been scheduled. We have no record of IRB discussions of research risks to these fetuses to be aborted or about the frame of reference used to discuss such risks. No report in the literature attempts to justify such research as meeting the test of minimal risk. Any application for federal funds would have required EAB review because CVS was nontherapeutic research with a risk of added fetal loss and maternal complications that clearly exceeded minimal risk.

The equality test was not rigorously applied by IRBs to these feasibility studies. To do so would have required randomizing the procedure in a series of wanted pregnancies at higher risk for chromosomal abnormalities due to maternal age and pregnancies to be ended by first-trimester elective abortion. In fact, the unknown risks of research with CVS at this stage were selectively assigned to pregnancies before abortion. If the aim was to prevent unknown added risks of fetal loss in continuing pregnancies, the IRBs took the correct approach. However, this strategy raises serious questions about the cogency of the equality argument. The same problem would arise in studying the feasibility of any new approach to prenatal diagnosis.

If an EAB had been able to advise on an application to DHHS to fund a CVS feasibility study, how would it have evaluated the risks of CVS to the fetus to be aborted and the value of the information to be gained? Data were scanty in the United States at the time, but publications about use in diagnostic cases were available from China,[29] the Soviet Union,[30] Great Britain,[31] and Italy.[32] At this stage of development, CVS would have added a 2% to 5% risk of fetal loss to the natural risks of spontaneous abortion. At week 10 of pregnancy, the risk of natural loss is about 6% for an under-30 age group. If the frame of reference was that risks of harm of experimental CVS are not to be greater than those ordinarily encountered in the daily life of wanted fetuses (at this stage) to be delivered, then CVS research clearly posed greater than minimal risk. However, the risk of fetal loss was probably well below what a previous EAB had approved in fetoscopy research. An EAB recommendation for DHHS Secretarial waiver would have been based on the prospect of an earlier, safer method of prenatal diagnosis to benefit the health of pregnant women in the future and to enable more wanted pregnancies at higher genetic risk to be saved. Another significant consideration would have been the likelihood that earlier prenatal diagnosis could lead to more effective fetal therapy.

In tandem with a request for a waiver of the requirement for minimal risk for CVS feasibility studies, an EAB could have also recommended an *early* randomized clinical trial comparing the safety and efficacy of CVS and amniocentesis that could have partially satisfied the equality argument.[33] Such a trial did not occur in the United States, not the least because the climate for support for such trials by federal funds is hostile. In the mid-1970s, NICHD supported the costs of a case-controlled study of the safety and efficacy of aminocentesis. Federal funds did not reimburse the cost of the procedures but only paid for data collection. Similarly, through a cooperative agreement, NICHD is now supporting only the costs of data collection in a seven-center comparative study of the safety and accuracy of CVS and amniocentesis.[34] The trial began in 1985, many months after CVS was being used clinically. Researchers attempted to use randomization in the trial but failed. Almost all women who were offered randomization objected. Little can be done to persuade patients to accept randomization when patients already have a strong bias for CVS and when they pay for the procedures. Randomized trials in pregnancy are more accepted in societies with national health insurance and lines of authority between scientific expertise and reimbursement decisions. Our point is that randomization, if used in a timely manner, is needed for the best approach to health policy. Randomization also distributes the research risks equitably. Randomized trials are currently underway in Canada and Denmark.[35] However, this means that CVS research in the United States is suboptimal and that research risks are unfairly distributed across international lines.

Fetal Therapy

Since the early 1980s, some significant developments have occurred in fetal therapy. These include surgical management of fetal urinary tract obstruction, diagnosis and management of fetal hydrocephalus, treatment of immune and nonimmune hydrops, and selected medical and pharmacologic treatments of alterable states of fetal distress.[36] Other than one case of experimental fetal therapy for congenital adrenal hyperplasia,[37] the federal role in research on fetal therapy has been minimal. Initial plans for innovative fetal therapy have been approved by local IRBs but are financially supported by the institution or patient fees. Even though the regulations clearly permit this research, physicians perceive that seeking federal support for fetal research that entails significant risks is counterproductive, especially when there is no EAB to advise the DHHS Secretary on the ethical implications of experimental fetal therapy.

Support has not been requested for research in fetal therapy or for an early controlled clinical trial to compare the consequences of prenatal with postnatal treatment of fetal disorders. Fetal therapy is in an embryonic state, but it is not too early to answer some questions about its efficacy.

Transplantations of Fetal Tissues, Cells, and Organs

More investigative research is required to learn whether transplantations of fetal tissues, cells, and organs are modes of therapy for infants, children, and adults who will die unless treated. Some research involving fetal neuronal grafts in monkeys with chemically induced Parkinsonianism[38] has been reported; together with other animal data,[39] it suggests that fetal nerve cell transplantation might be a source of treatment for Parkinson's disease in humans. Hematopoetic stem cells from the liver of fetal donors have already been used to treat genetic diseases and radiation sickness.[40] Fetal organ transplantations, especially involving the anencephalic fetus diagnosed and delivered with an intent to donate organs, might be a life-saving source of therapy for infants and children dying of heart, liver, or kidney diseases.[41]

The regulations appear to restrict neither fetal tissue or cell transplants from abortuses nor transplants from anencephalic fetuses delivered with the intent of organ donation if (1) tissues and organs are obtained from fetuses after death has occurred and in accordance with state law, and (2) the fetus is considered a donor of cells or organs and not a research subject. The recipient of the cells or organs is properly the subject of the experiment. Donation should be based on a morally valid consent by parent(s) as required by the regulations and by the Uniform Anatomical Gift Act, which has been enacted by each state.[42]

If researchers acted prior to fetal death to obtain cells, tissues, or organs, they would violate regulations pertaining to the nonviable fetus ex utero that prohibit "experimental activities which of themselves would terminate the heartbeat or respiration of the fetus" [45 CFR 46. 209 (b) (2)].

We find that those developing these lines of research in animals widely believe that any involvement of human fetuses as donors of tissues, cells, or organs is viewed as unethical by federal authorities and prohibited by federal regulations. Their misunderstanding could have arisen because of the lack of a EAB to which such concerns could be directed for clarification. In fact, the regulations do not prohibit such research with human fetal tissues or organs, as long as the conditions cited above are met.

In Vitro Fertilization

Medically assisted fertilization by IVF and embryo transfer has resulted in the births of approximately 5000 infants around the world. More than 200 IVF programs have been established, perhaps 50 of them in the United States. No federal funds have been expended on research on the safety and efficacy of IVF except that NICHD has issued a contract for a detailed follow-up study of children born after IVF. An ethics committee of the American Fertility Society noted the negative consequences of federal nonsupport.[43] Clinical activity has expanded rapidly in the private sector with a widely variable level of efficacy and relatively low rate of success "somewhat below the success rate of natural reproduction." In the best of hands, implantation occurs in 20% to 25% per reproductive cycle in which a woman is sexually active. The report notes the possibility of improvement in efficacy if systematic observation and research guided such an effort. Despite some cautious clinical trials with the approval of local IRBs, "in the absence of general guidelines, there is considerable reluctance and uncertainty about how far and in what direction to proceed."

Feasibility of Chromosomal and Genetic Diagnosis in the Pre-Implantation Human Embryo

Some preliminary research on chromosomal and genetic questions in the pre-implantation human embryo has occurred in Great Britain, reviewed by Penketh and McLaren.[44] They foresee that evaluation of DNA, enzymes, and chromosome complement will be possible on cell biopsies taken from pre-implantation embryos fertilized by IVF. If feasible, this methodology would enable families at highest genetic risk to have a diagnosis at the earliest possible time and avoid the trauma and moral problems of later abortions for genetic indications. Any federal support for research involving the human embryo fertilized by IVF is prohibited by the regulations. An EAB report of 1979 anticipated this issue in allowing for research with fertilized embryos not used for embryo transfer (ET).[45] The report stated that "such research performed as a corollary to research designed primarily to establish safety and efficacy of IVF-ET, would also be acceptable from an ethical standpoint" [p. 108]. The scientific and medical potential of embryo research, as well as the social, ethical, and legal problems of fertilizing embryos for research alone, were broadly examined in a Ciba Foundation conference in 1985.[46]

WHEN DOES THE FETUS DESERVE EQUAL PROTECTION IN RESEARCH?

Although Walters intended the equality principle to be used as a "general test," it has been transmuted by Congress to public policy and federal law. Furthermore, Congress probably intends that the equality test be applied beginning with implantation. The legislative history of the Health Research Extension Act of 1985[47] defines circumstances under which research involving living human fetuses may be conducted and reflects the intent of Congress:

> In the case of living human nonviable fetuses ex utero or living human fetuses for whom viability has not yet been determined, the Secretary may support only those research projects that (1) may enhance the well-being or meet the health needs of the fetus, (2) enhance the probability of the fetus' survival to viability, or (3) whose purpose is to develop important biomedical knowledge that cannot be obtained by other means and that will pose no added risk of suffering, injury, or death to the fetus. This standard is to apply

equally to fetuses that are aborted spontaneously or by induced abortion. [p. 718]

In the case of living human fetuses in utero, the agreement requires that the Secretary administer regulations regarding the standard of risk in such a manner that a fetus that is intended for abortion is exposed to no greater risk than that to which a fetus that is intended to be carried to term may be exposed. [p. 719]

The premise that each post-implantation human embryo and first-trimester fetus deserves equal and absolute protection with other human subjects of research is based on a moral claim. This claim is part of the morality of some communities and religious traditions. However, should public policy be promulgated from a premise that is so debatable and that is not integral to the morality of many other communities and religious traditions? The dominant moral tradition, as is shown below, is not to accord the fetus at the earliest stage an equal moral status with that of living persons. McCormick acknowledged that "public policy must root in the deepest moral perceptions of the majority, or at least in principles that the majority is reluctant to modify."[48]

The commission used essentially the same definition of the fetus, beginning with implantation, as was later adopted in the regulations[1] [p. 5]. However, the commission did not directly address the issues of personhood or the civil status of the fetus[1] [p. 62]. The commission did not differentiate between stages of development of the fetus and levels of permissible risk, as did the British Advisory Group report. General statements were made that "moral concern should extend to all who share human genetic heritage, and . . . the fetus, regardless of life prospects, should be treated respectfully and with dignity"[1] [p. 62]. These claims are something less than a rigorous argument for equality. In adopting its recommendations, the commission did not explain why the prevailing morality regarding the fetus should be altered to permit the equality position to prevail throughout gestation, especially in the first trimester. In effect, the right-to-life position for equal protection of the first-trimester fetus is embodied in the commission's recommendations and the subsequent regulations. There it has remained, to be easily elevated by Congress to law and public policy.

Why is this premise so debatable? The view that the interests of the newly fertilized embryo are equal to those of living persons did not appear until the nineteenth century.[49] This view of fetal equality "from the beginning" differs markedly from an older moral tradition that "attempted to grace the protection accorded to the nascent human being according to the stages of its development," a tradition recalled in a notable article by Dunstan.[50] His argument focused on the merit of claims for equal protection of the newly fertilized human embryo after IVF, but it has relevance to research in the earliest stage of gestation. Dunstan showed that the claim to absolute protection for the human embryo "from the beginning" is a recent development in moral reflection, and especially in Roman Catholic moral theology. Further, he showed that neither Christian or Jewish morality nor English law gives human life absolute protection at any stage, since to do so would unfairly rule out other valid moral claims.

The older tradition has more in common with a contemporary view of a developmental moral status of the fetus than with a categorical view of equality, especially as applied to the very early embryo and the first-trimester fetus. A developmental view refers to, but is not determined by, biological milestones in embryonic and fetal development. This view of the moral status of the fetus does not permit indifference at any stage but heightens society's obligation to protect the fetus with each advancing stage of development. This view has been developed by Sumner,[51] Callahan,[52] and Grobstein.[53]

Sisela Bok, the philosopher, took this position in a paper submitted to the commission.[54] She argued for a higher level of research risk before 18 weeks in pregnancy, a view compatible with the earlier British Advisory Group report. She surveyed the reasons society must protect life: (1) prevention of harm, fear, anguish, loss of continued experience, and suffering to the victim; (2) prevention of brutalization and criminalization to the agent; (3) prevention of grief and loss for the family of the victim; (4) prevention of greater harm to society that would follow from permissive killing. Bok argued that up to a point well before viability such reasons have no moral relevance because claims for the "humanity" of the fetus in the early stages of pregnancy fail to make sense. Furthermore, it can be argued that at the earliest stages the embryo or fetus cannot feel pain or suffer. Early abortion or fetal research with abortuses is not brutalizing to those who do it or to those who consent to it, nor is it a grave threat to society. Protection of human life in later stages of pregnancy and after birth need not be diminished as a result of early abortion.

If the commission had favored Bok's position, it would have drawn a line to permit research involving higher risks with fetuses of earlier gestational age, and it would have restricted research risks to "minimal" at later stages. The British Advisory Group report drew the line at less than 20 weeks but at a weight less than 300 g to protect against any suggestion that "consciousness" could be present in the fetus. Bok reduced the age limit to 18 weeks because of the variability of viability. However, the commission took a different position, possibly due to an influential synthesis of positions prepared for it by Toulmin, a philosopher-consultant to the commission who recommended a moderate, restricted approach to nontherapeutic fetal research[55] [p. 10–1/26].

Toulmin gave priority to McCormick's arguments as the most weighty with respect to nontherapeutic research. McCormick had opened the way for those whose moral views gave primary rights to the fetus at any stage to find validation for nontherapeutic studies. However, Toulmin's preference for McCormick's arguments meant assuming McCormick's risk standard, beginning with implantation, which Toulmin defined as "no discernible risk, no notable pain, no notable inconvenience, and . . . promise of considerable benefit[55] [p. 10–8]. The reader will remember that McCormick developed this definition of *risk* in consideration of nontherapeutic research with *children* and extended it to the fetus.

Toulmin allowed McCormick's risk standard to remain, rather than draw "a hard-and-fast line" dividing one class of fetuses from another to be involved in nontherapeutic studies. He did so, foreseeing, as did the commission, that "actual practice" of IRBs in decisions about nontherapeutic fetal research would probably be based less on a "single, hard-and-fast index of permissibility," but rather on a more discriminating body of "case law" and "precedents" [p. 10–15].[55] Toulmin expected that if his recommendations were accepted and the ban on nontherapeutic research was lifted, local IRBs would develop the "body of case law and . . . precedents," and a national body like the commission would "keep a watchful eye" on the development of that "case law." He did not reckon with the possibility that the national forum for ethical reflection would be dismantled. In short, McCormick's position of "no discernible risk" at all stages of pregnancy is the source of the use of the standard of minimal risk in all nontherapeutic fetal research.

In retrospect, it is easy to understand how this situation occurred. To a commission working within the climate of a ban on nontherapeutic research imposed by NIH and Congress, it must have seem sufficient to lay an ethical foundation for nontherapeutic research. Further, the commission desired not to cause more conflict about the moral status of the early fetus and to assure those who, with McCormick, gave primary rights to the fetus that the commission would not permit exploitation of the fetus to be aborted. In allowing this premise to remain inflexibly unmodified for all stages of pregnancy, however, the commission not only departed far from the moral views of many communities and individuals but it helped to lay a foundation on which the most restrictive construction could be laid on early fetal research in future congressional debates and actions.

Dunstan's conclusions about embryo research readily apply to early fetal research:

> The motive prompting the restriction [of any research with embryos not to be implanted] is admirable: to resist the erosion of the value of human life, already savagely assailed by the world's present economic and political activities. But we have to choose. Uterine life must be protected at some point. If we put that point too early, forbidding observation and experimental use of pre-implantation embryos in the early stages of cell division, we shall inhibit much useful research of potential human benefit, including the improvement of the chances of successful pregnancy, for lack of which many extra embryos are sacrificed at present. [p. 43]

Indeed, a new start for public policy on when and to what degree society must protect fetuses in research is needed. In our view, the commission and the regulations drew the line too early in applying a standard of minimal risk. Significant social and individual benefits are now being sacrificed to a moral claim less weighty than the imperative to find new and earlier pathways to diagnose and treat fetal disorders and relieve great human distress and suffering.

Today's public policy about fetal and embryo research has the case morally backward. A public policy about nontherapeutic research rooted in the "deepest moral perceptions of the majority" would first permit meritorious research up to 14 days with the human embryo not to be implanted, as an EAB recommended in 1979.[56] Governmentally appointed commissions in the United Kingdom[57] and Australia[58] have since concurred with this position and so did the ethics committee of the American College of Obstetrics and Gynecology in July 1986.[59]

Next, some fetal research should be permitted in the first trimester of pregnancy that might be inappropriate in later stages of gestation. At least the same standard of risk should be allowed with the early fetus as is now permitted with children. Federal policy, however, now *bans* embryo research and requires that the minimal-risk standard be used in nontherapeutic research in all stages of pregnancy. Federal regulations for nontherapeutic research involving children permit an increment of *greater* than minimal risk, provided certain conditions are met [45 CFR 46.406]. Are pre- and post-implantation human embryos and first-trimester fetuses of higher value than children? Does it make moral sense that the research-risk standard is more restrictive for embryos and early fetuses than for other research subjects, provided that consent obtained from parent(s) is morally and legally valid?

The way out of this odd, morally self-defeating position is to reform the regulations by a compromise drawn from elements in the positions of McCormick and Bok. The compromise will preserve a major step in research ethics—the protection of the fetus to be aborted. On the other hand, it will enable more significant fetal research to help future children and families who are now being deprived of the benefits of systematic study of the early fetus and early trials of diagnostic and therapeutic techniques.

McCormick's main accomplishments were to ground fetal research in the same ethics of proxy consent and beneficence that he held to justify research in children. In effect, he helped to justify fetal research as a desirable social good. Secondly, with Walters, he helped to draw a clear line to protect the fetus to be aborted from exploitation in research. The commission's recommendations embodied much of this thought, especially in its view that "the woman's decision for abortion does not, in itself, change the status of the fetus for purposes of protection. . . . The same principles apply whether or not abortion is contemplated; in both cases, only minimal risk is acceptable" [p. 66]. The later regulations clearly protect the fetus to be aborted from opportunistic research, which was the main reason Congress asked the commission to study the issue.

Excluded from the commission's positions was a major element of Bok's position—the allowing of higher research risks in the early stage of pregnancy. Her advice to the commission relied on the dominant moral view that the closer fetal development is to the line of viability, the more protection society owes to the fetus. Bok held that exposure of fetuses to be aborted to greater research risks was justified because of the validity of maternal consent and the social benefits to be attained, and because claims based on the "humanity" of the first-trimester early fetus intended to prohibit abortion and fetal research did not make sense.

We recommend that the regulations be amended to permit an increment of higher research risk in nontherapeutic research in the first trimester. However, the requirement to protect the fetus to be aborted from excessive risks that one would not knowingly impose on a fetus to be delivered should not be relaxed. This reform would allow more flexibility in research in the first trimester, whether the context of the research is abortion, clinical prenatal diagnosis, or the earliest stage of learning to perform a new fetal therapy. Greater gains in research will occur, and the original intent of the regulations not to restrict research unfairly will be carried out.

The path to reform is to extend to fetal research in the first trimester what is presently allowed with children. Sections 46.404, 405, and 406 would serve as good models for revision of the fetal regulations. One section would state, as does Section 46.208, that DHHS will fund research involving minimal risk to the fetus at any gestational age, if the purpose of the activity is the development of important biological knowledge that cannot be obtained by any other means. However, an additional provision in fetal research, along the lines of Section 46.406, in regulations to guide research in children will be necessary. Proposed new language is:

> Research involving greater than minimal risk and no prospect of direct benefit to individual fetuses between implantation and 12 weeks of gestation but likely to yield generalizable knowledge about the fetal disorder or condition.
>
> DHHS will conduct or fund research in which the IRB finds that more than minimal risk to fetuses prior to 12 weeks gestational age is presented by an intervention or procedure that does not include the prospect of direct benefit for the fetus, or by a monitoring or diagnostic procedure which is not likely to contribute to the well-being of the fetus, only if the IRB finds that:
>
> (a) The intervention or procedure is likely to yield generalizable knowledge about a fetal disorder or condition which is of vital importance for the understanding or amelioration of that disorder or conditions. (b) The activity permitted may be conducted only if the mother and father are legally competent and have given their informed consent, except that the father's informed consent need not be secured if: (1) his identity or whereabouts cannot reasonably be ascertained, (2) he is not reasonably available, or (3) the pregnancy resulted from rape.

The line drawn at 12 weeks gestational age to separate greater than minimal from minimal risks in fetal research should be compatible with the morality of many communities, religious traditions, and individuals in this society. Under this construction, DHHS could have supported a randomized controlled trial comparing the safety and accuracy of approaches to first- and second-trimester prenatal diagnosis as well as other studies that may lead to improved methods of fetal therapy.

Greater flexibility of research allowed in early pregnancy will also reduce conflict about the required use of the DHHS Secretary's authority to waive minimal-risk requirements. Without reform, virtually every nontherapeutic fetal study of any significance would require Secretarial waiver. This provision discourages interest in fetal research. The procedure for Secretarial waiver should be unchanged in the regulations, to provide a recourse when exceptions are justified to the minimal-risk requirements or to the added increment of risk in the proposed regulation for first-trimester fetuses, on recommendation by an EAB.

DEFINITION OF MINIMAL RISK

The final aspect of the fetal regulations that requires improvement is a vague definition of *minimal risk*. The commission did not precisely define this term, although it required that all nontherapeutic fetal research be conducted within the scope of minimal risk. Its report stated that "the term 'minimal' is a value judgment." "Determination of acceptable minimal risk is a function of the review process"[1] [p. 66]. In its later considerations of research with children, however, the commission defined *minimal risk* with a frame of reference that applied to children:

> "Minimal risk" means that the risks of harm anticipated in the proposed research are not greater, considering probability and magnitude, than those ordinarily encountered in daily life or duing the performance of routine medical or psychological examinations or tests, of healthy children.[60]

Curiously, this definition was not adopted in federal regulations to protect children in research. A definition for *minimal research* in children is found in the first section on definitions, cited earlier [45 CFR 46. 102 (g)], that drops the "healthy children" frame of reference and substitutes "physical" for "medical" tests. However, the subpart on research with prisoners has its own definition, which reads:

> "Minimal risk" is the probability and magnitude of physical or psychological harm that is normally encountered in the daily lives, or in the routine medical, dental, or psychological examination of healthy persons. [46. 303 (d)]

Subpart B, the fetal regulations, uses "minimal risk" without referring the reader in its section on definitions (46.203) to any definition, leaving the impression that one must use Section 46. 102 (g), cited above, which has no frame of reference and substitutes "physical" for "medical" tests.

The regulations present researchers with an inadequate array of definitions of *minimal risk*. Whose "daily life" is supposed to be taken into account when the probability and magnitude of harm are being considered? An unfortunate impression is created that the risks of daily fetal and maternal life are comparable to those of the daily life of "healthy persons," that there are no "medical" tests of minimal risk for fetuses, and that federal regulations deliberately obscure the definition of *minimal risk* to discourage applications for funding.

The risks to the members of the fetal-maternal dyad in pregnancy are significantly higher than are the risks of daily life to nonpregnant, healthy individuals. However, risks in "normal" pregnancy vary greatly from stage to stage and are complex. The risk of spontaneous abortion in pregnancy is a clear example, found to be about 10% before week 6 of pregnancy and about 1.3% between weeks 18 and 20.[61] Amniocentesis is a "routine medical test" for fetuses at higher genetic risk because it is the policy of physicians to refer such cases to obstetricians for the procedure. Indeed, NICHD supported a clinical trial of amniocentesis that resulted in a finding that it did not add a statistically significant risk of fetal loss to that of the normal risk of fetal loss at mid-trimester. Amniocentesis could hardly be characterized as a "physical" test, however, and it has a finite risk of fetal loss.

The commission was correct to state that the final *determination* of minimal risk in fetal research was a task for research review. But a better definition can be offered to IRBs, providing a frame of reference within which concepts such as *probability*, *magnitude*, and *daily life* can be applied. If it can be done with healthy children, prisoners, or other adults, it can be done in pregnancy. Moreover, regulations that rely so heavily on a concept of *minimal risk* ought to define it in a framework relevant to the regulated activity. If a concept is ill defined but nonetheless heavily used to regulate an activity, suspicions are justly raised of unfounded obstruction of that activity.

The following definition of *minimal risk* is proposed for IRB considerations of minimal risk in the context of fetal research:

"Minimal risk" in Subpart B means that the risks of harm anticipated in the proposed research are not greater, considering probability and magnitude, than those encountered in the daily life of pregnant women and fetuses (receiving routine prenatal care) in the stage of gestation in which the activity is planned, or during the performance of routine obstetrical and other medical examinations or tests appropriate to that stage of gestation.

NOTES AND REFERENCES

1. National Commission for the Protection of Human Subjects of Biomedical and Behavioral Research: Report and Recommendations, Research on the Fetus. DHEW Publication No. (OS) 76–127, pp 61–88. Washington, DC, US Govt Printing Office, 1975
2. Title 45, Code of Federal Regulations, Part 46—Protection of Human Subjects, Subpart B—Additional Protections Pertaining to Research Development, and Related Activities Involving Fetuses, Pregnant Women, and Human In Vitro Fertilization (revised as of March 8, 1983). Available from Office of Protection from Research Risks, Building 31, Room 4B-09, NIH, Bethesda, MD 20892
3. Baron CH: Legislative regulation of fetal experimentation. In Milunsky A, Annas G (eds): Genetics and the Law III, pp 431–435. New York, Plenum Press, 1985
4. 45 Code of Federal Regulations 46. 103 (b) (1)
5. 45 Code of Federal Regulations 46. 203 (c)
6. Section 496. Fetal Research. Health Research Extension Act of 1984. Report 98–1155, p 55
7. Goodlin RC: Cutaneous respiration in a fetal incubator. Am J Obstet Gynecol 86:571–579, 1963
8. Adam PAJ, Raiha N, Rahiala EL et al: Cerebral oxidation of glucose and D-BOH-Butyrate by the isolated perfused fetal head (abstr). Pediatr Res 7:309, 1973
9. Ramsey P: The Ethics of Fetal Research, pp 1–20. New Haven, Yale University Press, 1975
10. Maynard-Moody S: Fetal research dispute. In Nelkin D (ed): Controversy: Politics of Technical Decisions, pp 197–211. Beverly Hills, Sage, 1979
11. Hellegers AE: Fetal research. In Reich WT (ed) Encyclopedia of Bioethics, pp 489–493. New York, Free Press, 1978. Levine RF: Ethics and Regulation of Clinical Research, pp 197–206. Baltimore, Urban & Schwarzenberg, 1981
12. Copsey D, Gold M: NIH ethics policy near on fetal research. Ob-Gyn News, p A1. Apr 15, 1973. Cases of objectionable fetal research were collected in a broad, objective review by Mahoney MJ: The nature and extent of research involving living human fetuses. In Appendix, Research on the Human Fetus. DHEW Publication No. (OS) 76–128, pp 1–1/1–48. Washington, DC, US Govt Printing Office, 1976
13. Roe v. Wade, 410 U.S. 113, 159, (1973). Doe v. Bolton, 310 U.S. 113, 179 (1973)
14. Cohn V: NIH vows not to fund fetus work. Washington Post, p A1. Apr 13, 1973
15. National Research Act, Public Law 93–348, July 12, 1974
16. Department of Health and Social Security: Report of the Advisory Group: The Use of Fetuses and Fetal Material for Research. London, Her Majesty's Stationery Office, 1972. The Peel Commission Report
17. National Institutes of Health: Protection of Human Subjects: Policies and Procedures. Federal Register 38:31738–49, Nov 16, 1973
18. Collected in Appendix, cited at ref 12
19. Jonsen A: Talk given at a conference called Ethical Aspects of Human Fetal Tissue Transplantation. Sponsored by Case-Western Reserve School of Medicine, Cleveland, Dec 4, 1986
20. Gaylin W, Lappe M: Fetal politics: The debate on experimenting with the unborn. Atlantic Monthly, pp 66–71, May 1975. Fletcher JF: Fetal research: An ethical appraisal. Appendix, pp 3–1/3–14, cited at ref 12
21. Ramsey P, cited at ref 9. Ramsey P: Moral issues in fetal research. Appendix, pp 6–1/6–14, cited at ref 12. Louisell DW: Fetal research: Response to the recommendations. Hastings Cent Rep 5:9–11, 1975
22. McCormick RA: Experimentation on the fetus: Policy proposals. Appendix pp 5–1/5–11, cited at ref 12. Walters L: Ethical and public policy issues in fetal research. Appendix pp 8–1/8–18. McCormick RA, Walters W: A good beginning. Hastings Cent Rep 5:13–14, 1975
23. McCormick RA: Proxy consent in the experimentation situation. Perspect Biol Med 18:2–20, 1974
24. McCormick RA: How Brave a New World? p

25. Walters L: Appendix, esp p 8–10, cited at ref 12
26. Ethics Advisory Board of the US Department of Health, Education, and Welfare: Report and conclusions: DHEW support of research involving in vitro fertilization and embryo transfer, May 4, 1979. Federal Register 44:35, 1979
27. Steinfels M: At the EAB, same members, new ethical problems. Hastings Cent Rep 5:2, 1979
28. Fletcher JC, Schulman JD: Fetal research: The state of the question. Hastings Cent Rep 15:6–12, 1985
29. Anshan Department of Obstetrics and Gynecology: Fetal sex prediction by sex chromatin of chorionic villi cells during early pregnancy. Clin Med J 1:117–126, 1975
30. Kazy Z, Rozovsky IS, Bakharev V: Chorion biopsy in early pregnancy. Prenat Diag 2:39–45, 1982
31. Ward RHT, Modell B et al: Method of sampling chorionic villi in first trimester of pregnancy under guidance of real time ultrasound. Brit Med J 286:1542, 1983
32. Simoni G, Brambati B, Danesino C et al: Diagnostic application of first trimester trophoblast sampling in 100 pregnancies. Hum Genet 66:252–259, 1984
33. Fletcher JC: Ethical aspects of a controlled clinical trial of chorion biopsy approach to prenatal diagnosis. In Berg K (ed): Medical Genetics: Past, Present, and Future, pp 213–248. New York, Alan R. Liss, 1985
34. Cowart V: NIH considers large-scale study to evaluate chorionic villi sampling. JAMA 252:11–15, 1984
35. Jackson L: CVS Newsletter, p 1, Dec 1, 1986
36. Schulman JD (ed): Fetal therapy. Clin Obstet & Gynaecol 29:481–614, 1986
37. Evans MI, Chrousos GP, Mann D et al: Pharmacologic suppression of the fetal adrenal gland in utero: Attempted prevention of abnormal external genital masculinization in suspected congenital adrenal hyperplasia. JAMA 253:1014–1020, 1985
38. Redmond DE et al: Fetal neuronal grafts in monkeys given methylphenyltetrahydropyridine. Lancet 1:1124–1127, May 17, 1986
39. Fishman DS: Neural transplantation: Scientific gains and clinical perspectives. Neurol 36:389–392, 1986
40. O'Reilly RJ, Pollack MS, Kapoor N et al: Fetal liver transplantation in man and animals. In Gale RG (ed): Recent Advances in Bone Marrow Transplantation, pp 799–830, New York, Alan R. Liss, 1983
41. Fletcher JC, Robertson JA, Harrison M: Primates and fetuses as sources of organs: Medical, ethical, and legal issues. Fetal Therapy 1:150–164, 1986
42. Uniform Anatomical Gift Act: Table of jurisdictions wherein act has been adopted. 8A Unif Laws Annot 8A:15–16, 1983
43. Ethics Committee of the American Fertility Society: Ethical Considerations of the New Reproductive Technologies, Fertil Steril (Supp 1) 46:74, 1986
44. Penketh R, McLaren A: Prospects for prenatal diagnosis during pre-implantation human development. In Rodeck C (ed): Balliere's Int Obstet & Gynec. Philadelphia, WB Saunders (in press)
45. Ethics Advisory Board: Report on in vitro fertilization, cited at ref 26
46. Ciba Foundation: Human Embryo Research Yes or No? London, Tavistock, 1986
47. Legislative History, Public Law 99-158, Health Research Extension Act of 1985, pp 718–719
48. McCormick RA: How Brave a New World? p 79, cited at ref 24
49. Council on Science and Society: Report of a working party. Human Procreation, p 3. Oxford, Oxford University Press, 1984
50. Dunstan GR: The moral status of the human embryo: A tradition recalled. J Med Ethics 1:38–44, 1984
51. Sumner LW: Abortion and Moral Theology. Princeton, NJ, Princeton University Press, 1981
52. Callahan D: Abortion: Law, Choice, and Morality, p 377. New York, Macmillan, 1970
53. Grobstein C: From Chance to Purpose, p 102. Reading, Mass, Addison-Wesley, 1981
54. Bok, S: Fetal research and the value of life. Appendix, pp 2–1/2–18, cited at ref 12
55. Toulmin S: Fetal experimentation: Moral issues and institutional controls. Appendix pp 10–1/10–26, cited at ref 12
56. Ethics Advisory Board: Report on in vitro fertilization, p 108, cited at ref 26
57. Department of Health and Social Security: Report of the Committee of Inquiry into Human Fertilization and Embryology, p 84. London, Her Majesty's Stationery Office, 1984
58. Victorial, Committee to Consider the Social, Ethical, and Legal Issues Arising from In Vitro Fertilization: Report on the Disposition of

Embryos Produced by In Vitro Fertilization, p 60. Melbourne, FD Atkinson Government Printer, August 1984

59. Ethics Committee, American College of Obstetrics and Gynecology: Ethical issues in in vitro fertilization and Gynecology: embryo placement. July 1986

60. National Commission for the Protection of Human Subjects of Biomedical and Behavioral Research: Research Involving Children: Report and Recommendations. DHEW Publication No. (OS) 77–0004. Washington, DC, US Govt Printing Office, 1977; specific reference to the earliest definition of *minimal risk* is in Federal Register 40:33529, Aug. 8th, 1975

61. Harlap S, Shiono PH, Ramcharan S: A life table of spontaneous abortions and the effects of age, parity, and other variables. In Porter IH, Hook EB (eds): Human Embryonic and Fetal Death, p 148. New York, Academic Press, 1980

17

Primates and Anencephalics as Sources for Pediatric Organ Transplants: Medical, Legal, and Ethical Issues

John C. Fletcher,

John A. Robertson, and

Michael R. Harrison

In October 1984, doctors at Loma Linda Hospital in California transplanted the heart of a 7-month-old baboon into a newborn infant with hypoplastic left heart syndrome.[4] Baby Fae survived for 20 days and engendered controversy on several grounds. Animal-rights activists saw the transplantation as an abuse of animal rights.[49] Others raised questions about subjecting a nonconsenting subject to a novel heterograft experiment that had little chance of success.[2]

Although a review team from the National Institutes of Health found the institutional review process to have been adequate,[17] a question can be raised about how adequately the institution had planned to search for a human heart prior to the decision to subject a newborn to such invasive experimental xenografting. Obtaining cadaver organs for children is extremely difficult. In our view, such difficulty did not relieve the institution from the responsibility for a systematic search for a human heart in advance of the experimental xenograft. Clear evidence that a well-planned search had failed would have created a more compelling ground to take added and unknown risks.

The Baby Fae case has focused attention on pediatric organ transplantation, a problem that has been to a large extent ignored in the public policy debate about transplantation. A large and increasing number of children with otherwise fatal childhood diseases may have health and a potentially full life restored by transplantation of a variety of whole organs, tissues, and cells.

The supply of organs is a major problem. Even if research demonstrates the viability of pediatric transplantation, serious supply problems will remain. Proposals have been made to use chimpanzees and anencephalic abortuses and newborns to increase the supply of transplantable organs.[43,27]

This chapter discusses some of the medical, legal, and ethical issues involved in transplanting organs from primates and the anencephalic newborn and fetus. Serious ethical issues are involved that must be considered before proceeding with further research. We find that anencephaly is the most promising source of pediatric organs, but major ethical and legal problems must be overcome.

THE NEED FOR ORGANS FOR DYING CHILDREN

The need for small organs is acute and is likely to grow because of the potential benefits to so many children who will otherwise die. An increasing number of children with otherwise fatal childhood diseases may have a potentially full life restored by transplantation of vital organs: kidney, liver, heart, bone marrow, and in the near future "selective" transplants, such as pancreatic islets, endocrine tissues, and stem cells.[39,42,56,31,51] Each year in the United States, from 400 to 500 infants and children with end-stage renal disease could be taken off expensive dialysis regimens by renal transplantation.[55] An estimated 500 to 1000 children with biliary atresia, cholestatic syndromes, and some inherited metabolic defects have only one hope for survival—liver transplantation.[38,25,48,52,29] As many as 500 children born with hopeless forms of congenital heart disease, such as hypoplastic left heart syndrome, are potentially curable by heart transplantation.[3,13] For many childhood hematopoietic and malignant diseases, the only hope is bone marrow transplantation.[57,6] Enzymatic, immunologic, and endocrine deficiencies may be corrected using cellular (rather than whole organ) grafts—hematopoietic stem cells, islet cells, and so on.[53,20,48,9,59] Transplantation of fetal neural tissues is research with great therapeutic potential.[22,30,26,15,24,23] If such selective transplantation proves feasible, a large number of children could benefit.

Biologic tissue replacement may be the only satisfactory solution for failing organ function in the very young, for three reasons. (1) The new organ must grow with the recipient and adapt to increasing functional demand, making "half-way" technologies such as mechanical replacement inappropriate. (2) The long potential life span of the young recipient renders use of a biologically older tissue less desirable. (3) Rapid organ failure and the lack of interim support measures make the "time window" for transplantation extremely narrow.

Other than transplantation of livers and bone marrow, pediatric transplantation is not well developed. However, there is a severe shortage of livers. Children die on waiting lists. Because comparatively few children die in circumstances allowing organ donation (only 1200 in auto accidents), finding an appropriate cadaver organ during the limited time when the sick child is salvageable is unlikely. When livers are donated, ethical and logistical problems in allocation arise, which a greatly increased supply would alleviate. Ironically, pediatric heart and kidney donations are sometimes refused because of the dearth of pediatric transplantation programs.

Supply problems, costs, and shortages will increase as pediatric organ transplantation programs start up and research in whole organ, selected tissue, and cell transplants continues. The first apparently successful heart transplant in a newborn has occurred at Loma Linda University, although a scientific and medical report has yet to be published. Development of additional transplant therapies, such as pancreatic,[1,40,9] will increase demand for organs for newborns and lead to the supply and distributional problems that now exist with pediatric livers and adult organs.

We now consider two potential sources of pediatric organs suggested by the Baby Fae case: primates and anencephalics.

PRIMATES AS ORGAN SOURCES

The resort to a baboon heart in the Baby Fae case focused attention on the need for organs for very small infants. Although the experiment was unsuccessful, other attempts to pierce the species barrier will no doubt occur. Dr. Thomas E. Starzl of the University of Pittsburgh recently proposed that chimpanzees be used for experimental transplant in infants with serious liver disease and has sought permission from his Institutional Review Board to do so.

The close phylogenetic relationship to humans makes the chimpanzee an invaluable source of study of disease in humans generally and an obviously preferred option among animals as a source of organs. If primates are to be used, they are likely to be chimpanzees. There are, however, several reasons why chimpanzees will not meet needs for pediatric organs and why research should proceed in other directions.

One important reason is the poor chance medically that the graft and patient will survive. The American Medical Association's Council on Scientific Affairs recently reviewed the status of xenografts and concluded that there is little basis for expecting success in such cases.[16] Jonasson and Hardy,[32] in commenting on a medical report of the Baby Fae case, argue that graft survival is impossible until "lesions caused by preformed antibodies can be prevented by immunologic or pharmacologic manipulation of the recipient or of the donor organ."

The scientific foundations of xenografting need much more development. More information is needed about the degree of similarity between the genetic constitution of chimpanzees and humans and the degree to which the immune response to xenografts is impaired in infants. More understanding is needed of the immunology of rejection of transplants between near relatives, such as sheep and goats, and distant relatives, such as cats and dogs. Also, a data base on primate xenotransplantation needs to be assembled, the development of which would be a major undertaking. No evidence exists now to support an expectation that a xenograft would continue to function for 2 to 6 months even with maximum blockade of immune response. Moreover, little is known about immunosuppression of xenografts or whether cyclosporine will be as effective as it is with homografts. At best, xenografts might serve as a bridge to homografts. But temporary transplants merely change the distribution of recipients and do not increase the number of organs available for homografts.

If this account of the scientific unknowns and medical uncertainties is accurate, major ethical problems confront further research with xenografts. These facts suggest that primates are not likely to become an important source of pediatric organs. In a recent review of the ethical issues in the Baby Fae case, Caplan[10] concludes that parents should be free to consent to experimental xenografts when the alternative is death, as long as they are adequately informed that "nothing" is known about the long-term viability of xenografts in human beings. However, this position may be questioned. Proxies are not always permitted to subject nonconsenting subjects to research with greater than minimal risks, even as a last resort. Some chance of benefit, however small, must be clearly shown before offering an experiment to subjects. If chances of success are vanishingly small, a very intrusive experimental procedure may be unethical, even if the patient will die.

The low chance of medical success with xenografts also gives some credence to the animal-rights claim. The demonstrations at Loma Linda probably hurt the animal-rights cause more than they helped it, for they seemed to elevate the welfare of a baboon above the welfare of a dying newborn. However, most (even staunch) defenders of animal rights recognize that animals may be sacrificed if necessary to save a human life. If sacrificing chimpanzees to obtain organs allowed people to live, some animal protectionists might accept the practice. Yet they would object vociferously if the sacrifice of the chimpanzee were unlikely to produce significant medical benefit. On this point the ethics of animal and human experimentation converge.

Suppose, however, that chimpanzee hearts could be transplanted with the efficacy of human liver or adult heart transplants (60% to 80% survival for one year). Objections on the basis of the ethics of human or animal research would be overcome. A major practical problem—the problem of supply—would remain.

In April 1985, the National Institute of Arthritis, Diabetes, and Digestive and Kidney Diseases convened an ad hoc group of consultants to advise the Institutional Review Board at the University of Pittsburgh on Dr. Starzl's request to use chimpanzees as an organ source. Although their report did not prescribe any action, it called attention to serious supply problems.[43]

Supply shortages alone make chimpanzees an unlikely source of organs even if their organs could be transplanted successfully. Only about 50 or 60 experimentally naive chimpanzees are available for all research in this country annually. The entire population of chimpanzees residing in colonies that support biomedical research in the United States is approximately 1200. However, very few of these animals will contribute to a dedicated breeding colony. The majority (approximately 680) are aging wild-born animals, and very few of the remaining captive-born population are proven breeders and parents. Many suitable breeders have also been compromised by hepatitis research.

According to a National Chimpanzee Management Plan recently approved by the director of the National Institutes of Health, the population on which the survival of the American chimpanzee depends is 300 or less.[44] The plan calls for the formation of a self-perpetuating 350-animal colony to provide approximately 35 individuals annually for research, the rest being reserved for continued breeding. Using even a few animals as organ sources would create a direct trade-off with other research needs, including some research that is already in place and that could reasonably be viewed to be as important as or more important than research into heterografts. Studies that rely heavily on the chimpanzee include viral hepatitis and certain other viral diseases, transplantation immunology, and comparative behavioral studies. Currently, the greatest demand for use is in hepatitis and acquired immunodeficiency syndrome (AIDS) research. Young animals are not being used in AIDS research.

More seriously, even if chimpanzee liver transplantation were successful on a pilot basis, the anticipated therapeutic demand could not be met from this source. Multiple xenografts to the same individual while awaiting human transplant would only exacerbate those problems.

Chimpanzees are also quite expensive, perhaps more expensive than other research animals.[62] Because of the ten-year generation time, managing a chimpanzee colony is more similar to propagating a forest than to breeding other laboratory animals. Maintenance for each animal costs about $15 a day or almost $200,000 during its 35-year life span. Because of the cost of maintaining the breeders, the real cost of producing an infant is approximately $20,000. Since the ratio of animals killed to humans benefited would be 1:1, the use of chimpanzee organs would be very expensive.

Doubts about efficacy, ethical concerns, cost, and supply are reasons to believe that primates are not likely soon to be a major source of pediatric organs. We also believe that the transplant field, including pediatric transplantation, ought to invite creative suggestions to reduce these difficulties, so that the potential supply of organs from xenografts might not be such a forbidding barrier to this route. Further experimentation in xenografting ought not to be ruled out because of the serious limitations on supply at present. Perhaps embryo transfer and surrogate gestation will eventually provide a new direction. In the meantime, careful review of the ethical acceptability of any xenograft research should continue, with attention paid to the problems of cost and supply.

ANENCEPHALICS AS ORGAN SOURCE

Another possible source of organs for infants with end-stage organ disease is anencephalic newborns. The vast majority of severely handicapped dying newborns are not suitable sources for organ donation. Many preterm infants have metabolic derangements that render organs unusable. Either the underlying disease or infection that afflicts them or the life supports and drugs routinely administered in neonatal intensive care (NICU) to save their lives render their vital organs unsuitable for transplantation. For example, infants born with severe chromosomal malformations like trisomy 18 or trisomy 13 are not suitable organ sources because the abnormality in each cell heightens the potential for tumor development after transplant.

However, anencephaly is a fatal condition of newborns that is compatible with organ donation. Anencephaly is a neural tube defect that occurs in 1 in 2000 of the 3.7 million live births annually, producing about 1850 cases per year.[8] Anencephaly is a massive abnormality that results in an absent cranium and the virtual absence of the forebrain. The frontal, parietal, and occipital bones are present only in their basal portions. However, there is brain stem activity, which can sustain heart and lung action for a period. Nevertheless, most anencephalics will be stillborn or die in a few days.[37,18] Rarely, an anencephalic infant will live for two or more weeks.[61,5]

Two factors limit the number of anencephalics that may be donors. First, not all anencephalic infants are delivered in a condition suitable for organ retrieval. Fetal death and maceration occur before delivery in some cases. Second, prenatal diagnosis of anencephaly after screening for elevated levels of maternal serum alpha-fetoprotein now result in more mid-trimester elective abortions of anencephalic fetuses. For example, in a population of about 2.9 million in the west of Scotland, the rate of anencephalic and spina bifida live births and stillbirths declined 60.5% in five years, that is, from 4.3 per 1000 in 1976 to 1.7 per 1000 in 1981.[19] Prenatal diagnosis of anencephaly is also made in the third trimester of pregnancy by ultrasonography. Termination of the third trimester pregnancy for anencephaly is an acceptable option that is discussed below.[13]

If an anencephalic child is born, most pediatricians and neonatologists, with parental concurrence, would keep the infant warm, help the parents mourn, and allow the infant to die without procedures that unduly prolong life. At a time of great controversy over nontreatment of handicapped newborns, it is noteworthy that federal Baby Doe law specifically allows treatment to be withheld from anencephalics, though it is unclear whether nutrition and hydration might also be withheld. A 1984 federal law that forbids the withholding of medically indicated treatment from handicapped infants has three exceptions, any of which would cover the anencephalic child: (1) the infant is chronically and irreversibly comatose; (2) treatment would merely prolong dying and not be effective in correcting the life-threatening condition; (3) the provision of treatment would be virtually futile in terms of survival.[14] The law also states that the expression "withholding of medically indicated treatment" does not include "appropriate nutrition, hydration, or medication." By definition, an anencephalic infant can neither feel nor experience pain. In this case it is reasonable to argue that nutrition, hydration, and medication are not "appropriate" and therefore are not required by the law. However, the administration of medication and hydration could occur without unduly prolonging the life of the newborn or compromising organs for transplant.

Since anencephaly is a disease of the brain and not the rest of the body, vital organs will be intact. The expected high quality of the organs has led anencephalic newborns (whether from abortion or term delivery) to be considered as organ sources. Reports of kidney transplants from anencephalic newborns to recipients from 8 to 44 years old have already appeared.[35,45,34] Since the child with failing renal function can be supported by dialysis, transplantation of kidneys from newborn anencephalics has proven feasible. Those that have not failed for technical reasons have shown remarkable growth in size and function in a matter of weeks.

Much remains to be learned about the feasibility of pediatric transplants using organs from anencephalics. Whether tissues from anencephalics would always be metabolically or histologically sound for transplantation remains to be proven, since anencephalics are known to have hypoplastic cells in tissues.[41] The pituitary deficit and absence of hypothalamus result in endocrine problems such as hypothyroidism and other endocrine deficiencies. These may result in abnormal organ development and function.

A full discussion is available elsewhere of the technical feasibility of transplants of immature vital fetal organs as auxiliary heterotopic grafts, rather than as orthotopic total replacements.[27] If fetal organs prove suitable, transplantation for children may be greatly simplified biologically, technically, and logistically. The use of fetal organs may confer an immunologic advantage that will decrease the need for immunosuppressive drugs that compromise the recipient's growth and resistance to infection. Since histocompatibility antigens are expressed early in fetal life, the hope that fetal organs would be less "antigeneic" and thus less subject to rejection has proven naive. However, fetal grafts in general enjoy longer survival than more mature grafts, and the use of fetal donors makes possible immunologic manipulations that improve graft survival. The tissue type of the fetus can be determined from amniotic fluid or fetal blood, and the best possible recipient chosen by cross-matching. In addition, recipients can be pretreated with donor cells (amniotic fluid or blood) using the same strategy that has produced significant improvement in graft survival in clinical renal transplantation.

The advantages of HLA matching and donor-specific pretreatments are available now. In the future, it is possible that the unique immunologic relationship between mother and fetus may be the avenue to facilitate graft acceptance. In the few cases in which the need for transplantation can be predicted before birth (e.g., hypoplastic left heart, thalassemia), it may be possible to induce specific unresponsiveness in the potential recipient before birth for transplantation either before or after birth. Although transplantation immunity develops early in all mammals, there is a period in early gestation when the fetus is uniquely susceptible to induction of tolerance by donor cell suspensions. Also, graft rejection and graft-versus-host disease may be ameliorated if grafting is performed before the recipient becomes immunocompetent or the donor organ becomes populated by "passenger" leukocytes.

Legal and Ethical Issues in Obtaining Organs from Anencephalics

Although anencephalics appear to be a viable source for newborn organs, their use raises legal and ethical issues concerning the definition of personhood and death and the acceptability of actions that hasten death when nontreatment occurs. Analysis of these issues shows that organs could not be retrieved from anencephalics under existing law until brain stem function ceases, but there is no legal or ethical barrier to retrieval upon total brain death. As with adult organ procurement, reasonable efforts to preserve anencephalic organs prior to retrieval at brain death should be ethically and legally acceptable.

Organ Retrieval from Anencephalics Before Total Brain Death

When an anencephalic infant dies, the parents have legal rights under the Uniform Anatomical Gift Act to donate organs, tissues, or the entire body for purposes of research or transplantation.[60] The Uniform Anatomical Gift Act requires that the parents consent. Together with homicide and wrongful death laws, it also requires that the organ source be dead when organs are removed. The parents' right to donate anencephalic organs exists whether delivery is spontaneous or the result of an abortion.

Retrieval of organs from anencephalics would pose problems under existing law if the organs were removed before total brain death occurred, as would be necessary if viable organs could not be obtained when brain stem activity stops. Although the anencephalic is born without an upper brain and has just brain stem function, the anencephalic would probably be considered a legal subject under the law. The brain death concept of death adopted in 42 states rejected a partial or cortical standard of death in favor of a total brain death concept.[12]

Under this definition, the law might regard as homicide the removal of a heart from an anencephalic showing brain stem activity, for the removal would have directly caused brain death. This rule seems less directed at protecting the rights or interests of the anencephalic than at making a symbolic statement about active killing, for allowing the anencephalic to die is clearly permissible.

Should the law be changed to permit organ retrieval from anencephalics? Some might argue that since anencephalics have had no past cerebral function and possess no natural anatomical basis for future cortical function, they are in a different category from persons who had cognitive function and irreversibly lost it. This argument would favor amending the law to say that "individuals with congenital absence of upper brain and skull are dead," thus permitting organs to be removed. One could further argue that if nontreatment of anencephalics is permitted, organ removal before brain stem activity ceases should be as well. No moral subject will be injured, and the life of another will be saved.

This argument requires adopting a cognitive view of personhood and viewing the irreversible absence of cortical or cognitive function as the absence of a moral subject. Since retrieving vital organs will not harm or wrong the anencephalic and will provide great good to others, it should be permitted with parental consent. An ancillary consideration of these premises is the morality and legality of active euthanasia. Among some philosophers, the cognitive definition of personhood creates a basis for limited use of active killing, with parental consent, in the most severe and untreatable cases of handicapped newborns.[58,54]

The counterargument accepts some main premises of the foregoing argument but is hesitant about the need to change the law in the interest of drawing a line before active killing. Cognition clearly must be a major element in any rational definition of personhood. However, a strictly cognitive approach to personhood is vulnerable to variability and biases of culture and class. Further agreement is found in that organ retrieval does no essential harm to anencephalics and clearly benefits children who will otherwise die. But the counterargument denies the conclusion that the law should be changed to permit organ retrieval from anencephalics before total brain death. Although there is no need to protect the patient, this position holds that there is a social need to maintain a firm line against active killing and to have a clear definition of legal personhood that is not too vulnerable to the disagreements that understandably arise about a strictly cognitive approach to personhood.[7,21,50] Furthermore, such a line represents a symbolic commitment to human life generally and to prevention of the disputes likely to arise from a strictly cognitive definition of death and personhood.

Amending the brain death law to include anencephalics as dead would be a major change in legal policy. Since it is likely to generate controversy, the issue should not be pursued if viable anencephalic organs can be retrieved at total brain death. However, if postmortem anencephalic donations will not yield viable organs, then proposals to define anencephalics as dead should be seriously addressed. It may be that a majority of the community would give a higher priority to the life of persons needing transplants than to symbolic commitments that do not directly protect other persons.

Retrieval and Preservation of Organs from Brain-dead Anencephalics

The need to define anencephalics as dead arises only if viable organs cannot be retrieved from anencephalics with total brain death. The problem is that waiting for total brain death to occur might impair the organs that are then retrieved. Warm ischemia is a major risk to organ viability. To retrieve viable organs after total brain death without warm ischemia would require cooling the anencephalic newborn, by surface applications of cooling media or by cool intravenous solutions.

Here another ethical issue arises. Cooling the anencephalic patient to preserve organs might hasten cardiorespiratory and brain stem cessation, making total brain death occur somewhat sooner than it would have without cooling. Is cooling to preserve organs acceptable even if it might hasten total brain death?

An argument in favor of cooling anencephalics to preserve organs draws on precedents in widely accepted organ procurement practices and the doctrine of double effect, for cooling is very similar to a common donor maintenance procedure in organ procurement. Consider a potential organ donor who has suffered a major head trauma. After aggressive treatment with vasopressors, mannitol, and the withholding of fluids, the patient remains in deep coma with some brain stem activity. The patient is not yet brain dead but appears to be rapidly progressing toward that state. Cognitive death has clearly occurred. At that point the doctors, with family consent, may cease all aggressive treatment and allow the patient to become brain dead.

If the family also consents to organ donation, it is good procurement practice to institute aggressive hydration in order to assure the perfusion necessary for viable organs. The Postmortem Organ Procurement Protocol of a leading transplant center notes[46]:

> In caring for a patient who has been recognized as a potential donor, the attending physician of course will initially want to avoid any treatment which is incompatible with optimal care of the patient's primary condition. When the attending physician determines that the patient's condition is hopeless . . . the emphasis in the care of the potential donor should shift toward maintaining the viability of the kidneys, heart and liver for transplantation.

The switch to hydration to preserve organs, however, might contribute to cerebral swelling and thus hasten the total brain death that the previous therapies had tried to prevent. We think it unreasonable to construe legal and ethical doctrines against direct, active killing so broadly as to prohibit organ preservation in such cases and believe that reasonable people would agree with such a conclusion. Aggressive hydration does not injure the patient, since a patient with severe, irreversible brain injury rapidly degenerating into total brain death is beyond the point of injury. Similarly, cooling anencephalics, though it might hasten the total brain death that is imminent, does not injure them.

Such actions can also be justified under the argument of double effect. This approach holds that three criteria should be applied to weighing whether an action causing good effect A and evil effect B is acceptable. (1) The actor must sincerely intend not to cause the evil effect. (2) The good and evil effects must be caused simultaneously, so the evil is never a sequential means to the good. (3) A proportionately grave reason must exist to permit the evil effect.

An instructive parallel is morphine analgesia in terminally ill patients. In addition to relief of pain, morphine reduces respiration and causes death sooner than it would have occurred without the morphine. Although the physician has knowingly and actively hastened death, the actions are morally and legally accepted under the argument's three criteria. The physician's sincere intent is not to kill the patient but to relieve pain and reduce suffering. Further, the two effects are caused simultaneously, and the analgesic rather than the death of the patient is the means to the relief of suffering. Finally, the proportionately grave reason of great pain and suffering lends weight to permitting the effect of the death of the patient. Since the purpose of the morphine is to control pain and not cause death, the morphine is acceptable even though it hastens death, although an action undertaken for the purpose of causing death would be unacceptable.

Similarly, organ preservation techniques are done in order to preserve organs for transplantation once brain death occurs, not for the purpose of causing death (which is inevitable and soon expected). Hastening death is an acknowledged but unintended effect of a primary intent to preserve organs. True, morphine hastens death as an effect of benefiting the patient, and organ preservation is for the good of recipients. But this difference should not matter morally, for the patient cannot be harmed by the cooling procedures because of the devastating harm already done by the anomaly. The patient cannot feel or experience the cooling procedures. Further, the effect of preserving organs and the effect of hastening brain death are caused simultaneously by the cooling procedure. The death of the infant is not the means to the well-being of the organs. A very grave reason, saving the lives of children who will surely die, lends moral weight to permitting the hastening of total brain death. Thus, hydration and cooling to preserve organs for transplant should be permitted in near-brain-dead patients and anencephalics when the family consents to organ donation.

The argument of double effect could not be used satisfactorily to justify removing organs before total brain death occurs, even though it might be argued that the sincere intent is not to kill but to obtain life-saving organs. The death of the infant would be the sequential means to the organs, and one would be open to the charge of causing death to benefit others. A proportionately grave reason exists, but the act of causing death to benefit others would clearly be ethically less acceptable than an act that benefited others but hastened an already irreversible process of inevitable brain death. It is true that the anencephalic lacks interests in either case and cannot be hurt by organ removal before total brain death. Yet the effect is different in each case. The crux of the ethical problem is the symbolic meaning associated with actively hastening death when life-sustaining treatment is justly withheld. We think that reasonable people would read a different symbolic meaning in each case and would find hastening death indirectly by organ preservation more acceptable than directly causing total brain death by organ removal.

In sum, ethical concern about organ procurement from totally brain-dead anencephalic newborns is similar to concerns that arise in organ procurement generally. If organ preservation procedures that hasten death are acceptable in organ procurement generally, they should be acceptable for anencephalic donors as well.

Future experience may show that cooling will not adequately preserve organs or will prevent medical determinations that brain stem activity has ceased, since the usual tests of total brain death do not apply in the case of hypothermia. If that is so, the question of amending the law to define anencephalics as dead should be reopened, although the road to this goal would be impeded with obstacles.

Management of Pregnancies Involving Anencephalic Donors

In many respects the use of anencephalic donors raises the same ethical issues that arise in organ procurement generally. These concerns will require careful planning and sensitive management of the case, but they themselves would not prevent the donation if three ethical considerations of transplantation are followed. (1) The medical care of the potential donor must be separated from those who are interested in transplantation.[28] (2) Consent from the parents for donation must be obtained by persons other than those on the transplant team.[11] (3) The donor must be determined to have died.[47]

Once the prenatal diagnosis of anencephaly is confirmed, the family can choose to continue to carry a fetus who will die in utero and be stillborn or who will be delivered alive and die shortly after birth. Or the family can choose to terminate the pregnancy. Even when the diagnosis is made in the third trimester, most physicians accommodate the family's desire for abortion rather than force the mother to continue a hopeless pregnancy. Cases of anencephaly are discussed by Chervenak et al.[13] as the only clear exception to a moral presumption against abortion in the third trimester, because it is a disorder that is incompatible with postnatal survival for more than a few weeks and is marked by the total absence of cognitive function. Abortion of third-trimester anencephalic fetuses is clearly legal in 25 states and arguably so in the remainder.*

The ethical issue in management in the context of abortion is to allow organ retrieval without adding risk to the mother. If the parents choose to abort and consent to organ donation, the time and method of delivery should not be altered to facilitate organ recovery if the risk to the mother is increased. Cesarean section, for example, should not be done merely to obtain organs of better quality. In addition, steps to prevent the prospect of donation from influencing the abortion decision should be taken. The physician attending the mother should not request organ donation, although she or he might inform the mother that she will be asked. Nor should a riskier or more intrusive abortion procedure be chosen to improve the prospects for donation.

Although any method of evacuating the uterus poses some risk, maternal safety and reproductive potential are the primary concerns. Fetal organ procurement is a secondary consideration. The best approach is vaginal delivery by the usual techniques (cervical dilation with laminaria, ripening with prostaglandin, induction with pitocin, etc.) rather than the more violent techniques of intraamniotic saline or prostaglandin, which are often used to assure stillbirth in late abortions.[33,36] Although some anencephalic fetuses may not tolerate labor and die in utero before the organs can be procured, fetal monitoring would not be appropriate in most cases because obstetric management (i.e., method of delivery) should not be changed simply to save fetal organs for transplantation.

---

* While the states may under *Roe v. Wade*, 410 U.S. 113 (1973) prohibit abortion after viability, there is an exception for abortions necessary to preserve the life or health of the mother. It is arguable that a third-trimester abortion of an anencephalic fetus would be constitutionally permissible on this basis, if state law prohibited third-trimester abortions.

Management of the Anencephalic After Delivery

When anencephaly is not detected until delivery, management focuses on verifying the diagnosis and determining the course of action without regard to transplantation. Only after a decision to withhold treatment has been made should the parents be approached about organ donation. The possibility of organ donation should not be a factor in the decision to withhold treatment. The attending neonatologist should not be involved in the request for removal of organs. As with organ donation from any source, the physician treating the donor cannot have an interest or be directly involved in the transplant. However, if the infant survives long enough to make organ donation possible, the attending physician may inform the family that they will be approached and give the family information if asked.

Fortunately, in most cases anencephaly is now diagnosed before birth. Although the possibility of organ donations should not be a factor in the decision about when and how to end the pregnancy, once the decision for termination has been made, the family may be approached about the possibility of organ donation or may even ask about it spontaneously. If the family chooses to pursue the possibility of organ donation, they should be allowed to arrange the timing and place of delivery to facilitate transplantation. In many cases this will mean delivering in a transplant center.

Prenatal diagnosis allows time for the mother and family to make important decisions beforehand about whether they wish the newly delivered anencephalic to be resuscitated, whether they wish to see or hold the newborn as part of their grieving experience, whether they wish to allow organ donation, and how the organ retrieval will be accomplished. This is far preferable to discussion of these important decisions in the hurried and dramatic period after birth.

Management of the prenatally diagnosed potential organ donor should be carefully planned in advance with the family. If consent has been given before birth, management of the neonate after birth can be dictated by the wishes of the family and by the logistics of organ transplantation. For instance, the family may choose not to see the baby, or they may choose to hold and grieve over the body. The removal of organs from the brain-absent cadaver can then be carried out in the operating room as is presently done for brain-dead heart-beating cadavers. Needless to say, it must be done with compassion, sensitivity, and respect for the body of the anencephalic donor and the sensibilities of the donating family.

REFERENCES

1. Anderson A: Transplantation of the endocrine pancreas. Acta Paediatr Scand (Suppl)270:127–132, 1977
2. Annas GJ: Baby Fae: The "anything goes" school of human experimentation. Hastings Cent Rep 15:15–17, 1985
3. Bailey LL, Jang J, Johnson W, Jolley WB: Orthotopic cardiac xenografting in the newborn goat. J Thorac Cardiovasc Surg 89:242–247, 1985
4. Bailey LL, Nehlsen-Cannarella SL, Conception W, Jolley WB: Baboon-to-human cardiac xenotransplantation in a neonate. JAMA 254:3321–3329, 1985
5. Baird PA, Sadovnick AD: Survival in infants with spina bifida. Clin Pediatr 23:268–271, 1984
6. Barranger JA: Marrow transplantation in genetic disease. N Engl J Med 311:1629–1630, 1984
7. Beauchamp TL, Childress JF: Principles of Biomedical Ethics, pp 115–126. New York, Oxford University Press, 1983
8. Berendes HW: Personal communication, June 1, 1985
9. Brown J, Danilovs JA, Clark WR, Mullen YS: Fetal pancreas as a donor organ. World J Surg 8:152–157, 1984
10. Caplan AL: Ethical issues raised by research involving xenografts. JAMA 254:3339–3343, 1985
11. Caplan AL, Bayer R: Ethical, legal and policy issues pertaining to solid organ procurement: Report of project on organ transplantation, pp 11–12, Hastings-on-Hudson, NY, Hastings Center, Oct 1985
12. Cases and statutes are collected in President's Commission for the Study of Ethical Problems in Medicine and Biomedical and Behavioral Research: Defining Death, pp 109–166. Washington, DC, US Gov Printing Office, 1981
13. Chervenak FA, Farley MA, Walters L et al: When is termination of pregnancy during the third trimester morally justified? N Engl J Med 310:501–504, 1984
14. Child Abuse Amendments of 1984, Public Law 98–457
15. Cotman CW, Nieto-Sampedro M, Gibbs RB: Enhancing the self-repairing potential of the CNS after injury. CNS Trauma 1:3–14, 1984
16. Council on Scientific Affairs: Xenografts: Review of the literature and current status. JAMA 254:3353–3357, 1985
17. Dommel FW, Lanman R, McCormick RA et al: The NIH report of its review of the Baby Fae case. IRB 8:1–4, 1986. See Levine C: NIH approves the consent for Baby Fae or does it? Hastings Cent Rep, 15:2, 1985. Knoll E, Lundberg GD: Informed consent and Baby Fae. JAMA 254:3359–3360, 1985
18. Elwood JM, Elwood JH: Epidemiology of anencephalus and spina bifida, pp 253–299. New York, Oxford University Press, 1980
19. Ferguson-Smith MA: The reduction of anencephalic and spina bifida births by maternal serum alpha-fetoprotein screening. Br Med Bull 39:365–372, 1983
20. Fleischman RA, Mintz B: Development of adult bone marrow stem cells in H-2-compatible and incompatible mouse fetuses. J Exp Med 159:731–745, 1984
21. Fletcher JC: Abortion, euthanasia, and care of defective newborns. N Engl J Med 292:75–78, 1985
22. Freed WJ, Perlow MJ, Karoum F et al: Restoration of dopaminergic function by grafting of fetal rat substantia nigra to the caudate and nucleus: Long-term behavioral, biochemical, and histochemical studies. Ann Neurol 8:510–517, 1980
23. Freed JW, Wyatt RJ, de Medinacel L: Promoting functional plasticity in the damaged nervous system. Science 227:1544–1552, 1985
24. Gage FH, Bjorklund A: Intracerebral grafting of neuronal cell suspensions into the adult brain. CNS Trauma 1:47–56, 1984
25. Gartner JC, Zatelli BJ, Starzl TE: Orthotopic

liver transplantation: Two-year experience with 47 patients. Pediatrics 74:140–145, 1984
26. Harris EW, Cotman CW: Brain tissue transplantation research. Appl Neurophysiol 47:9–15, 1984
27. Harrison MR: Organ procurement for children: A fetal solution. Commentary, the anencephalic newborn as organ donor. Hastings Cent Rep 16:21–22, 1986
28. Howard RJ, Najarian JS: Organ transplantation: Medical perspective. In Reich WT (ed): Encyclopedia of Bioethics, Vol 3, p 1163. New York, Free Press, 1978
29. Iwatsuki S, Shaw BW, Starzl TE: Liver transplantation for biliary atresia. World J Surg 8:51–56, 1984
30. Jaeger CVB, Lund RD: Transplantation of embryonic occipital cortex to the brain of newborn rats: An autoradiographic study of transplant histogenesis. Exp Brain Res 40:265–272, 1980
31. Jamieson SW: Recent developments in heart and heart-lung transplantation. Transplant Proc 17:199–203, 1985
32. Jonasson O, Hardy MA: The case of Baby Fae. JAMA 254:3358–3359, 1985
33. Karim SMM, Ratnam SS, Hutabarat H et al: Termination of pregnancy in cases of intrauterine fetal death, missed abortion, molar and anencephalic pregnancy with intramuscular administration of 2a,2b-dihomo-15(s), 15-methyl-PGF2-alpha-methylester: A multicentre study. Ann Acad Med Singapore 11:508–512, 1982
34. Kinnaert P, Persijn G, Cohen B, Geertruyden J: Transplantation of kidneys from anencephalic donors. Transplant Proc 16:71–72, 1984
35. Kinnaert P, Vereerstraeten P, Van Asperen de Boer F et al: Transplantation of both kidneys of an anencephalic newborn to a 23-year-old patient. Eur Urol 7:373–376, 1981
36. Lawson J: Delivery of the dead or malformed fetus: Intrauterine death during pregnancy with retention of fetus. Clin Obstet Gynaecol 9:745–756, 1982
37. Lemire RJ: Anencephaly, p 3. New York, Raven Press, 1978
38. Lloyd-Still JD: Mortality from liver disease in children: Implications for hepatic transplantation programs. Am J Dis Child 139:381–384, 1985
39. Lum CT, Wassner SJ, Martin DE: Current thinking in transplantation in infants and children. Pediatr Clin N Am 32:1203–1232, 1985
40. McEvoy RC, Hegre OD: Syngeneic transplantation of fetal rat pancreas: III. Effect of insulin treatment on the growth and differentiation of the pancreatic implants after reversal of diabetes. Diabetes 28:141–146, 1979
41. Mills J: Personal communication, Jan 3, 1986
42. Monoco AP: Clinical kidney transplantation in 1984. Transplant Proc 17:5–12, 1985
43. National Institute of Arthritis, Diabetes, and Digestive and Kidney Diseases: Summary notes of ad hoc meeting on liver heterotransplantation, Apr 23, 1985
44. National Institutes of Health: National Chimpanzee Management Plan, Aug 30, 1985
45. Ohshima S, Ono Y, Kinukawa T et al: Kidney transplantation from an anencephalic baby: A case report. J Urol 132:546–547, 1984
46. Pittsburgh Transplant Foundation: Postmortem Organ Procurement Protocol. 1038 J Scaife Hall, Pittsburgh, PA 15261
47. President's Commission for the Study of Ethical Problems in Medicine and Biomedical and Behavioral Research: Defining Death, p 119. Washington, DC, US Gov Printing Office, 1981
48. Prummer O, Raghavachar A, Werner C et al: Fetal liver transplantation in the dog. Transplantation 39:349–355, 1985
49. Regan T: The other victim. Hastings Cent Rep 15:8–13, 1985
50. Robertson JA: Involuntary euthanasia of defective newborns: A legal analysis. Stanford Law Rev 27:213–268, 1973
51. Russell PS: Selective transplantation: An emerging concept. Ann Surg 201:255–262, 1985
52. Schmid R, Berwick DM, Combes B et al: Liver transplantation. National Institutes of Health Consensus Development Conference Summary. Vol 4, No 7, 1983
53. Simpson, TJ, Golbus MS: In utero fetal hematopoietic stem cell transplantation. Semin Perinatol 9:68–74, 1985
54. Singer P: Practical Ethics, pp 122–138. Cambridge, Cambridge University Press, 1979
55. So SKS, Nevine TE, Chang PN et al: Preliminary results of renal transplantation. Transplant Proc 17:182–183, 1985
56. Starzl TE, Iwatsuki S, Shaw BW et al: Orthotopic liver transplantation in 1984. Transplant Proc 17:250–258, 1985
57. Thomas ED: Marrow transplantation fro non-

malignant disorders. N Engl J Med 213:46–47, 1985
58. Tooley M: Abortion and infanticide, p 414. Oxford, Clarendon Press, 1983
59. Tulipan NB, Zacar HA, Allen GS: Pituitary transplantation I. Successful reconstitution of pituitary-dependent hormone levels. Neurosurgery 16:331–335, 1985
60. Uniform Anatomical Gift Act. See, for example, Vernon's Texas Statutes Annot, 4909(a)–(d)
61. Warkany J: Congenital Malformations, p 199. Chicago, Year Book Medical Publishers, 1972
62. Wolfle TL: Personal communications, Apr 22, 1985; May 27, 1986

18

Allowing Babies to Die

SECTION 1: MEDICAL ISSUES

Anne B. Fletcher

Since the late 1960s, modern technology has revolutionized the treatment of newborns in the United States. Thousands of infants who, in earlier decades, would have died or survived with severe handicaps are leading normal, healthy lives. However, because technology also allows the survival of children with severe physical and mental handicaps, ethical and moral dilemmas have arisen. Major questions need to be addressed as technology advances and costs spiral. Is it always correct to employ our vast technology for each infant? Once we start, should we ever stop? If so, who is going to make the decision that an infant be allowed to die? Does there come a time when it is more humane to stop therapy, or is life in itself of such supreme value that quality can never be an issue? Who is going to pay for this highly sophisticated care and provide continued financial support if the result is a handicapped child?

Eighteen years ago, neonatologists began to realize that their responsibilities as physicians no longer merely entailed caring for a sick infant until recovery or death. Technology had become so advanced that at times it merely prolonged dying and resulted in extended suffering for both infant and family. Fully aware that "not to decide is to decide," some of us began to see that our real responsibility as child advocates was to ensure that decisions to give care or to withhold or withdraw treatment were made actively in the best interests of the infant. This chapter discusses some milestones in decision making on behalf of handicapped newborns, medical aspects of decision making, and problems in decision making, such as the effects of government legislation on physicians who have tried to deal with the decision-making process.

MILESTONES IN DECISION MAKING

Certain milestones in ethical and moral decision making have profoundly influenced present-day thinking. In 1971, Lorber reported the results of his treatment of infants with myelomeningocele. He stated that certain criteria, if seen at birth, could be used to exclude some infants from treatment.[6] These criteria included gross paralysis of the legs, thoracolumbar or thoracolumbosacral lesions, kyphosis or scoliosis, intracerebral birth injury, and other gross congenital anomalies. The article provoked widespread discussions in the literature in the United States and abroad—discussions that continue. The same year, physicians and parents at Johns Hopkins University made the decision to allow an infant with Down's syndrome and duodenal atresia to die of starvation. A film, *Who Should Survive,* based on the story of this infant and made by the Kennedy Foundation in Washington, D.C., contributed to the early discussion of life-and-death decisions in neonatal units.

In 1973, Duff and Campbell wrote that of 299 infants who had died in their nursery, 43 or 14% had been allowed to die. The deaths included eight infants with a trisomy (unspecified) and three with meningomyelocele.[1] It is interesting to note that those who were allowed to die had a longer mean survival rate than those who died of "natural causes." Duff and Campbell stressed that pediatricians had become distressed with the severe handicaps that resulted from the preservation of life at all costs. These physicians opened a Pandora's box, and an explosion of journal and newspaper articles followed in which physicians, lawyers, and ethicists joined in discussions of whether life-and-death decisions were ethical and moral and by what process such decisions could be made.

Not until 1974 was any specific discussion of decision making concerning other than malformed infants initiated. At this time, the issue of the small premature infant on prolonged ventilation was raised. A conference convened by the University of California, San Francisco, asked individuals from many disciplines the following questions: (1) Is it ever right to withdraw life support from a clearly diagnosed poor-prognosis infant? (2) Is it ever right not to resuscitate an infant at birth? (3) Is it ever right to displace poor-prognosis infant A in order to provide intensive care for better-prognosis infant B? (4) Is it ever right to intervene directly to kill a dying infant?[5] Most participants answered "yes" to all four questions. However, they realized that theoretical considerations were very different from making difficult decisions at the bedside. Moreover, they chose to ignore the legal aspects of the questions. Procedural guidelines were recommended, which included better coordination of research efforts in neonatology, refinement of clinical criteria on which decisions could be made, better delivery-room policies regarding nonresuscitation, regionalization of neonatal care, better education of parents, and decision making with parents only after adequate time for observation and assessment. Finally, the conference concluded that advisory boards should be formed to discuss difficult cases, suggest criteria for withholding care, and even perform retrospective review of cases in which decisions had been made.[5] Had neonatologists heeded these recommendations, the present state of indecision might have been avoided.

From 1975 to 1982, newspaper articles were written regularly about infants with multiple congenital anomalies from whom care was being withheld. Debate continued in the professional literature. Some hospitals developed limited policies concerning nonresuscitation of patients. Minimal numbers of ethical review boards or committees were started. The President's Commission for the Study of Ethical Problems in Medicine was also examining these issues. Meanwhile, life-and-death decisions continued to be made in nurseries around the country.

Finally, on April 2, 1982, a term male infant with Down's syndrome and esophageal atresia was born in Bloomington, Indiana. The decision not to correct the atresia was made by the parents and physician. The hospital petitioned the state court for guidance, and a guardian *ad litem* was appointed. Ultimately, no judicial intervention occurred; the records were sealed; and the infant died six days later.

Although the infant was not fed and was

said to have died of starvation, it is more likely that death resulted from complications secondary to the esophageal atresia. The intent of starvation was there; society was finally shocked. It became apparent that physicians and parents could no longer proceed privately with their decision making. President Reagan resurrected Section 504 of the Rehabilitation Act of 1973 and instructed the Department of Health and Human Services (DHHS) to send a "notice" to health care providers reminding them that it was illegal for hospitals receiving federal financial assistance to withhold medical or surgical treatment and nutritional sustenance from handicapped infants. If care was withheld, federal assistance would be withdrawn.

During the next months, many physicians were interviewed about how the DHHS notice would affect the decision-making process. Some questioned the applicability of Section 504 to the care of infants and wondered what the government meant by the term *handicapped*. Did it refer only to infants with Down's syndrome and spina bifida, or did it apply to all infants in an intensive care unit? No answers were forthcoming.

Before physicians and parents could respond adequately to this intrusion, the Interim Final Ruling was issued March 7, 1983. It required institutions to post conspicuous (14" × 17") signs in each pediatric unit, delivery room, and pediatric and neonatal intensive care unit stating that "Discriminatory failure to feed and care for handicapped infants in this facility is prohibited by law."[8] Any person having information that this "failure" was occurring could call a "Handicapped Infant Hotline" 24 hours a day, seven days a week. Instead of the usual 30- to 60-day period during which the public could comment, a period of 14 days was allowed.

Medical groups filed suit against the DHHS, stating that the Interim Final Ruling was an unnecessary intrusion into a very sensitive area of medicine. Three weeks later, Judge Gerhard Gessell declared the ruling invalid on the basis of the short comment period. Subsequent rulings have come and gone; the new Child Abuse and Neglect Act of 1984 has been passed and awaits further action by DHHS. It appears likely that physicians, parents, and the decision-making process will remain under the aegis of government for quite some time.

MEDICAL ASPECTS OF DECISION MAKING

All infants admitted to an intensive care nursery are, by definition, either handicapped or have the potential to become so as a result of physiologic immaturity or birth injury. These infants can be classified into three general categories. The first includes infants whose prognosis is so poor that any therapy will only prolong dying. Examples of this group include infants with anencephaly, holoprosencephaly, trisomy 13 and triosomy 18, premature infants weighing less than 500 g, and those with multiple, severe congenital anomalies. The second group consists of infants whose prognosis is good to excellent, such as larger premature infants and those with correctable congenital anomalies. The final group includes infants whose prognosis is unknown at the time of admission; this group consists mainly of premature infants weighing from 500 to 1000 g. All infants admitted to an intensive care nursery receive maximum therapy until there has been enough assessment to provide a basis for decision making.

Decision Makers and Aids for Decision Making

Since newborns are unable to decide for themselves, others must make decisions for them. The best decision can be made by the team of individuals involved in the overall care of the infant. This team usually consists of the responsible attending physician and fellow in training; the resident or nurse practitioner caring for the infant; the nurse at the bedside; personnel who support the family, such as a social worker or chaplain; and, most importantly, the parents or legal guardians. All are considered to be advocates for the child who will act in the child's best interest.

Certain aids for decision making are essential. A monthly departmental care conference allows in-depth examination of each chronically ill infant and helps to ensure continuity of care and communication with the parents. It also encourages an exchange of views on the management of each infant. Readily available consultations within the department as well as with other departments may be of great value when the prognosis of an infant is in question. Individual conferences are called by nurses and physicians to resolve questions about patient care and to indicate when decisions must be made about prognosis. Disagreements can be raised and are usually resolved. Frequent conferences with parents regarding the care and prognosis of their infant establish and maintain communication, making life-and-death decisions more easily approached should the need arise. Finally, the advent of Infant Bioethical Review Boards has made it possible for the team to seek help with particularly difficult cases and when disagreements cannot be resolved. A board can provide great support to physicians and parents, helping to alleviate the stress imposed on those who make the final decision.

Making the Decision

Decision making is complex. It takes a great deal of time and skill; it often takes a toll on the decision makers: parents, nurses, and physicians. In our nursery, we have attempted to make decision making an active process from the moment of admission to the time of death or discharge. We have tried to combine decision making with sound ethical and moral reasoning. As previously mentioned, there are two groups of infants about whom decisions may have to be made. In the first group, where the prognosis is known and is poor, a decision may be made quite early in the hospitalization. In the group where the prognosis is uncertain, infants are given maximal care until the prognosis can be more clearly defined. The most difficult problems exist in the group in which the prognosis remains uncertain. A decision may come only after many weeks or even months. Most infants in this group are premature infants who were born with the potential of being normal but with immature organs on which present methods of intensive care have imposed their toll.

Because each infant and set of parents are distinct individuals, the decision-making process is unique for each infant. Informed decisions can be made only after a thorough evaluation of each particular problem. The physician's personal experience and knowledge of the relevant literature are important. Decisions rarely need to be made in haste. In most cases, there is adequate time to assess each infant and to educate the parents. Because the decision makers look after the best interests of the child, their hope is that each child will have a reasonable life without prolonged pain and suffering and a good chance for pleasurable interaction within the family and society. In addition, it is expected that care will be beneficial and will not merely prolong dying. Discussions are often lengthy, but eventually recommendations must be made to the parents, who in turn must make the final decision supported by a caring team. All appropriate information is documented in the medical record.

Parents are essential to the decision-making process. It has been suggested that parents may not be the best advocates for their children. After the birth of a deformed or premature infant, parents are emotionally overwhelmed and in varying states of shock, denial, depression, and anger. Indeed, they must mourn the loss of the normal child they expected. They need intense and continuing support from the whole team involved in the care of their infant. As the initial emotion subsides, parents have concerns about how they will cope with a handicapped infant, the stability of their marriage, the effects on other siblings, their careers, and lifestyles, as well as the huge costs involved, which they may not be able to meet. Despite these very real concerns, most parents are the best advocates for their children. With appropriate understanding and help, parents can participate in and make decisions with which they can live comfortably.

Most parents want the very best for their child. They want their child to love and be loved and to participate in activities that they themselves have taken part in. They want their child to be accepted as an independent individual in society. Almost invariably, parents accept their child and want to participate in all care decisions, including those dealing with life and death. Sometimes they initiate discussions about stopping aggressive care when physicians cannot call a halt.[10] Even the President's Commission for the Study of Ethical Problems in Medicine and Biomedical and Behavioral Research suggested that when the infant's prognosis is ambiguous or uncertain, parents should be allowed to make the final decision.[9]

Sometimes the best interests of the infant and the parents coincide; sometimes they do not. However, the parents—not the physicians, the government, or the pro-life or handicapped-advocacy groups—are certainly the ones who will bear the fruits of technological advances in neonatology, bitter or sweet, for the rest of their lives. Can anyone really know what is in the best interest of a child? The parents are probably closest to knowing. On the rare occasion that parents make a poor decision on an infant's behalf, there is protection under existing laws, and physicians or the hospital can go to court as the infant's advocate.

PROBLEMS IN DECISION MAKING

Some of the problems related to making decisions are due to difficulties inherent in the process; others are related to external influences. In the former category is the factor of an uncertain outcome for a given infant. The physician's personal experience and statistics from the literature may give a reasonably clear picture. However, follow-up studies may be short-term and not reflective of the ultimate prognosis of the child, or they may be long-term and not reflective of current methods of therapy. Thus, in decision making, with rare exceptions, a small degree of uncertainty is inevitable.

A second problem in the process is that of the potential "miracle." The physician easily remembers the one very small infant who did well. Parents also hear of unusual survivals, and sometimes they are called to the nursery to see their dying infant, only to have the child survive for a while longer. It is never possible to predict the exact time of death.

A third problem lies with the parents. Some are very young, children themselves, unmarried and without much support. They cannot be expected to handle such difficult decisions. Parental attitudes are changing as increasing numbers of people join fundamentalist religious groups. Although they accept death, they cannot take part in a decision to stop prolonging life. Thus, at times, physicians painfully proceed with nonbeneficial care. Moreover, many parents seem to accept the care of their severely handicapped child initially, not realizing the magnitude of their undertaking until later, when the full manifestation of the handicap becomes apparent.

A fourth problem exists with some physicians, who can never make decisions to withdraw life support, even if there are distinct ethical, moral, and clinical guidelines. Physicians enter medicine to preserve life, not to end it. Some fear death and cannot see it as a part of life. Their feelings of guilt and helplessness in the face of a dying patient are at times overwhelming. Legal liability and malpractice play an increasing role in determining the extent and type of care patients receive. Medical schools are just beginning to offer major education in moral philosophy and ethics. Finally, many physicians view technology as something to be used for its own sake, whether or not it is beneficial to the patient.

In the last few years, two external forces have profoundly influenced the decision making of physicians, parents, and hospitals: the Baby Doe regulations and the Child Abuse and Neglect Act of 1984. The lack of clear definitions of terms used in the regulations has compounded the problems of decision making. Prolongation of dying and suffering, rather than preservation of life and prevention of wrong decisions, may be the result of government intervention into the practice of medicine. The days in which parents and physicians could decide to end an infant's life without the advice, support, and appraisal of representatives of society are past.

In addition, physicians are being forced to consider the enormous costs of intensive care and care of handicapped infants. Medicaid has already begun to limit the duration of hospitalization for all children; DRGs (diagnosis-related groups) established by third-party payers are looming to reduce the cost of medical care. These may be inadequate for the sickest infants. There have already been decreases in financial support for programs for the handicapped. Adequate institutional care, chronic care programs, and special education in schools are lacking. New programs for the chronically ill are needed. At the present time, the cost of care is never an issue considered in the decision-making process. If the present national trend of cost containment continues without due thought to the generation of handicapped children who are being saved, the cost of care may become a major factor in decision making.

A NEONATOLOGIST'S VIEWPOINT

In 1988, there were 3.7 million births in the United States. Of these infants, 250,000 were at risk of dying or of having lifelong handicaps and were admitted to neonatal intensive care units. The cost of this care approximated that allotted to cardiac bypass or renal dialysis. Neonatologists have been placed in an untenable position. We have been told that care for infants who weigh less than 900 or 1000 g is not yet cost-effective[2,11] and that occasionally we give too much care.[10] Nevertheless, proposed agreement among handicapped groups and the American Academy of Pediatrics tells us to give medical care "without regard to quality of life or anticipated or actual limited potential or underlying handicap."[4]

Although every infant deserves a chance to live and discrimination against any group or class of infants is wrong, the current regulations create some real difficulties. The first problem involves the use of the term *handicap*. The word is defined as "a deficiency, especially an anatomical, physiological or mental deficiency that prevents or restricts normal achievement."[7] To say that decisions should not be made on the basis of handicap is unrealistic. Normal infants do not require a decision; degree of handicap must be defined if the regulations are to have any meaning.

The second problem has to do with the expression "quality of life." We are told that it should not be used because it is vague and subject to individual interpretation and because the quality of life of someone other than the infant may be under consideration. Yet the phrases that are used instead—"irremedial handicap," "reasonable life," "child's best interest," "pain and suffering," and "futile care"—are equally vague and defy definition, except as applied in an individual case.

The third problem is the failure to delineate general and specific guidelines under which to operate. General criteria may be useful in some categories of abnormalities, such as anencephaly or Down's syndrome, but they are useless when applied to the very small, immature infant with multiple difficulties. Education, awareness, and consultative help would be more helpful than individual criteria for such cases. Specific guidelines are difficult to define and do not take into account different circumstances surrounding infants in different environments.

The final problem has to do with the decision makers. The ideal would be to have an observer who is consistent, omniscient, omnipercipient, disinterested, and dispassionate.[3] The nursery team in conjunction with the parents and an Infant Review Board should aim to achieve this ideal, even though no group of human beings with their inherent imperfections and prejudices can attain it.

There is no doubt that erroneous decisions have been made and that infants must be protected under the law. Enlightened government regulations may accomplish this protection, or they may improve decision making for a few while harming many more. Concerns about government control may influence physicians to practice medicine even more defensively and perhaps turn away from decision making altogether. Furthermore, pressure from the federal government to treat all neonates equally may improve survival statistics. It will take decades, however, to understand the full emotional and economic impact of caring for thousands of severely handicapped individuals who otherwise would have died in the neonatal period.

Neonatologists must continue making decisions in their nurseries. We must make them carefully and with as much input as possible, thus regulating ourselves. We must continue to support and educate parents. It is equally important that we try to set guidelines for the use of technology so that it is used only when there is likely to be true benefit. There may even be times when we go to court as advocates to allow an infant to die against the parents' wishes. We must demand that the government provide adequate support to handicapped children and their families so that their physical as well as emotional needs are met. We have to avoid the possibility of a lack of resources, lest one day potentially normal children die because of the limited availability of care.

During a recent discussion of a very difficult case, a resident physician said to me sadly, "We treat our pets more humanely than we treat our infants." I was reminded that laws for the prevention of cruelty to animals preceded those outlawing child abuse and neglect. My hope is that in the arena of decision making we continue to treat infants humanely. In conclusion, to those who write, talk, or make regulations about these issues, I say, "Come to the bedside and suffer with us, for only then will you know what actually happens." To those who say they have talked to the handicapped about whether they would rather be alive or dead, I say, "You have only talked with the ones who can speak."

REFERENCES

1. Duff RS, Campbell AGM: Moral and ethical dilemmas in the special care nursery. N Engl J Med 289:890, 1973
2. Executive summary of the cost effectiveness of neonatal intensive care. In Budetti P, McManus N, Heinen L: The Cost Effectiveness of Neonatal Intensive Care, pp 79–86. Performance for the Office of Technology Assessment, United States Congress, Contract No 933-22-600, June 20, 1980
3. Fost N: Ethical issues in the treatment of critically ill newborns. Pediatr Ann 10:16, 1981
4. Healy A: Treatment of disabled infants (commentary). Pediatrics 73:563, 1984
5. Jonsen AR, Phibbs RH, Tooley WH, Garland MJ: Critical issues in newborn intensive care: A conference report and policy proposal. Pediatrics 55:756, 1975
6. Lorber J: Results of treatment of myelomeningocele: An analysis of 524 unselected cases with special reference to possible selection treatment. Dev Med Child Neurol 13:279, 1971
7. Morris W (ed): The American Heritage Dictionary of the English Language. Boston, Houghton Mifflin, 1981
8. Nondiscrimination on the basis of handicap (45CFR Part 84). Federal Register 48:9630, March 7, 1983
9. President's Commission for the Study of Ethical Problems in Medicine and Biomedical and Behaviorial Research: Deciding to Forego Life Sustaining Treatment, p 218. Washington, DC, US Gov Printing Office, 1983
10. Stinson R, Stinson P: The Long Dying of Baby Andrew. Boston, Atlantic Monthly Press, 1983
11. Walker DB, Feldman A, Uohr BR, Oh W: Cost-benefit analysis of neonatal intensive care for infants weighing less than 1000 grams at birth. Pediatrics 74:20, 1984

SECTION 2: LEGAL ISSUES

Leonard H. Glantz

For more than a decade there has been a stream of articles in the medical, legal, and ethics literature regarding the appropriateness of withholding and withdrawing care from seriously handicapped newborns. This is partly a result of the advances in medical science and technology that have provided interventions that can keep alive newborns who previously had been doomed to a certain death. There are now at least 7500 neonatal intensive care unit beds in about 600 hospitals in the United States, and over 1000 neonatologists have been certified. The number of infants who die in the first 28 days of life was halved between 1970 and 1980.[31] These advances now force parents and physicians to make choices where none was previously available. But the new technologies do not give parents and physicians purely free choices. The difficult question is "Are there circumstances in which physicians and parents *must* use the new technologies available to them?"

The advances in knowledge and technique, however, are not sufficient reasons to explain the explosion in interest in the difficult area of treatment decisions for newborns. For many years, relatively simple surgical techniques to treat ill newborns have been withheld. In 1977, a published study indicated that substantial numbers of physicians would respect the wishes of parents who declined medically beneficial treatment for newborns.[38] In that study, 76.8% of pediatric surgeons and 49.5% of pediatricians said they would acquiesce to the parents' decision to refuse to consent to surgery to repair an intestinal atresia if the child had Down's syndrome. Remarkably, 7.9% of the surgeons and 2.6% of the pediatricians would acquiesce to the same decision even if the child were perfectly normal aside from the atresia. The authors also found this "surprising" and ascribed some, but not all, of these responses to misreading the question.

Studies like this provide documentation of attitudes that are disturbing regardless of the advances in the treatment of newborns. It would appear that newborns who could be treated and live perfectly happy lives might not be receiving those treatments. From a legal and ethical perspective, it is also disturbing to realize that the decisions regarding which newborns receive treatment, and which do not, may be determined not on any principled basis, but according to the desires and inclinations of the particular parents or physicians who are making the decision. Furthermore, two studies published in the *New England Journal of Medicine* in 1973 documented that nontreatment decisions were in fact being made in regard to certain newborns.[8,37] These studies resulted in a congressional hearing in which testimony indicated that each year "several thousand" newborns die as a result of lack of treatment, although it was not known how many would have survived with treatment.[28]

While this activity was occurring in the medical community, other societal forces were at work that help explain concern about nontreatment decisions for newborns. Not until the mid-sixties did child abuse and neglect by parents become widely recognized, with all states ultimately passing child abuse laws. These laws not only permitted state intervention into the parent-child relationship but *mandated* reporting by physicians and others. Furthermore, these laws were formal recognition of the fact that parents can injure their children and that children sometimes need protection from their parents. Similarly, a children's rights movement gained momentum; it argued that children should be recognized as human beings who have rights separate from their parents.[33] Finally, the advent of the patient's rights movement, the expansion of the bioethics field, and court actions, such as the *Quinlan* case,[26] directed our attention to the rights of both competent and incompetent seriously ill and dying patients. All these forces came together, and as a result increased attention was focused on determining the needs and rights of the newborn, the authority of the parent to make treatment decisions, and the appropriate role of the physician.

Remarkably, with all the attention paid to the legal issues regarding the seriously handicpapped newborns—including a number of articles that hypothesize the causes for legal action, including criminal liability[34,36]—few cases have been brought to court. This is particularly surprising given the comparatively large number of cases regarding incompetent adults that have come to court. However, court rulings in cases that deal with incompetent adults provide guidance because the issues they present are identical to those presented by newborns, who are, after all, incompetent patients too. This entire body of case law provides substantial guidance on when it is appropriate to terminate or withhold treatment from seriously ill newborns.

CASE LAW

In 1974, a Maine trial court was presented with the issue of nontreatment of a newborn.[24] In that case a child was born without a left eye, with a rudimentary left ear lacking an ear canal, with a malformed left thumb, and with a tracheal-esophageal fistula. The physicians recommended surgery to repair the fistula; the parents refused to consent and asked for cessation of intravenous feeding. The hospital sought court authorization for the surgery. While the case was pending, the child's condition deteriorated. He had periods of apnea and suffered several convulsions. It was determined that the right eye did not respond to light, that there were several unfused vertebrae, and that there was "some brain damage." As a result of these findings, the doctors no longer recommended surgery but rather recommended that all life-support systems be withdrawn. At this stage of the proceedings, one is confronted by an unusual situation: all the parties (who started out in adverse positions) now agreed on the outcome they desired—termination of care. This was of no consequence to the court because the case was still within its jurisdiction, and it felt it had to decide on the legality of the requested actions. It is also noteworthy to see why the physicians changed their position. At the outset of the case there was no indication of brain damage. Rather there was a deformed child whose parents were refusing life-saving treatment. Although the deformities were sufficient for the parents to refuse further care, they were not sufficient for the physicians to acquiesce in their decision. Once it was established that there was the certainty of "some" brain damage, the physicians, invoking their own value judgments, then felt that acquiescence with the parents' decision was appropriate. In its decision mandating treatment, the court provided criteria for such decision making. First, the negative emotional impact that this had, and will continue to have, on the parents is not relevant to the treatment decision. Such considerations, the court said, are relevant only to the issue of permanent custody. Second, the court decided that "the doctor's qualitative evaluation of the value of the life to be preserved is not legally within the scope of his expertise." Third, the court found that it was the doctor's opinion that the child would certainly die without surgery and that with the surgical correction the "child can survive but with some degree of permanent brain damage." The court therefore concluded,

> In the court's opinion, the issue before the court is not the prospective quality of life to be preserved, but the medical feasibility of the proposed treatment compared with the almost certain risk of death should treatment be withheld. Being satisfied that corrective surgery is medically necessary and medically feasible, the court finds that the defendants herein have no right to withhold such treatment and that to do so constitutes neglect in the legal sense.[24] [p. 4]

This court was presented with a pure quality-of-life question. The nature of the surgery, its risks, and its chances for success were identical before and after the determination of the existence of brain damage. Indeed, as is often the case with newborns, the extent and significance of the brain damage could not be determined—it was referred to as "some" brain damage. Thus the physicians were asking the judge to permit the withholding of treatment not because they believed the treatment was risky, unusually painful, or futile, but because they did not think that the child possessed a life worth saving. The court was unwilling to approve such judgments. Indeed, how would a court that was sympathetic to this position set forth the principles on which it was basing its decision? How poor would the quality of life have to be before nontreatment on this basis would be justified.?

This court established the criterion of "medical feasibility" as the standard by which these decisions should be made. What this seems to mean in the context of this case is that a procedure is medically feasible if it is possible to perform, would cure the life-threatening condition, and would be done on a child absent the perception of poor quality of life.

Courts in deciding cases are very concerned with establishing criteria that can be applied in the future. The goal is to try to reduce the arbitrariness of future decisions. Whether a child lives or dies should not, ideally, be determined by who the decision maker happens to be. Fairness and justice require that similarly situated newborns should be treated similarly, if at all possible. It is this search for criteria that has so baffled the courts and federal regulators.

In 1976 the New Jersey Supreme Court decided the first case regarding the termination of high-technology life-sustaining treatment. In the Quinlan case,[26] the court was faced with deciding the lawfulness of the parents' request to withdraw the use of a respirator that was keeping their comatose 22-year-old daughter alive. Karen Quinlan had suffered two 15-minute periods in which she had stopped breathing. After ineffectual attempts at mouth-to-mouth resuscitation, she was taken to a hospital where she was placed on a respirator. Her physicians eventually determined that she was in a chronic vegetative state from which she would never recover and that if the respirator were removed she would die. After a great deal of soul searching, her parents asked her physicians to remove the respirator, a request that the physicians refused to grant.

The physicians claimed that their refusal was based on their conception of what medical ethics, standards, and practice required. It was claimed that because Quinlan was not brain dead it would be improper to remove the life-sustaining respirator. However, it also appeared that the physicians would not transfuse her if she hemorrhaged, provide surgery if it became necessary, or resuscitate her if needed. It appears that the physicians were drawing a distinction between performing an "act" (removing the respirator) and withholding a necessary treatment, a distinction the court kindly referred to as "elusive to the nonmedical lay mind."

Although the Quinlan case may seem like an "easy" case today, it must be remembered that the law was not known at the time the case was commenced. Indeed, it is often forgotten that the trial court ruled that the respirator could not lawfully be removed from Quinlan.[22]

Unlike the court in the Maine case discussed earlier, the New Jersey Supreme Court explored the right that Quinlan would have to refuse such treatment. It determined that the constitutional right of privacy was broad enough to encompass a patient's right to refuse life-sustaining treatment. The court said that there was "no doubt" that if Karen were miraculously lucid for an interval, she could effectively decide on discontinuation of the life-support apparatus "even if it meant the prospect of a natural death." It further held that the state's countervailing interest in the "preservation and sanctity of human life" would not be sufficient in this instance to authorize overriding her wishes. The court indicated that if one were dealing with a case involving a procedure that encompassed "minimal bodily invasion," and the chances of recovery and return to a "functioning life" were "very good," the outcome might be otherwise. But the state's interest in the preservation of life weakens "and the individual's rights to privacy grows as the degree of bodily invasion increases and the prognosis dims." Here the court described her prognosis as "very poor—she will never resume a cognitive life." The court also described the bodily invasion as very great—requiring 24-hour nursing care, antibiotics, a catheter, tube feeding, and the assistance of a respirator.

Since Karen could not make her wishes known, the court found that the only way to "prevent the destruction of the right" is to permit her guardian and family to render their best judgment about what she would want in those circumstances. It is important to note that the court explicitly held that it is *not* the parents' rights that the court is recognizing. Rather it is the parents and guardian who are to exercise *Karen's* right on her behalf. In explaining its decision, the court argued that physicians distinguish between "curing the ill and comforting and easing the dying" and implied that courts should likewise make this distinction. The court also stated that "therapy" (the court put this word in quotation marks) that "offers neither human nor humane benefit" is not required to be administered. It then explicitly held that removing the life-sustaining machinery would not constitute homicide because such an act would be pursuant to the lawful exercise of a constitutional right. Finally, the court concluded that if the guardian, family, and physicians conclude that there is no "reasonable possibility" of Karen's ever emerging from her comatose condition to a "cognitive, sapient state" and a hospital "ethics committee" agrees, then all life-support systems may be withdrawn and such action should be without civil or criminal liability on the part of any participant. The court also alluded to the possibility that its ruling would apply to other "terminal" conditions not involving the loss of cognitive or sapient life.

Although there are some serious flaws in the *Quinlan* case,[15] it provides us with many important lessons. The first is that the law does permit nontreatment even when such nontreatment will hasten a person's death. The second is that patients have a constitutional right not to be treated. The third is that this right may be exercised on behalf of an incompetent person by a surrogate. The importance of these points to the nontreatment of newborns is readily apparent, since the court's analysis has nothing to do with Karen's age. If she were a newborn suffering from the same irreversible condition, the reasoning of this case would be identical.

The other point, which is never spoken in this case but which comes through time and time again, is that this court is in large part basing its decision on Karen's poor quality of life. The fact is that termination of treatment is permissible because she will never return to a "cognitive, sapient state," because she has no chance of returning to a "functioning life," because her prognosis is "dim," because she leads a "vegetative" existence, because she has lost "human qualities." Although this court never mentioned the expression "quality of life," it is a factor that had significant impact on its analysis and outcome. Indeed, it is the primary reason that the state's interest in the preservation of Karen's life was so diminished. It is also clear that the court believed that as a result of her condition, Karen herself had no interests. She could not suffer pain, know her condition, or comprehend any benefit from her care. As a result, her parents and physicians could have made a decision either to continue to treat her or to withhold treatment, and either decision would have been sustained by the court.

The *Quinlan* case involved terminating life-support systems from a comatose person; the next state supreme court case involved the withholding of a recognized therapy from a conscious though severely retarded man. *Superintendent of Belchertown State School v. Saikewicz*[39] involved a 67-year-old man with an I.Q. of 10 who lived in a state facility his entire life and who had no family. He was diagnosed as suffering from acute myeloblastic monocytic leukemia, and the issue was whether his physicians' and guardian's decision to withhold chemotherapeutic treatment from him was lawful. Testimony in the case indicated that if chemotherapy was administered, he would have a 30% to 50% chance of remission that would increase his life from between two to thirteen months. The testimony also indicated that he might have to be restrained in order for treatment to be administered and that as a result of treatment he might become anemic, need transfusions, and suffer nausea and other unpleasant side effects. If left untreated, he could live for a matter of weeks or several months, and he would likely die without discomfort.

In its decision, the court adopted much of the reasoning of the *Quinlan* court. It held that competent people have both a constitutional and a common law right to refuse life-sustaining treatment and that this right must be extended to incompetent individuals because "the value of human dignity extends to both." The primary criterion for determining what treatment decision is to be made on behalf of an incompetent person is the doctrine of "substituted judgment." This means the surrogate decision maker must try to ascertain the incompetent person's "actual interests and preferences." The decision should be "that which would be made by the incompetent person if that person were competent, but the decision should take into account the present and future incompetency of the individual as one of factors that would necessarily enter into the decision-making process of the competent person"[39] [p. 431]. This is a subjective test: What would this person choose if competent? The court recognized that in some instances this may be difficult to ascertain, in which case it would be necessary to rely on "objective criteria."

Weighing the burdens of the treatment proposed against the benefits, and relying in part on Mr. Saikewicz's inability to comprehend the reasons for the severe disruptions of his formerly secure and stable environment, the court affirmed the trial court's decision authorizing the withholding of chemotherapy treatment. However, one of the factors the trial court relied on in authorizing nontreatment was the "quality of life possible for him even if the treatment does bring about remission." The Massachusetts Supreme Court responded to this by saying, "To the extent that this formulation equates the value of life with any measure of the quality of life, we firmly reject it." In essence the court said that the fact of Mr. Saikewicz's profound retardation was not a permissible criterion for nontreatment. On the other hand, the court said it believed that this was not what the trial judge was referring to when he used the "ill chosen term 'quality of life.' . . ." Instead the court interpreted the trial court's use of that term to refer to the "continuing state of pain and disorientation precipitated by the chemotherapy treatment" and said that this was a permissible factor to take into account when making such decisions.

In this case, a court permitted the withholding of a widely used, life-prolonging treatment because it concluded that given the limited benefits versus the significant (although not overwhelming) burdens of treatment, it would be reasonable to conclude that this individual would refuse the treatment if he were in a position to do so.

Four years later the same court authorized the termination of kidney dialysis of a 79-year-old man suffering from chronic organic brain syndrome and kidney disease. The decision was based in large part on his wife's testimony that he would not wish to receive such treatment.[19] Although the court four years earlier had decried the use of "quality of life" judgments, in this case it noted that the dialysis treatments would not restore him even temporarily to a "normal, cognitive, integrated, functioning existence, but simply kept him alive." Much of this case was spent explaining some ambiguous portions of the *Saikewicz* case, and much of it was dedicated to allaying physicians' fears of legal action. At one point the court noted that physicians may refuse to follow the wishes of patients because of fear of potential criminal liability. The court said, "Little need be said about criminal liability: there is precious little precedent, and what there is suggests that the doctor will be protected if he acts on a good faith judgment that is not grievously unreasonable by medical standards." This statement demonstrates substantial regard for the medical profession and the court's understanding that doctors cannot be asked to practice with the fear that some court will second-guess them and send them to jail. Indeed, this has never happened. But the court's statement demonstrates the importance of the medical profession's establishing some standards of practice, because such standards are what the court will look to for guidance. Criminal liability, according to the Massachusetts court, can be established only if a doctor's acts are *"grievously* unreasonable by *medical standards."*

There are a few cases in which these principles set forth by the courts have been applied to infants. *In re L.H.R.*[20] required the Georgia Supreme Court to decide who, if anyone, could authorize the termination of life-support systems sustaining the life of an infant. Fifteen days after her birth, L.H.R. suffered a "medical catastrophe" that left her in a chronic vegetative state with 85% to 90% of her brain tissue destroyed. The child's neurologist, parents, and guardian *ad litem* concurred that all life-support systems should be removed. The hospital sought a declaratory judgment from a court regarding the lawfulness of such removal. The court limited its ruling to resolving the issue of who can exercise the constitutional right to refuse treatment "on behalf of a terminally ill infant who is in a chronic vegetative state with no reasonable possibility of attaining cognitive function." The court ruled that in this circumstance the right to terminate treatment may be exercised by the parent or legal guardian with no need to seek a legal guardian or court approval. The court said, "We conclude that the decision whether to end the dying process is a personal decision for family members or those who bear a legal responsibility for the patient"[20] [p. 723].

A Massachusetts Supreme Court case involved the treatment of a 4½-month-old child who suffered from untreatable deformities of his heart and circulatory system.[7] There was no treatment available for him, nor any hope of treatment becoming available, and the prognosis was death within one year. The child's parents abandoned him shortly after birth, and the child became a ward of the state within the legal custody of the Department of Social Services (DSS). The child contracted a bacterial infection and was placed on a respirator. Because of the child's condition, his physician recommended that a "do not resuscitate" (DNR) order be entered. DSS "as a matter of policy" declined to consent to the DNR order, and the hospital sought court authorization. The testimony in the case indicated that resuscitation would be "invasive and traumatic" and would cause the child substantial pain and possible brain and liver damage. Medical testimony further indicated that a resuscitation attempt would not be in the child's best interest. On the basis of this testimony, the Juvenile Court authorized the entry of a DNR order. In an unusual twist, the hospital returned to court two weeks later seeking a revocation of the DNR order. The bacterial infection had disappeared, although the underlying cardiac condition and life expectancy estimates remained unchanged. The Juvenile Court judge refused to revoke his earlier order, finding that the disappearance of the bacterial infection had no relevance to his earlier findings regarding the child's best interests and substituted judgment. The Massachusetts Supreme Court affirmed the Juvenile Court's finding based on the child's dim prognosis and the substantial degree of bodily invasion, accompanied by discomfort and pain, that the child would suffer if resuscitation were attempted.

It should be noted that these cases involve decisions for the care of extremely ill infants for whom there is essentially no treatment. The authority of parents to make nontreatment decisions for less sick children is much more problematic. As a general rule, parents cannot refuse routine life-saving treatment for children. For example, all courts confronted with the issue have held that parents may not withhold necessary blood transfusions from their children on religious grounds.[16] Such treatment is routine and necessary to save the child's life, and refusal to consent to such care is technical child neglect. Clearly the benefits of transfusion outweigh the burdens to the child. Courts are more wary in overruling parental refusal to consent to more serious, dangerous, or invasive procedures but will do so when the child's life can be saved. Thus, one court overrode the parents' refusal to continue to consent to chemotherapy to treat their 2-year-old's leukemia when the medical testimony indicated that the therapy is life saving in 50% of all cases and was effective in this particular instance, that the child was suffering no serious side effects, and that death was certain without the treatment.[6]

On the other hand, what the courts consider a nontreatment decision is not always clear. In *Matter of Hofbauer*,[25] a 7-year-old was diagnosed as suffering from Hodgkin's disease. Left untreated, the disease is invariably fatal. The parents rejected the proposed radiation and chemotherapy treatments and chose instead to take their son to a physician who used "nutritional and metabolic therapy" including injections of laetrile. A proceeding was commenced alleging that the child was neglected because he was not receiving "adequate medical care." Numerous physicians testified that the proposed nutritional treatment was inadequate, but the court found that where, as here, a parent sought "accredited medical assistance" and provided their child with care recommended by a physician that has not been "totally rejected by all responsible medical authority," the parents have done all that is required of them. The outcome of this case may also be predicated on the parents' stated willingness to obtain established care if the proposed therapy did not succeed. This case is indicative of courts' unwillingness to intervene in treatment decisions in which a licensed physician has recommended a course of treatment to a parent and the parent has accepted it. Courts are not prone to arbitrate medical disputes, even in cases as extreme as this one.

At times, courts have erred by going too far in the direction of parental autonomy when it comes to treatment decisions for children. For example, the case of Phillip B.[21] involved a 12-year-old with Down's syndrome who required surgery to repair a congenital heart defect. At birth his parents placed the child in residential care. The reparable heart defect would cause progressive loss of energy, resulting in a bed-to-chair existence and ultimately death by the age of 20. The operation had a mortality rate of 5% to 10%, although Down's syndrome children have a higher than average rate of complications.

A petition was filed with the Juvenile Court alleging that the child was not being provided with the "necessities of life." The trial judge dismissed the petition, citing the inconclusiveness of the evidence. The Appeals Court sustained the ruling. In view of the approach courts generally take in resolving these issues, one can only conclude that these courts failed in their duty to protect this child. To reject an operation with even a 10% mortality rate and thereby let a child confront worsening debilitation and certain death is unjustifiable.[35] It is inconceivable that these courts would have come to the same conclusion if the child had not had Down's syndrome, and the existence of this condition is simply not enough to deprive a child of life-saving surgery.

The more typical case is exemplified by *Application of Cicero*.[2] In that case, a child was born with a meningomyelocele. Failure to repair this defect can lead to infection and death. The father refused to consent to surgery when the "potential enormity of the disorder" was fully explained to him. In this case, the baby was born with a relatively low lesion. Its deficits were determined to be likely below the ankle. She should be able to walk with short leg braces, and her lack of sphincter control could be medically and surgically ameliorated. She had no signs of hydrocephalus, and she was predicted to have normal intellectual development. The court, in mandating the treatment said, "This is not a case where the court is asked to preserve an existence which cannot be a life. What is asked is that a child born with handicaps be given a reasonable opportunity to live, to grow and hopefully to surmount those handicaps"[2] [p. 967].

When courts do not exercise their duty to

protect those infants who can benefit from medical treatment, it should be expected that other agencies will attempt to provide that protection. This is in fact what happened in the Baby Doe controversy, which ultimately demonstrated the futility of federal intervention.

THE BABY DOE EXPERIENCE

The case of Baby Doe that arose in April 1982 in Bloomington, Indiana, was the impetus for the federal government's action to try to enforce treatment of handicapped newborns. In one sense, it is surprising that this particular case caused such a reaction because little is known of its legal aspects, since all the court records were sealed. On the other hand, this very secrecy would indicate to some that more accountability is desirable, since such secrecy may lead to abusive decisions. Baby Doe was born with Down's syndrome, esophageal atresia, and suspected tracheoesophageal fistula. There was also a suspicion that the heart was abnormally enlarged. The family's pediatrician strongly recommended that the child be transferred to a children's hospital for surgical repair of the esophagus and further testing. The obstetrician painted a gloomier picture, informing the couple that a number of surgeries might be required, that nothing could be done about the Down's syndrome, and that the child would be retarded. He explained to the parents that they could refuse to consent to the surgery, in which case the baby would die in a few days. The parents decided to refuse the surgery. Additionally, it was ordered that the baby not receive any intravenous feedings, and no food or water could be given by mouth. The nursing staff was so distraught by these orders that the baby had to be removed from the nursery and placed in a private room. There also continued to be substantial discord between the pediatrician, who favored treatment, and the obstetrician, who did not.

The hospital's lawyer, aware of this discord, recommended judicial intervention. He called a judge at 10 P.M. and briefly described the situation. The judge agreed to go immediately to the hospital, where a hearing was held at about 10:30 P.M. Testimony was concluded at 1:00 A.M., and the judge rendered his decision upholding the nontreatment decision about a half-hour later. A number of additional legal proceedings were held as a result of a local district attorney's dismay at the outcome of the hospital hearing, but all the judges who heard the case noted that the parents' decision was lawful. The baby died as the local prosecutor was en route to the U.S. Supreme Court to appeal the state supreme court's decision.[9,23,30]

As a result of the public argument of this case in the state supreme court, the story was published in newspapers around the country. One month after Baby Doe's death, the U.S. Department of Health and Human Services (DHHS) issued a notice to all hospitals (apparently at the insistence of the White House) "reminding" hospitals that Section 504 of the Rehabilitation Act of 1973[42] makes it

> unlawful for a recipient of Federal financial assistance to withhold from a handicapped infant nutritional sustenance or medical or surgical treatment required to correct a life-threatening condition, if: (1) the withholding is based on the fact the infant is handicapped: and (2) the handicap does not render the treatment or nutritional sustenance medically contraindicated.[14]

This "reminder" caused serious concern in some portions of the medical community because it was far from clear that Section 504 had anything to do with specific treatment decisions and because it was unclear how these sweeping generalizations could be applied. One commentator asked why a handicap could *never* be grounds for nontreatment. He gave the example of a newborn with a major malformation of the brain resulting in complete absence of cortical function who was blind, deaf, and completely incapable of ever engaging in social interaction. He asked, if this child has no kidneys, does Section 504 outlaw the withholding of dialysis?[14]

In the apparent belief that this "reminder" was not sufficient to protect handicapped newborns, on March 7, 1983, DHHS published a rule requiring every hospital to post "in a conspicuous place in each delivery ward, each maternity ward, each pediatric ward, and each nursery, including each intensive care nursery," the following notice:

DISCRIMINATORY FAILURE TO FEED AND CARE FOR HANDICAPPED INFANTS IN THIS FACILITY IS PROHIBITED BY FEDERAL LAW

Section 504 of the Rehabilitation Act of 1973 states that no otherwise qualified handicapped individual shall, solely by reason of handicap, be excluded from participation in, be denied the benefits of, or be subjected to discrimination under any program or activity receiving federal financial assistance.

Any person having knowledge that a handicapped infant is being denied food or customary medical care should immediately contact:
Handicapped Infant Hotline
U.S. Department of Health and Human Services
Washington, D.C. 20201
Phone 800-____ ____ Available 24 hours a day

or

Your State Child Protective Agency

Federal law prohibits retaliation or intimidation against any person who provides information about possible violations of the Rehabilitation Act of 1973.

Identity of callers will be held confidential.

Failure to feed and care for infants may also violate the criminal and civil laws of your state.[10] [Emphasis in original]

The reason DHHS gave for publishing this rule without first publishing a proposed rule and providing for a comment period was that it was "necessary to protect life from imminent harm. Any delay would leave lives at risk."

This rule caused an immediate outcry from the medical profession. It was felt that it was a direct accusation of widespread child abuse by health professionals and that the notice would leave the impression in the minds of parents that hospitals did not adequately care for handicapped children. Additionally, it provided a specter, correctly it turned out, of federal officials descending on hospitals in an attempt to second-guess difficult treatment decisions. The American Academy of Pediatricians filed suit in federal court to enjoin the federal government from enforcing this rule.[1] Judge Gesell struck down the rule on the technical ground that DHHS had violated the Administrative Procedure Act, but the judge made it clear that he had even deeper concerns. He pointed out that any "anonymous tipster" could trigger a very disruptive investigation. He also excoriated DHHS for totally ignoring the importance of any parental role in treatment decisions. The judge also felt that this rule was a simple-minded approach to a very complex problem and that it was unlikely that Congress meant Section 504 to apply to individual treatment decisions. The decision noted that there was no evidence of widespread denial of proper care to newborns that would justify the rule and further noted that although the rule requires that there be no denial of "customary medical care," there was no evidence that there was such a thing as a customary standard of care for these children.

Instead of appealing this ruling, DHHS issued new proposed regulations[11] and, on January 12, 1984, new final regulations.[12] In many respects, these regulations were similar to the original rule. Notices still had to be posted, although they were somewhat smaller in size, and they had to be posted where nurses and other medical professionals who provide health care to infants would see them. In addition, state child protective services were required to institute procedures for quickly investigating these cases, and the use of Infant Care Review Committees was encouraged by DHHS. The rule now said that "nourishment and medically beneficial treatment (as determined with respect for reasonable medical judgments) should not be withheld from handicapped infants solely on the basis of their present or anticipated mental or physical impairments." Although this rule is less dogmatic than the previous ones, it merely restates the controversy that has plagued this discussion for years rather than even beginning to answer questions such as these: What is "medically beneficial treatment?" What is a "reasonable medical judgment" in this area, and is it different from the "customary medical care" that was required by the earlier rule?

While this was going on in Washington, a second case developed in New York. On October 11, 1983, a child who came to be known as Baby Jane Doe was born with a number of disorders including myelomeningocele, microencephaly, and hydrocephalus. The child was transferred to Stony Brook Hospital with the intention of having surgery performed to close the lesion and treat the hydrocephalus. However, after lengthy discussions with doctors, nurses, and social workers, the parents chose not to consent to the surgery but rather to opt for conservative treatment involving antibiotics and covering the lesion so that skin could grow over it. There was apparently no dissension from this choice by the hospital staff. However, a self-styled "right-to-life" lawyer in Vermont received an anonymous tip about this child's treatment and brought suit in New York to have the baby receive surgery.[9] The trial court judge ruled there was an immediate need for surgery and ordered the procedures. An immediate appeal was filed, and the appellate court reversed, siding with the parents.[43] The court found that there was no support for the finding that the child's life was in imminent danger and that the only physicians who testified both agreed that the parents' choice of treatment was "well within accepted medical standards." It also found that although the mortality rate is higher when conservative treatment is used, in this case surgery would involve a great risk of depriving the infant of what little function remained in her legs and would also likely have other negative repercussions. The court concluded that "These concededly concerned and loving parents have made an informed, intelligent and reasonable determination based upon and supported by responsible medical authority." Thus, the parents did make a *treatment* decision; and although their decision did not maximize the child's sense of survival, it satisfied the parents' legal obligation. This ruling was in accordance with the *Hofbauer* case, discussed above, which holds that parents are not obliged to provide *maximal* medical care.

The decision was appealed by the guardian *ad litem*, and New York's highest court also supported the parents.[44] This court was not shy about expressing its displeasure with the way the case had come to court. It pointed out that the Vermont attorney had no relationship with the child, parents, family, or medical professionals treating the child. The petitioner also had no first-hand knowledge of the facts regarding the child's condition, the treatment she was receiving, or the factors that had led to the parents' decision. In essence, the court concluded that these parents had been put through three continuous weeks of litigation in three levels of courts by a stranger with no stake in the outcome. The court found this "distressing" and "offensive" and made it clear that the proceedings should never have been allowed to go forward on this basis.

It should come as no surprise that DHHS, in the era of the Baby Doe hotline, received a hotline complaint that Baby Jane Doe was being denied medical treatment. The complaint was referred to New York's Child Protective Services, which performed an investigation and concluded that the child was being appropriately treated. During the state litigation, DHHS had obtained copies of the infant's medical records through October 19. These were personally reviewed by Surgeon General Koop, who decided he needed later records to decide whether the denial of treatment had been based solely on handicap. On October 23, DHHS made repeated demands for these medical records so it could determine whether Section 504 had been violated.

These requests demonstrated to the medical community the massive disruption the Baby Doe regulations would bring. Up to this point, there had been a decision made by parents to consent to what the treating physicians deemed to be appropriate, if not maximal, care. This case had been reviewed by three levels of courts, including the state's highest court, and the state's Child Protective Services. With the exception of the trial court judge, who profoundly misconstrued the facts and the law, all the higher courts and the child protective agency had found the treatment to be legally acceptable. After all this, a federal bureaucrat in Washington made it apparent that he believed the final judge of the appropriateness of the treatment decision was to be him. Given this, the hospital could only decide to fight. It refused to turn over the records, and DHHS went to court to compel their disclosure. This was the first chapter in the ultimate legal fight that would bring down the Baby Doe regulations.

The District Court supported the hospital's refusal to release the records by demonstrating the major flaw in DHHS' regulations.[40] Section 504 pertains only to discriminatory activity by a recipient of federal funds, which is the hospital in this instance. At all times the hospital and its employees were willing to perform the surgery. It was the *parents'* decision, not the hospital's decision, not to perform the surgery, and therefore the hospital could not conceivably have violated the federal law. The law does not apply to the parents, and therefore the records need not be disclosed because it was impossible for the federal law to have been violated given the facts of this case. The court was also clearly convinced of the appropriateness of the parents' decision.

The government appealed and for the first time offered a new argument, which claimed that the hospital's failure to seek a court order to override the parental decision to choose a more conservative treatment constituted a violation of Section 504.[41] This, of course, ignored the plain fact that the various decisions of the New York courts and child protection agency demonstrated without a doubt that the hospital was correct in its decision not to seek such an order.

The Court of Appeals affirmed the District Court's ruling. It pointed out that until DHHS sent its "reminder" to hospitals, it had been the position of that agency that Section 504 did not authorize it to be involved in specific treatment decisions. Furthermore, the court found that the federal legislative history supported this point of view. Thus, the court concluded that DHHS had no authority in this area.

Ultimately, the Supreme Court decided the issue based on cases brought by the American Medical Association and American Hospital Association to strike down the final Baby Doe regulations.[4] The court held that nontreatment of an infant based on a parental refusal to consent cannot be the basis for a violation of Section 504. First, in the absence of parental consent, the hospital could not legally treat such an infant. Second, such nontreatment would, by definition, not be "solely by reason of the handicap" but solely by reason of lack of parental consent. Last, in the absence of parental consent, the child would not be "otherwise qualified" for treatment.

In addition, the government's lawyer conceded that DHHS had never been able to find a case in which a hospital refused to treat an infant whose parents had consented to such treatment. Indeed, while the hotline was operational, DHHS never found one case of discriminatory nontreatment among the 49 it investigated. Thus the need for federal regulations was unsupported by the factual record. The court also rejected the government's contention that Section 504 could require hospitals to report parents' treatment refusals to state agencies and maintained that Section 504 does not give the government authority to "commandeer" state agencies to enforce compliance of federal laws. The court concluded that Section 504 did not authorize the federal government to give "unsolicited advice either to parents, to hospitals or to state officials who are faced with difficult treatment decisions concerning handicapped children." Having been stymied by trying to apply an inappropriate statute to this circumstance, the advocates of the Baby Doe regulations had to rely on congressional action.

The Child Abuse Prevention and Treatment Act was originally passed to make federal funds available to states that met certain conditions. In 1984, in the wake of the Baby Doe controversy, this act was amended to require state child protection agencies to adopt procedures for rapidly responding to reports of "medical neglect," including the "withholding of medically indicated treatment" from disabled infants with life-threatening conditions.[32] The term "withholding of medically indicated treatment" was defined as

> the failure to respond to the infant's life-threatening conditions by providing treatment (including appropriate nutrition, hydration, and medication) which, in the treating physician's or physicians' reasonable medical judgment, will be most likely to be effective in ameliorating or correcting all such conditions, except that the term does not include the failure to provide treatment (other than appropriate nutrition, hydration or medication) to an infant when, in the treating physician's or physicians' reasonable medical judgment, (A) the infant is chronically and irreversibly comatose; (B) the provision of such treatment would (i) merely prolong dying, (ii) not be effective in ameliorating or correcting all of the infant's life-threatening conditions, or (iii) otherwise be futile in terms of the survival of the infant; or (C) the provision of such treatment would be virtually futile in terms of the survival of the infant and the treatment itself under such circumstances would be inhumane.

As a close reading of this statute indicates, it resolves none of the difficult problems inherent in making treatment decisions on behalf of handicapped newborns. For example, the law prohibits the withholding of "*appropriate* nutrition, hydration and medication." Of course, the difficult issue is to determine what is appropriate in a given circumstance. But what is clear is that by using the modifier "appropriate," the legislation does not always require the provision of nutrition, hydration, or medication. Indeed, one can ask, who would advocate the withholding of *appropriate* nutrition, hydration, or medication? The legislation also explicitly permits the withholding of care from certain classes of infants, such as the irreversibly comatose. This, in and of itself, is a significant departure from the original Baby Doe rules.

It is far from clear what it means for a treatment to be "virtually futile" or "inhumane." What is a treatment that merely prolongs dying? The regulations and interpretive guidelines issued by DHHS provide almost no clarification.[13] It is important to keep in mind what the law and regulations apply to. Unlike the rules promulgated under Section 504, these rules do not apply to either hospitals or physicians. Nor do they give the federal government authority to investigate or interfere in any individual treatment decision. Rather, they are conditions that state governments must meet to receive certain federal funding. Thus, child abuse and neglect enforcement is back in the hands of the states, where it belongs and where it has always resided. It is really quite remarkable that, given the years, manpower, and dollars that have gone into this federal litigation and legislation, we are in essentially the same position we were in prior to all this activity. In many ways, this is confirmation of just how difficult it is to set forth criteria that would cover the wide range of circumstances these cases present.

Conclusion

Since the demise of the Baby Doe rules and the creation of the federal child abuse statute and regulations, there has been little activity in this area. Scholarly commentary continues to be written, but there has been little if any action in the courts. There is also no indication that the child protection agencies in the various states have been any more active in this area than in the past.

What is certain to happen is a continuation of the slow, case-by-case adjudication of the difficult or contested cases. Although judicial decisions have been relatively scarce in the infant nontreatment area, many major decisions dealing with incompetent adults have application to newborns. The trend of these decisions indicates that a number of principles have been or are in the process of being established. The courts have consistently decided that medical treatments that would serve to prolong life may be withheld or discontinued. The continuation of life at any cost is not legally required. That is particularly evident in the case of irreversibly comatose individuals. Furthermore, since *Quinlan* in 1976, there has been no appellate case in which physicians and families agreed that nontreatment was the most desirable and appropriate course of action but a court mandated treatment. Courts have also become increasingly sophisticated in handling nontreatment cases. Thus, several courts have held that in such cases one must weigh the burden and benefits of the treatment that might be provided, regardless of how such treatments are classified.[3,17] For example, the courts have not been impressed with the distinction between "ordinary" and "extraordinary" treatment.[17] They find the distinction impossible to define and also find that "ordinary" as well as "extraordinary" treatments can be withheld. Similarly, courts have not been impressed with the distinction of withholding versus withdrawing treatment.[5,17] If a treatment is not appropriate for a particular person, it does not make any difference if it is to be withheld or withdrawn as long as it is not inflicted on the patient. Finally, and somewhat surprisingly, the courts that have heard cases involving the administration of artificial nutrition have unanimously held that in appropriate circumstances such artificial nutrition can be withheld or discontinued.[3,5,17,18] This is surprising because of the powerful, emotional aspects involved in depriving one of nutrition and thereby "starving" someone to death. However, the courts have recognized that artificial nutrition is more akin to a medical procedure that has risks and benefits than to providing someone with a meal. Thus, courts have not stood in the way of families and physicians making nontreatment decisions on behalf of incompetent patients. Indeed, it could be argued that if anything the courts that erred have done so too much in the direction of permitting nontreatment.[21,35]

One case in New York seems to indicate that nontreatment decisions may not be made on behalf of incompetent persons including infants. *Matter of Storar*[27] involved a 52-year-old resident of a state facility who had a mental age of about 18 months. An only child, he was visited daily by his 77-year-old mother. In 1979, he was diagnosed as suffering from cancer of the bladder. He received radiation therapy with his mother's consent. In 1980, cancer of the bladder was again diagnosed, and it was deemed to be terminal regardless of the treatment that was rendered. The cancer had spread to his lungs and other organs, and it was estimated that he would die within three to six months. Lesions in the bladder were cauterized in an unsuccessful attempt to stop the bleeding. As a result of the bleeding, Mr. Storar required transfusions every 8 to 15 days. Mrs. Storar initially consented to the transfusions but then withdrew her consent when she concluded that her son disliked the transfusions and tried to avoid them.

The director of the state institution Mr. Storar resided in sought a court order authorizing the transfusions. The trial court denied the petition, noting that the transfusions would not cure his fatal disease and involved some pain and that the patient submitted to them reluctantly. New York's highest court reversed. The court said that Mr. Storar suffered from two conditions—terminal cancer and bleeding. Although his death from the terminal cancer could not be averted, death from blood loss could. The court also noted that the transfusions did not cause "excessive pain" (and indicated that if they did, then a different outcome might be appropriate) and that with the transfusions he could continue to live life as he had been doing prior to the diagnosis of the fatal disease. The court, analogizing this case to Jehovah's Witnesses cases involving a parent's denial of blood to a child, ruled that in a case such as this courts may not allow an incompetent patient to "bleed to death" because of a parent's belief that it would be in his best interest.

One can question the logic and reasoning of this case (it is not at all like the Jehovah's Witness cases), but it is important to note that this court seems to conclude that one person cannot make a best-interest determination on behalf of an incompetent if it will lead to nontreatment. As it said in a later case, "a third party has no recognized right to decide that the patient's quality of life has declined to a point where treatment should be withheld and the patient should be allowed to die"[29] [p. 446]. If this is in fact the standard this court will apply, it is hard to see how nontreatment decisions can be made for handicapped newborns in this jurisdiction. However, there are two provisos that are important regarding this court. First, it stands alone in its belief that surrogate decision making is unauthorized unless one actually knows the incompetent person's desires. Second, this court has never been confronted with an "easy" case. In *Storar*, the blood transfusions provided the patient with a quality of life identical to his quality of life prior to the diagnosis of his fatal illness. One wonders if the result would have been the same if Mr. Storar had been comatose and on a respirator that his mother wished to have withdrawn, or if he had suffered great pain as a result of the transfusions and had to be regularly and forcibly restrained to get the painful treatment that could only extend his life three to six months.

It is important to realize that courts have not changed the process of medical decision making in this area. If anything, the courts have looked to medical practice to help them sort out many of these difficult issues. The cases are replete with references to the medical literature. Indeed, the AMA's Council on Judicial Affairs' position that there are appropriate circumstances for withholding even nutrition and hydration has already been cited by the courts as one basis for upholding the lawfulness of such action[18] [p. 17].

The medical community cannot expect the courts to provide answers to all the difficult questions posed by nontreatment decisions for handicapped newborns. The profession itself must continue to engage in the process of adopting standards for determining when medical care provides insufficient benefits to justify the burdens treatment presents. The courts can only answer the question about the lawfulness of such decisions, and with history as our guide, the courts will uphold humane decisions that are made to help the alleviation of suffering.

REFERENCES

1. American Academy of Pediatrics v. Heckler, 561 F. Supp. 395 (D.D.C. 1983)
2. Application of Cicero, 421 N.Y.S.2d 965 (Sup. 1979)
3. Bartling v. Superior Court, 209 Cal. Rptr. 220 (Cal App. 2 Dist. 1984)
4. Bowen v. American Hospital Association, 90 L.Ed.2d 584 (1986)
5. Brophy v. New England Sinai Hospital, 497 N.E.2d 417 (Mass. 1986)
6. Custody of a Minor, 379 N.E.2d 1053 (Mass. 1979)
7. Custody of a Minor, 385 Mass. 697 (1982)
8. Duff R, Campbell A: Moral and ethical dilemmas in the special care nursery. N Engl J Med 289:890, 1973
9. Elias S, Annas G: Reproductive Genetics and the Law, chap 7. Chicago, Year Book Medical Publishers, 1987
10. 48 Federal Register 9630 (Mar 7, 1983)
11. 48 Federal Register 30846 (July 5, 1983)
12. 49 Federal Register 1622 (Jan 12, 1984)
13. 50 Federal Register 14878 (Apr 15, 1985)
14. Fost N: Putting hospitals on notice. Hastings Cent Rep 12:5, 1982
15. L. Glantz, The role of personhood in treatment decisions made by courts. Milbank Mem Q 61:76, 1983
16. A. Holder, Legal Issues in Pediatric Medicine, 2nd ed, p 102. New Haven, Conn, Yale University Press, 1985
17. In the matter of Claire Conroy, 486 A.2d 1209 (N.J. 1985)
18. In the matter of Hilda Peter, case No. A-78 (N.J. Sup. Ct. 1986)

19. In the matter of Spring, 405 N.E.2d 115 (Mass. 1980)
20. In re L.H.R., 321 S.E.2d 716 (Ga. 1984)
21. In re Phillip B, 156 Cal. Rptr. 48 (App. 1979)
22. In re Quinlan, 137 N.J. Super. 227 (Ch.Div. 1975)
23. Lyon, J: Playing God in the Nursery, chap 1. New York, Norton, 1985
24. Maine Medical Center v. Houle, Civil Action No. 74-145 (Superior Ct. 1974)
25. Matter of Hofbauer, 47 N.Y.2d 648 (1979)
26. Matter of Quinlan, 355 A.2d 647 (N.J. 1976)
27. Matter of Storar, 52 N.Y.2d 363 (1981)
28. Panel told defective infants are allowed to die, New York Times, p 18. June 12, 1974
29. People v. Eulo, 482 N.Y.S.2d 436,446 (Ct. App. 1984)
30. Pless J: Letter to the Editor. N Engl J Med 313:664, 1983
31. President's Commission for the Study of Ethical Problems in Medicine and Biomedical and Behavioral Research: Deciding to Forego Life-Sustaining Treatment, chap 6, 1983
32. Public Law 98-457, amending 42 U.S.C. 510(a)
33. The right of children—Parts I and II. Harvard Educational Review, Nov 1973, Feb. 1974
34. Robertson J: Involuntary euthanasia of defective newborns: A legal analysis. Stanford Law Rev 27:213, 1975
35. Robertson J: Legal aspects of withholding treatment from handicapped newborns: Substantive issues. J of Health Politics, Policy and Law 11:215,224, 1986
36. Robertson J, Fost N: Passive euthanasia of defective newborn infants: Legal considerations. Pediatrics 88:833, 1977
37. Shaw A: Dilemmas of "informed consent" in children. N Engl J Med 289:885, 1973
38. Shaw A, Randolph J, Manard B: Ethical issues in pediatric surgery; a national survey of pediatricians and pediatric surgeons, Pediatrics (Suppl)60:588, 1977
39. Superintendent of Belchertown State School v. Saikewicz, 370 N.E.2d 417 (Mass. 1977)
40. U.S. v. University Hospital, 575 F.Supp. 607 (E.D.N.Y., 1983)
41. U.S. v. University Hospital, 729 F.2d 144 (2d Cir., 1984)
42. 29 U.S.C. 794
43. Weber v. Stony Brook Hospital, 467 N.Y.S.2d 685 (A.D.2 Dept. 1983)
44. Weber v. Stony Brook Hospital, 456 N.E.2d 1186 (N.Y. 1983)

SECTION 3: ETHICAL ISSUES
Albert R. Jonsen

In this book, the noun "baby" appears for the first time in the title of this chapter in the part of the book entitled "Fate of Fetuses." Sometimes, the fate of a fetus is to become a baby. Some fetuses, however, never become babies. They die in the womb and are ejected dead from it either spontaneously or by the deliberate or accidental intervention of another. Still others are "untimely ripped from mother's womb" and come into the world as living but unfinished beings. Once in the world, they are babies; certain protections of the law attach to them unequivocally; and many human emotions are directed toward them. The question is, what are the moral obligations incumbent on parents and health professionals to sustain premature babies alive in the world?

The perspective of this chapter is limited: I speak only of the fetus who enters the world in an essentially fetal condition. Strictly speaking, it is improper to call such a being a "fetus" once it is outside the womb. If dead, it should be called an abortus; if living, an infant. Yet in a certain sense, it is proper to refer to the premature infant as a "born fetus." The fetus extracted from its usual life-support system, the maternal body, is physiologically very much like the fetus still in the uterus. Its lungs are still fetal: they are unprepared to accept the task of breathing ambient oxygen. Circulation of blood may persist in a partly fetal pattern. The immune system is weakly responsive to infection, and certain organs, such as the liver, are slow to initiate essential functions. Thus, it is not too much of an exaggeration to describe the premature infant as physically and physiologically a born fetus. Such beings are the object of my reflections about moral responsibility.

The scope of these reflections is further limited to life sustained by medical intervention. Only the relatively recent practice, found in developed nations, of applying science, technology, and clinical skills to the premature infant in order to sustain its life is considered here. This chapter also excludes the Baby Doe cases, in which the infants were not premature but did suffer from some physical anomaly calling for medical or surgical attention. In the publicized cases, one infant with Down's syndrome had a correctible intestinal defect, and the second was born with spina bifida. The literature of medical ethics is filled with discussions of these cases. Unfortunately, the discussions are often generalized as "the ethics of newborn intensive care." The Baby Doe cases, however, differ in significant ways from the most common ethical problem in newborn intensive care—namely, the appropriate treatment of the small premature infant whose only deficit is its immaturity. The ethical aspects of this sort of intensive care have received less attention than, or have been confounded with, the Baby Doe cases. This chapter deals exclusively with the premature newborn infant.

The majority of infants in need of neonatal intensive care are not afflicted with genetic or congenital anomalies. Most infants admitted to the intensive care nursery are term or near-term babies—that is, babies who have reached the end of a complete gestation. They have relatively simple cardiopulmonary problems that require only a few days of care. A segment of infants admitted to the nursery are notably premature and of low birth weight (defined as less than 38 weeks gestation and below 2500 g, or 5½ lb). Some 230,000 infants born in the United States each year, 7% of all live births, weigh less than 2500 g. Infants weighing less than 1500 g are classified as very low birth weight. Low birth weight infants suffer a 10% mortality at the upper weight range to almost 100% at the lower.

Low birth weight is almost always associated with prematurity. The primary medical problem of these infants is that their lungs are not yet mature enough to breathe oxygen from the ambient air. Thus prematurity may result in severe deprivation of oxygen and subsequent acute and chronic lung disease. Although prematurity causes a variety of problems, respiratory disease and its consequences are the most serious. About 200,000 infants receive intensive care each year. Of these, about 75,000 suffer the problems attending prematurity. Twenty-five thousand will die from respiratory problems, even with the best of care. Only a very small number of infants admitted to the intensive care nursery suffer from the congenital anomalies that afflicted the so-called Babies Doe. About 5000 babies are born with spina bifida, and a notable but still small portion of the 4000 Down's syndrome babies require life-saving surgery.[3,5]

Against this background, how should the moral issue be formulated? What is the moral meaning of these questions: Is there an obligation to sustain neonatal life? Is it morally permissible to allow babies to die? When can life-sustaining measures be withheld or withdrawn? In recent years, these questions have been discussed at great length in many books and articles. In the particular case of the born fetus, these questions must be seen in light of one essential reality: the born fetus, extracted from its natural environment into a hostile environment, is an unfinished creature. It lacks the integration requisite to living successfully in a world of atmospheric oxygen, invading microbes, variable temperatures, and alien nutrients. The goal of the science and technology of neonatal medicine is to provide time and support while organic integration takes place.

The way we describe a disease or condition often colors our view of it and shapes our ethical attitudes. Characterizing a disease as "fatal" or "lethal" or an infection as "communicable" or "preventable" suggests much about attitudes, values, and plans of action. The phrase "terminal illness" does not specify a particular diagnostic entity, like peptic ulcer or viral pneumonia. Rather, it refers to the identification in a particular patient of some disease known to lead eventually and inevitably to early death, or it refers to the presence of a clinical condition that presages the initiation of the dying process. "Terminal illness" points toward death: the use of the words suggests that medical options are limited and that the sufferer should expect decline and death.

Death, as commonly understood in Western culture, is the disintegration of the living organism. As the President's Commission for the Study of Ethical Problems in Medicine stated in its report *Defining Death*,

> The functioning of many organs—such as the liver, kidneys and skin—and their integration, are vital to individual health in the sense that if any one ceases and that function is not restored or artificially replaced, the organism as a whole cannot long survive. All elements in the system are mutually interdependent, so that the loss of any part leads to the breakdown of the whole, and eventually, to the cessation of functions in every part.[4]

Death, then, takes place "at the moment when the body's physiological system ceases to constitute an integrated whole."[4]

The born fetus is not yet an integrated whole. It is inchoate, which is defined in the *Oxford English Dictionary* as "just begun, incipient; in an initial or early stage; hence, elementary, imperfect, undeveloped, immature." If the fetus had remained in its natural environment, it would have become an integrated whole, ready to move into its next world. If it leaves the womb sufficiently mature but still imperfect, it may survive in the new environment with little or no assistance. But if it emerges still quite immature, it is either doomed to die or must depend on the elaborate but only partially adequate technologies of neonatal care. Thus, some born fetuses, unable to attain integration, die; others survive with help; still others survive but are irreversibly damaged by the help they receive or by the concomitants and sequelae of the illnesses of immaturity.

In view of the ethical judgments that must be made about treatment, I wish to offer a neologism to describe the condition of the premature infant: "inchoate illness," the condition of being not yet physically and physiologically integrated to the degree sufficient to sustain life function without technical support. The neonate, for whatever reason, has been cut loose from its natural life-support system. Its deficit is its physiological inability to function. The fetus in utero is quite satisfactorily situated in its life-support system. Unless it suffers from a lethal defect in its uterine condition, it has no illness. Absent such a defect, from the viewpoint of medical ethics, there is no obligation to intervene in its life. A sick infant born after birth is wholly different, relative to medical ethics, from a developing fetus in utero.

Ethicists have discussed at length the moral relevance of being in the world and in the human community, and they have come to different conclusions about the moral differences between infanticide and abortion. I recognize the complexity of this argument but will rely less on philosophical analysis than on intuitive perception and judgment: the premature infant does engender, by the fact of its living presence, moral duties based on beneficence, respect, justice, and compassion. The specific ways in which these duties are fulfilled depends on the severity of its inchoate illness.[1]

What is the value of defining a new illness and creating a neologism to describe it? It is to reveal the analogy with terminal illness. An analogy is a reference that reveals a basic similarity and an important difference between two entities. The similarity between terminal and inchoate illness lies in the absence of organic integration. The difference lies in the fact that for the born fetus, integration has not been achieved; in the mature organism, integration has been achieved and is beginning to break down. Thus, at death, the mature organism disintegrates, and the born fetus has failed to integrate.

The analogy between inchoate illness and terminal illness suggests an important consideration for the resolution of the ethical problem. One crucial implication of designating a person "terminally ill" is the effect on the obligations that others have toward that person. Obligations incurred by kinship, friendship, or professional role that would otherwise require helping the person overcome illness or sustain its burdens are modified in the presence of terminal illness. Those obligations no longer urge interventions aimed at survival but rather encourage emotional and physical comforting. It is possible, then, for the physician who up to that point has been battling against death to leave off therapeutic efforts and turn to palliative ones. There is no obligation to perform what one honestly suspects will be futile.[2]

Historically, the initial goals of neonatal intensive care seem to have acknowledged this form of the ethical imperative. In the earliest years, the effort was inspired by the hope that infants born mature enough to survive even without treatment could be treated in ways that would prevent the devastating effects of prematurity, particularly the damage to the brain that would impair mental development and physical capabilities. There was little urgency to save every life; indeed, it was then common to place explicit limits of weight and gestational age on resuscitation. Thus, the obligation to provide medical intervention was premised on the assumption that technology could support the infant's own struggle for integration and at the same time produce a healthier infant than would have been possible without intervention. As the technology and skills were perfected, the class of patients grew to include infants who, in earlier days, would have had no chance of survival. This class of very small prematures now shows many of the deficits from which their elder siblings in the nursery had been protected.

The point of introducing the concept of "inchoate illness" as an analogy to "terminal illness' is to suggest that very small prematures can be excluded from life-saving interventions without moral opprobrium. The concept also suggests that born fetuses who do have better initial potentiality for integration should be treated until it begins to appear that the efforts are failing or are causing deleterious physical effects. Thus, the 1200-g newborn baby may have severe lung disease that does not resolve after several months of ventilatory support; at the same time, it begins to suffer from the devastating problems that attend inchoate illness and the "iatrogenicity" of neonatal intensive care. This course cannot be predicted in advance; it is sometimes recognized only slowly and tragically late. When this begins to happen, ethical perplexity about the right action is compounded by the uncertainties of how long one should wait before deciding. Still, the complex of clinical signs that failure to integrate is continuing despite intensive efforts places the baby in the class of patients for whom the obligation to save is transformed into the obligation to comfort until the end.

The small compass of this chapter makes it impossible to argue this thesis in detail. Many questions can be raised. In particular, we must acknowledge a notable difference between terminal and inchoate illness—namely, that the likelihood of the former reversing itself and resolving seems much smaller than that the latter might do so. "Terminal," as a concept, seems much more final than "inchoate," though both are empirically and clinically complex. In the presence of even a minute probability of integration, does a stringent obligation to utilize every technical effort remain? The relationship between clinical probability and ethical futility is perplexing. Greater clarity in conceptualization and argument is needed before any set of principles for the care of the inchoately ill can be set forth. Nevertheless, the thesis is offered in the hope that those who care for born fetuses will recognize its relevance to their work and that those who look on neonatology from without will appreciate the uniqueness of the ethical questions posed by inchoate illness.

REFERENCES

1. Fletcher, JC: Abortion, euthanasia and the care of defective newborns. N Engl J Med 292:75, 1975
2. Nelson, L: Primum esse utile. Yale J Biol Med 51:655, 1978
3. Oh W, Stern L: Diseases of the respiratory

system. In Behrman RE (ed): Neonatal and Perinatal Medicine. St Louis, CV Mosby, 1977

4. President's Commission for the Study of Ethical Problems in Medicine: Defining Death, pp 32–33. Washington, DC, US Gov Printing Office, 1981

5. Public Health Service: Antenatal Diagnosis. Washington, DC, National Institutes of Health, 1979

PART VII
NONMEDICAL ISSUES

19
Government Involvement in the Doctor-Patient Relationship

Ruth S. Hanft and

Wendy J. Evans

Traditionally physicians in the United States have placed a high value on their professional autonomy and the sanctity of the physician-patient relationship. Until quite recently, most physicians practiced as individual entrepreneurs with few constraints on their professional decisions. The constraints that did exist were generally imposed either by peer regulation from within the profession or by widely accepted public health measures such as immunization and drug safety. When government did intervene, the intervention was based on professional standards, such as licensure, determined by physicians themselves or by peer judgments, such as research funding applications, which are granted on a peer-review basis. Most drug and device safety and efficacy studies are conducted by physicians.

Government intervention in health care—beyond epidemic control, research, and care for certain special populations such as the military—is relatively recent. The rapid increase in government intervention in other areas of health care in the last two decades reflects the weakening political power of the physician. For many decades, organized physicians' groups successfully either prevented public intervention in many areas of the health field or controlled areas of the field in which government intervention provided economic or social benefit to the profession, such as licensure and accreditation. Only when the public demand for equity, safety, and distributive justice became overwhelming did government enter the health field in a major way. Thus, the changes in the extent and degree of government intervention over the past 20 years have occurred in large measure as a result of the emergence of the government's role as a purchaser of health care. In addition, other political pressures based on ethical, moral, or religious concepts have had an increasing impact on government intervention as reflected by the introduction of requirements for informed consent and by anti-abortion legislation.

HISTORIC OVERVIEW

Political and Economic Theories

Political and economic theories augmented by ethical concepts of autonomy, justice, and liberty provide the bases for debate on the roles of the public and private sectors in society. Most democratic, capitalist societies have varying and shifting proportions of public- and private-sector activities. The concept of a social contract provides a political basis for the discussion of public- and private-sector roles whereby the population of a society enters into a contract with government, and a constitution defines the rights and responsibilities of the two parties.[2] Utilitarian theory bases public intervention on achieving the greatest good for the greatest number.

In economic theory, the concept of public good provides the rationale for governmental allocation intervention. Adam Smith, the father of laissez-faire capitalism, cites four areas of government activity: (1) the protection of society from violence and invasion; (2) the protection of members of society from injustice; (3) the establishment and maintenance of beneficial public institutions and public works "which are of such a nature that the profit they could earn would never repay the expense to any individual"; (4) meeting the expenses to support the sovereign.[10] The second and third obligations provide the rationale for government intervention in health care.

John Stuart Mill wrote that under certain circumstances the public sector is required to intervene and that almost all areas are amenable to public-sector intervention when the private sector fails to provide the needed goods or services. John Maynard Keynes phrased this concept as "the public doing what is not done at all."[11] Public finance theory yields further economic factors that stimulate public-sector intervention, including imperfect markets, joint consumption or indivisibility of benefits, external barriers to market distribution, and imbalances in supply. Application of these theories provides justification for public health regulation, the provision of or requirement for immunization, providing health benefits when the market does not provide equity, and supporting increases in the supply of health workers.

Equally important in a democratic society are the social choices or decisions made by the electorate concerning the allocation of functions and resources to the public and private sectors. Obviously the resources and power of specific electoral interest groups are reflected in these choices, and the structure of the government can influence the power of electoral interests. During the New Deal and the following 40 years, public choice increased government intervention in a number of areas, most notably social welfare policy. Public choice has consistently led to increased federal funding of biomedical research and the development of new NIH institutes, such as the Arthritis Institute. A major public intervention to require new taxation to finance or absorb what were private or state functions requires broad consensus across society, as does the decision to reverse the public-private balance.

"The vector of public goods is a vector of differences between the goods and services the private economy is motivated to provide and the goods and services the 'public' wants, is willing to pay for, and expects its government to assist in achieving."[27] Resources are finite. The way a society distributes these resources is a complex combination of political structure and philosophy, concepts of justice, personal freedom and equality, and economic philosophies.

Ethics, morals, and religion also influence public intervention. Concepts of rights, obligations, virtue, and responsibility influence societal decisions that may or may not be enforced by public action. Moral codes can govern whole societies or specific professions. For example, the principle of autonomy or individual liberty can generate numerous conflicts between the professional and patient, such as parental refusal of treatment for children, and informed consent for new procedures. The principle of justice can also lead to conflicts between professionals and society on micro-decisions that command scarce resources.

Health as a Public Good

In most nations public efforts in health care predate other social insurance and social welfare programs. The early health-related programs were the forerunners of what is now known as public health, as distinguished from personal health services. The rationale for public health interventions differs from the rationale for public intervention in the provision of personal health services today. Public health in its classic context is an indivisible good, fraught with numerous externalities. An individual alone cannot control exposure to epidemics, unsafe water, or air.

Until the late eighteenth century, personal health services were largely the responsibilities of families, religious orders, and fraternal societies. The major entry of the public sector in financing and providing health care did not occur until the late 1800s in Europe and from approximately the same period but only at the state and county levels in the United States.[25] Public-sector involvement in personal health care and in institutions training health care personnel and providing care is a relatively recent phenomenon. Notable exceptions are the care for the military or the merchant marine, the mentally ill, and lepers, which has historically been provided by many nations.

The rationale for public support of personal health services is complex and includes issues of rights, equity, justice, societal productivity, and avoidance of other social costs. Complicating these issues are externalities such as the relationship between environment and illness—for example, the issue of cause and effect between asbestos exposure and certain types of cancer, heredity, and, more recently, the influence of personal behavior, lifestyles, and choice on health status. In addition, the interaction among genetics, environment, and lifestyle with the provision of personal health care cannot be adequately disaggregated as to their separate influence on the health status of a specific individual. The end result is that most nations have underwritten or provided access to care.

Government Intervention in Providing Personal Health Care

Public intervention on a *national* level began in Europe in 1883 when Germany established the first system of compulsory sickness insurance. Over the years, Austria, Hungary, Norway, Serbia, Britain, Russia, and the Netherlands followed suit. Other countries subsidized private voluntary benefit societies.[26] To date, the United States is the only major industrialized nation (other than South Africa) without a national health insurance program. Public health measures such as pure air, water, and sewage have largely been state and local rather than federal activities, although federal intervention has increased in the last 20 years. In the areas of epidemic control and the purity and safety of food and drugs, the federal government has been preeminent.

In the United States, the first federal intervention in personal health care for the general population was in the area of maternal and child health, although the states still played the major role in the program. Direct federal involvement in personal health care did not begin until the enactment of Medicare and Medicaid in 1965. Prior to 1965, federal involvement was indirect, through grants to public and private institutions. Specifically, from the 1930s onward the federal government indirectly subsidized or stimulated the delivery of health services by means of two major mechanisms. The Hill-Burton Act of 1968 provided grants and loans for construction of hospitals and clinics and required beneficiaries of the act to provide some charity care. Federal support of biomedical research provided indirect financing for the education of physicians and an unintended stimulus for the development of specialized faculty and, secondarily, a large pool of specialty physicians.

Historically, states and counties played a larger role in both the financing and the delivery of personal health services and in the support of institutions. Direct personal health care services have been provided by states and counties for many decades through state-owned university academic health center hospitals, state mental hospitals, tuberculosis hospitals (in earlier years), and county and municipal hospital and clinic systems caring for the indigent. In addition, licensure of health professionals is nominally a state function, although the health professions, primarily physicians, set the standards to be enforced by the states. Numerous critics of this essentially private regulatory process define private regulations as "guilding," supply control, and market control. In the United States, the accrediting, credentialing, and licensure processes for health professionals and for institutions are controlled by private-sector interest groups.

During the 1960s the concept of health care as a "right" for all citizens was implicitly and explicitly accepted by a majority of the population. The federal government's role in personal health care services changed dramatically with the advent of the Great Society programs and the enactment of Medicare and Medicaid.[19] A plethora of federal health programs evolved, expanding health care expenditures and shifting the sources of support for health care from the private to the public sector and from states and localities to the federal government. Programs included both increased federal investment in biomedical research and several new types of programs including direct federal support for health professional education, community mental health centers, community health centers, migrant health centers, and, above all, the Medicare and Medicaid programs.

Physicians as a group fought many of these programs, with the notable exception of the expansion of biomedical research. They feared government control and interference in the practice of medicine. However, at that time, the major federal financing programs adopted existing private regulatory standards as federal standards and further did not constrain or limit existing payment practices of usual and customary fees or interfere in medical practice beyond establishing rarely imposed standards to assure that care was "reasonable and necessary."

By the late 1960s, the escalation in federal health expenditures began to stimulate efforts to check their growth. At the end of the Johnson administration, Secretary of Health, Education, and Welfare Wilbur Cohen froze increases in physicians' fees under Medicare. This had the perverse and unintended effect of transferring payment from the Medicare program to beneficiaries. The freeze was intended only to affect the physician group; however, physicians passed extra costs on to the consumer. Regulatory approaches such as health planning were imposed. President Nixon's wage and price control program remained in effect for the health industry after the controls had been lifted from other sectors of the economy. The net result was increased utilization of services and total costs. The Nixon administration proposed a series of regulatory changes in Medicare, including prospective payment experiments, utilization review through Professional Standards Review Organizations, and prior approval of capital expenditures, which culminated in the Social Security Amendments of 1972.[20] Market approaches were tried as solutions to the cost problems. Efforts to stimulate competition in the health industry were made, including the development of health maintenance organizations (HMOs).[21] It is interesting to note that organized physicians' groups opposed the development of HMOs. Successful efforts were also made to expand physician supply by providing support for the expansion of medical schools and student positions.

During the Carter administration, further efforts were made to slow the growth of federal health care expenditures. These included a major but unsuccessful attempt to control hospital costs by regulatory cost capping. Funding for health profession education programs was reduced, and the growth in biomedical research funding halted.

With the change in administration in

1981, public policy efforts focused on stimulating the operation of supply-and-demand market forces in the health care arena. Major budgetary and legislative changes were made, many using both defederalization and regulatory approaches. Although many attempts to cut federal expenditures were blocked by Congress, several proposals that had a major impact on the health sector were enacted. These changes included efforts to constrain demand, reduction of federal Medicaid expenditures, increases in cost sharing for Medicare beneficiaries, and a constant-dollar funding decline in federal categorical health programs such as maternal and child health and community health centers. A mix of market and regulatory approaches on the supply side was adopted—major changes in hospital reimbursement, physicians' fee freeze (with transfer effects from the public to the private sector), and reduction in support for and a concomitant proposal to eliminate health-planning legislation. The most far-reaching, long-term changes were made in the Medicare program. ERTA and TEFRA legislation dramatically altered Medicare hospital reimbursements[22] and were followed by the 1983 Social Security Amendments, which mandated a totally new reimbursement system for hospitals.

Government Involvement in the Doctor-Patient Relationship

The extreme libertarian view of the appropriate government role in the doctor-patient relationship is a hands-off policy. This is best portrayed in economic terms as a market approach. The dominant thrust of current public health care policy is to enhance market forces by removing demand and supply barriers and to deregulate or ease regulations. Operation of a true economic market requires buyers and sellers to be unconstrained—that is, autonomous—in striking a bargain. A market is generally perceived as freedom for the buyer to purchase a product and a seller to sell or not to sell. Free entry into the market for buyers and sellers is a fundamental requirement. However, in health care the third-party payer, whether public or private, is interposed between buyers and sellers. Pure markets are rare. In certain arenas of society and life there are severe limitations on the ability of markets alone to protect the public from harm or to allocate goods and services. In health care these factors are as follows.

Constraints on the Entry of Sellers or Providers or Products

Because of the life, death, or disability consequences of providing health care services, barriers of entry for professionals and institutions have been established, ostensibly for qualitative reasons. Although authors such as Friedman and Havighurst have criticized the severity of limitations imposed by accreditation, licensure, and credentialing requirements,[6] some entry barriers are considered necessary to protect the public in matters of life and death. Similarly, the potential of harm to individuals provides the basis for the development of FDA drug and device safety requirements.

Consumer Sovereignty and Consumer Information

The life, death, and disability consequences of many medical decisions and the complexities underlying many of these decisions limit the individual's ability to participate fully in the decision-making process at the physician-patient micro-level.[9] The physician, to a greater or lesser extent, acts as agent for the patient (paternalism) or as an autonomous provider, deciding the range and scope of services to be provided and the particular technology or technologies to be utilized. Although patients are involved in this decision-making process, the technical expertise required in medicine is such that the consumer must frequently rely on the judgment of the provider. The ethos of the physician is to consider the patient's welfare first and do all he or she can to save life and reduce morbidity, disability, and pain. The combination of lack of precision in medical decision making and concern for the individual patient drives the decision-making process toward providing more rather than less care. Cumulative micro-decisions exert a major impact on the cost of care. The agent/physician controls a large proportion of demand and, except for certain salaried types of practice or risk contracts, derives economic benefits from added services.[8] When the consumer does not pay directly for the services, the consumer has no direct financial stake in the decisions. Both government and private employers as prudent buyers therefore seek to assure that only necessary care is provided. In the market context, they impose limits on what they will purchase through the design of health benefit plans, economic incentives, and direct intervention such as utilization and peer review.

Externalities

Externalities are endemic in health care. The effects of environment, employment, geography, climate, and epidemics on health status and health care costs cannot be fully measured but are regarded as considerable. Examples of federal attempts to control or quantify some externalities are found in communicable disease control, reportability of certain diseases, and some occupational health and safety provisions.

Social Good

The social values of health care services are considered greater than individual values. Mushkin describes these as "extra buyer benefits" in an individual's purchase of medical services to control infectious disease.[17] Beyond this, decisions based on the individual's ability to purchase care or other barriers to care can affect productivity, disability, and other social costs—a further rationale for public intervention in purchasing care.

Postponability of Care

The purchase of certain types of health care cannot be delayed as can most consumer purchases. For example, treatment for a closed head injury, diagnosed cancer, or myocardial infarction cannot be delayed without serious consequences to individuals, families, and ultimately society; lack of care for infectious diseases places others in society at risk.

Unevenness of Risk

Individual risk cannot be predicted with certainty because of heredity and environmental influences. The need for services is also related to age, sex, and income. Many nations have tried to spread these risks, using some private or public insurance mechanism, because without some form of risk sharing, the costs of illness could potentially impoverish individuals, families, and local communities.

Virtually all economists and analysts in the field believe that there must be some public-sector underwriting and control of health care. The market alone cannot protect citizens against harm, allocate resources, and achieve social justice; the issue is the degree of market control and public intervention.

METHODS OF INTERVENTION AND THEIR EFFECTS

Illegality and Legality

The laws of a democratic society reflect its basic social and ethical standards and its social compact or constitution. In a pluralistic society like the United States, conflicts over basic values are frequently resolved in the courts. The balance between individual liberty or autonomy and societal interest is a source of recurrent and fundamental conflict. In addition, the United States has a federal government, in which certain spheres of government activity are reserved to the states. The abortion issue provides a clear example of state versus federal preeminence and a clash of social values. It is also an example of how changing medical technology—in this case, advances in the care and salvage of very low birth weight infants—forces a continual updating of political compromises on such issues.

On the issue of abortion, the federal courts have ruled in favor of individual freedom of the mother to decide and have struck down the more restrictive state laws. However, the federal government as a purchaser of care has through congressional action restricted this individual choice for the poor and dependents of the military by denial of payment for abortions under Medicaid and CHAMPUS.

The United States is a litigious nation, and malpractice suits and liability awards determined through the courts have interfered with the autonomy or decision-making freedom of physicians. Fear of suits may encourage the overuse of health care resources even when the results of "extra" care may have marginal or no effect on health outcomes. The widespread use of fetal monitoring and high cesarean section rates are attributable in part to substantial malpractice awards.

Protection of the Population

A number of laws and regulations that intervene between the physician and patient are based on safety and protection of the *population* from illness, disability, and death beyond *individual* control. The clearest example of general protective laws are those related to clean water and air and exposure to toxic substances. However, several types of protective laws that intervene in the physician-patient relationship represent the balance between individual interests and societal interests. The reportability of certain communicable diseases and the recent controversy surrounding the reporting of individuals with positive HIV virus antibody tests affect both the rights and the privacy of the individual patient and the confidentiality of the doctor-patient relationship.

Nonefficacious procedures and drug and device legislation designed to protect patients from harmful effects intervene in both physician and patient autonomy by limiting physicians' judgment to use certain techniques. Although there is little controversy regarding the need to assure safety, the approval processes and the length of the processes have been questioned. A prime example of unnecessary delay in the introduction and release of a useful technology is provided by the case of maternal serum alpha-fetoprotein (MSAFP) kits, as discussed in Chapter 4. The United Kingdom and all Europe began MSAFP screening in the mid-1970s, but the FDA refused to act on applications for RIA kit release in the United States in 1977. In 1980, the FDA proposed stringent limitations on AFP testing that were unacceptable to large segments of the medical community. Despite considerable data showing the efficacy of AFP measurements, not until 1983 did the FDA withdraw the restrictions and allowed widespread AFP testing. New and useful drugs have repeatedly appeared on European markets years before becoming available in the United States. Conversely, federal protections have avoided such disasters as thalidomide-deformed babies. Recently the issue of the use of new and unapproved drugs in patients with terminal illnesses has been revived in the case of experimental drugs for AIDS patients.

Supply Control

Supply control falls into two categories, control of manpower and control of facilities and equipment. The federal government, although frequently blamed for problems of medical manpower supply, plays a very minor role in this area. In fact, the health care professions by and large control the supply and use of manpower. Although state licensure and federal and state reimbursement policies enhance the power of these private regulatory bodies, government generally influences supply only indirectly through economic incentives and disincentives. The standards for admission to medical schools are set by the medical schools, the American Medical Association, and the Association of American Medical Colleges. Accreditation is a private process controlled by the Liaison Committee on Medical Education. Residency accreditation and specialty certification are also private processes controlled by the profession. Federal and state roles are limited to providing financing incentives or disincentives to increase or decrease enrollment and to assure conformity with civil rights legislation, as in all education programs.

However, federal and state governments have played a much more substantial role in controlling the diffusion of facilities and equipment, by means of regulations such as certificates of need and health planning such as is done by health systems agencies. As in most jurisdictions, laws governing facilities and equipment are directed at institutions such as hospitals rather than at physicians, with virtually no interference in the physician-patient relationship. Individual access to certain types of equipment is frequently more a function of hospital privileges, a private-sector decision, than of government planning activities.

Allocation of Research Resources

Obviously the quantity and allocation of research resources ultimately affects the advancement of knowledge and technology, the type of medical care, and the diagnostic and treatment modalities available to physicians for care of their patients. In the United States the allocation of resources occurs through a complex process. The federal government is dominant in the financing of fundamental or basic biomedical research. Industry, notably drug and device manufacturers, plays a major role in applied and developmental research and diffusion. The allocation of public resources involves numerous interests: the executive branch of government, including government research scientists; Congress; disease-specific interest groups such as the American Cancer Society; industry that may benefit from basic research findings; universities that derive indirect costs and faculty support from research; academic researchers; physicians; and the public. A considerable body of literature exists on the political interplay of these diverse interest groups.[4,12,15,28]

Once gross allocations of resources have been made, resources are distributed to programs, projects, and investigator-initiated grants through peer-review processes. Although governmental in nature, these processes are dominated by university academicians and physicians rather than by bureaucrats. There is a considerable literature concerning problems with the present peer-review process—constraints on unconventional ideas, bias against less-than-established researchers and institutions, and so on. Furthermore, NIH advisory committees composed of scientists from the private sector play a major role in establishing research priorities.

In recent years, ethical controversies have arisen about human experimentation and, particularly, informed consent.[3] The newer informed-consent requirements were enacted in response to public revulsion at the findings of the Nuremberg trials on Nazi human experiments and the Public Health Service syphilis experiments.[13,16,23] Debates about informed consent and human experimentation frequently pit concepts of individual rights of patients and autonomy of research physicians against each other. However, most of the controversies arise at the periphery of a societal consensus on the need for a certain amount of human experimentation and the concomitant need for informed consent by research subjects. Controversial areas include what constitutes and who can provide informed consent for individuals who are severely impaired, children, and the comatose; how much information should be provided to patients about risk; and the timing of the human experiment vis-à-vis research results in animal experimentation.[1,4,5,7,14,18,24,29,30,31]

A relatively new phenomenon is the moratorium on the conduct of certain types of research—notably, in vitro fertilization research and fetal research. Although this moratorium could be regarded as a limitation on human experimentation, the source of the ban is less an issue of protection of individuals than the imposition of the religious and moral sensibilities of certain groups. These bans are political in origin and represent an extension of the forces that oppose abortion in any form, for any reason.

Direct Intervention in Doctor-Patient Relationships

With the exception of the requirement of reporting communicable diseases, direct government intervention in the doctor-patient relationship is very new. Since the early 1980s, a number of issues related to the care of the newborn have arisen. The courts struck down the efforts of the Department of Health and Human Services to intervene in decisions between parent and physician on the care of newborns. Following the highly publicized introduction of regulations requiring a hotline posting in all labor and delivery suites to "ensure" the equal treatment of "damaged" infants, a considerable legal battle ensued. In numerous decisions, the strength of such guidelines and warnings has been progressively diluted, reaffirming the prerogative of the patient-physician relationship. This can only be seen as a major victory for the preservation of individual rights. The ethical aspects of the life-and-death decisions often required following the birth of a malformed baby have been discussed in Chapter 18, Section 3. From a purely political perspective, we find it unlikely that the Reagan administration, which purports to support less government interference, would advocate such an invasive approach to the doctor-patient relationship.

The fundamental issue in these cases is the appropriate role of government in intervening in parent-physician decision making and the intervention of government in the normal interchange between patient and physician, physician and hospital. In addition, the issue of decision making by adolescents and the role of government in intervening in the adolescent-physician relationship is of current concern. Here again, strong moral views of subgroups of the population, most notably associated with the right-to-life movements, have been most active in influencing government interposition between patient, parent, and physician. It should be noted that in the case of government intervention in neonatal care, the issue is interposing government between parent and physician for the infant. In the case of adolescents, it is interposing the parent between child and physician.

The reporting of communicable diseases has been widely accepted. In our society and in most other democratic societies, strict protections of privacy are maintained. However, with the development of recent, widespread paranoia about AIDS, concerns are being raised about the use and reporting of the HIV antibody test and the implications of breaches of privacy for those who test positive. The Justice Department has ruled that the protection against discrimination in employment of the disabled does not apply to persons who have AIDS.

Indirect Intervention Through Public and Private Insurance Programs

There are two types of influences on physician-patient relationships in private and public health care financing. The design of health insurance benefit packages, while influencing the site of service and the scope of services covered, is not intended to interfere directly in the physician-patient relationship. Rather the benefit structure is usually either a reflection of the historic shape of traditional insurance or the result of negotiations between management and labor or payers and insurers. In the case of programs like Medicare, benefits for hospital care, medical care services, and skilled nursing homes are defined in law. Durational limits, such as covered days of home health care, are also defined by law based on a political consensus patterned after private insurance.

Clearly, however, the design of health insurance benefits has influenced and continues to influence physician-patient relationships. For example, when laboratory and diagnostic tests were fully covered on an inpatient basis but not on an outpatient basis, physicians and patients were encouraged to use the site where fuller payment would be made. Included in this category of design of benefits is the denial of payment for experimental or investigational procedures, such as the artificial heart. These provisions have always been part of private and public insurance programs under the rubric of reasonable and necessary, medically necessary, or widely accepted practices. However, insurance carriers have historically been extremely reluctant to promote new modes of treatment from experimental "uncovered" to customary and "covered."

The second type of program influences physician-patient relationships more directly and is relatively recent. Contrary to popular belief, many techniques now used to intervene between physician judgment and actions and the patient, except for retrospective utilization review, are private-sector measures instituted by large employers, unions, or private insurers. Second surgical opinion programs, preadmission certification, and concurrent review were all pioneered by the private sector and are prospective constraints. The Medicare requirement of professional or peer review, which superseded the current utilization review, was initially limited to hospital admissions and lengths of stay. A number of state Medicaid programs now require preadmission certification, second surgical opinions, and the use of generic drugs.

Falling between these two categories are a series of payment policies specifically designed to influence behavior. In 1983, Medicare reimbursement for hospitals was changed from retrospective reasonable costs to prices set by diagnosis-related groups. The rationale was to end open-ended payment and to thereby provide incentives to decrease hospital utilization, to contain hospital inflation, and to use out-of-hospital services. Hospitals now have incentives to question the practice patterns of physicians who exceed norms of practice established around averages. Various review processes have been instituted by hospitals and their medical staffs.

No efforts have yet been made directly by the government to use physicians' fees in a similar manner, although there is widespread belief that the usual customary and reasonable method of determining fees encourages the use of high technology and procedure-oriented services versus cognitive services. For example, some policy analysts believe that the high rate of cesarean sections in the United States is partially a function of the higher fees for this procedure than for a normal delivery or a forceps delivery. However, the government is promoting enrollment in comprehensive health plans paid on a capitation basis, to reduce these incentives.

This trend is emerging in the public sector and affects physician-patient relationships. Encouragement of enrollment in health maintenance organizations (HMOs) and preferred provider organizations (PPOs) is designed to put both the physician and the patient at some financial risk in order to encourage prudent use of health services. The incentives for the physician are the reverse of traditional fee-for-service practice, in which the physician who uses services prudently benefits financially. The out-of-pocket cost is reduced for consumers if they agree to enter an HMO and PPO arrangement, but consumers then limit their choices of physicians and hospitals to providers who are part of the organization.

CONCLUSION

Few experts on the health care scene hold that either consumers or physicians should have full autonomy and freedom as individuals to make decisions that affect society as a whole. Issues of safety, unnecessary disability, premature death, distributive justice and use of social resources, and freedom, individual rights, and autonomy frequently come into conflict. The issue is the balance and dominance of each of these concepts.

REFERENCES

1. Annas GJ: Sterilization of the mentally retarded: A decision for the courts. Hastings Cent Rep 11:18–19, 1981
2. Bawden DL: The Social Contract Revisited: Aims and Outcomes of President Reagan's Social Welfare Policy, p xi. Washington, DC, Urban Institute Press, 1984

3. Brandt AM: Racism and research: The case of the Tuskegee syphilis study. Hastings Cent Rep 6:21–29, 1978
4. Epstein SS: Politics of Cancer. San Francisco, Sierra Club, 1978
5. Eth S, Eth C, Edgar H: Can a research subject be too eager to consent? Hastings Cent Rep 11:21–21, 1981
6. Friedman M: Capitalism and freedom. In Clark Havighurst: Regulating Health Facilities Construction. Washington, DC, American Enterprise Institute for Public Policy Research, 1974
7. Gaylin W: The competence of children: No longer all or none. Hastings Cent Rep 12:33–38, 1982
8. Ginzberg E: Medical economics: More than curves and computers. In The Economics of Health and Medical Care. Ann Arbor, University of Michigan Press, 1964
9. Hanft RS: Monitoring medical technology: Shall technology be regulated? In The Technology Explosion in Medical Science: Implications for Health Industry and the Public. New York, SP Medical and Scientific Books, 1983
10. Herber BP: Modern Public Finance, pp 23–24. Homewood, Ill, Irwin, 1983
11. Herber BP: Modern Public Finance, p 25
12. Jaffe FS et al: Abortion Politics: Private Morality and Public Policy. New York, McGraw-Hill, 1987
13. Jones J: Bad Blood. New York, Free Press, 1981
14. Lipsett MB, Fletcher JC: Do vitamins prevent neural tube defects (and can we find out ethically)? Hastings Cent Rep 13:5–8, 1983
15. McKinlay JB et al: Politics and Health Care. Cambridge, Mass, MIT Press, 1982
16. Mitscherlich A, Mielke F: The Death Doctors. London, Elar Books, 1962
17. Mushkin S: "Why health economics?" In The Economics of Health and Medical Care. Ann Arbor, University of Michigan Press, 1964
18. Pattulo EL: Social scientists and research reviews: Two views—who risks what in social research? Hastings Cent Rep 10:15–19, 1980
19. Public Law 89–97
20. Public Law 92–603
21. Public Law 93–222
22. Public Law 97–35 and Public Law 97–248
23. Rothman D: Were Tuskegee and Willowbrook "studies in nature"? Hastings Cent Rep 12:5–7, 1982
24. Silverman WA: Mismatched attitudes about neonatal death: Medical "rescue" vs parental automy. Hastings Cent Rep 11:3–7, 1981
25. Starr P: The Social Transformation of American Medicine p 235. New York, Basic Books, 1982
26. Starr P: The Social Transformation of American Medicine, p 237
27. Steiner PO: The public sector and the public interest. In Haverman RH, Margolis J (eds): Public Expenditure and Policy Analysis, p 8. Boston: Houghton Mifflin, 1983
28. Strickland PC: Politics, Science and Dread Disease: A Short History of the United States Medical Research Policy. Cambridge, Mass, Harvard University Press, Commonwealth Fund Publication Service, 1972
29. Swazey JP: Protecting the "animal of necessity": Limits to inquiry in clinical investigation. Daedalus 107:129–143, 1978
30. Veatch RM: Two views of the new research regulations: 1. Protecting human subjects: The federal government steps back. Hastings Cent Rep 11:19, 1981
31. Wigodsky HS: Two views of the new research regulations: 2. New regulations, new responsibilities for institutions. Hastings Cent Rep 11:14, 1981

20

What About the Children? The Dilemma of Prematernal Liability

Lynn D. Fleisher

At eight months, "Aaron" is about the size of an infant half his age. Listless and uncoordinated, he has yet to learn to sit up on his own. His huge brown eyes, rheumy and red-rimmed, roll in his pale face, incapable of focusing on anything for more than a split second. . . . Aaron (not his real name) is part of a tragic national trend. He is the child of an addict who not only injected heroin during her pregnancy but also used cocaine, a drug that may have even more serious consequences for the developing fetus.[10]

In October 1984, the American Society of Law and Medicine sponsored an international symposium on the legal, social, and ethical implications of new reproductive and prenatal techniques entitled "What About the Children?" Recognizing the explosion of new technology in the area of human reproduction, the symposium looked to the interests of the child who is born as a result of "alternate" or "artificial" methods of reproduction. As the quotation above indicates, however, perhaps it is appropriate to take a step backward and explore the interests of the child who is born as a result of more "natural" reproductive processes. Such an exploration is not painless. It is fraught with justifiable fears of the devastating effects that restrictions on a woman's behavior during pregnancy may have on the civil liberties of all women. There are, however, other rights that hang in the balance. Courts and commentators already have begun to ask, "What about the children?" This chapter does not purport to provide an answer but merely attempts to make clear the validity of the question.

Pregnancy, whether achieved naturally or by means of one of the new reproductive technologies, is a unique biological situation. In no other circumstance does one person's treatment of *her own body* so directly and so dramatically affect the future life and health of another human being. For the very same reason, pregnancy is a unique legal situation. Rapid advances in our understanding of the importance of responsible prenatal care and

520

the dangers inherent in certain prematernal* behavior raise complex ethical and legal questions concerning the rights and the obligations of the pregnant woman vis-à-vis her future child. In the unique circumstances of pregnancy, the conflicts inherent in the recognition of a prematernal duty are compelling; they encompass the right of the child to be born free of any negligently induced injury and the constitutionally guaranteed right of the pregnant woman to personal privacy and bodily integrity.

PREMATERNAL INFLUENCES: FROM OLD WIVES' TALES TO THALIDOMIDE—AND BEYOND

Until about the turn of the century, many people—including physicians—believed that fetal malformations could be caused by prematernal "experiences," especially those that frightened a woman during the early stages of pregnancy. Typical of this belief are the following cases, reported by a physician to the editor of the *Lancet* on November 26, 1850:

> The first case was the wife of a ganger at Bramford, to which place she had recently removed, and in which a dwarfish woman had resided for many years, remarkable for the smallness of her arms. I delivered this man's wife, in due time, of a full-grown healthy babe, with the exception of the absence of both arms from the shoulder-joint. On seeing the child, the mother explained the matter by acknowledging the surprise the first appearance of the above dwarf made on her mind in the early stage of gestation.
>
> The second case, was a Mrs. J., residing in a neighbouring village, whom I delivered of a full-grown babe alive, but which died a few hours after birth. To my surprise I found, on separating the cord, the whole or a greater part of the small intestines protruding through a circular aperture adjoining the umbilicus. These bowels exhibited a singular convoluted appearance, forming two or three circles round the opening, and held in their position by adhesion to the skin of the abdomen. The mother on seeing the child immediately explained the matter by expressing the surprise she experienced one night in placing her hand on a cold plate of sausages in the dark pantry in the early stage of pregnancy. The resemblance was so complete as at once to strike the female attendant.
>
> The third case was a Mrs. H., a neighbour, confined of a healthy female child, in due time, without a right arm, having merely a rounded stump at the end of the scapula. This she explained to me arose from the fright she experienced by a mendicant coming into her shop, holding up the stump of the right arm. Mrs. H. gave him alms immediately to get rid of the sight; but felt so poorly that she was obliged to take a little brandy to recover the shock, accusing herself at the time for being so simple. This lady now informs me that this occurred during the first month of gestation while suffering from gastric irritation.[21]

It was another letter to the editor of the *Lancet*, however, published just a little over 100 years later, that actually documented the significant and potentially tragic effects of prematernal behavior on the developing fetus. In that letter, McBride first reported what turned out to be an epidemic of limb-reduction malformations in newborns resulting from prematernal ingestion of the sedative thalidomide early in pregnancy.[28] Between 1959 and 1962, the births of at least 2000, and possibly more than 3000, thalidomide babies were reported in West Germany, and it is estimated that over 10,000 babies were damaged worldwide.

During the next quarter of a century, we came to recognize a large number of genetic conditions and predispositions, environmental exposures, and behavioral characteristics of the pregnant woman that contribute to the 3% of all newborn children who are born with major congenital abnormalities. Initial

---

* The author has coined the term *prematernal* to distinguish the status of a woman during pregnancy from the maternal status that arises on the birth of a child.

concerns focused on the potential induction of major structural malformations. It has become clear, however, that functional deficits, such as growth retardation and impairment of mental capacity, also may result.

Many factors determining the present and future health of the newborn child are beyond the control of the pregnant woman and her physician—and often beyond their knowledge. There is substantial evidence, for example, that factors related to the pregnant woman's own childhood growth and development and, perhaps, to her intrauterine existence, are important in determining the outcome of her pregnancies. "[H]ealthy babies become healthy children who grow up to be healthy adults who become healthy parents who produce healthy babies."[5] In addition, from 13% to 14% of the observed anomalies result from mutant genes or chromosomal abnormalities that are transmitted from the pregnant woman or from the child's father to the child. These conditions are beyond the control of the woman to prevent, other than by avoiding the birth of the child or, in a small number of cases, by submitting to fetal therapy.

Approximately 5% of all major congenital anomalies seen in newborns result from environmental causes, and in some cases they may be *prevented* by behavior that the pregnant woman chooses to engage in or not to engage in. These causes include prematernal and prepregnancy illnesses that may be amenable to treatment, prematernal exposure to infectious agents, environmental chemicals encountered as a result of occupational activities, and substances intentionally ingested or utilized as a result of the pregnant woman's personal habits.

For pregnant women, there may be "no such thing as 'recreational' drug use."[10] For example, it is estimated that 5 million Americans now use cocaine regularly. "Cocaine kids" began to appear in the early 1980s, and they now may make up more than half of the drug-affected babies born. "Because the drug produces dramatic fluctuations in blood pressure, it apparently can deprive a fetal brain of oxygen or cause fragile vessels within it to burst, the prenatal equivalent of a stroke. Such strokes can leave the infant with permanent physical and mental damage."[10]

One of the most serious risks to the fetus is prematernal use of the drug alcohol. Alcohol has been recognized as a pregnancy risk since ancient times.[1] The association between prematernal alcoholism and abnormal fetal development was recognized by the Greeks, and in Carthage a bridal couple was not allowed to drink wine on their wedding night, in order to prevent the conception of defective offspring. Concerns about drinking during pregnancy were expressed during England's "Gin Epidemic" of 1720–1750, and in 1834 a report to the House of Commons noted that infants born to alcoholic women had a "starved, shrivelled and imperfect look."[1]

Modern recognition of alcohol's true teratogenic potential, however, awaited the 1973 publication of two articles by Jones and Smith, which clearly established the potential for fetal damage from prematernal alcohol use.[26] These papers described 11 children, born to alcohol-abusing women, who were affected with growth retardation, craniofacial and cardiac defects, and developmental delay. These authors also coined the term "fetal alcohol syndrome," which has served effectively to focus interest on the devastating effects of this avoidable pregnancy risk.[3] "There is no longer any doubt that alcohol can act as a teratogen in both humans and animals."[2] Over 400 cases of full-blown fetal alcohol syndrome have been reported in the literature. It has been estimated that from 2% to 13% of American women drink heavily during pregnancy, with the result that 50% to 70% of them deliver abnormal infants. The fetal alcohol syndrome is seen with a frequency of 1 to 3 per 1000 births, and other nonspecific "alcohol-related birth defects" are even more frequent. There is no cure for the prenatal injuries caused by prematernal alcohol abuse; the only hope lies in prevention.

The in utero environment provided by the pregnant woman clearly plays a crucial role in the development of the fetus and thereby may ultimately determine the health and abilities of the child. Are we therefore compelled to recognize a *duty* on the part of the pregnant woman to refrain from behavior that runs an unreasonable risk of damaging the fetus? And, if we accept the concept of prematernal negligence, how far are we willing to go to prevent negligent prematernal behavior?

THE LEGAL BACKGROUND FOR RECOGNITION OF A PREMATERNAL DUTY

Recognition of a prematernal duty implies that recovery for a breach of this duty would be available to an injured child. It is within this context of personal liability between a parent and a child, rather than between a parent and the state, that the question of a prematernal duty is most appropriately addressed. In the past there were two legal barriers to the acceptance of such a cause of action by a child—barriers that no longer exist today.

Rejection of Parent-Child Immunity

At common law there was no immunity between parents and their children; parents and children could sue each other. The American-born doctrine of parent-child tort immunity had as its goals the preservation of parental authority and family harmony and the avoidance of fraudulent claims. Recently, however, some courts have recognized that once a tort has been committed, the family relationship already has been damaged, and prohibiting reparations will not aid in restoring familial harmony. Finding that the possibility of fraud is not a sufficient reason to avoid recognition of the strong interests of the injured child and society, many courts now attempt to balance the child's interest in compensation against the parent's interest in maintaining autonomy and authority.[48]

An increasing number of states have abrogated the parent-child tort immunity doctrine in all cases except those in which the tortious conduct arises out of the parent-child relationship. At least 20 states have either rejected the doctrine completely or more strictly limited its application (to parental disciplinary acts and legal duties), holding the parents to a "reasonable parent" standard in other areas of behavior.

Recognition of Third-Party Liability for Prenatal Torts

Whereas the recognition of the right of the child to recover for injuries resulting from the negligent acts of his or her parent is still evolving, the child's right to recovery against third parties for prenatal injuries is firmly established. American jurisdictions today are unanimous in recognizing a child's right to maintain a cause of action against a third party for intentionally or negligently inflicted prenatal injury. This, however, has not always been the case.

In *Dietrich* v. *Inhabitants of Northampton*,[14] which appears to be the first reported case on the subject of prenatal tort action, the Massachusetts Supreme Court denied a cause of action in tort for prenatal injuries, basing its decision on a lack of precedent and on the concept that the unborn child was a part of the mother at the time of the injury and any damages that were recoverable at all were recoverable by her. *Dietrich* was uniformly followed for the next 60 years. Justifications for denying this cause of action included the absence of any duty owed to an unborn child who existed only as a part of the mother, the difficulty of showing a causal relationship between the wrongful act and the injury to the child, the danger of spurious or fraudulent claims, and the possibility that to allow such an action would pave the way for a cause of action by a child against his or her mother for negligent behavior during pregnancy.

The modern trend toward recognition of a cause of action for prenatal injury began in 1946, when *Bonbrest* v. *Kotz* held that a child could recover for negligently induced prenatal injuries if the fetus was viable at the time of injury and subsequently born alive. "It is but natural justice that a child, if born alive and viable should be allowed to maintain an action in the courts for injuries wrongfully committed upon its person while in the womb of its mother."[7] The court reasoned that blind adherence to prior authority could not be justified in light of current medical knowledge and that the law had to parallel the progress that had been made in medicine since 1884. In "the most spectacular abrupt reversal of a well-settled rule in the whole history of the law of torts,"[32] uniform and eventually unanimous acceptance of the *Bonbrest* decision followed.

A number of jurisdictions have based their recognition of the cause of action on the strength of the child's interest in being born in a healthy condition. In *Womack* v. *Buchhorn*, the Michigan Supreme Court followed the "overwhelming weight of judicial authority" in holding that an action lies at common law for the negligent infliction by third parties of prenatal injury. The *Womack* court held that

> [J]ustice requires that the principle be recognized that a child has a legal right to begin life with a sound mind and body. If the wrongful conduct of another interferes with that right, and it can be established by competent proof that there is a causal connection between the wrongful interference and the harm suffered by the child when born, damages for such harm should be recoverable by the child.[51]

Although the case law in many jurisdictions still appears to limit the action for prenatal injury to circumstances in which the fetus was viable at the time of the wrongful act, when actually faced with the issue, almost all courts have allowed recovery even though the injury occurred prior to viability.

Moreover, several jurisdictions recognize a cause of action for injury occurring prior to conception. In *Renslow* v. *Mennonite Hospital*,[34] the Illinois Supreme Court found that an infant could recover damages for injuries sustained as a result of her mother having been sensitized, many years prior to conception, by a negligently administered Rh-positive blood transfusion. Preconception torts also are recognized in the wrongful life cause of action. The California Court of Appeals, in *Curlender* v. *Bio-Science Laboratories*,[11] determined that a child born with a genetic disease has a cause of action against the laboratory that negligently determined that her parents were not at risk for having an affected child, thereby precluding their option of avoiding the child's conception or birth. Some jurisdictions limit recovery for a prenatal tort to cases in which the fetus is subsequently born alive, although the majority rule today does not require live birth.

CHILD VERSUS MOTHER FOR PRENATAL INJURY: A PAUCITY OF PRECEDENT AND AN ABUNDANCE OF POLICY CONSIDERATIONS

Grodin v. *Grodin*: The Question of Liability for Prematernally Induced Injury

The acceptance of prenatal tort liability raises the issue of whether the legal right of a child to begin life with a sound mind and body encompasses the right to be born free of any *prematernally induced* injury. The Michigan Court of Appeals appears to have answered this question in the affirmative. In *Grodin* v. *Grodin*,[20] the mother, without knowledge that she was pregnant, had taken the antibiotic tetracycline. As a result, the child developed tooth discoloration. The child asserted that the mother had been negligent in failing to seek appropriate prenatal care, by not requesting a pregnancy test, and by not informing her obstetrician that she was taking the drug. The Michigan Court of Appeals held that a finding that the mother had been unreasonable in her exercise of parental discretion could give rise to liability for negligently inflicted prenatal injury.

The *Grodin* holding relied on the determination by the Michigan Supreme Court in *Womack* v. *Buchhorn* that "a child has a legal right to begin life with a sound mind and body. If the wrongful conduct of another interferes with that right . . . damages for such harm should be recoverable by the child."[51]

Noting that the holding in *Womack* referred only to the negligent conduct of "another" without limiting the parties who might be held liable for the negligently inflicted injury, the *Grodin* court found that a child's mother would bear the same liability for negligent prenatal conduct as would a third person. The court found that a woman's decision to take drugs during her pregnancy is an exercise of her discretion and that the focal question in determining liability is whether her behavior represents a reasonable exercise of parental discretion.

Grodin v. *Grodin* represents the first attempt by a court to dovetail the rule for parental liability and the rule for liability for negligent infliction of prenatal injury to encompass *prematernal* liability. No prior court had extended either the "reasonable parent standard" or the "wrongful conduct of another," which gives rise to liability for a prenatal tort, to include liability for the behavior of a woman toward her fetus during pregnancy. However, although *Grodin* stands as the first case to recognize the possibility of a civil remedy for the child who has been injured by prematernal negligence, the court totally neglected to address the difficult but crucial policy considerations that arise with the attempt to hold a pregnant woman liable for her prematernal behavior. Moreover, in reliance on *Grodin*, the Illinois Appellate Court recently found that a 5-year-old girl could maintain a tort action against her mother for prenatal injuries suffered in a car accident that occurred during pregnancy. The court devoted a total of one paragraph to the issue.[47]

Recognition of a Prematernal Obligation

The recognition of a child's right to be born free of any prematernally induced injury appears to be in direct conflict with the constitutionally protected rights of a woman to autonomy, privacy, and bodily integrity. In *Roe* v. *Wade*,[39] the United States Supreme Court established that a woman's right of personal privacy, grounded in the fourteenth amendment, has "some extension to activities relating to marriage; procreation; contraception; family relationships; and child rearing and education."[40] *Roe* found that interference with, or regulation of, such fundamental rights as the decision to avoid childbirth can be justified only by a "compelling" state interest. A state may recognize a significant interest in protecting the "potential for life" in the fetus; as this potential increases with gestation, the state's interest correspondingly grows in importance, and it becomes compelling at the moment of viability of the fetus.

The privacy right is not, therefore, absolute. "[T]he pregnant woman cannot be isolated in her pregnancy."[41] *Roe* held, however, and recent Supreme Court decisions have reaffirmed, that up until viability, a state's interest in protecting the potential life of the fetus is not strong enough to override the fundamental privacy right of the pregnant woman to have an abortion.[4]

Several states have determined, however, that this right of privacy is limited, not only by the state's prerogative to proscribe post-viability abortions, but also by an enforceable duty to protect the health of a viable fetus. In *Raleigh Fitkin–Paul Morgan Memorial Hospital* v. *Anderson*,[33] a blood transfusion was ordered against the religious beliefs of a pregnant woman, to save her life and that of her 32-week-old fetus. The New Jersey Supreme Court, joining its recognition of a *parens patriae* power to order blood transfusions for an infant over the religious objections of its parents, to its determination that a child could recover for injuries negligently inflicted on it prenatally by a third party, found that the right of the unborn child deserved the protection of the state.

In *Jefferson* v. *Griffin Spalding County Hospital Authority*,[25] the Georgia Supreme Court found that the state's compelling interest in protecting the life of a 39-week-old fetus outweighed the pregnant woman's right to refuse treatment on religious and privacy grounds and ordered the woman to submit to a cesarean section and other necessary medical treatments. The *Jefferson* court found that the mother was due to begin labor at any moment and that the unborn child was a human being fully capable of independent life. The court then concluded that the child was lacking the proper prenatal care necessary for life and health. Finding as a matter of law that the child was entitled to the protection of the Juvenile Court Code of Georgia, the court granted temporary custody of the child to the state and county agencies, giving them full authority to make all necessary medical and surgical decisions.

To date, at least 22 court orders for forced obstetrical intervention have been sought, with the result that courts in 11 states have ordered cesarean sections, courts in 2 states have ordered hospital detentions, and at least 1 court has ordered an intrauterine transfusion—against the pregnant woman's wishes.[22,27] In the most recent case, a terminally ill woman was forced to have a cesarean section in an attempt to save her 26-week-old fetus, even though the court recognized that the surgery was likely to shorten the woman's life.[22] The woman and the fetus both died after the surgery.

THE NATURE AND SCOPE OF A PREMATERNAL DUTY

The specific legal obligations that a woman may have toward her child-to-be and the potential liability that could attach to a failure or a refusal to meet these obligations are yet to be explored. The scope of this unique obligation must be delineated and the expedient standard of care established, in order to avoid unjust and substantial invasions of the pregnant woman's rights to privacy and bodily integrity and also to assure protection of the future child's quality of life. As medical technology increases our ability to enhance prenatal health and thereby the future health of the child, exploration of these issues becomes prerequisite to any rational attempt to establish such a prematernal obligation.

Conflicting Rights

The conflicts that may arise between the state's interest in the fetus and the pregnant woman's rights of privacy and bodily integrity, in contexts other than abortion, have not been addressed by *Roe* or its progeny. The Supreme Court has not spoken on the means a state may use to protect its interest in the fetus, other than prohibiting abortion after viability. *Roe* also left unanswered the question of what rights, if any, the fetus has vis-à-vis the prematernal interests of a pregnant woman. What *Roe* clearly does proclaim, however, is that the fetus is not a *person* as recognized by the fourteenth amendment. The Supreme Court found that "the fetus, at most, represents only the potentiality of life. [T]he unborn have never been recognized in the law as persons in the whole sense."[42]

Generally, personhood is established at birth. "Fetuses are not counted as U.S. citizens in the decennial census; there is no income tax exemption for the unborn or the stillborn; states are under no legal obligation to provide welfare funds or food stamps for fetuses."[45] Although the laws of property, crime, and torts do evidence some degree of protection over the interests of the unborn, such law is of little assistance in ascertaining the existence of a prematernal duty to the fetus or in delineating the scope of that duty, should it exist.

Recognition of a prematernal duty necessarily would abridge the pregnant woman's freedom to control her own body and would infringe on her constitutionally protected right of privacy. It is her body, however, and her behavior toward it prior to and during a pregnancy that plays so crucial a role in the future of her child. The general health and nutrition of the pregnant woman, her exposure to various environmental agents, and even her emotional state will influence profoundly the physical and mental development of the child. May it not, therefore, be argued that a woman's freedom of bodily control can be somewhat restricted during pregnancy? As our Supreme Court recognized while upholding a mandatory vaccination statute, "[r]eal liberty for all could not exist under the operation of a principle which recognizes the right of each individual person to use his own, whether in respect of his person or his property, regardless of the injury that may be done to others."[24]

Instead of searching for elusive and vague fetal rights, the critical question in determining liability for premature behavior is what rights *the child*, if born, has vis-à-vis the premature interests of its mother-to-be. If a child does have the right to be born with a sound mind and body, does this right impose a correlative prematernal duty on the pregnant woman to refrain from negligent behavior toward her fetus? The courts have not addressed the issue directly, but cases such as *Grodin*, *Jefferson*, and *Anderson* appear to recognize this obligation. Some legal commentators agree that such a prematernal duty does exist.[29,35] Margery Shaw, for example, argues that "once a pregnant woman has abandoned her right to abort and decided to carry the fetus to term, she incurs a 'conditional prospective liability' for negligent acts toward her fetus if it should be born alive."[46]

The Prematernal Duty: An Attempt to Resolve the Conflict

The medical profession has begun to concentrate its efforts on primary prevention of poor pregnancy outcomes, rather than on expensive, complicated, and perhaps inadequate therapies. Advances in obstetric and neonatal intensive care have resulted in dramatic improvement in infant mortality rates. Prevention is medicine's primary strategy for providing the newborn with the optimal quality-of-life prognosis. Perhaps in an attempt to keep up with the progress that medicine has made in this area, the courts have responded by recognizing the child's "right to be born healthy" in a variety of legal contexts. Such a broad principle, however, provides few guidelines in ascertaining the *relative rights* of the child and the mother. "Whatever parents' moral obligations to their children, at the beginning of life and thereafter, the principle of a right to a healthy birth is too far-reaching to establish a legal rule."[8] It is often not within the power of parents or physicians to produce a "healthy" child, or to prevent the birth of an nonhealthy one. Their capacity to intervene and to affect the health of the unborn child is limited. Their duty to *try*, however, is determined by the standard of behavior imposed on them by society.

The law recognizes a duty on the part of *every person*, pregnant or not, to act according to a certain standard of conduct in order to protect others from unreasonable risk of harm—that is, to act nonnegligently. The newborn child clearly is entitled to this protection, and courts since *Bonbrest* have recognized that the child's right includes the right to be born free of any negligently induced injury. It is this more limited birthright that must be evaluated in ascertaining the scope of a prematernal obligation. Such a right, however, would be meaningless if it did not protect against negligence by the person whose behavior posed the greatest potential risks to the life of the child.

The fact that the pregnant woman carries an unborn child within her own body does not give her the right to act negligently toward it. However, the unique circumstances of pregnancy do require a careful evaluation of the appropriate standard of care to be applied in establishing a prematernal duty. In other words, we must determine what behavior, if any, would constitute "negligence" by a pregnant woman toward her unborn child.

Ascertaining the Appropriate Standard of Care for a Pregnant Woman

Negligent behavior falls below a standard established by law for the protection of others against an unreasonable risk of harm. Thus, in light of a recognizable risk, for conduct to be negligent it must be *unreasonable*. A reasonable standard of conduct is determined by balancing the risk and the extent of the harm threatened, in light of its social value, against the value of the interest the actor is seeking to protect.[50] The question is whether "the game is worth the candle."[31]

The question of prematernal negligence, therefore, must be decided, in each individual case, by a careful balancing of the risk to the particular fetus of the harm threatened, and the potential severity of that harm, against the fundamental right of the pregnant woman to privacy in her choice of conduct. The pregnant woman is not, by any stretch of the imagination, a third party. Nor, however, is she a mother. Her unique status demands the application of a unique standard of care.

Any standard of reasonableness must, in fairness, be qualified according to the special circumstances of pregnancy. Just as a blind person must take the special precautions, be they more or less, that an ordinary reasonable person would take if she or he were blind, so should the standard of conduct applicable to a pregnant woman be sufficiently flexible to take the biological and emotional factors of pregnancy into consideration. A woman's decision to take a drug during pregnancy is an exercise of her discretion. It is not, however, an act of maternal discretion; the woman is not merely deciding whether to administer a drug to her child. A woman's decision to take a drug, in light of her pregnancy, should be based on her need for the drug and also upon the potential for injury to which she is exposing her future child. It is an exercise of prematernal discretion. The standard of conduct by which a pregnant woman's treatment of her own body is to be assessed, therefore, can be determined only within the unique context of pregnancy. She must behave as a *reasonable pregnant woman* would.

Reasonable Prematernal Behavior

Roe v. *Wade*, while proclaiming that a pregnant woman has a fundamental right to privacy, recognized that this right is not absolute. It can be limited by the state's assertion of compelling interests in safeguarding health, maintaining medical standards, and protecting potential life. The right of privacy is limited by the fact that the pregnant woman carries a fetus within her; it is only logical that this limitation somehow encompasses the right of the child to be born free of prematernally induced injury.

For meaningful benefits to result, however, the prematernal duty must arise at the time the woman knows, or should know, of her pregnancy and decides to carry the fetus to term. Viability, so crucial in the decision to terminate a pregnancy, may be invalid as the temporal landmark for determining when the prematernal obligation begins. Some of the most devastating fetal effects may be caused by prematernal behavior during the first trimester of pregnancy. Nor is it necessarily inconsistent to hold a pregnant woman liable for her behavior toward a pre-viable fetus that she had the option of aborting. In fact, the availability of the abortion option argues even more strongly for some measure of responsibility once the choice not to abort has been made.

Moreover, the child's interest in her health is different from the state's interest that is recognized in the abortion context and, as such, requires different standards for protection. The pre-viable fetus does *not* have a right to be born. The courts have proclaimed, however, that the child who is born does have a right to be born whole. "While the right to abortion recognized in *Roe* v. *Wade* means that a woman has no legal duty to ensure that a fetus is born alive, this does not necessarily preclude the law from imposing on the woman who does go to term, a duty to assure that the fetus is born as healthy as possible."[38]

A few obvious examples illustrate the application of the reasonable prematernal behavior standard. The reasonable prematernal behavior standard would support a finding that a pregnant woman's use of heroin or cocaine, or her consumption of large quantities of alcohol, was negligent. Both types of behavior have been shown conclusively to cause severe injury in the newborn child. The use of heroin or cocaine is illegal. There is no "fundamental right" to use psychoactive drugs.[36] Although alcohol abuse is not illegal and clearly is not as socially unacceptable as heroin use, the effects on the child of a chronic alcohol abuser are well known and far more devastating and permanent than neonatal heroin withdrawal symptoms. The right of the child to be born free of the fetal alcohol syndrome could justify a finding of liability on the part of the woman whose chronic alcohol abuse during pregnancy caused injury to her child.

A different result, however, may be called for in the application of the reasonable prematernal behavior standard to smoking during pregnancy. Long-term follow-up studies on the children of women who smoked during pregnancy have not produced definitive results. Also relevant is the fact, unfortunate though it may be, that a large number of pregnant women continue to smoke despite frequent mention in the media of potential adverse effects on the fetus. Because the standard to be applied would be a community standard, such evidence of the usual and customary behavior of other pregnant women would be admissible as an indication of what the community regards as proper, or at least acceptable, behavior.

In all applications of the reasonable prematernal behavior standard, the magnitude of the infringement on the fundamental rights of the pregnant woman must be considered carefully. Liability for prematernal negligence should *not* be found where her behavior represented a reasonable, although in retrospect unwise, exercise of judgment, even though the child was severely injured by her behavior.

Once prematernal negligence has been established, however, there is no valid reason to deny the injured child the right to damages. Any policy objections based on the possibility of intrafamily disharmony, fraud, or collusiveness would be no greater than those the courts have dealt with adequately in rejecting parent-child tort immunity in other contexts.[47] Further, the specter of women aborting just to avoid liability for prematernal negligence is untenable. Such personal human decisions generally are not based on the presence or absence of a legal cause of action. And, if the pregnant woman's behavior has been so negligent as to present a real threat to the future life of her child, abortion may be a reasonable choice.

TROUBLESOME IMPLICATIONS OF A PREMATERNAL DUTY

It seems reasonable on medical, ethical, and legal grounds to require that a pregnant woman act nonnegligently toward the fetus that she intends to carry to term. If we do recognize a duty on the part of the pregnant woman to refrain from certain conduct, a breach of this duty could give rise to a cause of action by the child for prenatal injury. Some would say, however, that this is not enough—that the real goal is to actively *prevent* such fetal mistreatment. One commentator has opined that "[t]here is no question that a state could prohibit behavior by a pregnant woman [such as using tobacco, alcohol, or drugs] that might reasonably be thought to kill a viable fetus *in utero* or cause it to be born in a damaged state."[36] Another anticipates that a statute requiring Breathalyzer tests of pregnant women would be upheld because of endangerment of the fetus.[44] But how far are we willing to go—and how do we protect against *abuses* that may unreasonably deny the woman her rights to privacy, autonomy, and bodily integrity?

The rapidly increasing ability to diagnose disorders prenatally and to treat them in utero with drugs or with a variety of surgical interventions raises myriad questions and policy considerations.[16,19,35,37] If the pregnant woman refuses prenatal diagnosis and/or beneficial maternal or fetal therapy, can she be held liable for the resultant injury or the wrongful death of the child? It has been suggested that under certain circumstances, "parents may be found to have a duty to receive genetic counseling and carrier testing, to use contraceptives, to be sterilized, to reveal a genetic risk to a spouse or a relative, to protect their gonads against adverse effects, and to consider whether they have a 'right' to knowingly pass on deleterious genes."[43]

The potential for abuse of the pregnant woman's rights seems inordinate under such a broad theory of duty. Consider, for example, the maternal PKU syndrome. Affected women have been put on an extremely distasteful and highly restricted low-phenylalanine diet before conception or as soon as possible thereafter, in an effort to decrease the toxic concentration of phenylalanine in their amniotic fluid and thereby to avoid the maternal PKU syndrome. If appropriate dietary restriction is found to prevent maternal PKU effectively, should civil liability arise or perhaps mandatory dietary therapy be enforced if treatment is refused? Note that for therapy to be successful, it is likely to be necessary *prior* to conception. Would this justify mandatory screening of high-risk women?

Will surgical interventions to correct fetal abnormalities merely be "available" to the pregnant woman, or will they become mandatory, through civil liability or state intervention, to protect the health of the future child? In 1985, pediatric surgeons in California removed a 23-week-old fetus from the womb, successfully operated to correct a blocked urinary tract, and returned the unborn child to the uterus. Nine weeks later, the baby boy, who would have died in utero without the surgery, was born alive and well.[19] Early intervention in cases such as this may well mean the difference between life and death or between a normal infant and one suffering from a severe abnormality. What if the pregnant woman carrying such a fetus refuses to consent to this surgical procedure and is not planning to terminate the pregnancy? Should the state intervene and compel fetal surgery?

Can such procedures be imposed on the pregnant woman against her will and in disregard of her own interests in privacy and bodily integrity? Cases such as *Anderson* and *Jefferson*, by ordering prematernal medical treatment to protect the life of the pregnant woman and her viable fetus, against the woman's will, suggest an affirmative duty on the part of the pregnant woman to take such steps as are necessary to ensure the health of the future child. Commentators disagree about the complex ethical and legal justifications for forcing prematernal surgery. One has suggested that, in the context of fetal surgery, "the patient's status as fetus and its position within the mother do not lead to results different from those which arise with similar conflicts in pediatric practice, where the moral and legal status of the patient is clear and the mother's body is not invaded."[37] And yet, society does *not* require parents to donate a kidney, or even a pint of blood, to save a dying child. "[I]f we do not ask people to risk their health for an *actual* life, have we any right to require such a sacrifice for a *potential* life?"[49] Indeed, the real question posed by treatment refusals during pregnancy is "whether doctors or the government may usurp patients' decision-making rights and appropriate or invade their bodies to advance what they perceive to be the therapeutic interests of a second patient, the fetus."[11,27]

If the pregnant woman refuses prenatal diagnosis or refuses to abort an affected but untreatable fetus, can she be held liable for the wrongful life of the defective child? A child has the right to be "born free of any negligently induced injury." Does such a right include the addendum "or not to be born at all?" The wrongful-life cause of action appears to encompass this interest by recognizing the right of a defective child to recover damages for the actual pain and suffering it will endure during its lifetime.[12] With respect to the possibility of a wrongful life suit against the parents of an affected child, one court has said that there is "no sound public policy which should protect those parents from being answerable for the pain, suffering, and misery which they have wrought upon their offspring."[13] The courts that have recognized the wrongful-life action also have based their findings on the need to foster societal objectives by encouraging responsible use of new medical technology, such as genetic counseling and prenatal diagnosis. It could be argued that a pregnant woman has as much of a responsibility to utilize these techniques to prevent her child from being born in a defective condition as does a physician. The courts, however, are not likely to recognize an action that imposes on a pregnant woman the obligation to abort an affected fetus.

Child abuse statutes may be written or interpreted to encompass prematernal negligence and, perhaps in extreme cases, a refusal to submit to fetal surgery. The Federal Child Abuse Act expressly authorizes intervention if the child is "threatened with harm."[17] The Michigan Court of Appeals, in neglect proceedings concerning a heroin-addicted newborn, has held that the behavior of a woman toward her fetus during pregnancy could constitute abuse and neglect under the relevant child protection statute.[23] Recently, a San Diego woman whose son was born brain-dead with amphetamines in his system was charged with criminally contributing to his death by disregarding doctors' orders to stay off her feet and away from drugs and to seek medical care immediately if she began to hemorrhage.[18] She was charged under a 1926 section of the California penal code that made it a crime for a parent to fail to furnish necessary medical attention for a child. The case was dismissed when a San Diego Municipal Court judge ruled that the law, which was intended to assure that fathers paid child support, did not apply to the facts before him.[9] However, a heated debate was provoked throughout the country over whether denying care to a fetus should be a crime.[49]

Legal recognition of a prematernal duty also has implications for the role of the obstetrician. No longer will it be only the pediatrician who faces the problem of dual—and possibly conflicting—professional obligations, for instance, in a case where parents want to withhold care from a seriously ill newborn. How, for example, is the obstetrician to respond when he or she has knowledge of prematernal behavior that may have deleterious effects on fetal development? The obstetrician may have to face the dilemma of violating the pregnant woman's confidentiality by testifying against her in an action brought by the state or by the child after birth—or by reporting her behavior to state authorities in an effort to prevent damage to the fetus. A Maryland physician recently went to court in an effort to force a pregnant woman to stop taking the narcotic drugs that allegedly injured her first child and threatened the health of her 28-week-old fetus.[15] The fetus showed retarded growth, and the physician claimed that continued drug use would further retard and prevent its growth and development in a life-threatening manner. The court ordered the woman to enroll in a drug rehabilitation program and to submit to weekly urine testing until the child was born.

"Concern" for the health of a future child could allow pregnant or even merely fertile women—or men—to be excluded from certain types of employment. The United States Court of Appeals for the Fourth Circuit found, in *Wright* v. *Olin Corp.*, that under appropriate circumstances an employer may, as a matter of business necessity, impose otherwise impermissible restrictions on employment categories for women if the restrictions are reasonably necessary and effective to protect the health of unborn children of female employees from work-related hazards.[52] Employers could use this type of rationale to exclude fertile women from work environments, rather than cleaning up the toxic situation or attempting to provide some type of protection for them. Clashes between interests in fetal health, equal employment opportunity, and women's rights are inevitable in these situations.

Thus, although *preventing* prematernally induced fetal injury undoubtedly would be preferable to merely compensating an affected child, state-enforced standards of prematernal behavior would provide an unacceptable potential for abuse of the pregnant, and perhaps even the fertile, woman's rights. In addition, any standard of conduct prescribed for the pregnant woman by legislative enactment could not take into account the unique and intimate factors encompassed by each individual case. And it is these personal, individual considerations that tort law is able—in fact is designed—to balance. This is not to say that societal concerns may not be involved in these essentially private disputes. "[T]he twentieth century has brought an increasing realization of the fact that the interests of society in general may be involved in disputes in which the parties are private litigants."[6] Public policy inevitably becomes part of the balancing process. However, it is the balancing process itself—

the "process of weighing the interests for which the plaintiff demands protection against the defendant's claim to untrammelled freedom in the furtherance of his own desires"[30]—that is essential to so serious a finding as that of prematernal negligence.

CONCLUSION

The recognition of a prematernal duty to refrain from negligent behavior toward the fetus, and to take whatever affirmative steps are reasonably necessary to insure the health of the future child, raises numerous ethical and legal questions. The next few years will witness a multitude of tentative approaches to these questions as the courts struggle to define the parameters of prematernal liability. A just determination of tort liability for prematernal negligence necessitates a thoughtful balance between the woman's constitutionally protected right to privacy and bodily integrity during her pregnancy and the right of the child, if born, to be born free of negligently inflicted injury.

Future courts must delineate the boundaries of the prematernal duty—hopefully, with due regard for the fundamental rights that hang in the balance. Although *Roe* v. *Wade* does not establish that prohibition of postviability abortion is the only means a state may use to protect its interest in the potential life of the fetus, or that other compelling interests may not be recognized, any attempt to limit the personal privacy and autonomy of a woman during her pregnancy is made under the watchful eye of *Roe*.

NOTES AND REFERENCES

1. Abel EL: Consumption of alcohol during pregnancy: A review of effects on growth and development of offspring. Hum Biol 54:421, 1982 ("Behold, you are barren and have no children; but you shall conceive and bear a son. Therefore, beware, and drink no wine or strong drink. . . . Judges 13:3–4")
2. Abel EL, *id.* at 443
3. Abel EL, Sokel RJ: Preventing alcohol-related birth defects. In Gleicher N, Roux J (eds): Principles of Medical Therapy in Pregnancy, 198X, contains an excellent review of the association between prematernal alcohol use and birth defects and has contributed to much of the discussion in the text
4. Akron v. Akron Center for Reprod. Health, Inc., 462 U.S. 416 (1983); Planned Parenthood Ass'n of Kansas City, Mo. v. Ashcroft, 462 U.S. 476 (1983); Simopoulos v. Virginia, 462 U.S. 506 (1983)
5. American Association of University Affiliated Programs for Persons with Developmental Disabilities: Developmental Handicaps: Prevention and Treatment 62, 1983
6. Bohlen FH: Fifty Years of Torts. Harv L Rev 50:725, 1937
7. Bonbrest v. Kotz, 65 F. Supp. 138, 142 (D.D.C. 1946) (quoting the Supreme Court of Canada in Montreal Tramways v. Leveille, 4 D.L.R. 337, 345 [1933] [emphasis omitted])
8. Capron AM: The continuing wrong of "wrongful life." Genetics and the Law II: 81,91, 1980
9. Case against woman in baby death thrown out, p B5. New York Times, Feb 27, 1987
10. Cocaine babies: Addicts bear ailing infants, p. 50. Time, Jan 20, 1986
11. Curlender v. Bio-Science Laboratories, 106 Cal.App.3d 811, 165 Cal. Rptr. 477 (1980)
12. Curlender, *id.*, 106 Cal.App.3d at 829, 165 Cal. Rptr. at 488
13. Curlender, *id.* Shortly after this decision, however, the California legislature provided that "no cause of action arises against a parent of a child based upon the claim that the child should not have been conceived, or if conceived, should not have been born alive." Cal. Civil Code § 43.6 (West Supp. 1983)
14. Dietrich v. Inhabitants of Northampton, 138 Mass. 14 (1884)
15. Drug case stresses fetus rights, p. A18. New York Times, Apr 27, 1983
16. Elias S, Annas GJ: Perspectives on fetal surgery. Am J Obstet Gynecol 145:807, 1983, offers an excellent discussion of the policy considerations raised by the new fetal therapy techniques.
17. Federal Child Abuse Act, 42 U.S.C. § 5102 (1982)
18. Fetal abuse charged in son's death, §1, p 3. Chicago Tribune, Oct 2, 1986
19. Fetal surgery methods join ranks of medicine

laced with social issues, §1, p 5. Chicago Tribune, Oct 7, 1986
20. Grodin v. Grodin, 102 Mich. App. 396, 301 N.W.2d 869 (1980)
21. Hamilton: Letter to the Editor. Lancet II:621, 1850 (reported in Pediatrics 71:128, 1983)
22. In re A.C., No. 87-609, slip op. (D.C.Ct.App. June 16, 1987)
23. In re Baby X, 97 Mich. App. 111, 293 N.W.2d 736 (1980), recognized "fetal abuse" for heroin use during pregnancy under a child protection statute.
24. Jacobson v. Massachusetts, 197 U.S. 11, 26 (1905)
25. Jefferson v. Griffin Spalding County Hospital Authority, 247 Ga. 86, 274 S.E.2d 457 (1981)
26. Jones KL, Smith DW, Ulleland CN, et al: Patterns of malformation in offspring of chronic alcoholic mothers. Lancet I:1267, 1973; Recognition of the fetal alcohol syndrome in early infancy. Lancet II:99, 1973
27. Kolder VFB, Gallagher J, Parsons, MT: Court-ordered obstetrical interventions. N Engl J Med 316:1192, 1194, 1987
28. McBride WG: Thalidomide and congenital abnormalities. Lancet II:1358, 1961
29. Parental liability for prenatal injury. 14 Colum J L & Soc Probs 14:47,81, 1978 ("Duties of parenthood should not commence upon the birth of the child; they should commence when the parents know or have reason to know of the pregnancy.")
30. Prosser WL: Handbook of the Law of Torts, 15 (4th ed 1971)
31. Prosser, id. at 148.
32. Prosser, id. at 336.
33. Raleigh Fitkin–Paul Morgan Memorial Hospital v. Anderson, 42 N.J. 421, 201 A.2d 537 (1964)
34. Renslow v. Mennonite Hospital, 67 Ill.2d 348, 367 N.E.2d 1250 (1977)
35. Robertson JA: Procreative liberty and the control of conception, pregnancy and childbirth. Va L Rev 69:405,441, 1983 ("The mother who chooses not to abort has the same duty as an outsider to avoid prenatal actions injurious to a child who would otherwise be born healthy.")
36. Robertson, id. at 442.
37. Robertson JA: The right to procreate and in utero fetal therapy. J Leg Med 3:333,350, 1982
38. Robertson, id. at 352
39. Roe v. Wade, 410 U.S. 113 (1983)
40. Roe v. Wade, id. at 152
41. Roe v. Wade, id. at 159
42. Roe v. Wade, id. at 162
43. Shaw MW: Conditional prospective rights of the fetus. J Leg Med 5:63,93, 1984
44. Shaw, id. at 103 (suggesting liability of a pregnant woman for "furnishing alcohol to a 'minor,' her fetus, which is prohibited by law")
45. Shaw MW: The potential plaintiff: Preconception and prenatal torts. Genetics and the Law II:225, 1982 (footnotes omitted)
46. Shaw, id. at 228
47. Stallman v. Youngquist, 152 Ill.App.3d 683, 504 N.E.2d 920 (1987). The Stallman court spent most of its opinion on a reevaluation of parental tort immunity in Illinois. Finding that the "major justifications for parental immunity do not withstand analysis in light of modern conditions," the court held that "an unemancipated minor child may recover damages in an action brought against a parent for personal injuries caused by the negligence of the parent in the operation of a motor vehicle." 152 Ill.App.3d at 692, 504 N.E.2d at 925
48. The reasonable parent standard: An alternative to parent-child tort immunity. U Colo L Rev 47:795,796,798–799, 1976
49. The troubling question of "fetal rights," pp 87–88. Newsweek, Dec 8, 1986
50. United States v. Carroll Towing Co., 159 F.2d 169 (2d Cir. 1947) ("If the probability be called P; the injury L; and the burden [of adequate precautions] B; liability depends upon whether B is less than PL.")
51. Womack v. Buchhorn, 384 Mich. 718, 725, 187 N.W.2d 218,222 (1971) (quoting Smith v. Brennan, 31 N.J. 353, 157 A.2d 497 [1960])
52. Wright v. Olin Corp., 697 F.2d 1172 (4th Cir. 1972)

21
Government Funding of Abortions: The Constitutional Issues

David C. Sobelsohn

Controversy has surrounded the topic of abortion from antiquity. Today many remember the Hippocratic proscription[1] (cf ref. 51); few recall Hippocrates' minority status—on the subject of abortion, most other Greek philosophers disagreed with him.[2]

So did a majority of Western philosophers through the Middle Ages,[3] including those claiming allegiance to the Catholic church.[4] For these Western philosophers, abortion triggered no moral sanction, as long as it preceded fetal "ensoulment" or "animation."[5] Disagreement as to the precise time at which this occurs led legal authorities to focus on "quickening"—the first intrauterine movement of the fetus[6]—as the critical point.[7] As a result, Anglo-American common law imposed no criminal penalties on abortion prior to fetal quickening.[8]

So matters stood until the early part of the 19th century. In 1828, New York enacted the first American law prohibiting abortion of an unquickened fetus; the law made an exception for abortions needed to save the pregnant woman's life.[9] By 1840, eight American states had statutes dealing with abortion,[10] while the other states continued to follow the common-law principle leaving abortion before quickening outside the criminal law.[11]

The American Medical Association (AMA) became involved in the issue when in 1857 it established its Committee on Criminal Abortion. The committee issued its report in 1859.[12] Stressing the "inherent rights of the fetus,"[13] the report deplored abortion, blaming the practice on a widespread belief that the fetus was not alive until quickening, and on the "grave defects of our laws," which failed to criminalize abortion before quickening.[14] The AMA promptly adopted a resolution calling upon state legislatures to revise their abortion laws.[15]

A few states soon followed the AMA's recommendation.[16] But it was only after the carnage of the Civil War that the AMA position swept a nation anxious to rebuild. The war ended in 1865; by 1868—the year the states ratified the 14th amendment to the U.S. Constitution—every state in the Union had criminal laws prohibiting abortion, regardless of the period of pregnancy.[17]

Despite widespread disobedience and inconsistent enforcement,[18] these and similar laws remained on the books through the middle of the 20th century. By the mid 1960s, virtually every American jurisdiction banned abortions, whenever performed, unless needed to save the pregnant woman's life.[19]

The 1960s saw the start of a liberalizing trend.[20] That trend received a major impetus in 1962 when the respected American Law Institute (ALI) published its draft Model Penal Code.[21] The ALI proposal, adopted by 14 states during the late 1960s and early 1970s,[22] decriminalized abortions of pregnancies resulting from "rape, incest, or other felonious intercourse," or that threatened to "gravely impair" the woman's "physical or mental health" or to produce a child with "grave physical or mental defect."[23] The Conference of Commissioners on Uniform State Laws (in 1971) and the American Bar Association (in 1972) approved an even more lenient position, based largely on a New York law enacted several years earlier.[24] This statute essentially followed the Model Penal Code for abortions after 20 weeks' gestation, but generally removed criminal sanctions completely from abortions performed during the first 20 weeks.[25]

The United States Supreme Court entered the area of abortion regulation in 1971.[26] A District of Columbia criminal abortion law made an exception for abortions necessary to preserve the woman's "health." To avoid problems of vagueness,[27] the Court construed the term "health" to include psychological as well as physical well-being.[28]

In its 1973 decision in *Roe v. Wade*[29] the Supreme Court finally dealt with the issue of abortion directly. For 50 years previously, Supreme Court decisions had recognized a constitutional right of family privacy. In these decisions, the Court had invalidated laws forbidding teaching schoolchildren any language other than English,[30] requiring all children to attend public school,[31] requiring the sterilization of certain "habitual" criminal offenders,[32] and prohibiting the use of artificial contraceptives.[33]

Citing these and other precedents,[34] the Supreme Court ruled that the right of family privacy "is broad enough to encompass a woman's decision whether or not to terminate her pregnancy."[35] But, as the Court noted,[36] the state can limit even fundamental constitutional rights if necessary to further sufficiently strong state interests.[37] The state in *Roe v. Wade* claimed two such interests: protecting the health of the pregnant woman and preserving the life of her fetus.[38]

Neither interest justified the law at issue in *Roe*. First, even as of 1973, first-trimester abortions were safer than carrying a pregnancy to term.[39] Of course, the state retained an interest in maintaining certain medical standards.[40] But in the first trimester, the Court ruled, the state could satisfy that interest by requiring the reasonable supervision of a licensed physician.[41] During the second trimester, mortality in abortions approached that in normal childbirth; thus, beginning with the second trimester, the state could impose additional "regulation[s] reasonably relate[d] to the preservation and protection of maternal health."[42]

Nor did the state's interest in fetal life justify the law at issue in *Roe*. The Court acknowledged that, if the fetus had equal constitutional status with its carrier, the state could interfere with the pregnant woman's constitutional right of privacy in order to preserve the fetus's constitutional right to life.[43] But only "persons" have a constitutional right to life,[44] and the law had never recognized fetuses as "persons in the whole sense."[45] Nevertheless, at viability—the point at which the fetus can live outside the womb[46]—the fetus closely resembles a prematurely born infant,[47] clearly a constitutional "person."[48] Thus, the Court ruled that, after viability, the state could ban abortions, except when necessary to preserve the pregnant woman's life or health.[49]

The Court's decision in *Roe v. Wade* sparked a firestorm of protest.[50] Within a year after the decision, almost 30 constitutional amendments were introduced in Congress to overturn the case[51] (cf ref. 1); ultimately some members of Congress attempted to overturn *Roe* by simple legislative action.[52] Nevertheless, when the Supreme Court was asked, 10 years later, to overrule *Roe*, the Court refused, citing the doctrine of "stare decisis."[53]

By far the most successful attack on the right to abortion has been the denial of public funding.[54] Such laws have come in several varieties.[55] An early restriction eliminated funding for "elective" or "nontherapeutic" abortions.[56] Later enactments limited funding to abortions necessary to prevent "severe and long-lasting physical health damage" to the pregnant woman, or of pregnancies resulting from rape or incest.[57] Some statutes have included funding for abortions needed to prevent the birth of "severely defective infants."[58] The most severe restrictions prohibit funding for all abortions not needed to preserve the life of the pregnant woman.[59] All of these limitations coexisted with state readiness to fund medical expenses associated with childbirth.[60]

Initial decisions on such limitations generally found them unconstitutional.[61] Indeed, in a case decided the same day as *Roe v. Wade*,[62] the Supreme Court had invalidated procedural limitations[63] on the right to abortion, in part on the grounds that the state imposed no such procedural limits on the performance of any other surgical procedures.[64] Restrictions on government funding, applicable only to abortions, would seem to fall under the same analysis. Moreover, a well-established constitutional doctrine prohibits the government from conditioning public benefits on the recipient's waiver of a constitutional right.[65] Medicaid schemes that pay medical expenses associated with pregnancy, but only if the recipient agrees to give up her right to an abortion, would seem invalid under this "unconstitutional conditions" doctrine.[66]

Nevertheless, when the funding issue reached the U.S. Supreme Court, the Court upheld the limitations. In *Maher v. Roe*,[67] the Court considered a Connecticut regulation limiting abortion funding to abortions deemed "medically necessary."[68] The lower court had invalidated the regulation, reasoning that "abortion and childbirth . . . are simply two alternative medical methods of dealing with pregnancy," that the Constitution protects the choice of either method, and that this protection prohibits discriminatory state funding that favors one choice over the other.[69]

But the Supreme Court reversed.[70] The Court acknowledged that "when a State decides to alleviate some of the hardships of poverty by providing medical care, the manner in which it dispenses benefits is subject to constitutional limitations."[71] But the Court found "a basic difference between direct state interference with a protected activity"—such as a criminal law banning that activity—"and state encouragement of an alternative activity."[72] There was simply nothing in the Constitution limiting "the authority of a State to make a value judgment favoring childbirth over abortion, and to implement that judgment by the allocation of public funds."[73]

Three years later, the Supreme Court faced the issue in its starkest form.[74] Congress had prohibited the use of any federal funds to reimburse the cost of Medicaid abortions except under certain narrowly defined circumstances. In its narrowest form, the Hyde Amendment—named after its original congressional sponsor, Representative Henry Hyde of Illinois—prohibited all federal funding of abortions "except where the life of the mother would be endangered if the fetus were carried to term."[75] An Illinois state law was to the same effect.[76] The lower courts invalidated the restrictions,[77] reasoning that the case differed from *Maher v. Roe*[78] in that these laws eliminated funding even for abortions deemed medically necessary.[79]

But the Supreme Court again reversed.[80] Like the restriction upheld in *Maher*, the Hyde Amendment "places no governmental obstacle in the path of a woman who chooses to terminate her pregnancy."[81] The Constitution, the Court ruled, leaves the state free to refuse to "subsidize" constitutionally protected conduct[82] in order to "encourage[ ] alternative activity deemed in the public interest."[83] The state's interest in protecting the fetus, deemed insufficient to support a criminal law in *Roe v. Wade*,[84] nevertheless sufficed here to justify disparate funding of childbirth.[85]

Refusal of government to fund abortions raises a number of complex constitutional questions. Even if there is no absolute constitutional right to funding, government action taken deliberately to discourage exercise of a protected constitutional right seems at war with fundamental premises underlying our constitutional system. Moreover, each state has its own constitution. Indeed, a number of state supreme courts have rejected the U.S. Supreme Court's approach to the constitutional question of state abortion funding. The rest of this chapter will explore these issues.

THE CONSTITUTIONAL ISSUES

Federal

Absolute Right to Funding

Some constitutional rights carry with them an apparent right to government financial assistance and support. For instance, the Constitution protects the right to vote,[86] and the Supreme Court has ruled that the state may not require citizens to pay a fee in order to exercise that right.[87] Thus, one may say the right to vote carries with it a corollary right to state financial support for the electoral process.

Another example is the right to a fair hearing, guaranteed by the due-process clauses of the fifth and 14th amendments.[88] Under certain circumstances, a fair hearing may require the assistance of an attorney, and the right to an attorney may include the right to compel the state to provide an attorney at its own expense.[89]

A third example comes from the area of family relations. Many years ago, the U.S. Supreme Court recognized a right to marry.[90] A case then arose challenging a statute requiring the payment of fees and costs for the granting of a divorce—thereby effectively precluding the poor from obtaining a divorce.[91] The Court held the law unconstitutional, ruling that, because of the "basic position of the marriage relationship" in American society, the state could not deny divorces solely on the basis of inability to pay.[92]

Yet, despite many years of urging from academics[93] and members of the judiciary,[94] the Constitution has not been read generally to require government funding of constitutional rights.[95] There are several good reasons for this.[96] First, the structure of our Federal Constitution reflects a classic liberal philosophy. Such a philosophy sees the major threat to liberty coming from government action, not from a refusal of government to act. The Constitution's text reflects this philosophy in various prohibitions against certain types of government action[97] (cf ref. 1 and 51); by contrast, the Constitution contains few provisions requiring affirmative support for personal liberties. Imposing a constitutional requirement on government to provide financial support for constitutional rights thus would be inconsistent with the Constitution's very framework.

A second reason cautions against recognizing a general constitutional requirement of affirmative government support for constitutional rights. Enforcing such a requirement would involve the courts in delicate areas of government financing. Courts would have to decide how much support was "enough," and might well become involved in ordering tax increases to provide funds for such support. These areas require reconciliation of many competing values, and often the establishment of extensive government mechanisms to administer. Establishment and supervision of these bureaucracies, in the name of the Constitution, is a task for which judges are ill-trained and ill-suited.[98]

Finally, the areas in which, arguably, the Constitution does require affirmative government support can all be explained as either proscriptions against government intrusion or as strictly limited to their contexts.[99] For instance, the Supreme Court has never required that a state set up and fund an electoral machinery; it requires only that access to that machinery, once the state has set it up, must be equalized for all interested parties. The Constitution, strictly speaking, does not guarantee a right to a fair hearing; it guarantees against certain deprivations if undertaken by the state without a fair hearing. Thus, rather than a right to require government action, the right to a fair hearing—and the right to a government-paid attorney—are really limitations on the power of the state to take action. Finally, the right to obtain a divorce differs significantly from other constitutional rights, in that a divorce, under law, cannot be obtained without government action—the state has a monopoly on the granting of divorces. By contrast, most constitutional rights are simply variations of what Justice Brandeis once called "the right to be let alone—the most comprehensive of rights and the right most valued by civilized men."[100] Consequently, the weight of argument seems to counsel against recognizing an absolute right to government funding of abortions.

Conditional Right to Funding

However, no one seeking government funding of abortion has had to make the argument that the Constitution absolutely requires funding.[101] This results from the decision of virtually every state in the union to provide, through participation in the federal Medicaid program,[102] for compensation for expenses associated with pregnancy and childbirth. This compensation obviously encourages pregnant women to bring their pregnancies to term. Such a choice is protected by the Federal Constitution,[103] but so is the contrary choice, to abort a pregnancy.[104] Thus, a state's refusal to fund abortion, because it accompanies full funding of a woman's contrary choice, raises a significantly different issue from a hypothetical refusal by the state to fund either choice—namely, whether, by disparate funding of constitutional choices, the state can attempt to induce recipients of government largesse to make constitutional choices in conformity with state policy.

At one time, the U.S. Supreme Court easily resolved this question. The Court simply followed an 1892 opinion by then Chief Judge Oliver Wendell Holmes, speaking for the Massachusetts Supreme Judicial Court, who had summarily rejected the petition of a police officer dismissed for his political activities by saying, "The petitioner may have a constitutional right to talk politics, but he has no constitutional right to be a policeman."[105] In Holmes's view, a recipient of government largesse—such as employment—had no cause to complain of conditions accompanying that largesse. He had a simple choice: he could turn the job down or "take[ ]the employment on the terms which are offered him."[106]

This distinction between constitutionally protected rights and unprotected government privileges was applied to defeat a wide variety of claims associated with government largesse. For instance, in one case, public-school teachers lost their jobs for membership in one of a list of allegedly "subversive" organizations.[107] Echoing Justice Holmes, the Court upheld the teachers' dismissal, ruling that, although they had the right "to assemble, speak, think, and believe as they will," no one had any right "to work for the state in its school system on his own terms." If they did not agree with the terms laid down by the state, they could retain their beliefs and associations and seek employment elsewhere; state employment was a mere "privilege."[108] Similar reasoning led to upholding suspension of a physician's license for refusing to produce certain papers for the House of Representatives Committee on Un-American Activities: "The practice of medicine," said the Court, "is lawfully prohibited by the State except upon the conditions it imposes. Such practice is a privilege granted by the State . . . ," and thus can be withheld upon violation of any "reasonable" conditions.[109]

This approach has some intuitive appeal. The maxim "the greater includes the lesser" has longstanding status in American law.[110] It is generally true that most largesse, particularly private largesse, brings with it certain conditions, conditions that the entity providing the largesse has a perfect right to impose. Indeed, some of those conditions provide the very purpose for the largesse, as in, for example, a farm subsidy program whose condition and purpose is to limit production in order to maintain prices.

And a right-privilege distinction may present little danger in a society in which the government plays a minor role. Having no "constitutional right to be a policeman" or to receive other forms of government largesse may have little significance if work as a government employee represents a very small fraction of the available employment opportunities or if government plays only a very minimal role in distributing other kinds of benefits.

But if our society ever fit that mold, it has long ceased. Today, "[t]he greatest force of a modern government lies in its power to regulate access to scarce resources."[111] For more than 45 years, government in the United States has employed over 15% of the available workforce.[112] Government today provides financial support for virtually every aspect of our lives, from housing[113] and food[114] to education[115] and transportation.[116] And if one analyzes use of tax deductions as a form of government largesse, the power of government to influence our constitutional choices through manipulation of government largesse appears overwhelming. Indeed, by thorough manipulation of the "right-privilege" distinction, all our constitutional rights could be effectively lost. Certainly we would hardly accept a tax law limiting charitable deductions to contributions made to politically approved charities, or a city's refusal to provide police and fire protection to churches of a particular disfavored denomination. Yet the Supreme Court has never held either the charitable deduction or police and fire protection to be a constitutional right; they are mere "privileges." As Justice Sutherland noted in 1926, "If the state may compel the surrender of one constitutional right as a condition of its favor, it may, in like manner, compel a surrender of all. It is inconceivable that guarantees embedded in the Constitution may thus be manipulated out of existence."[117]

But an even deeper principle requires rejection of the "right-privilege" distinction. The recognition of a constitutional right carries with it some implications about the status of a choice protected by that right. If the concept of a constitutional right means anything, it means that decisions as to the morality of choices protected by that constitutional right are to be left to the individual—shielded from state coercion.[118] Recognition of a constitutional right means that we, as a society, have decided to allocate decisionmaking authority with regard to that right to the individual, not to the state.[119] The state may suppress exercise of that right, but only with reference to competing state interests of equal or compelling weight. The state may *not* attempt to discourage exercise of that right simply out of naked hostility to the right, or based on the view that exercise of that right in a certain way is not morally justified.[120]

Following these arguments, the Supreme Court long ago abandoned the "right-privilege" distinction. In one case, for example, several states imposed durational residency requirements for the receipt of welfare benefits. To the argument that, since there was no constitutional right to welfare, there should be no constitutional barrier to a condition on the receipt of welfare benefits, the Court responded that the question "cannot be answered" by reference to a distinction between a " 'right' and a 'privilege.' "[121] The Court went on to analyze the justifications for the law. One argument the states made was that the limitation served "to discourage the influx of poor families in need of assistance." To this the Court responded that "the nature of our Federal Union and our constitutional concepts of personal liberty" required recognition of a federal constitutional right of interstate travel; once such a right was recognized the deliberate attempt to discourage exercise of that right was "constitutionally impermissible."[122] In another case, despite the state's desire to discourage membership in a particular political organization, the Court ruled that a state college could not deny official recognition and the accompanying privilege to distribute literature on campus to a student organization on the grounds that such recognition itself was not a constitutional right but merely a state-granted privilege.[123]

A final case illustrating the principle that the state may not act deliberately to discourage the exercise of a constitutional right comes from the area of abortion regulation. The city of Akron, Ohio required that, before abortions could be performed, attending physicians had to inform their patients of the development of the fetus, the date of possible viability, the physical and emotional complications that might result from an abortion, and the availability of agencies to provide information about adoption and childbirth. The Court declared this requirement unconstitutional; rather than a neutral regulation aimed at securing "informed consent," the regulation was "designed to *influence* the woman's informed choice between abortion or childbirth" so as to "persuade her to withhold [her consent] altogether."[124] Consequently, the restriction violated the constitutional principle protecting a woman's right to choose.

This principle should require invalidating Medicaid schemes funding childbirth but failing to fund abortions. No colorable argument can be made that these limitations proceed from anything other than a desire to discourage abortions—from a bare hostility to exercise of a constitutional right.[125] Such hostility is an invalid basis for laws touching on constitutional rights.[126]

What explains the Supreme Court's refusal to invalidate these funding laws? The Court's own explanation is unpersuasive. The Court claimed that laws refusing to fund abortions "imposed no restriction on access to abortions that was not already there."[127] But this language seems reminiscent of the now-discredited right-privilege distinction. Using the same rationale, one could justify a scheme of disparate financial support for favored political groups, or for longtime residents instead of newcomers. In both instances, the failure to provide support for the disfavored activity or group would "impose[ ] no restriction" that was not "already there" before adoption of the funding scheme. And yet both statutes would violate the principle that the government must not act deliberately to discourage the exercise of constitutional rights, and would undoubtedly be declared unconstitutional.

An explanation can be found for the Supreme Court's apparent inconsistency on the issue of abortion funding. To do so, however, one must investigate the derivation of the constitutional right to abortion, a right whose derivation differs markedly from that of the right of political organization or of interstate travel.

The prevailing political principle of our government is majoritarian democracy. With some exceptions, if a political majority, acting through its elected representatives, wishes a particular result expressed in positive law, the courts' role is to respect that result. The U.S. Supreme Court has articulated this principle in the rule that most laws, to satisfy the Constitution, need have no more than a "rational" relation to a "legitimate" government interest.[128] In practice, this requirement is virtually toothless; most laws satisfy it without difficulty.[129]

The law at issue in *Roe v. Wade*—proscribing abortion except to save the pregnant woman's life—easily satisfied this requirement.[130] The state claimed its law furthered interests in the pregnant woman's health and in the life of her fetus.[131] Whether the law best furthered these interests was not at issue; as the Court admitted, they were clearly "legitimate" state interests,[132] and the means chosen were plainly not "irrational."[133]

Over at least the last 50 years, however, the Court has developed an exception to the general principle of judicial deference to majority will.[134] If the law interferes with a "fundamental" constitutional right, or uses "suspect" classifications, the state must demonstrate the law to be "necessary" to fulfill a "compelling" state interest.[135] The government interest furthered by the law must be not only "legitimate" but "compelling"[136] (cf ref. 51); the law must not only further that interest but do so by the least offensive means.[137]

The Court's confrontation with the abortion issue in *Roe v. Wade* took place against a backdrop of decades of Supreme Court decisions recognizing a "fundamental" constitutional right of family privacy. For example, in 1923 the Court invalidated a law forbidding the teaching in school of any language, other than English, before the ninth grade.[138] "[T]he individual has certain fundamental rights which must be respected," the Court said; these included the rights of teachers to teach and of parents to obtain instruction for their children.[139] In a later case the Court invalidated a law requiring all children to attend public school; the law interfered "with the liberty of parents and guardians to direct the upbringing and education of children under their control."[140]

It was a small step from a right to direct the upbringing of children to a right to retain the capacity to have children. So in 1942, the Court rejected a law requiring the sterilization of certain "habitual" criminal offenders; the Court called procreation "one of the basic civil rights of man."[141] And a right to have children logically implies the right to choose not to have children. Thus, in 1965, citing the "right of privacy," the Supreme Court invalidated a law prohibiting the use of artificial contraceptives.[142]

In recognizing the right to an abortion, the Court relied on the above decisions and others.[143] But, as the Court admitted, the Constitution "does not explicitly mention any right of privacy."[144] From where had the Court derived such a right? The Court almost casually referred to "the Fourteenth Amendment's concept of personal liberty and restraints on state action."[145] But the only mention of "liberty" in the 14th amendment is in a clause forbidding the state to deprive any "person" of "liberty" without "due process of law."[146] No one in any of the Court's family-privacy decisions had complained about the "process" by which the state had enacted the law or enforced it against them.[147] Thus it seems that in recognizing either the right to an abortion or the more general right of family privacy from which it derives, the Supreme Court could rely on no specific textual provision of the U.S. Constitution.

This matters for at least two reasons. First, it is not intuitively obvious that the proper body for articulating constitutional norms in a majoritarian democracy is an unelected court of life-tenured judges.[148] Other countries have systems of constitutional review of legislation that rely not on the courts but on a branch of the legislature.[149] When the U.S. Supreme Court first arrogated to itself the power to declare laws unconstitutional, it relied on the greater skill of law-trained judges in interpreting the words of a legal document, such as the Constitution.[150] This rationale vanishes to the extent that the judge fails to find a constitutional value in the words of the Constitution itself.

Fidelity to the constitutional text matters for a second reason. Words confine choice. Disregard for the constitutional text raises the spectre of unlimited judicial license to invalidate legislation, turning our democracy into little more than an appointive aristocracy of life-tenured autocrats. Without a specific textual provision providing the source for a constitutional value, one must look elsewhere for a source that both supports that value and can confine courts in their selection of values to something other than the judges' own subjective preferences.

Structural implications of the document itself provide one possible source.[151] For example, the Constitution sets up a federal system, leaving power largely in state governments[152] while delegating specific national powers to a central government.[153] States may regulate behavior, as long as they refrain from interfering with the basic constitutional purpose of turning a loose confederation of states into one nation.[154] And thus the Court has inferred, from this aspect of the governmental structure established in the Constitution, rights of interstate travel[155] and of interstate trade[156] (cf ref. 51); state interference with such rights would seriously threaten our federalism.

But this source of values provides little assistance for recognition of a constitutional right of family privacy. Traditionally, matters of family law have been left to state government[157]; thus, state regulation of such matters poses little threat to the federalistic structure. Indeed, to the extent that the constitutional design reserves family-law matters to the states, interference with such matters by any branch of the federal government—including the Supreme Court—upsets the structure of federalism.[158]

All other possible sources for a constitutional right of family privacy promise, at best, uncertain restraints on judicial discretion.[159] For example, some have sought to find a right to privacy in American tradition.[160] But this approach poses several problems. First, nothing in the constitutional text or structure establishes the federal judiciary as a Court of Historical Review. But even assuming the legitimacy of such a judicial role, a reliance on historical analysis raises several unanswerable questions.[161] Whose history must the courts consider? This country consists of diverse ethnic groups, each with its own heritage,[162] and diverse geographic regions, each with its own traditions.[163] And what is the relevant time period? Does a practice become "so rooted in the traditions and conscience of our people as to be ranked as fundamental"[164] so long as it has survived 10 years? Fifty? Finally, by manipulating the level of generality of the tradition one can derive virtually any right: a right of privacy "surrounding the marriage relationship"[165] quickly becomes a right to "mak[e] choices about the most intimate aspects" of one's life.[166]

Other scholars have suggested that courts interpreting constitutions should seek to reflect "contemporary norms."[167] But, to the extent that any discoverable consensus even exists as to what constitute "contemporary norms,"[168] articulating those norms is precisely the task of a democratically elected legislature[169]; life-tenured appointed judges are far more likely "to express the points of view of the class to which they belong rather than that of the whole community."[170] Still others have pointed to a supposed future consensus as the appropriate source for constitutional values.[171] But "prediction is a risky enterprise for anyone,"[172] let alone appointed judges, and any decision based on a "prediction" of a future consensus will inevitably influence the reaching of that consensus.[173] As for finding constitutional values in works of philosophy, philosophers do not all agree,[174] and the Constitution gives little warrant for choosing one school of philosophy over another.

If the Supreme Court had no better warrant for recognizing a constitutional right to privacy in *Roe v. Wade* than that it had done so before, perhaps that can suffice.[175] Previous judicial decisions have long served as an appropriate source for values in areas other than constitutional law.[176]

But, as the Supreme Court itself has repeatedly pointed out, precedent has much less weight in constitutional law than in other areas of law.[177] In other areas, erroneous judicial decisions can be overruled by the legislature[178]; but erroneous decisions of constitutional dimensions—unless overruled by the Court itself—remain law until altered by constitutional amendment, a long and arduous process.[179] Thus, as Justice Felix Frankfurter pointed out, "[T]he ultimate touchstone of constitutionality is the Constitution itself and not what we have said about it."[180]

As a result, one may analyze the Supreme Court's decisions in the abortion-funding cases as proceeding from a profound discomfort with constitutional rights based primarily on precedent. This discomfort has led the Court to provide only limited constitutional protection for such rights—protection only against the most coercive type of state interference, such as criminal sanction, but not against interference through other forms of government action, such as limitations in government spending programs. As the Court itself has noted, "The Court is most vulnerable and comes nearest to illegitimacy when it deals with judge-made constitutional law having little or no cognizable roots in the language or design of the Constitution."[181] In the abortion-funding area, the U.S. Supreme Court has taken this admonition to heart.

State

In our system of government, states may, under their own constitutions, provide their citizens with rights not found in the Federal Constitution.[182] This appears most obviously when the state constitution expressly protects rights recognized neither in the federal text nor anywhere in federal constitutional doctrine.[183] But even when the constitutions have similar provisions, and the U.S. Supreme Court has interpreted a provision in the Federal Constitution not to provide certain protection, the state supreme court may interpret the parallel provision in the state's own constitution to provide that protection.[184]

Many sound reasons support this approach. First, the state constitutional provision may have broader language than the parallel federal provision. For example, the U.S. Constitution protects the right not "to be a witness" against oneself.[185] By contrast, some state constitutions protect the right not "to give evidence" against oneself.[186] Consequently, some state supreme courts have protected a witness's refusal to yield written evidence in that witness's possession; such a refusal is unprotected under the Federal Constitution.[187] Similarly, an examination of the records of the state constitutional convention may reveal a specific—and possibly broader—intent different from that underlying a parallel federal constitutional guarantee.[188]

Structural concerns on the state constitutional level may differ from those on the federal level. For example, the U.S. Supreme Court may limit the scope of a federal guarantee in part out of concern for values of federalism—the importance of leaving certain decisions in the hands of state authorities.[189] A state supreme court, as one of those state authorities, would have no such concern.[190] On the other hand, the specific mention, in many state constitutions, of particular governmental agencies and offices poses structural problems wholly absent under the Federal Constitution.[191]

Finally, although doubt may exist as to the relevance and importance to constitutional interpretation of such sources as tradition, precedent, and public attitudes, each of those sources may well provide different guidance on the state level as compared with the federal. A state may, for instance, have its own peculiar traditions, distinct from whatever traditions exist in the nation as a whole.[192] In short, most of the various sources of constitutional meaning may yield a different answer when the subject of the inquiry is a different constitution.[193]

Other basic differences between state and federal constitutional law relate to the nature of service on the state and federal bench. While federal judges are appointed for life,[194] and thus have limited political accountability, state judges typically are elected for a term of years, and thus are subject to the demands of a democratic electoral process.[195] Moreover, although amendment of the Federal Constitution is difficult, state constitutions are amended relatively easily and frequently.[196] Finally, unlike federal judges, state judges are typically invested with broad policymaking powers, covering both state common law and the operation of the state judicial system.[197] Thus, state judges may have more expertise and are subject to more popular control in their constitutional decisionmaking. As a result, there may be far more room, on the state as opposed to the federal level, for judicial protection of rights not explicitly derived from the constitutional text or structure.

So it has been with the issue of government funding of abortions. The courts of five states—California, Connecticut, Massachusetts, New Jersey, and Oregon—have used their own constitutions to invalidate state laws eliminating Medicaid abortion funding.[198] Only one state supreme court has ruled to the contrary.[199]

For example, the Massachusetts Supreme Judicial Court found its state constitutional right to privacy in provisions of the state constitution paralleling the federal "due process" clause.[200] The statute before the court mirrored that upheld, as against a federal constitutional attack, by the U.S. Supreme Court in *Harris v. McRae*[201]—it provided funding for childbirth but limited abortion funding to abortions "necessary to prevent the death of the mother."[202]

But the Massachusetts court found that its state constitution "affords a greater degree of protection" for abortion rights than the Federal Constitution.[203] In particular, the court ruled that the state constitution, in the context of family privacy, imposed a requirement of state neutrality: "the State . . . may not use criteria which discriminatorily burden the exercise of a fundamental right."[204] Because the state's purpose was to discourage abortion, the state had violated its obligation to act with "genuine indifference" towards constitutional choices.[205] The state's interest in protecting fetal life could not justify this discrimination; the court therefore invalidated the limitation.[206] The court did, however, accept a lower-court distinction between "nontherapeutic" and "medically necessary" abortions, reasoning that the Medicaid statute established a single standard of "medical necessity," and provided no funds generally for services—whether or not related to pregnancy—failing to meet that standard.[207]

The New Jersey statute resembled that of Massachusetts in funding all costs of childbirth but only those abortions "necessary to preserve the woman's life."[208] New Jersey's constitution protects "certain natural and inalienable rights," including "those of enjoying and defending life and liberty" and of "pursuing and obtaining safety and happiness."[209] This language, the court declared, includes the right of privacy.[210] The court also discussed state precedent, some of it antedating *Roe v. Wade*, protecting rights of family privacy.[211] From these cases, the court derived the same principle cited by the Massachusetts court: "[o]nce [the state] undertakes to fund medically necessary care attendant upon pregnancy, . . . [it] must proceed in a neutral manner." Because it was "not neutral" to fund childbirth but not abortion, the state's refusal to fund "medically necessary" abortions was unconstitutional.[212] Like the Massachusetts court, however, the New Jersey court distinguished between "medically necessary" and "nontherapeutic" abortions, upholding the state's refusal to fund the latter on the ground that "the essential purpose of Medicaid" is "to provide necessary medical care for the indigent," and nontherapeutic abortions by definition are "unnecessary."[213]

The distinction between "therapeutic" and "elective" abortions, drawn by the New Jersey and Massachusetts courts, is somewhat elusive. Pregnancy is a physical condition requiring medical supervision and treatment. That treatment can take the form of assistance with childbirth or termination of the pregnancy by abortion.[214] Childbirth always carries a risk to a pregnant woman's health—indeed, recent research indicates that abortion through the 16th week of gestation may pose less risk to the patient than even "normal" childbirth.[215] As a result, many authorities have doubted the validity of a separate category of "therapeutic" abortions.[216] After all, an abortion is never "elective" in the same sense as cosmetic surgery. Moreover, both the New Jersey and Massachusetts courts adopted a constitutional principle of "neutrality." Under such a principle, it should have sufficed simply to rule that the state had to make abortions available on the same basis as other medical procedures. Yet both courts went further, expressly distinguishing "elective" from "therapeutic" abortions.[217]

Faced with a different statute and a different constitutional provision, the California Supreme Court took a different approach.[218] While providing comprehensive funding for medical expenses related to childbirth, California's Medicaid statute also funded many "therapeutic" abortions.[219] In addition, by contrast with the Federal Constitution and those of Massachusetts and New Jersey, the California Constitution provides explicit protection for a right of privacy.[220]

In issuing its decision, the California Supreme Court noted that, previously, it had found the state right broader than the parallel right of family privacy under the Federal Constitution, and thus had refused to follow federal precedent in interpreting the state right.[221] The court also found that its previous decisions diverged from the federal doctrine in the context of government benefits.[222] Thus, the absence of any additional "governmental obstacle in the path" of a woman's right to choose, which the U.S. Supreme Court had found determinative in upholding an abortion-funding cut-off,[223] the California court deemed irrelevant.[224] Considering the "practical importance of many government benefits" and the risk "that a discriminatory benefit program will effectively nullify important constitutional rights,"[225] the court compelled the state to justify its discriminatory funding of childbirth over abortion. But discriminatory funding did not conserve the state's fiscal resources,[226] and the interest in "protecting the potential life of the fetus" could not prevail when weighed against a pregnant woman's right of procreative choice.[227] Thus, the court invalidated the limitation, as applied either to "medically necessary" or to "elective" abortions.

Perhaps one can trace the California court's more expansive ruling to the presence in the California Constitution of an express right of privacy.[228] Even state supreme courts may feel a need to pay attention to the constitutional text.[229] The remaining two cases in which state courts overturned restrictive abortion-funding limitations[230] both resemble the Massachusetts and New Jersey examples. Neither Connecticut's nor Oregon's state constitution has express protection for a right of privacy. Both state Medicaid schemes denied funding for at least some "therapeutic" abortions,[231] and each court limited its ruling to those abortions deemed "medically necessary."[232] Both courts followed the state courts of Massachusetts, New Jersey, and California in proclaiming the right to interpret the state constitution to provide broader protection for constitutional rights than does federal constitutional doctrine.[233] Both courts ultimately adopted some version of a state constitutional requirement of "neutrality."[234]

There is no requirement that a state supreme court interpret its own constitution's provisions differently from parallel provisions of the U.S. Constitution. Some state courts have taken the position that, while U.S. Supreme Court decisions do not control on the meaning of state constitutional provisions, state supreme courts "should be guided by the same principles" in interpreting state constitutions.[235] Thus, the only state supreme court following the federal lead on the issue of abortion funding, the Supreme Court of Pennsylvania—whose constitution contains no explicit right of privacy—also followed the federal doctrines in reaching its conclusion. There was no constitutional obstacle, said the court, to the state's subsidy of "alternative constitutional rights"; in the context of abortion funding, preserving fetal life was a sufficiently "important" governmental interest to warrant state refusal to fund abortions.[236]

CONCLUSION

The recognition of a woman's federal constitutional right to terminate her pregnancy has provoked much controversy and raised many troubling legal issues. One of the most troubling issues has arisen from the refusal of the federal government and many state governments to provide poor women who choose abortion with the same access to medical care those women receive when they choose to bring their pregnancies to term. The U.S. Supreme Court, in a series of cases, has upheld such disparate governmental funding, even though motivated by a deliberate hostility to exercise of the constitutional right to abortion. A plausible explanation for these rulings is that, in contrast with such constitutional rights as free speech, the Federal Constitution nowhere explicitly protects either the right to abortion or the right to family privacy from which it derives. For institutional reasons, the U.S. Supreme Court may be moving toward limiting the scope of constitutional rights derived neither from the Constitution's text nor its general framework.

State courts, interpreting state constitutions, operate under a different set of constraints. As a result, state courts feel free to recognize rights under their own state constitutions despite the U.S. Supreme Court's refusal to recognize such rights under the Federal Constitution. Most of the state courts dealing with the issue of government funding of abortions have rejected the federal approach and required government neutrality in the area of family planning.

Such diversity is one of the benefits of our federal system. As Justice Brandeis noted years ago, "It is one of the happy incidents of the federal system that a single courageous State may, if its citizens choose, serve as a laboratory; and try novel social and economic experiments without risk to the rest of the country."[237] If the U.S. Supreme Court's abortion-funding decisions eventually are to be overruled, it will be the state supreme courts that will have shown the way.

NOTES AND REFERENCES

1. Edelstein L: The Hippocratic Oath 3 (1943) ("I will not give to a woman an abortive remedy"); see also Castiglioni A: A History of Medicine 154 (2d ed, 1947): cf refs. 13, 37, 46, 51, 53 (translating oath as "I will not give to a woman a pessary to produce abortion")
2. Edelstein L: supra n.1, at 12, 15–18; accord Lader L: Abortion 75–77 (1966); Mohr J: Abortion in America: The Origins and Evolution of National Policy, 1800–1900, at 35 (1978)
3. Roe v Wade, 410 U.S. 113, 133 n.22 (1973)
4. Callahan D: Abortion: Law, Choice, and Morality 409–447 (1970)
5. Id. cf refs. 13, 15, 64, 72, 73, 82, 83, 92, 108, 126, 131–33 & 139 et al. at 133
6. Stedman's Illustrated Medical Dictionary 1183 (24th ed, 1982)
7. Lader L: supra n.1, at 78; Mohr J: Abortion in America: The Origins and Evolution of National Policy, 1800–1900, at 3. (1978). Quickening generally occurs during the fourth or fifth month of gestation. Id.
8. Blackstone W: Commentaries on the Law of England *129–130, Vol 1; Coke E: Institutes III *50; Mohr J: Abortion in America: The Origins and Evolution of National Policy, 1800–1900, at 4. (1978). Historians disagree about the existence and severity of common-law sanctions for abortion after quickening. See Lader L: supra n.1, at 78–79. See generally Roe v. Wade, 410 U.S. 113, 134–136 (1973)
9. N.Y. Rev. Stat., pt. 4, c. 1, tit. 2, art. 1, § 9, p. 661 and tit. 6, § 21, p. 694 (1829). On the origins of this law, see Mohr J: Abortion in America: The Origins and Evolution of National Policy, 1800–1900, at 26–32, 38, (1978)
10. Quay E: Justifiable Abortion—Medical and Legal Foundations (pt. 2), 49 Geo. L. J. 395, 435–438 (1961)
11. Roe v. Wade, 410 U.S. 113, 135–136 (1973)
12. 12 Trans. of the AMA 73–78 (1859)
13. See id. at 76. A later report by the Committee described those opposing criminalization as having "perverted views of morality." See 22 Trans. of the AMA 39 (1871). Neither report emphasized the health risks to women of having abortions. See generally Mohr J: Abortion in America: The Origins and Evolution of National Policy, 1800–1900, at 18–19 (1978); Tribe L: American Constitutional Law § 15–10, at 1356 (2d ed, 1988)
14. 12 Trans of the AMA 75–76 (1859)
15. Id. at 28, 78. For extensive discussion of the "physicians' crusade against abortion" from 1857–1880, see Mohr J: Abortion in America: The Origins and Evolution of National Policy, 1800–1900, at 147–170 (1978)
16. See, e.g., Conn. Pub. Acts, c. 71, § 1 (1860)
17. See statutes cited in Roe v. Wade, 410 U.S. 113, 175 n.1 (1973) (Rehnquist J, dissenting). See generally Mohr J: Abortion in America: The Origins and Evolution of National Policy, 1800–1900, at 200–225 (1978)
18. See Mohr J: Abortion in America: The Origins and Evolution of National Policy, 1800–1900, at 254–255 (1978); Luker K: Abortion and the Politics of Motherhood 48–54 (1984). Estimates of illegal abortions range from 48,000 to 1.2 million annually. Compare Louisell D, Noonan J: Constitutional Balance, in Noonan J (ed): The Morality of Abortion 220, 241–243 (1970) with Lucas R: Federal Constitutional Limitations on the Enforcement and Administration of State Abortion Statutes, 46 N.C. L. Rev. 730 (1968). See also Tietze C: The Effect of Legalization of Abortion on Population Growth and Public Health, in Alan Guttmacher Institute, Planned Parenthood Fed'n of America: Abortion 1974–1975: Need & Services in the United States, Each State & Metropolitan Area, at 110 (1976)
19. See Quay E: supra n.10, at 447–520; Note, Abortion: The Five-Year Revolution and Its Impact, 3 Ecology L.Q. 311, 313 (1973). For an effort to explain the lack of legal change on the issue of abortion for nearly a century in the United States, see Luker K: Abortion and the Politics of Motherhood, 40–65 (1984)
20. This trend has led to substantial modifications of abortion law in most Western countries since the 1960s. See Glendon M: Abortion and Divorce in Western Law 11 (1987).

21. See American Law Institute, Model Penal Code § 230.3 (Proposed Official Draft 1962)
22. See Roe v. Wade, 410 U.S. 113, 140 n.37 (1973)
23. American Law Institute, Model Penal Code § 230.3(2) (Proposed Official Draft 1962)
24. See N.Y. Penal Code § 125.05, subd. 3 (Supp. 1972–1973)
25. See Uniform Abortion Act § 1 (b)(2), reprinted in 58 A.B.A. J. 380 (1972)
26. United States v. Vuitch, 402 U.S. 62 (1971)
27. See generally Note, The Void-for-Vagueness Doctrine in the Supreme Court, 109 U. Pa. L. Rev. 67 (1960)
28. United States v. Vuitch, 402 U.S. at 72
29. 410 U.S. 113 (1973)
30. Meyer v. Nebraska, 262 U.S. 390 (1923)
31. Pierce v. Society of Sisters, 268 U.S. 510 (1925)
32. Skinner v. Oklahoma *ex rel.* Williamson, 316 U.S. 535 (1942)
33. Griswold v. Connecticut, 381 U.S. 479 (1965)
34. Roe v. Wade, 410 U.S. at 152–153
35. *Id.* at 153 cf refs. 13, 15, 64, 72 & 73, 82 & 83, 92, 108, 126, 131–33, 139, et al
36. See *Id.* at 155
37. See generally Nowak J, Rotunda R, Young J: Constitutional Law §§ 11.4, at 351, & 14.3, at 530–531 (3d ed, 1986); Note, Of Interests, Fundamental and Compelling: The Emerging Constitutional Balance, 57 B.U. L. Rev. 462 (1977)
38. 410 U.S. at 148–151
39. See, *e.g.*, Lamm R, Davison S: Abortion Reform, Yale Rev. L. & Soc. Action, Spring 1971, at 55, 56; Tietze C: United States: Therapeutic Abortions, 1963–1968, 59 Studies in Family Planning 5, 7 (1970), cited in Roe v. Wade, 410 U.S. at 149 n.44
40. Roe v. Wade, 410 U.S. at 149
41. *Id.* at 164–165; see Connecticut v. Menillo, 423 U.S. 9 (1975) (upholding criminal-abortion law as applied to nonphysician); Tribe L: The Supreme Court, 1972 Term—Foreword: Toward a Model of Roles in the Due Process of Life and Law, 87 Harv. L. Rev. 1, 4 n.20 (1973)
42. Roe v. Wade, 410 U.S. at 163, 164. The Supreme Court later interpreted this standard to require it to decide, on an ad hoc basis, the medical efficacy of various state abortion regulations. See, *e.g.*, Akron v. Akron Center for Reproductive Health, 462 U.S. 416 (1983) (invalidating second-trimester hospitalization requirement); Planned Parenthood of Missouri, Inc. v. Danforth, 428 U.S. 52 (1976) (invalidating ban on saline amniocentesis); Doe v. Bolton, 410 U.S. 179 (1973) (invalidating requirement that two additional physicians certify need for abortion)
43. 410 U.S. at 156–157; see Note, Of Interests, Fundamental and Compelling: The Emerging Constitutional Balance, 57, B.U. L. Rev. 462, 485 (1977). But see Regan D, Rewriting *Roe v. Wade*, 77 Mich. L. Rev. 1569, 1641 (1979) (decision in Roe supportable even if fetus a "person")
44. See U.S. Const. amend. V ("No person shall be . . . deprived of life, liberty, or property, without due process of law"); *id.* amend. XIV, § 1 ("nor shall any State deprive any person of life, liberty, or property, without due process of law")
45. 410 U.S. at 162; see *id.* at 158. But see Epstein R, Substantive Due Process by Any Other Name: The Abortion Cases, 1973 Sup. Ct. Rev. 159, 183 (claiming that, "in other legal contexts," fetuses "are regarded as persons")
46. See Stedman's Illustrated Medical Dictionary 1556 (24th ed, 1982). See also Planned Parenthood of Missouri, Inc. v. Danforth, 428 U.S. 52, 63–65, 83 (1976) (upholding identical statutory definition of "viability")
47. See Perry M: Abortion, the Public Morals, and the Police Power: The Ethical Function of Substantive Due Process, 23 U.C.L.A. L. Rev. 689, 735 (1976); Tribe L: The Supreme Court, 1972 Term—Foreward: Toward a Model of Roles in the Due Process of Life and Law, 87 Harv. L. Rev. 1, 18–19, 28–29 & n.132 (1973)
48. *Cf.* Planned Parenthood Ass'n of Kansas City v. Ashcroft, 462 U.S. 476 (1983) (upholding requirement of second physician to care for fetus at post-viability abortions). But see Colautti v. Franklin, 439 U.S. 379 (1979) (invalidating, as overly vague, law requiring particular standard of care for abortions performed when doctor has "sufficient reason to believe that the fetus may be viable"). See generally Macklin R: Personhood and the Abortion Debate, *in* Garfield J, Hennessey P (eds): Abortion: Moral and Legal Perspectives 80 (1984)
49. 410 U.S. at 163–164
50. See, *e.g.*, Cox A: The Role of the Supreme Court in American Government 113–114 (1976); Lusky L: By What Right? 16–17, 20 (1975); Ely J: The Wages of Crying Wolf: A Comment on *Roe v. Wade*, 82 Yale L. J. 920 (1973); Epstein: Substantive Due Process by Any Other Name: The Abortion Cases, 1973 Sup. Ct. Rev. 159. See generally Rubin E: Abortion, Politics, and the Courts: *Roe v. Wade* and Its Aftermath 89–95, 117–183 (1987)
51. See [1974] Rep. on Human Reproduction and

the Law (Legal-Medical Studies) at I-A-3; see also Gunther G: Constitutional Law 532–533 & n.17 (11th ed, 1985). At least 19 states have called for a constitutional amendment to overturn the case. See Comment, The Establishment Clause and Religious Influences on Legislation, 75 Nw. U.L. Rev. 944, 944 n.5 (1980)

52. See S. 158 & H.R. 900, 97th Cong., 1st Sess. On the constitutionality of such a law, compare Galebach S: A Human Life Statute, Human Life Rev., Winter 1981, at 5, reprinted in Garfield J, Hennessey P (eds): Abortion: Moral and Legal Perspectives 123 (1984) with Estreicher S: Congressional Power and Constitutional Rights: Reflections on Proposed "Human Life" Legislation, 68 Va. L. Rev. 333 (1982) and Emerson T: The Power of Congress to Change Constitutional Decisions of the Supreme Court: The Human Life Bill, 77 Nw. U.L. Rev. 129 (1982). For an argument that the Court's ruling on the "personhood" of the fetus made an extreme political reaction inevitable, see Calabresi G: Ideals, Beliefs, Attitudes, and the Law 95–97 (1985)
53. See Akron v. Akron Center for Reproductive Health, 462 U.S. 416 (1983). The doctrine of "stare decisis" requires courts "[t]o abide by, or adhere to, decided cases." Black's Law Dictionary 1261 (rev. 5th ed, 1979)
54. Medicaid in 1976 financed nearly one third of all legal abortions. See 35 Cong. Q. Wkly. Rep. 1199, 1200 (1977). For a discussion of the background of early attempts to limit federal funding of abortions, see Rubin E: Abortion, Politics, and the Courts: Roe v. Wade and Its Aftermath 163–165 (1987)
55. See generally Note, Abortion, Medicaid, and the Constitution, 54 N.Y.U. L. Rev. 120, 135 (1979); 3 Fam. Plan. Pop. Rep. 113 (1974) (charting early restrictions)
56. See, *e.g.*, Conn. Welf. Dep't Pub. Assis. Prog. Man., vol. 3, ch. III, § 275 (1975); 3 Pa. Bull. 2207, 2209 (1973). A "therapeutic" abortion has been defined as one "necessary to ameliorate a condition that is deleterious to a woman's physical and/or psychological health." See Doe v. Maher, 515 A.2d 134, 135 n.4 (Conn. Super. 1986). See also Planned Parenthood Ass'n, Inc. v. Department of Human Resources, 63 Or. App. 41, 663 P.2d 1247, 1252 (1983) (defining "medically necessary" abortion as any abortion required because "specified medical problems may be caused or aggravated by the pregnancy"), affirmed on other grounds, 297 Ore. 562, 687 P.2d 785 (1984)
57. See, *e.g.*, Act of Oct. 18, 1978, Pub. L. No. 95–480, § 210, 92 Stat. 1567 (federal "Hyde Amendment")
58. See, *e.g.*, statutes quoted in Committee to Defend Reproductive Rights v. Myers, 29 Cal. 3d 252, 625 P.2d 779, 782 n.1, 172 Cal. Rptr. 866, 869 n.1 (1981)
59. See, *e.g.*, Pub. L. No. 94–439, § 209, 90 Stat. 1434 (1976) (another version of federal "Hyde Amendment"); Ill. Ann. Stat. ch. 38, § 81–21 (Smith-Hurd Supp. 1980)
60. See, *e.g.*, Right to Choose v. Byrne, 91 N.J. 287, 450 A.2d 925, 927 (1982); Fischer v. Department of Public Welfare, 509 Pa. 2d 293, 502 A.2d 114, 116 (1985); Doe v. Maher, 40 Conn. Super. 394, 515 A.2d 134, 152 (1986). See generally Johnson C, Bond J: Coercive and Noncoercive Abortion Deterrence Policies, 2 Law & Pol. Q. 106, 115–116 (1980)
61. See, *e.g.*, Wulff v. Singleton, 508 F.2d 1211, 1215 (8th Cir. 1974), rev'd on other grounds, 428 U.S. 106 (1976); Doe v. Rose, 499 F.2d 1112, 1116–1117 (10th Cir. 1974). See also Tribe L: The Supreme Court, 1972 Term—Forward: Toward a Model of Roles in the Due Process of Life and Law, 87 Harv. L. Rev. 1, 42 (1973); Comment, Abortion on Demand in a Post-*Wade* Context: Must the State Pay the Bills?, 41 Fordham L. Rev. 921, 928–931 (1973)
62. See Doe v. Bolton, 410 U.S. 179 (1973)
63. In particular, state law required advance approval of all abortions by an "abortion committee" of at least three members of the hospital staff. See *id.* at 184
64. *Id.* at 197–198
65. See, *e.g.*, Shapiro v. Thompson, 394 U.S. 618 (1969); Elfbrandt v. Russell, 384 U.S. 11 (1966); Sherbert v. Verner, 374 U.S. 398 (1963); Speiser v. Randall, 357 U.S. 513 (1958). See generally O'Neil R: Unconstitutional Conditions: Welfare Benefits with Strings Attached, 54 Calif. L. Rev. 443 (1966); Van Alstyne W: The Demise of the Right-Privilege Distinction in Constitutional Law, 81 Harv. L. Rev. 1439 (1968); Note, Unconstitutional Conditions, 73 Harv. L. Rev. 1595 (1960)
66. See Committee to Defend Reproductive Rights v. Myers, 29 Cal. 3d 252, 625 P.2d 779, 172 Cal. Rptr. 866 (1981), discussed in Note, *Committee to Defend Reproductive Rights v. Myers*: Abortion Funding Restrictions as an Unconstitutional Condition, 70 Calif. L. Rev. 978 (1982). See also Brudno B: Wealth Discrimination in the Supreme Court: Equal Protection for the Poor from *Griffin* to *Maher*, in Collins R (ed): Constitutional Government in

America 229, 237 (1980) (calling scheme a "classic case of an 'unconstitutional condition' "); The Supreme Court, 1976 Term, 91 Harv. L. Rev. 70, 143–145 (1977)
67. 432 U.S. 464 (1977); cf. Poelker v. Doe, 432 U.S. 519 (1977) (upholding municipal hospital system's refusal to provide most abortion services)
68. Conn. Welf. Dep't Pub. Assis. Prog. Man., vol. 3, ch. III, § 275 (1975). When Connecticut later eliminated all state abortion funding except of abortions "necessary because the life of the mother would [otherwise] be endangered," the restriction was invalidated under the state constitution. See Doe v. Maher, 40 Conn. Super. 394, 515 A.2d 134 (1986)
69. See Roe v. Norton, 408 F. Supp. 660, 663–664 & n.3 (1975) (three-judge court)
70. Maher v. Roe, 432 U.S. 464 (1977). In a companion case, the Court decided that nothing in the Federal Social Security Act, establishing the Medicaid program, required states participating in the program to fund nontherapeutic abortions. Beal v. Doe, 432 U.S. 438 (1977)
71. 432 U.S. at 469–470
72. Id. at 475
73. Id. at 474
74. Harris v. McRae, 448 U.S. 297 (1980); Williams v. Zbaraz, 448 U.S. 358 (1980)
75. Pub. L. No. 94-439, § 209, 90 Stat. 1434 (1976). For a discussion of the various versions of the Hyde Amendment, see Rubin E: Abortion, Politics, and the Courts: Roe v. Wade and Its Aftermath 169–171 (1987)
76. Ill. Ann. Stat. ch. 38, § 81–121 (Smith-Hurd Supp. 1980)
77. See McRae v. Califano, 491 F. Supp. 630 (S.D.N.Y. 1980); Zbaraz v. Quern, 596 F.2d 196 (7th Cir. 1979) (statutory grounds)
78. 432 U.S. 464 (1977), discussed supra
79. See McRae v. Califano, 491 F. Supp. at 737; Zbaraz v. Quern, 596 F.2d at 198–199 (statutory grounds); see also Harris v. McRae, 448 U.S. 297, 315 (1980) (recognizing distinction)
80. See Harris v. McRae, 448 U.S. 297 (1980); Williams v. Zbaraz, 448 U.S. 358 (1980)
81. 448 U.S. at 315
82. Id. at 316 n.19
83. Id. at 315
84. See Roe v. Wade, 410 U.S. 113, 162 (1973)
85. See 448 U.S. at 324
86. See U.S. Const. art. I, § 2, cl. 1, & id. amend. XVII, cl. 1 (election of members of Congress); id. IV, § 4 (guaranteeing to each state a "Republican form of government"); Reynolds v. Sims, 377 U.S. 533, 554 (1964). But see Minor v. Happersett, 88 U.S. (21 Wall.) 162 (1874) (U.S. Constitution does not guarantee right to vote)
87. Harper v. Virginia State Board of Elections, 383 U.S. 663 (1966)
88. U.S. Const. amend. V; id. amend. XIV, § 1
89. See Gideon v. Wainwright, 372 U.S. 335 (1963)
90. See Loving v. Virginia, 388 U.S. 1, 12 (1967)
91. Boddie v. Connecticut, 401 U.S. 371 (1970)
92. Id. at 376
93. E.g., Michelman F: In Pursuit of Constitutional Welfare Rights: One View of Rawls' Theory of Justice, 121 U. Pa. L. Rev. 962 (1973); Michelman F: Welfare Rights in a Constitutional Democracy, 1979 Wash. U.L.Q. 659
94. E.g., Dandridge v. Williams, 397 U.S. 471, 508 (1970) (Marshall J, dissenting); Right to Choose v. Byrne, 91 N.J. 287, 450 A.2d 925, 944–946 (1982) (Pashman J, concurring in part and dissenting in part)
95. See, e.g., San Antonio Independent School Dist. v. Rodriguez, 411 U.S. 1, 44 (1973); Lindsey v. Normet, 405 U.S. 56 (1972); Dandridge v. Williams, 397 U.S. 471, 508 (1970)
96. See Bork R: The Impossibility of Finding Welfare Rights in the Constitution, 1979 Wash. U.L.Q. 695
97. See, e.g., U.S. Const. art. I, § 8 (prohibiting enactment of a "Bill of Attainder or ex post facto Law"); id. amend. I ("Congress shall [not] abridg[e] the freedom of speech"); id. amend. VIII (prohibiting imposition of "cruel and unusual punishments")
98. See Winter R: Poverty, Economic Equality, and the Equal Protection Clause, 1972 Sup. Ct. Rev. 41, 93–97
99. See generally Tribe L: American Constitutional Law § 16–51, at 1647 (2d ed, 1988)
100. Olmstead v. United States, 277 U.S. 438, 478 (1928) (dissenting opinion)
101. But see Right to Choose v. Byrne, 91 N.J. 287, 450 A.2d 925, 944–946 (1982) (Pashman J, concurring in part and dissenting in part) (making such an argument)
102. Social Security Act Tit. XIX, 42 U.S.C. §§ 1396–1396k
103. Cf. Skinner v. Oklahoma ex rel. Williamson, 316 U.S. 535, 541 (1942) (constitutional right to procreate)
104. See Roe v. Wade, 410 U.S. 113 (1973) (constitutional right to abort)
105. McAuliffe v. Mayor of New Bedford, 155 Mass. 216, 220, 29 N.E. 517, 517 (1892)
106. 155 Mass. at 216, 29 N.E. at 518

107. Adler v. Board of Education, 342 U.S. 485 (1952)
108. *Id.* at 492
109. Barsky v. Board of Regents, 347 U.S. 442, 451 (1954)
110. See Doyle v. Continental Ins. Co., 94 U.S. 535, 542 (1876). See generally Kreimer S: Allocational Sanctions: The Problem of Negative Rights in a Positive State, 132 U. Pa. L. Rev. 1293, 1304–1314 (1984)
111. Kreimer S: Allocational Sanctions: The Problem of Negative Rights in a Positive State, 131 U. Pa. L. Rev. 1293, 1296 (1984) (footnote omitted)
112. See Stanbeck T, Bearse P, Noyelle T, Karasek R: Services: The New Economy 12–13, table 1.2 (1981)
113. See, *e.g.*, 42 U.S.C. §§ 1437–1440 (United States Housing Act of 1937)
114. See, *e.g.*, 7 U.S.C. §§ 2011–2030 (Food Stamp Act)
115. See Brown v. Board of Education, 347 U.S. 483, 493 (1954) (calling the providing of free education "perhaps the most important function of state and local governments")
116. See, *e.g.*, 49 U.S.C. § 1604 (urban mass transit grant program)
117. Frost & Frost Trucking Co. v. Railroad Comm'n, 271 U.S. 583, 593–594 (1926)
118. See Perry M: The Abortion Funding Cases: A Comment on the Supreme Court's Role in American Government, 66 Geo. L.J. 1191 (1978)
119. See Tribe L: The Supreme Court, 1972 Term—Forward: Toward a Model of Roles in the Due Process of Life and Law, 87 Harv. L. Rev. 1 (1973)
120. See Committee to Defend Reproductive Rights v. Myers, 29 Cal. 3d 252, 625 P.2d 779, 794 n.26, 172 Cal. Rptr. 866, 881 n.26 (1981)
121. Shapiro V. Thompson, 394 U.S. 618, 627 n.6 (1969); *accord, e.g.*, Sherbert v. Verner, 374 U.S. 398, 404 (1963) ("too late in the day" to rely on distinction for resolving constitutional questions)
122. Shapiro v. Thompson, 394 U.S. at 627–628
123. Healy v. James, 408 U.S. 169 (1972)
124. City of Akron v. Akron Center for Reproductive Health, Inc., 462 U.S. 416, 444 (1983)
125. See Perry M: The Abortion Funding Cases: A Comment on the Supreme Court's Role in American Government, 66 Geo. L.J. 1191, 1196, 1200 (noting that, under Medicaid, states refusing abortion funding must pay far greater costs of childbirth)
126. *Id.*; see Committee to Defend Reproductive Rights v. Myers, 29 Cal. 3d 252, 625 P.2d 779, 794 n.26, 172 Cal. Rptr. 866, 881 n.26 (1981)
127. Maher v. Roe, 432 U.S. 464, 474 (1977)
128. See, *e.g.*, McDonald v. Board of Election, 394 U.S. 802 (1969); Williamson v. Lee Optical Co., 348 U.S. 483 (1955). See generally Nowak J, Rotunda R, Young J: Constitutional Law §§ 11.4, at 351, & 14.3, at 530 (3d ed, 1986)
129. See generally Gunther: The Supreme Court, 1971 Term—Foreward: In Search of Evolving Doctrine on a Changing Court: A Model for a Never Equal Protection, 86 Harv. L. Rev. 1 (1972)
130. See Roe v. Wade, 410 U.S. 113, 173 (1973) (Rehnquist J, dissenting)
131. See *i.d.* at 156 (majority opinion)
132. *Id.* at 162
133. See *id.* at 148–150
134. See generally Nowak J, Rotunda R, Young J: Constitutional Law §§ 11.4, at 351, & 14.3, at 530–531 (3d ed, 1986); Note, Of Interests, Fundamental and Compelling: The Emerging Constitutional Balance, 57 B.U. L. Rev. 462 (1977)
135. See, *e.g.*, Shapiro v. Thompson, 394 U.S. 618, 630–631 (1969) ("fundamental rights"); Palmore v. Sidoti, 466 U.S. 429 (1984) ("suspect classifications")
136. See, *e.g.*, Shapiro v. Thompson, 394 U.S. 618, 634 (1969)
137. See Shelton v. Tucker, 364 U.S. 479, 488 (1960)
138. Meyer v. Nebraska, 262 U.S. 390 (1923)
139. *Id.* at 400–401
140. Pierce v. Society of Sisters, 268 U.S. 510, 534–535 (1925)
141. Skinner v. Oklahoma *ex rel.* Williamson, 316 U.S. 535, 541 (1942)
142. Griswold v. Connecticut, 381 U.S. 479, 486 (1965)
143. See Roe v. Wade, 410 U.S. 113, 152–153 (1973) (citing Meyer, Pierce, Skinner, Griswold, and decisions ranging from Union Pacific R. Co. v. Botsford, 141 U.S. 250 (1891) to Eisenstadt v. Baird, 405 U.S. 438 (1972)). See generally Heymann P, Barzelay D: The Forest and the Trees: Roe v. Wade and its Critics, 53 B.U. L. Rev. 765, 772–776 (1973) (finding Roe to fit well within prior cases)
144. 410 U.S. at 152
145. *Id.* at 153
146. U.S. Const. amend. XIV, § 1
147. See Roe v. Wade, 410 U.S. 113, 173 (1973) (Rehnquist J, dissenting); *cf.* Ely J: Democracy and Distrust 18 (1980) ("there is simply no

avoiding the fact that the word that follows 'due' is 'process' "). But see Tribe L: Constitutional Choices 10–11 (1985) (stressing phrase "of law")
148. See Bickel A: The Least Dangerous Branch 4 (1962); Tribe L: American Constitutional Law § 3-2, at 25 (2d ed, 1988)
149. See Cappelletti M: Fundamental Guarantees of the Parties in Civil Litigation: Comparative Constitutional, International, and Social Trends, 25 Stan. L. Rev. 651, 654–659 (1973)
150. See Marbury v. Madison, 5 U.S. (1 Cranch) 137 (1803)
151. See generally Black C: Structure and Relationship in Constitutional Law (1969)
152. See U.S. Const. amend. X
153. See U.S. Const. art. I, § 8
154. See Zobel v. Williams, 457 U.S. 55, 61 (1982) (Brennan J, concurring)
155. See, *e.g.*, Shapiro v. Thompson, 394 U.S. 618 (1969)
156. See, *e.g.*, Southern Pacific Co. v. Arizona, 325 U.S. 761 (1945)
157. See DeSylva v. Ballentine, 351 U.S. 570, 580–581 (1956); *In re* Burris, 136 U.S. 586, 593–594 (1890). See generally Areen J: Family Law (2d ed, 1985)
158. See Sandalow T: Federalism and Social Change, 43 Law & Contemp. Prob. 35, 38 (1980) (Roe decision illustrates development of unitary system of government in United States)
159. See generally Ely J: The Supreme Court, 1977 Term—Foreword: On Discovering Fundamental Values, 92 Harv. L. Rev. 5 (1978)
160. See, *e.g.*, Moore v. City of East Cleveland, 431 U.S. 494, 503 (1977) (plurality opinion); Developments in the Law—Family Law, 93 Harv. L. Rev. 1156 (1980)
161. See generally Ely J: Democracy and Distrust 60–63 (1980)
162. See, *e.g.*, People v. Woody, 61 Cal. 2d 716, 40 Cal. Rptr. 69, 394 P.2d 813 (1964) (constitutional protection for use of peyote by American Indians)
163. See, *e.g.*, Ravin v. State, 537 P.2d 494, 504 (1975) (constitutional protection for home use of marijuana by residents of Alaska)
164. Palko v. Connecticut, 302 U.S. 319, 325 (1937) (quoting Snyder v. Massachusetts, 291 U.S. 97 (1934))
165. Griswold v. Connecticut, 381 U.S. 479, 486 (1965)
166. Bowers v. Hardwick, 478 U.S. 186, 199–200 (1986) (Blackmun J, dissenting); see Tribe L: American Constitutional Law § 15–21, at 1428 (2d ed, 1988) (deeming it "crucial," in historical analysis, to "define the liberty at a high enough level of generality")
167. Sandalow T: Judicial Protection of Minorities, 75 Mich. L. Rev. 1162, 1193 (1977); *accord, e.g.*, Deutsch J: Neutrality, Legitimacy, and the Supreme Court: Some Intersections between Law and Political Science, 20 Stan. L. Rev. 169, 196–197 (1968); Perry M: Substantive Due Process Revisited: Reflections On (And Beyond) Recent Cases, 71 Nw. U.L. Rev. 417, 419–421 (1976); Wellington H: Common Law Rules and Constitutional Double Standards: Some Notes on Adjudication, 83 Yale L.J. 221, 284 (1973). See also Lupu I: Untangling the Strands of the Fourteenth Amendment, 77 Mich. L. Rev. 981, 1040–1041 (1979) (reflect contemporary norms in light of American history); Tushnet M: The Newer Property: Suggestions for the Revival of Substantive Due Process, 1975 S. Ct. Rev. 261, 271 (to same effect)
168. See Ely J: Democracy and Distrust 63–64; (1980); Perry M: The Constitution, the Courts, and Human Rights 94 (1982)
169. See Ely J: Democracy and Distrust 67 (1980)
170. Griffith K: Judge Learned Hand and the Role of the Federal Judiciary 90 (1973) (quoting Judge Learned Hand); *accord* Fairman C: Mr. Justice Miller and the Supreme Court 374 (1939)
171. See Chayes A: The Role of the Judge in Public Law Litigation, 89 Harv. L. Rev. 1281, 1316 (1976)
172. Ely J: Democracy and Distrust 70 (1980)
173. See *id.*
174. Compare Rawls J: A Theory of Justice (1971) with Nozick R: Anarchy, State, and Utopia (1974)
175. See Bennett R: Objectivity in Constitutional Law, 132 U. Pa. L. Rev. 445, 486 (1984); Michelman F: Commentary, 56 N.Y.U. L. Rev. 525, 532 (1981); Sedler R: The Legitimacy Debate in Constitutional Perspective, 44 Ohio St. L.J. 110, 119 & n.167 (1983) See generally Monaghan H: Taking Supreme Court Opinions Seriously, 39 Md. L. Rev. 1 (1979)
176. See generally Levi E: An Introduction to Legal Reasoning (1946); Llewellyn K: The Common Law Method (1961); White G: The American Judicial Tradition (1976)
177. See, *e.g.*, Edelman v. Jordan, 415 U.S. 651, 671 n.14 (1974); *accord, e.g.*, Eakin v. Raub, 12 S. & R. 330 (Pa. 1825) (Gibson CJ, dissenting) ("ab-

solutely" no weight); Boys Markets, Inc. v. Retail Clerks Union, 398 U.S. 235, 259–260 (Black J, dissenting); see Lusky L: By What Right? 292 (1975) ("the Court has flatly repudiated the doctrine of *stare decisis* on constitutional issues"); see generally Maltz E: Some Thoughts on the Death of Stare Decisis in Constitutional Law, 1980 Wis. L. Rev. 467
178. See, *e.g.*, Portal-to-Portal Act of 1947, 61 Stat. 84, 29 U.S.C. § 252 (1979) (overruling Anderson v. Mt. Clemens Pottery Co., 328 U.S. 680 (1946))
179. See Kurland P: Politics, the Constitution and the Warren Court 176–177 (1970); Berger R: Congress v. The Supreme Court 207 (1969)
180. Graves v. O'Keefe, 306 U.S. 466, 491–492 (1939) (concurring opinion); *accord, e.g.*, Coleman v. Alabama, 399 U.S. 1, 22–23 (1970) (Burger CJ, dissenting); Douglas W: Stare Decisis, 49 Colum. L. Rev. 735, 736 (1949). See also Tribe L: Constitutional Choices 272 n.2 (1975) (noting that "Those who justify what they do today by calling it a small step beyond what they did yesterday may soon wander far indeed from their original commitments")
181. Bowers v. Hardwick, 478 U.S. 186, 194 (1986)
182. Pruneyard Shopping Center v. Robbins, 447 U.S. 74 (1980)
183. See, *e.g.*, Fla. Const. art. I, § 21 (guaranteeing access to court "for redress of any injury"); compare Duke Power Co. v. Carolina Env. Study Group, 438 U.S. 59 (1978) (upholding, against federal due process challenge, statutory limitation of nuclear power plant liability) with Kluger v. White, 281 So. 2d 1 (Fla. 1973) (invalidating, under state access-to-court provision, statutory limitation of right to sue for automobile property damage)
184. See, *e.g.*, Pruneyard Shopping Center v. Robbins, 447 U.S. 74 (1980). See generally Williams R: In the Supreme Court's Shadow: Legitimacy of State Court Rejection of Supreme Court Reasoning and Result, 35 S.C. L. Rev. 353 (1984)
185. See U.S. Const. amend. V
186. See, *e.g.*, Utah Const. art. I, § 12
187. See Hansen v. Owens, 619 P.2d 315 (Utah 1980)
188. See State v. Miyaski, 62 Hawaii 269, 281–282, 614 P.2d 915, 922–923 (1980) (Hawaii constitution's self-incrimination provision was meant to incorporate then-current interpretation of federal provision, but not subsequent elaborations)
189. See, *e.g.*, San Antonio Independent School Dist. v. Rodriguez, 411 U.S. 1, 44 (1973)
190. See Serrano v. Priest, 18 Cal. 3d 728, 557 P.2d 929, 135 Cal. Rptr. 345 (1976), cert. denied, 432 U.S. 907 (1977) (rejecting San Antonio Ind. School Dist. v. Rodriguez)
191. See, *e.g.*, Florida Department of Natural Resources v. Florida Game & Fresh Water Fish Commission, 342 So. 2d 495 (Fla. 1977) (attempt to strip Commission of power held unconstitutional because inconsistent with Commission's status as agency expressly created by state constitution)
192. See, *e.g.*, Ravin v. State, 537 P.2d 494, 504 (1975) (noting that Alaska "has traditionally been the home of people who prize their individuality," court interprets state constitution to protect the right to ingest marijuana at home). As to precedent, see, *e.g.*, State v. Sheridan, 121 Iowa 164, 96 N.W. 730 (1903) (finding, in state constitution, rule barring introduction of illegally seized evidence; decided 58 years before similar ruling by United States Supreme Court). As to public attitudes, compare District Attorney v. Watson, 411 N.E.2d 1274, 1282 (Mass. 1980) (death penalty violates prevailing standards of decency in Massachusetts) with Gregg v. Georgia, 428 U.S. 153 (1976) (death penalty constitutional under federal standard)
193. See generally State v. Hunt, 450 A.2d 952, 964–967 (N.J. 1983) (Handler J, concurring); Developments in the Law—The Interpretation of State Constitutional Rights, 95 Harv. L. Rev. 1324, 1359–1362 (1982). See also Carson W: Last Things Last, 19 Willamette L. Rev. 641, 653–662 (1983) (listing sources for state constitutional analysis)
194. U.S. Const. art II, § 2; *id.* art. III, § 1
195. See Galie P: State Supreme Courts, Judicial Federalism and the Other Constitutions, Judicature 71:2, at 108 (1987)
196. See Developments in the Law—The Interpretation of State Constitutional Rights, 95 Harv. L. Rev. 1324, 1354 & n.106 (1982)
197. See Baar C: Judicial Activism in State Courts: The Inherent Powers Doctrine, in Porter M, Tarr G: State Supreme Courts: Policymakers in the Federal System 142 (1982)
198. See Committee to Defend Reproductive Rights v. Myers, 29 Cal. 3d 252, 625 P.2d 779, 172 Cal. Rptr. 866 (1981); Doe v. Maher, 40 Conn. Super. 394, 515 A.2d 134 (1986); Moe v. Secretary of Administration & Finance, 382 Mass. 629, 417 N.E.2d 387 (1981); Right to Choose v. Byrne, 91 N.J. 287, 450 A.2d 925 (1982); Planned Parenthood Association v. Department of Human Resources, 63 Ore. App. 41, 663 P.2d 1247 (1983), affirmed on other grounds, 297 Ore. 562, 687 P.2d 785 (1984)

199. See Fischer v. Department of Public Welfare, 509 Pa. 2d 293, 502 A.2d 114 (1985) (upholding funding cut-off)
200. See Superintendent of Belchertown State School v. Saikewicz, 373 Mass. 728, 370 N.E.2d 417 (1977); compare Roe v. Wade, 410 U.S. 113, 153 (1973) (finding federal right of privacy in federal due process clause). See generally Wilkins H: Judicial Treatment of the Massachusetts Declaration of Rights in Relation to Cognate Provisions of the United States Constitution, 14 Suffolk U. L. Rev. 887, 909–910 n.135 (1980)
201. 448 U.S. 297 (1980)
202. Moe v. Secretary of Administration & Finance, 382 Mass. 629, 417 N.E.2d 387, 390 n.3 (1981)
203. Moe v. Secretary of Administration & Finance, 417 N.E.2d at 400
204. Id. at 400, 401
205. Id. at 402
206. Id. at 404
207. Id. at 394 n.12
208. N.J.S.A. 30:4D-6.1 (1981); see Right to Choose v. Byrne, 91 N.J. 287, 450 A.2d 925, 927 (1982)
209. N.J. Const. art. I, par. 1
210. Right to Choose v. Byrne, 450 A.2d at 933
211. Id. at 935
212. Id.
213. Id. at 935 n.6
214. See Butler P: The Right to Medicaid Payment for Abortions, 28 Hastings L.J. 931, 955 (1977) (defining "necessary medical services" as that care "which is responsive to the problem for which it is offered")
215. LeBolt S, Grimes D, Cates W: Mortality from Abortion and Childbirth: Are the Populations Comparable?, JAMA 248–188, 191, 1982
216. See, *e.g.*, Roe v. Norton, 522 F.2d 928, 935 (2d Cir. 1975); Right to Choose v. Byrne, 91 N.J. 287, 450 A.2d 925, 942 (1982) (Pashman J, concurring in part and dissenting in part); cases cited in Note, Abortion, Medicaid, and the Constitution, 54 N.Y.U. L. Rev. 120, 124 n.40 (1979)
217. Moe v. Secretary of Administration & Finance, 382 Mass. 629, 417 N.E.2d 387, 394 n.12 (1981); Right to Choose v. Byrne, 91 N.J. 287, 450 A.2d 925, 935 n.6 (1982)
218. Committee to Defend Reproductive Rights v. Myers, 29 Cal. 3d 252, 625 P.2d 779, 172 Cal. Rptr. 866 (1981). See generally Note, Committee to Defend Reproductive Rights v. Myers: Abortion Funding Restrictions as an Unconstitutional Condition, 70 Calif. L. Rev. 978 (1982)
219. These included abortions when continued pregnancy would cause either death or severe physical health damage, when pregnancy resulted from illegal intercourse, or when pregnancy would result in the birth of a severely defective infant. See Committee to Defend Reproductive Rights v. Myers, 625 P.2d at 782 n.1, 172 Cal. Rptr. at 869 n.1
220. Cal. Const. art. I, § 1
221. City of Santa Barbara v. Adamson, 27 Cal. 3d 123, 130 n.3, 164 Cal. Rptr. 539, 610 P.2d 436 (1980)
222. Committee to Defend Reproductive Rights v. Myers, 625 P.2d at 787, 172 Cal. Rptr. at 874
223. See Harris v. McRae, 448 U.S. 297, 315 (1980)
224. Committee to Defend Reproductive Rights v. Myers, 625 P.2d at 787–788, 172 Cal. Rptr. at 874–875
225. Committee to Defend Reproductive Rights v. Myers, 625 P.2d at 788, 172 Cal. Rptr. at 875
226. Id. at 794, 172 Cal. Rptr. at 881
227. Id. at 796, 172 Cal. Rptr. at 883
228. Cal. Const. art. I, §1
229. See Galie P: State Supreme Courts, Judicial Federalism and the Other Constitutions, Judicature 71:2, at 110 (1987)
230. Doe v. Maher, 40 Conn. Super. 394, 515 A.2d 134 (1986); Planned Parenthood Association v. Department of Human Resources, 63 Ore. App. 41, 663 P.2d 1247 (1983), affirmed on other grounds, 297 Ore. 562, 687 P.2d 785 (1984). The state in Doe v. Maher failed to appeal the adverse decision. See Doe v. Heintz, 204 Conn. 17, 526 A.2d 1318, 1320 (1987)
231. 3 Manual, Conn. Department of Income Maintenance Medical Assistance Program, c. III, policy 275, cited in Doe v. Maher, 515 A.2d at 135; Ore. Admin. Rule 461-14-052, cited in Planned Parenthood Association v. Department of Human Resources, 663 P.2d at 1249
232. Doe v. Maher, 515 A.2d at 135; Planned Parenthood Association v. Department of Human Resources, 663 P.2d at 1252
233. Doe v. Maher, 515 A.2d at 152; Planned Parenthood Association v. Department of Human Resources, 663 P.2d at 1256
234. Doe v. Maher, 515 A.2d at 152; Planned Parenthood Association v. Department of Human Resources, 663 P.2d at 1258
235. *E.g.*, Kroger v. O'Hare Township, 481 Pa. 101, 117, 392 A.2d 266, 274 (1978)
236. See Fischer v. Department of Public Welfare, 509 Pa. 2d 293, 502 A.2d 114, 121–122 (1985)
237. New State Ice Co. v. Liebmann, 285 U.S. 262, 311 (1932) (dissenting opinion)

22
Sociologic Implications

*Dorothy C. Wertz and
James R. Sorenson*

Recent years have seen extraordinary societal value and monetary expenditure placed on a small number of select fetuses. There appear to be few limits to the heroic medical efforts that have been or will be undertaken to ensure that would-be parents with sufficient resources receive not only a healthy child but a "perfect" child. Few realize that these heroic efforts on behalf of prospective parents are the culmination of long-term social trends that have greatly increased the value of a fetus, provided that its parents decide to carry it to term. The current availability of choices regarding parenthood, family structure, and the fate of the fetus has resulted from a combination of recent social trends. In this chapter, we describe long-term and recent social trends affecting the value placed on fetuses. We argue that several trends—especially voluntary or planned parenthood through use of contraception, smaller families, and changes in gender roles—have combined to produce a system in which fetuses are divided into two categories, the "wanted" and "unwanted." Increasingly complicated technological resources are brought to bear on conceiving, saving, and perfecting the wanted fetus; the unwanted fetus may be aborted without regard to its health or genetic characteristics.

LONG-TERM TRENDS

Long-term social trends are those of at least 40 years duration (traceable to the end of World War II), in contrast to more recent trends originating in the 1960s and 1970s. Several long-term trends, such as family limitation and use of contraceptive devices, go back to the nineteenth century, at least among the middle class. Other important trends, such as parents' desire for each child to be perfect—a virtual work of art—and the increased use of medical technology in normal birth in the interest of producing that perfect child, go back to the beginning of this century. Somewhat more recent changes in gender roles associated with women's movement into the work force—a steady though not always acknowledged trend since World War II—have intensified already strong trends toward viewing parenthood as optional, toward smaller families, and toward the demand that children be perfect. We discuss each of these trends as it has affected the value placed on the fetus.

Limitation of Family Size

In the United States, for several generations before reliable contraceptives became available, middle-class families desirous of upward social mobility attempted to limit the size of their families. The results of their efforts became clearly visible in a trend toward smaller families after the Civil War. Historical demographers have discerned the trend even earlier among some groups, notably Philadelphia Quakers,[14] and some historians and economists claim that the trend toward family limitation in the United States can be traced back for 200 years.[8] By the beginning of this century, the principle of having smaller families had become firmly established among the middle class, even though the means of contraception used were not always reliable.[16]

The estimated birthrate for women aged 15 to 44 years decreased from 278 per 1000 in 1800 to 130 per 1000 in 1900, 115 per 1000 in 1920, and 77 per 1000 in 1940. Although there was a reversal of this trend during the twenty years between 1945 and 1965, during which birthrates climbed as high as 123 per 1000, historical demographers have regarded this as a temporary aberration, or a cyclical rebound from the low birthrates during the Great Depression of the 1930s.[5,20]

In the 1970s and 1980s, birthrates per 1000 women aged 15 to 44 continued to decline, to 68.4 per 1000 in 1980, following the historical long-term trend. The larger number of women in this age group (a result of the 1945–1965 baby boom) meant a sizable increase in the *number* of children actually born. The average number of children per married couple, however, declined from 4.9 in 1900 to 1.8 in 1980.

Decline in Infant Mortality

The trend toward smaller families has gone hand in hand with a steady decline in infant mortality. In the past, parents were willing to limit the number of children born only after they could be reasonably certain that all children born would live to adulthood. Between 1870 and 1874, 170 of every 1000 children born in Massachusetts died before the age of 1 year.[20] By 1900–1904, the infant death rate had dropped to 141; by 1920–1924, it had reached 79; and by 1940–1944 (before the application of antibiotics to the civilian population), it was down to 34. U.S. Children's Bureau studies of infant mortality[2,21] have attributed the initial high mortality and its subsequent decline to economic conditions, infant feeding practices, and the presence or absence of government programs for infant care and nutrition, rather than to scientific advances in medical treatment. For many years, family income and race have been the best predictors of infant survival. In 1970, for example, infant mortality was 17.8 per 1000 live births for white infants and 30.9 per 1000 for black infants.[20]

The infant mortality rate affected not only the number of children that families believed they had to conceive in order for at least one child to live to adulthood, but also the value that they placed on the unborn fetus. As long as people perceived that a child was likely to die before reaching maturity, they placed a lower value on the life of a very small child, or a fetus, than on the life of an adult. Until the middle of the nineteenth century, the names of infants who died were routinely given to the nextborn child of the same sex; infants were seen as fragile objects to be replaced, rather than as unique and irreplaceable personalities. In difficult births, full-term fetuses were destroyed to save the lives of mothers who could live to bear other children. For most of human history, there was no question that the life of the mother was of greater value than that of an unborn child who might not survive to adulthood. This belief becomes easier to appreciate in view of the truly appalling infant mortality in Europe. For example, it is estimated that 277 of every 1000 babies born in seventeenth-century London died before the age of 1 year.[18] Destructive operations on the fetus ceased only after the cesarean operation became a viable alternative rather than a death sentence for the mother, sometime early in the twentieth century.[25] Ironically, the papal encyclical forbidding Catholic physicians to destroy the fetus to save the life of the mother (*Casti Connubi,* 1930) appeared only after this dilemma had virtually disappeared from modern obstetrics as a result of the successful use of the cesarean. By then the fetus had acquired higher societal value, as families conceived fewer children, each of whom was likely to survive to maturity.

Desire for the Perfect Child

As families became smaller, they also tended to be planned, in the sense that each child was wanted and its birth was timed to occur at an appropriate time in its parents' lives and at a desired interval after the birth of the previous child. Actual practice frequently fell short of these ideals, as many people failed to use contraceptives efficaciously. Nevertheless, the idea of having few children, all wanted, all perfectly timed, continues to dominate the plans of most families. Not only should children be planned, wanted, and timed, but each of the few born to a family should be perfect. Quality has replaced quantity in family ideals, and each child has become a work of art.

Parents' desire for perfection in their children became evident around the turn of the century. Middle-class families were willing to pay what they considered outrageous fees to obstetrical specialists to avoid possible damage to the baby's brain in birth. Obstetricians drastically altered procedures in routine, "normal" births, adding routine episiotomies and outlet forceps specifically to improve on nature in protecting the baby's brain. In the 1920s, physicians feared that if they left birth to nature, without intervening with instruments, the baby's brain would be damaged in its passage through the birth canal and the infant might be doomed to a life of crime.[4] Then, as now, there was much scientific and popular speculation about biological causes of crime[6] and the heritability of I.Q. and personality traits. Those parents who could afford to sought specialist skills and maximal technological intervention in order to be assured that their children would be as nearly perfect as possible.

A family that planned to have only two or three children was far less ready to accept one with a "defect," however minor, than were larger families in earlier generations. The problems of upwardly mobile families in accepting less-than-perfect children were compounded by society's increasing emphasis on successful performance in school and on academic credentials as requirements for employment. For many families, perfection came to be equated with the straight-A average.

Families who desired perfect children tended to see each child as an object of intense and extensive expenditure, both emotional and financial. They regarded the child as evidence of their own creativity and expected to spend large sums of money and time in enriching its life through cultural programs, sports, and recreation, in addition to providing the best education they could afford. In return for their efforts, it was no longer sufficient for the child to be born and grow up; the child had to reach its full potential and become "successful" in some measurable terms, as evidence of its parents' success as child raisers. Small wonder that parental anxiety about perfection and medical interventions on behalf of perfection were extended into fetal life as soon as technological developments permitted.

The desire for and standard of perfection are likely to increase as long as we live in a technological society that rewards mental activity and as long as families remain small and make great expenditures of effort on each child. The desire for perfection, more than any other long-term social trend, will increase the extraordinary scientific efforts and financial expenditure that are likely to occur in the next century to perfect fetuses that are "wanted" by the parents. The value placed on such fetuses has never been higher. The fate of the "unwanted" fetus, however, is another matter. The existence of choices about parenthood has led to medical extremes in the values placed on fetuses.

Changes in Gender Roles

Certain long-term changes in gender roles have contributed to parental desires for perfect children, largely through the expansion of women's roles and self-identities into the world of work. Married women's work outside the home, considered "deviant" at the turn of the century,[24] is now the accepted pattern. It has become necessary for many families to have two wage earners in order to reach or maintain a middle-class style of life. In 1940, approximately 15% of married women with husbands present were in the labor force. There was a slow but steady increase in the percent employed outside the home, even during the baby-boom years, when many women regarded their employment as a means of helping their families to enjoy a higher standard of living. By 1965, 35% of married women with husbands present were in the labor force; by 1980, over 50 percent were in the labor force.[20] A somewhat more recent trend is the employment of women with children under 6 years of age. Almost unheard of in 1948, when fewer than 3% of married women whose husbands were present and who had preschool children were in the labor force, the employment rate of married women with infants under 1 year is now over 50%. The trend toward women's employment is unlikely to reverse itself. Unless prices of houses, college tuition, and other goods and services undergo radical decline, women's earnings will be necessary to the support of most families. Even in a politically conservative climate, the percent of women employed, including married women with small children, will probably increase.[13,19] Conservative women may justify their employment in terms of providing for their families, and liberal women may justify their employment in terms of self-development or mental health; but women of all political stripes will continue to enter the labor force in greater numbers. Many women now define their identities primarily in terms of their work roles, as men have traditionally identified themselves, rather than in terms of their family roles. At the same time, a few men have begun to identify themselves primarily in terms of their family roles, rather than their work roles, though there is as yet no indication that this will become a major trend.

Increased acceptance of employment outside the home as the normal pattern for married women has meant that many couples, when planning their families, must now include in the potential costs of childbearing not only the mother's lost earnings but her lost opportunities for advancement in the job that she will pursue for most of her adult life. Faced with these costs, more couples have postponed childbearing until their late twenties or early thirties. Still others, using reliable means of contraception, have chosen voluntary childlessness or a one-child family, options that would have been considered "selfish" by the majority of Americans just a generation ago.[22] The expansion of women's roles, however, has meant that fewer women have the energy or time to devote exclusively to family roles.[1] In the absence of a large, readily available, inexpensive class of servants, unemployed grandmothers, or maiden aunts to help care for the children, and without adequate or easily affordable day care centers, couples are choosing to have fewer children or none at all.

The trend toward mothers' employment has further strengthened their desire to have perfect children, partly because the mother may see herself as giving up career advancement in order to have a child. In return for her own sacrifice of opportunities, she expects that the child will, at very least, be normal. The birth of a retarded or neurologically impaired child is a greater social and economic disaster in today's small family with an employed mother than it was in larger families in which the mother was a full-time homemaker. The birth of a defective child frequently means that the mother must leave the workforce, losing not only her economic gain but much of her hard-won identity as a worker. She is forced into the primary role of mother, perhaps for the rest of her life, often with little hope that her efforts will be rewarded by any significant "success" on the child's part. Her problems are compounded by the current beliefs of educators that retarded children are most likely to reach their full potential if kept at home and by the refusal of institutions in many states to accept even severely retarded infants and children until they have first spent some years at home. Large, traditionally oriented families with mothers who see their primary role as motherhood are better able to cope with the birth and rearing of such children than are small families with employed mothers who do not anticipate a lifetime of motherhood.[10] Families that adopt retarded children tend to be of the large, tradition-oriented type. The parents see their duty as providing a family setting for children to grow up in rather than providing expensive educational or personal growth opportunities for individual children. Frequently religion is central to the lives of these families; they accept birth defects as the will of God.

Families of the newer, smaller type, on the other hand, will go to great lengths to try to avoid the births of retarded children, using all possible techniques to be sure that nothing goes wrong. If they are to have only two children, and if they are to expend great emotional and financial resources helping each one to attain its full potential, they want to be sure that each child begins life as nearly perfect as possible.

Increased Medical Intervention in Reproduction

In the interest of producing perfect children, increasingly sophisticated medical technology has become routine in low-risk as well as in high-risk pregnancies and births. Our dependence on physicians and medical interventions in birth has a long history[25] that is peculiarly American in its reverence for science and medicine.[17] To a greater extent than families in England or western Europe, American families in the nineteenth century were willing to turn over control of pregnancy and birth to physicians, with their promise of superior science, and to abandon midwives, who relied on nature. Another way of saying this is that Americans lost touch with "nature" far earlier than citizens of other Western countries. For practical purposes, it is no longer possible for physicians or families to base their arguments on what "nature intended." Medicine has done so much to improve on nature, for so many years, that in most cases we either do not know what nature intended or we are unwilling to permit or accept an outcome in which medicine has not intervened.

A concomitant trend, also with a long history, is the preference of American physicians for sophisticated "high" technologies that help a few patients in unusual situations, as opposed to basic, "low" technologies that benefit many people. An example of this is the development, beginning in the 1920s, of elaborate and expensive methods of saving ever smaller, low birth weight babies, while at the same time failing to provide the maternal nutrition and prenatal care that could have prevented them from being low birth weight. In recent years, there have been cases where the health care system has expended over $150,000 on intensive neonatal care for one low birth weight baby. At the same time, the almost 2:1 ratio of black-to-white infant mortality, a measure of basic care, has remained almost unchanged since 1915. The preference for high technology over basic technology derives from the entrepreneurial roots of American medicine and from American admiration of doctors as heroes in the battle with death.

The two-class system of American medical care (private versus clinic) has helped to exacerbate physicians' preference for sophisticated technologies. Perhaps the most important thing to remember about most of the technologies described in previous chapters is that they will be used for the benefit of very few people. Most of these people will be middle class or above, able to seek out and pay practitioners with the most advanced technologies and able to demand certain types of services, such as in vitro fertilization. Although the desire for perfect children is not limited to the middle class, private patients are most likely to benefit from research on infertility and prenatal diagnosis, while clinic patients serve as research subjects.

The only technique described in previous chapters that is now used on many patients of all social classes is the cesarean section, whose alarmingly increased rates since 1975 have already become a problem for investigation by public health departments. Cesarean rates in the United States, when compared with rates in other countries, reflect a multitude of American cultural ideas about reproduction: desire for the perfect child, distrust of nature, admiration of intervention, particularly surgical intervention, and belief that a surgical delivery is somehow "neater" because time and place are controlled.

The trends described above—small families, desire for the perfect child, and women's employment—are all part of a long-term pattern of increased emphasis on the individual and on one-to-one interpersonal relationships within the nuclear family. For many people, traditional forms of larger community—religious, ethnic, geographical, or political—are no longer binding forces in American life.[23,26] To be sure, many families will continue to adhere to traditional value structures,[10] and some families of the future will resemble families of the past, particularly in regard to gender roles.[3] It is likely, however, that even families with traditional values will be affected by long-term trends that place a premium on having the perfect child.

RECENT TRENDS

Recently, especially within the last ten years, other social trends have gathered momentum: parenthood by choice, growing acceptance of alternatives to the nuclear family, postponement of childbearing, the virtual disappearance of healthy infants available for adoption, the feminist movement, the women's health movement. When combined with increased use of technologies during pregnancy, notably ultrasound, that tend to heighten the mother's awareness of the fetus,[7] most of these newer trends have further heightened the desire for perfection and the value placed on a wanted, potentially normal, fetus. Some of these trends are likely to endure; others may be reversed within a generation. In what follows, we consider the potential effects of each.

Parenthood by Choice

Although limitation of family size has had a long history in the United States, purposeful avoidance of parenthood by a married couple was considered deviant and usually described as "selfish." Few childless couples in the past were willing to admit that their condition might be voluntary; sociological researchers had difficulty locating participants for studies of "voluntary childlessness."[22] Even after the development and widespread acceptance of reliable contraceptive methods, the use of these methods to reject parenthood altogether was socially unacceptable in most circles. Within the last few years, however, nonparenthood has become an acceptable option. Another option that most couples formerly eschewed, the one-child family, is also gaining favor, as psychological research debunks traditional beliefs about the "loneliness" or "selfishness" of only children.

The appearance of the voluntarily childless family or the "one-child-by-choice" family suggests that parenthood itself is now an option, a choice that couples make rather than a general condition of humanity.[23] Those who *choose* to become parents may feel an additional weight of responsibility for the outcome of their choice, in that parenthood is a condition that they could have avoided altogether. In order to justify their choice, they set higher standards of health for their progeny than did couples who considered parenthood a *social* inevitability rather than a choice. If something is wrong with the child, those who regard parenthood as a condition of their own choosing are more likely to feel guilt than those who see parenthood as a universal condition ordained by God or nature. All the more reason for these "voluntary parents" to go to the utmost lengths to ensure that their child is perfect, thus reassuring themselves that they made the right choice.

Alternative Family Forms

Although variants of the traditional nuclear (husband and wife) and extended families have always existed and have affected large numbers of people, until recently most of these variants were considered "deviant" from middle-class norms. Those who became parents outside the bonds of matrimony were pressured to conform by either marrying or releasing the child for adoption by a married couple. Now, however, single parenthood, including *planned* single parenthood, is becoming an acceptable option, to the extent that it can be voluntarily chosen by some middle-class women without automatically incurring the penalties of rejection by family or loss of job. Increasingly, parenthood, both natural and adoptive, is becoming a socially accepted choice for women and men who do not wish to marry. A further development of this theme is lesbian and gay parenthood through artificial insemination. The emergence of single parenthood as a *planned* option among the middle class is indicative of what we might call a growing popular belief that there is a "right" to become a parent and that everybody who chooses to do so should be allowed to exercise this right, with the possible exception of a few severely retarded or institutionalized individuals.

Postponed Childbearing

The median age at marriage has increased to 24 for women and 26 for men, up from 18 and 22 during the baby boom of the 1950s. Later marriage is not new historically; our present averages are about the same as those in 1800. In earlier times, age at marriage fluctuated with economic conditions. It was usually not considered suitable for a couple to marry until the man had established himself financially. With industrialization, the age at marriage decreased, as a wage earner could support a family without waiting to inherit the farm. The recent increase in age at marriage reflects both the new morality made possible by oral contraception and the longer period of schooling necessary to become established in a technological society. Even after they marry, many couples are postponing childbearing until the woman is in her thirties, sometimes her middle or late thirties. Postponed childbearing is a concomitant of women's entry into the work force. For the most part, American business has not been willing to adjust its demands to women's life cycles by providing maternity leaves to fledgling career women; therefore, some women have adjusted their life cycles by postponing childbearing. This postponement sometimes appears necessary on account of the increasing costs of raising a child, now estimated to be close to $200,000, not counting college tuition. Another cause of late childbearing is the remarriage of divorced persons, who may start second families with the new spouse when in their thirties and forties.

One result of postponed childbearing is an increase in perceived infertility. For every year of postponement after a woman's early twenties, there is a slightly increased possibility that she may be unable to conceive. Although there is no firm evidence for a statistical increase in infertility since the 1930s (when almost 20% of couples were childless), earlier statistics cannot separate involuntary from possibly voluntary childlessness. Some previous causes of infertility, such as syphilis, have been largely eliminated by modern treatment. New causes, such as environmental pollution, chlamydia infections, or second marriages of previously sterilized persons, have appeared. It is far from clear whether there has been any actual increase in the rate of infertility. Nevertheless, people's perceptions of infertility have become more acute as parenthood has become a voluntary choice. Frequently those who *choose* to become parents feel that because they have chosen to do so, they therefore have a *right* to become parents. If they are unable to actualize their choice, they demand appropriate medical services to overcome infertility. Their desire for a medical solution is increased by the disappearance of adoption as a viable option for most families.

Unavailability of Healthy Infants for Adoption

One result of the social acceptance of single parenthood is the virtual disappearance of healthy white American infants for adoption. As the result of a revolution in mores about single parenthood in the early 1970s, most unwed teenagers who carry their pregnancies to term now keep their babies. Many of those who would formerly have given the child up for adoption now have legal abortions. Most American children now available for adoption are either physically, intellectually, or emotionally damaged. The time-honored option for infertile couples, adoption of a healthy child, is no longer possible for most, even if they are willing to endure the investigation by bureaucratic agencies and the years of waiting. Infertility treatment, in vitro fertilization, and even surrogate motherhood are frequently the least complicated options available and promise the best results in terms of a healthy child. For some couples, even an artificial placenta would appear as a simpler solution than negotiating the bureaucratic maze of adoption agencies or raising an emotionally damaged child. There are now national organizations of the infertile; these not only provide information and support but lobby that government funding of research on infertility be made a national priority.

The Feminist Movement

Not least among recent trends affecting the fetus is the revived feminist movement. Although feminism itself is a long-term trend in American culture, its strength has tended to wax and wane. The feminist movement so active early in this century, after winning the battle for suffrage, virtually disappeared from the 1930s through the 1950s, only to be reactivated in the 1970s. Its immediate future is uncertain; having achieved some of its goals, it appears once again to be waning. From its beginnings in the nineteenth century, feminism has always supported women's control over their own bodies. In the nineteenth century, feminists supported health education, women's entry into medicine, self-help, efforts at painless childbirth, and, somewhat more tacitly, limitation of family size and contraception.[9,25] In the twentieth century they have openly supported reproductive choice through contraception and, if necessary, abortion.[15] Feminists, though advocating healthy practices during pregnancy, support the woman's right to self-determination as paramount and would oppose any attempt at legal control over her health behavior during pregnancy and birth. Even if the feminist movement loses strength, the long-term trends in reproductive choice and changes in gender roles that it has supported will continue. The belief in women's control over reproductive choices is firmly rooted in a large segment of the population.

Self-Help

Movements for medical self-help in America go back to the early nineteenth century, when legitimate doctors were few and medicine was more likely to harm than help. Self-help advocates have usually appealed to principles of Jacksonian democracy and the rights of the common man (or woman) and have opposed the power of medical professionals.[17] Although there are self-help advocates of every political stripe, most have tended to cluster at the extreme radical or extreme conservative ends of the spectrum. Self-help advocates include feminists and anti-feminists, pro-choicers and pro-life advocates. In recent years, self-help advocates have received much publicity by demanding the right to free choice of medical treatments considered unorthodox by most of the profession, such as use of laetrile. Although such extreme measures are espoused by only a minority of Americans, many more are in agreement with the time-honored concept that patients should have the right to free choice of treatment and the right to reject medical dicta.

In reproductive medicine, self-help is most likely to take the form of a demand for natural childbirth or for home birth. Few home-birthers, however, wish to do away with reproductive technology entirely. Many are quite willing to have infertility treatments, genetic screening, prenatal diagnosis, and ultrasound, for example. For most, the desire for the perfect child outweighs ideas about self-help. They justify home birth on the grounds that it is safer for the baby than hospital birth because anesthesia is not used. Few techniques described in this book are amenable to self-help. Ironically, those that are—artificial insemination by donor (A.I.D.) and surrogate motherhood—are those most fraught with psychological, social, and legal difficulties. Given the current "megatrend" toward self-help,[12] it is likely that in the future some people will arrange A.I.D. and surrogate motherhood on their own, avoiding medical, legal, and bureaucratic control. Already, some women's health groups and other special-interest groups are establishing their own sperm banks. Some couples will find their own surrogates, avoiding screening restrictions and the $15,000 legal and agency fees. For some persons living in nontraditional families, including would-be single parents or gay parents, self-help arrangements may be the only alternatives.

The Anti-Abortion Movement

Although American physicians opposed abortion in the nineteenth century, in part to raise the moral image of their profession, there was no organized, grassroots anti-abortion movement as we know it today.[11] Luker[10] describes the origins of the popular anti-abortion movement as quite recent, dating from the 1973 Supreme Court decision that legalized abortion during the first two trimesters of pregnancy. Those who support this movement describe themselves as "pro-life"; their values about family roles are more traditional than those of pro-choice advocates. Although pro-life women frequently hold jobs, they regard these as secondary to their roles as mothers. Pro-lifers tend to have larger families, less education, and lower family incomes than pro-choice advocates. Some see themselves as a persecuted minority and identify with the fetus that pro-choicers wish to abort. According to Luker, pro-lifers place far less emphasis on perfection than do pro-choicers. They do not expect to make each child a work of art; for pro-lifers, it is sufficient that a child be born into an accepting family and community, whatever the child's capacity. Pro-lifers oppose abortion for reasons of genetic defect; the fetus with a potential birth defect becomes the symbol of all humans who differ from the majority and whose rights must be protected.

The outcome of the pro-choice, pro-life conflict will not be resolved in the near future. It may be that, as Luker's book implies, pro-lifers are fighting a rear-guard action, defending values that will be held by fewer persons as increasing numbers of women enter the workplace, postpone childbearing, and have smaller families or no families at all. On the other hand, sometime in the next century there may be technological breakthroughs that make possible fetal survival at gestational ages below 22 weeks, thereby calling into question any legally set limits of viability. If and when these breakthroughs occur, the pro-choice, pro-life controversy will erupt with renewed fury.

Permanence of Recent Trends

Some of the recent trends described above will probably become long-term trends: parenthood by choice and alternative family forms are likely candidates for permanence. On the other hand, the current trend toward postponement of marriage and childbearing could reverse itself, quite unpredictably, within a few years. It is virtually impossible to predict accurately whether couples will choose to begin their families earlier or later; many reproductive practices tend to follow cyclical patterns. Twenty years ago no one would have predicted that today most unwed teen-age mothers would keep their babies; twenty years in the future this pattern may change once again. The feminist movement may go into temporary eclipse, but it is likely to be revived again in changing political climates. Self-help is likely to remain as a permanent trend among a minority of families, with application to relatively few situations in a high-technology field.

RESULTS OF SOCIAL TRENDS: THREE EMERGENT BELIEFS ABOUT THE FETUS

The various social trends—long-term and recent—described above have combined to change our views of parenthood and of the fetus. Three popular beliefs have emerged, rarely stated explicitly, that influence many of the actions of researchers and medical professionals. The first of these beliefs is that people have a right to become parents, at all costs. This belief underlies demands that society spend money on infertility and new reproductive techniques. The "right to parenthood" is the pro-choice analog of the "right to life" because it also includes the "right *not* to be a parent."

The second emergent popular belief is that people have the right to have "perfect" children. Several long-term social trends have combined to make the birth of a retarded child a greater disaster to the middle-class family than ever before. The birth of such a child usually means the that mother has to leave the workplace, losing not only needed income but part of her hard-won identity as a worker. Frequently, the child is raised at home, not only because many institutions now refuse to accept children until their full potential has been elicited at home, but also because middle-class values require that families spend maximal emotional and financial resources on each child. Families will therefore attempt to prevent potential imperfections at all costs, while maintaining their belief that they have the right to have children. Increasingly, they will demand an array of high-technology services to ensure perfection. The demand for fetal surgery, for example, stems from beliefs that people have not only the right to be parents, but the right to be parents of the perfect child. For some parents, these two imagined "rights" have assumed the sanctity of those guaranteed by the Constitution.

The third emergent belief is that there is an implicit two-class system for fetuses: the wanted, for whom no expense should be spared, and the unwanted, which can be aborted with impunity. What differentiates one class from another is simply parental choice. Parental autonomy, already a dominant value among parents and medical professionals, will win out. In the future, we will see immense resources spent on salvaging one fetus while another of similar gestational age and condition is discarded at the parents' wishes. At present, we are spared such scenarios only because there is a biological limit on fetal viability at about 22 to 23 weeks gestational age; a fetus of less gestational age has no lung tissue and would require an artificial placenta to survive outside the mother. In the future, however, beliefs in the rights to parenthood and to perfect children may lead to consumer demand for research on heroic measures for survival of the (wanted) fetus, even if this means development of an artificial placenta or womb. Sometime within the next century, this research will breech the current lower limits of fetal viability. At that point, society will have to make a choice. Either the limit for legal termination of pregnancy will have to be set earlier in the pregnancy, to coincide with the new limits of viability (a step that would go counter to currently prevailing pro-choice trends), or some version of the two-class system for fetuses will take effect.

In time, it is possible that new scientific developments will advance the limits of fetal viability back to conception, but only at extraordinary expense. Long before this happens, it will become evident that what happens to a fetus depends not only on whether it is wanted or unwanted but on where it and its parents fit into the system of American medical care. Most of the technologies described in previous chapters will benefit the few rather than the many, not only because they are designed for unusual situations, but because they are expensive. In the absence of a national health service or other form of equalizing system, some parents and their fetuses will receive lavish outlays of resources, others will become research subjects, and others will not benefit from the new technologies at all.

We predict that prenatal diagnosis will become routinely used in all pregnancies, as a result of consumer demand. Although prenatal diagnostic procedures will make women more aware, early in the pregnancy, of the fetus as a separate being, this awareness will not prevent most of them from aborting a defective fetus. The use of prenatal diagnostic procedures will serve to keep pregnancy and birth firmly under medical control. Although a few families will have home births, these will usually occur after thoroughly medicalized, screened, and tested pregnancies. The new techniques will serve to enhance the prestige of obstetricians as purveyors of high technology. Popular beliefs about parents' rights to choose size, spacing, and quality of children will include acceptance of their right to sex preselection, with unforeseeable consequences to society. Above all, barring a revolutionary change in our values, beliefs in parental autonomy will continue to dominate our thinking about the fetus.

REFERENCES

1. Bernard J: The Future of Marriage. New Haven, Yale University Press, 1982
2. Bremner RH: Children and Youth in America: A Documentary History, Vol II, 1866–1932, Vol. III, 1933–1973. Cambridge, Mass, Harvard University Press, 1970–1974
3. Caplow T, Bahr HM, Chadwick BA, Hill R, Williamson MH: Middletown Families: Fifty Years of Change and Continuity. New York, Bantam, 1982
4. DeLee JB: The prophylactic forceps operations. Am J Obstet Gynecol 1:34–44, 1920
5. Easterlin RA: Population, Labor Force and Long Swings in Economic Growth: The American Experience. New York, Columbia University Press, for National Bureau of Economic Research, 1968
6. Fink AE: Causes of Crime: Biological Theories in the United States, 1800–1915. Philadelphia, University of Pennsylvania Press, 1938
7. Fletcher JC, Evans MI: Maternal Bonding in Early Fetal Ultra-Sound Examinations. N Engl J Med 308:392–393, 1983
8. Fuchs VR: How We Live: An Economic Perspective on Americans from Birth to Death. Cambridge, Mass, Harvard University Press, 1983
9. Gordon L: Woman's Body, Woman's Right: A Social History of Birth Control in the United States. New York, Penguin Books, 1977
10. Luker K: Abortion and the Politics of Motherhood. Berkeley, University of California Press, 1984
11. Mohr JC: Abortion in America: The Origin and Evolution of National Policy. New York, Oxford University Press, 1978
12. Naisbitt J: Megatrends: Ten New Directions Transforming Our Lives, 6th ed. New York, Warner, 1983
13. Oppenheimer VK: The Female Labor Force in the United States: Demographic & Economic Factors Governing its Growth & Changing Composition. Population Monograph Series, No 5. Westport, CT, Greenwood Press, 1976
14. Reed J: From Private Vice to Public Virtue: The Birth Control Movement and American Society Since 1830. New York, Basic Books, 1978
15. Ruzek SB: The Women's Health Movement. New York, Praeger, 1978
16. Sanderson W: Quantitative aspects of marriage, fertility, and family limitation in nineteenth-century America: Another application of the Coale specifications. Demog 16:339–358, 1979
17. Shryock R: Medicine and Society in America, 1660–1860. Ithaca, NY, Cornell University Press, 1962
18. Smith DS: The demographic history of colonial New England. J Econ Hist 32:177–187, 1972
19. Sweet JA: Women in the Labor Force. New York, Seminar Press, 1973
20. US Dept of Commerce, Bureau of the Census: Historical Statistics of the United States: Colonial times to 1970, Part 1. Washington, DC, US Govt Printing Office, 1975. See also Statistical Abstract of the United States, 1984

21. US Dept of Labor, Children's Bureau: Infant Mortality Series, nos 6, 7, 8, 9. Washington, DC, US Govt Printing Office, 1915–1918
22. Veevers JE: Differential childlessness by color: A further examination. Soc Biol 29:180–186, 1982
23. Veroff J, Douvan E, Kulka RA: The Inner American: A Self-Portrait from 1957 to 1976. New York, Basic Books, 1981
24. Wertz DC: Social science attitudes toward women workers, 1870–1970. Int J Wom Stud 5:161–171, 1982
25. Wertz RW, Wertz DC: Lying-In: A History of Childbirth in America. New York, Free Press, 1977
26. Yankelovitch D: New Rules: Searching for Self-Fulfillment in a World Turned Upside Down. New York, Random House, 1981

Conclusion

Duane F. Alexander

The changes in contemporary society resulting from medical discoveries are enormous and well known, but in no area have these changes been more dramatic and rapid than in the activities surrounding childbearing. Alan Dixler's comment in Part I-C that "The law is far from static and even the pace of change can vary" is true also of medical science, ethics, politics, and sociology as they are addressed throughout this book. It is clear, however, that the new capabilities brought by medical research are the driving actions that bring reactions from the other fields.

The rapidity with which we have had to cope with these changes can best be understood by remembering that the grandmothers or great-grandmothers of most of today's new parents had limited knowledge of reproduction and few choices of contraceptives (which were banned in some states as recently as the 1960s). Their families were large; most pregnancies were unplanned; prenatal care was minimal; fetal diagnosis was unknown; and there was limited access to abortion, which was illegal in most places. Pregnant women had a 1% chance of dying at each childbirth (today it is less than 0.01%), and their babies had a 10% chance of dying before 1 year of age (reduced today to 1%). If they could not become pregnant but wanted to have children, adoption was their only alternative.

The chapters in this book discuss the far-reaching changes in all aspects of pregnancy and childbirth brought about by the application of advances in medical research, along with the resulting societal changes and the struggle of the law and ethical thought to keep pace. It becomes clear that the only thing that has been unchanging with regard to contraception, new approaches to treating infertility, prenatal diagnosis, and abortion is the official doctrine of a few religious groups.

Although much of the legal basis for changes in the law that have officially sanctioned new medical practices rests on the right to privacy, these matters are, paradoxically, far more public than ever before. Whereas in the past issues of sexuality and reproductive behavior rarely received serious public discussion, these topics now fill our newspapers, legislatures, courts, and personal conversations. In many ways this new openness and public discussion of what formerly were taboo topics is healthy, but this benefit is lost if contentiousness and intolerance in the public debate become divisive. This book clearly points out this hazard in the age-old dilemma of, as John Fletcher describes it, balancing individual liberty and self-determination against accountability for following particular bodies of normative ethical guidance in everyday life. The dilemma is where to draw the normative line.

At least two things are certain: more changes in reproductive technology will come, and conflict over both current practices and the new technologies will continue in the legal, legislative, and ethical arenas. Scientists surely will develop a technique for prenatal diagnosis of fetal genetic disease from maternal blood samples, making such testing available on a broad basis. Gene replacement therapy will come far sooner than anyone would have predicted ten years ago. Congenital acquired immune deficiency syndrome (AIDS) and sexual transmission of AIDS are already posing new dilemmas in reproductive health. Imminent development of a pill to induce menses reliably to prevent implantation or in very early pregnancy will raise new questions about abortion. As the book points out, although the specific topics change, the basic issues in the debate remain the same. With the increasing prevalence and prominence of these issues, it becomes increasingly important for participants in the debate to seek ways to find common ground and work out differences. Such profound issues in society deserve a better means of resolution than periodic struggles over a "swing-vote" appointment to the United States Supreme Court. It is to be hoped that the multiple views from various professions brought together in this book will be a part of the process of discovering that common ground.

Index

A

Abdomen, fetal, ultrasound of, 77
Abdominal wall defects
  perinatal management of, 333
  prenatal diagnosis of, 77
  ultrasound presentation of, 77
Abetalipoproteinemia
  prenatal diagnosis of, 23
  prenatal therapy for, 410
Abortion, 6. *See also* Habitual abortion; Pregnancy termination
  in anencephaly, 56–57
    in third trimester, 472, 476–477
  criminalization of, 534–535
  decriminalization of, 535
  in Down's syndrome, 56–57
  elective vs. therapeutic, 544–545
  ethical issues in, 272–273
  and father's rights, 308–309
  fetal research using abortus after, 451–454
  fetus as source of therapy after, 438
  of fetus carrying Huntington's disease, 40
  first trimester, vs. second trimester, 17–18
  government funding of, 534–546
    absolute right to, 537–538
    conditional right to, 538–542
    constitutional issues, 537–545
    restrictions on, 536
    state regulation of, 542–545
  historical perspective on, 534–535
  immediate late, prevention of, 211
  imminent, diagnosis of, 73
  interests of father in, 315
  legal aspects of, 514–515
  for mentally retarded mother, 104–105
  and moral status of fetus, 314–315
  with open neural tube defect, 56–57
  and prematernal duty, 432, 434, 443
  presented as option in pre-amniocentesis counseling, 41
  public funding for, denial of, 515, 536
  regulation of, 540
  and rights of embryo, 356
  versus selective termination, 268, 272–273
Abortion pill, 567
Abortion techniques, relative risks of, 41
Abortus tissue, study of, 41, 451–454
Acardia, in twin gestation, 248–249
Acardiac monster, 249
Acatalesemia, prenatal diagnosis of, 25
Acetylcholinesterase, amniotic fluid
  and gestational age, 47
  in prenatal diagnosis, 46–47
Acetylsalicylic acid, teratogenicity, 129
Achondroplasia, prenatal diagnosis of, 25
Acid lipase deficiency, prenatal diagnosis of, 23
Acidosis, neonatal, with midforceps delivery, 319
Acid phosphatase deficiency, prenatal diagnosis of, 23
Acquired immunodeficiency syndrome, 517, 567
  experimental therapy for, 515
  research, primates used for, 471
  transmission of
    during artificial insemination, 374
    in leukocyte therapy, 392
Acrylonitril, mutagenicity, 163
Actinomycin D
  cytogenetic effects on meiotic chromosomes of oocytes, 164
  teratogenicity, 120
Acute intermittent porphyria, prenatal diagnosis of, 25
Adenine arabinoside, teratogenicity, 120
Adenosine deaminase deficiency
  gene therapy for, 421–422, 425
  prenatal diagnosis of, 25

569

Index

Adoption, 374, 375, 382
  commissioned, 383
  prenatal, 381
  unavailability of infants for, 561
Adrenal corticosteroids, teratogenicity, 121
Adrenocorticotropic hormone, teratogenicity, 121
Adrenogenital syndrome, prenatal diagnosis of, 24
Adrenoleukodystrophy, prenatal diagnosis of, 23
Adult polycystic kidney disease, prenatal diagnosis of, 26
Aflatoxin B_1, as transplacental carcinogen, 156
AFP. *See* Alpha-fetoprotein
Agammaglobulinemia, prenatal diagnosis of, 26
Agent Orange, teratogenicity, 131–132
Albinism, ocular, prenatal diagnosis of, 21
Alcohol
  abuse, as prematernal negligence, 528–529
  consumption in pregnancy
    data collection on, 140–141
    dose-response relations, 140–141, 145–146
    interviewing patient about, 145–146
    recommended levels for, 145–146
  and intrauterine growth retardation, 204
  teratogenicity, 124, 140, 417, 522
Alcohol-related disorders, adverse pregnancy outcomes, 142–143
Aliphatic hydrocarbon mixtures, reproductive toxicity, 161
Alkylating agents
  correlation of genotoxicity with epidemiologic findings, 165
  reproductive toxicity, 154
  teratogenicity, 117–118
Allura red AC, as perinatal behavioral toxin, 155
Alobar holoprosencephaly, ultrasound presentation of, 61, 62
Alpha-1 antitrypsin deficiency, 84–85
  prenatal diagnosis of, 25
Alpha-fetoprotein, 3
  amniotic fluid
    analysis of, 45–47
    concentration of, and gestational age, 45–46
    in diagnosis of neural tube defects, 45–46
    elevated
      disorders associated with, 47
      and negative ACHE, 47
  fetal plasma level, and gestational age, 45–46
  maternal serum, 4
    access to testing for, 58–59
    analysis, 47–50
    benefits of testing and screening for, 57–58
    California's statewide screening program for, 58–59
    in detection of chromosomal anomalies, 50–52
    elevated, causes of, 48–49
    ethical issues in testing, 54–59
    factors affecting, 49–50
    freedom and coercion issues related to, 59
    future application of testing of, 52
    and gestational age, 46
    as indication for amniocentesis, 40
    prenatal diagnoses made with, 77
    quality control concerns about testing for, 52, 57–58
    reduced, protocol for, 51
    resource allocation for testing for, 52, 58–59
    risks of testing and screening for, 57–58
    studies of screening of, in U.S., 54–55
    test kits for, 52, 54–55, 515
    threshold levels indicating further testing, 48–50, 57–58
    United Kingdom Collaborative Study of screening of, 54–55
  use for prenatal diagnosis, history of, 44
Alpha-fetoprotein testing, 220
  evolution of, 185–186
  public policy issues in, 189–190
  test kits for, historical perspective on, 189–190
Alpha-methyldopa, reproductive toxicity, 154
Alpha-thalassemia, prenatal diagnosis of, 26, 31
American College of Obstetrics and Gynecology, Ethics Committee
  recommendations on court-ordered actions, 444
  recommendations on surrogate motherhood, 381
  on research, 462
  statement on sterilization of mentally retarded women, 108, 110–113
American Law Institute, draft Model Penal Code, 535
American Medical Association, position on abortion, 534–535
Aminoglycosides, teratogenicity, 120
Aminopterin, teratogenicity, 118
Amniocentesis, 17, 20–27
  for assessment of lung maturity, 218
    in twin gestation, 256
  availability of procedure, 38–39
  early, for genetic analysis, 29
  for elective sex selection, 40–41
  in fetal heart disease, 419
  indications for, 38–40
  maternal age and, 18
  physician qualifications for performance of, 38
  in premature rupture of membranes, 216–217
  risks of, 38, 47
  in second and third trimester, 36–37
  sonar guidance in, 36–37
  spontaneous abortion after, 27
Amniotic band syndrome, 119
Amniotic fluid
  phospholipid content, significance of, 216, 217
  steroid concentrations in, in second trimester, 405
Amphetamines, teratogenicity, 127, 417
Amyloidotic polyneuropathy, prenatal diagnosis of, 25
Anderson's disease, type IV, prenatal diagnosis of, 21
Androgens, teratogenicity, 121–122
Anemia, and fetal hypoxia, 206
Anencephalics
  brain-dead, retrieval and preservation of organs from, 474–476
  management of, after delivery, 477–478
  as organ source, 469, 471–478
    legal and ethical issues in, 473–476
    management of pregnancies involving, 476–477
    before total brain death, 473–474
Anencephaly, 221
  incidence of, 472
  legal issues in, 33–34
  management of, 333
  maternal serum alpha-fetoprotein in, 48
  moral status of fetus or newborn afflicted with, 55–56
  organ harvest from fetus or newborn afflicted with, 55–56
  prenatal diagnosis of, 472, 477
  timing of, in embryogenesis, 155
  treatment of, ethical issues in, 56–57
  ultrasound presentation of, 61
Anesthetics. *See also* Dental anesthetics
  correlation of genotoxicity with epidemiologic findings, 165
  reproductive toxicity, 166–168
  teratogenicity, 129
Aneuploidy
  chemicals inducing, 155
  and maternal serum alpha-fetoprotein, 50–51
  parental, and risk to fetus, 18
Animal rights claims, about primates as organ sources, 470–471
Ankyloglossia, prenatal diagnosis of, 26

Anomalous fetus, cesarean delivery of, 332–334
Anti-abortion movement, 562
Antianxiety agents, teratogenicity, 126–127
Antibiotics, teratogenicity, 119–120
Anticoagulants, teratogenicity, 128–129
Anticonvulsants, teratogenicity, 127–128
Antidepressants, teratogenicity, 127
Antihistaminic drugs, teratogenicity, 129–130
Antihypertensives, teratogenicity, 130
Antimalarials, teratogenicity, 121
Antimetabolites, teratogenicity, 118
Antimicrobial agents, teratogenicity, 119–121
Antinausea drugs, teratogenicity, 129–130
Antineoplastic agents
  reproductive toxicity, 166
  teratogenicity, 117–119
Antinuclear antibody, 391
Antipsychotics
  reproductive toxicity of, 154
  teratogenicity, 125–127
Antipyrene, ratio of concentration in breast milk vs. maternal blood, 158
Antisperm antibodies, 388, 391
Antithrombin III, defect in, prenatal diagnosis of, 25
Antithyroid agents, teratogenicity, 123
Antituberculins, teratogenicity, 120–121
Apallic syndrome, 298
Apgar scores
  after breech presentation, 282
  of very low birth weight infants, 221, 223
Apolipoprotein C-II deficiency, prenatal diagnosis of, 23
Apolipoprotein loci, DNA polymorphisms at, 88
Application of Cicero, 494
Appropriate for gestational age infant
  prognosis for, 224
  survival of, 202
Arginase deficiency, prenatal diagnosis of, 21
Argininemia, prenatal diagnosis of, 21
Argininosuccinate lyase deficiency, prenatal diagnosis of, 21
Argininosuccinate synthetase deficiency, prenatal diagnosis of, 21
Argininosuccinic aciduria, prenatal diagnosis of, 21
Arnold Chiari malformation, 75
Arsenic
  mutagenicity, 163
  reproductive toxicity, 159, 161
Artificial insemination, 373–374
  as adultery, 357–358
  by donor, 361–363, 365, 372, 374, 379
    and information on parental lineage, 378
    legal status of, 357–358
    presumption of paternity in, 382
    self-help in, 562
    state statutes on, 379
  by husband, 374
Ascites, fetal, ultrasound presentation of, 63, 65
Aspartame, as perinatal behavioral toxin, 155
Aspartylglycosaminuria, prenatal diagnosis of, 23
Asphyxia
  after breech presentation, 282
  intrauterine, total, causes of, 406
  as issue in malpractice suits, 341–342, 344–345
  with midforceps delivery, 318
  perinatal, 206
    neonatal complications with, 205–206
    prevention of, 223
Aspirin, teratogenicity, 129
Assisted breech delivery, 280
Ataxia telangiectasia

diagnosis of, 20
inheritance of, 20
Atherosclerosis, premature, prenatal diagnosis of, 23
Autoimmune disease, fetal wastage in, 391
Autonomy
  maternal right to, 235, 236
  parental, 563
  physician and patient, limitation of, 515
  principle of, 5, 239, 274, 378–379, 510–511
Autosomal disorders, transmission of, from parent to offspring, 94–95
Autosomal dominant disorders, transmission of, from parent to offspring, 97
Autosomal dominant hypercholesterolemia, predictive genetic testing for, 85–86
Autosomal recessive disorders, transmission of, from parent to offspring, 97–98
Azathioprine, teratogenic risk of, 118
Azoethane, as transplacental carcinogen, 156
Azoxyethane, as transplacental carcinogen, 156

B

Baby, allowed to die. *See* Euthanasia
Baby Doe case, 444, 472, 485–486, 495–499, 502
Baby Fae, 468–471
Baby Jane Doe, 497
Baby M case, 377–379, 383–385
Baby selling, 380–381
  prohibition on, 383
Ballance v. Dunnington, 193
Barbiturates
  fetal addiction risk, 128
  reproductive toxicity of, 154
  teratogenicity, 128
Bardet-Bredle syndrome, 77
Becker muscular dystrophy, prenatal diagnosis of, 25, 27
Beckwith-Wiedmann syndrome, prenatal diagnosis of, 27
Bed rest
  benefits of, 213
  in higher-order multiple gestations, 261
  in prevention of premature delivery, 213–216
  in twin gestation, 255–256
Behavioral disorders, alcohol-related, 143–144
Behavioral toxins, perinatal, environmental agents as, 155
Bendectin, safety in pregnancy, 129–130
Beneficence, 378
  principle of, 5, 274, 313, 316
Benomyl, mutagenicity, 163
Benzene, mutagenicity, 163
Benzine hexachloride, ratio of concentration in breast milk vs. maternal blood, 158
Benzo(a)pyrene
  reproductive toxicity, 162
  as transplacental carcinogen, 156
Bermann disease, prenatal diagnosis of, 24
Beta-galactosidase deficiency, prenatal diagnosis of, 23
Beta HCG, serum level, and ultrasound detection of gestational sac, 72
11-Beta-hydroxylase deficiency, prenatal diagnosis of, 25
Beta-mannosidosis, prenatal diagnosis of, 23
Beta-sympathomimetic agents
  maternal complications with, 212
  in prevention of preterm delivery, 212
  in twin gestation, 254–255
Beta-thalassemia
  gene therapy for, 422–423
  prenatal diagnosis of, 26, 37

Biochemical disorders, diagnosis from CVS, 30
Biomedical ethics, principles in, 273–275
Biomedical Ethics Advisory Committee, 450
Biomedical technology. *See also* Reproductive technology; Technology
  effect on roles of women, 13
  and health beliefs, 13–14
  sociologic issues in, 11–12
Biophysical profile, 412
  in twin gestation, 253
Biopsy, in utero, of fetal tissue, 37
Biotin, prenatal administration of, 405–406
Biparietal diameter, in twin gestation, 250–253
Birth control pills. *See* Oral contraceptives
Birth weight
  effects of alcohol on, 142–143
  and neonatal survival, 200–202
1-3-Bis(2-chloroethyl) 1-nitrosourea, as transplacental carcinogen, 156
Blacks, maternal serum alpha-fetoprotein levels in, 49–50
Bladder, extroversion of, timing of, in embryogenesis, 155
Bladder exstrophy, prenatal diagnosis of, 77
Bladder obstruction, ultrasound presentation of, 77
Bladder puncture, in oocyte retrieval, 352
Blood disorders, prenatal diagnosis of, 25–26
Blood-forming tissue, disorders of, prenatal diagnosis of, 25–26
Blood sampling, fetal, in fetal heart disease, 419
Blood transfusions
  court-ordered, 235, 435, 493–494, 525
  intrauterine, 526
    court-ordered, 444
  legal issues concerning, 500–501
  Rh-positive, tort liability for, 524
Bloom syndrome
  diagnosis of, 20
  inheritance of, 20
Blue Cross and Blue Shield association of America, Technology Evaluation and Coverage Program, 191–192
Bonbrest v. Kotz, 523–524
Bone disorders, prenatal diagnosis of, 25
Bone dysplasia, 76
Bone marrow transplantation, 469
  as fetal therapy, 411
  in-utero, 426
Bone marrow transplantation/retroviral gene transfer, fetal, 426–427
Bony abnormalities, diagnosis of, 67–68
Bourn Hall, 350
Brachial plexus injury, and midforceps delivery, 318
Brain death
  cardiovascular collapse after, 296
  criteria for diagnosis, 298
  definition of, 296
  diagnostic criteria for, 311–312, 315
  legal implications of, 296
  maternal, during pregnancy, 296–305
    cardiovascular support in, 300, 301–302
    case report, 297–298, 307–308
    and consent of mother to heroic measures, 316
    cost of life-support after, 305, 313
    endocrine abnormalities in, treatment of, 300, 304
    ethical issues concerning, 311–316
    fetal care after, 299–304
    heparin prophylaxis in, 300, 304
    infection control in, 300, 304
    interests of father in, 315
    interests of fetus in, 314–315
    interests of mother in, 313–314
    legal issues related to, 307–311
    mother-fetus relationship in, ethical issues related to, 315–316
    nutritional support in, 300, 303–304
    obstetric strategies with, 304–305
    outcome for fetus, 298, 299, 308
    proposed solution to issues concerning, 310–311
    resource allocation in life-support after, 312–313
    respiratory support in, 299–301
    and rights of father and family, 308–309
    temperature lability in, treatment of, 300, 302–303
  retrieval of organs from anencephalics before, 473
  short-term maintenance after, 296, 298, 312
  somatic survival after, 298
Brain life, 367
Brandt maneuver, 280
Breast cancer, and age of first pregnancy, 392
Breech presentation
  anesthesia for, 281–282, 287
  assisted delivery with, 280
  augmentation of labor with, 286–287
  cesarean section for, 276–278
  cesarean section in, 284, 287, 332
    elective, 287–289
    in twin gestation, 258–259
  conduct of delivery in, 287
  congenital abnormalities observed in, 277–278
  definitions of, 278–279
  delivery method for, effect on outcome, 290–291
  delivery of aftercoming head, 280–281
  delivery procedures with, 280–281
  delivery team for, 281–282
  double footling, 279
  external cephalic version in, 283–284
  fetal injury in, 288
  forceps use with, 281
  frank, 278–279
  hyperextension of head with, 286
  incidence of, 276, 332
  incomplete, 278–279
  labor and delivery with, 278–283
  legal issues in, 342
  of low birth weight infant, 332
  management alternatives in, 276, 278, 283–289
  management of
    future goals for, 292–293
    impact of society and social mores on, 292
  mechanism of labor with, 279–280
  obstetric management of, 276–293
  outcome with, risk factors in, 276
  oxytocin in labor with, 286–287
  and pelvimetry, 282–283
  perinatal morbidity and mortality in, 276–278
  preterm, 282
    cesarean section with, 290
    management of, 289–291
    outcome with, 290–291
    vaginal delivery with, 289–290
  route of delivery with, 278
  selective trial of labor in, 284–288
    informed consent for, 284
    preparation for delivery, 284–286
  single footling, 278–279
  type of, by gestational age, 291
  vaginal delivery with, safety of, 284, 286
  in very low birth weight, and obstetric management, 222
  x-ray evaluation in, 282–283, 286
British Advisory Group on Use of Fetuses and Fetal Material for Research, 451, 460, 461
Brominated vegetable oil, as perinatal behavioral toxin, 155

Brown, Louise, 350, 374
Busulfan, teratogenicity, 117–118
Butylated hydroxyanisole, as perinatal behavioral toxin, 155
Butylated hydroxytoluene, as perinatal behavioral toxin, 155
n-Butylnitrosourea, as transplacental carcinogen, 156

C

Cadmium
  cytogenetic effects on meiotic chromosomes of oocytes, 164
  detection of toxic effects, 158
  mutagenicity, 163
  as perinatal behavioral toxin, 155
  reproductive toxicity, 159, 160, 161
Caffeine
  cytogenetic effects on meiotic chromosomes of oocytes, 164
  as perinatal behavioral toxin, 155
  ratio of concentration in breast milk vs. maternal blood, 158
Calcium channel blockers, in prevention of premature delivery, 212
Cancer, childhood, from prenatal toxicity, 155–157
Carbamazepine, effect on fetus, 103
Carbamylphosphate synthetase deficiency, prenatal diagnosis of, 21
Carbofuran, as perinatal behavioral toxin, 155
Carbohydrate metabolism, disorders of, prenatal diagnosis of, 21
Carbon disulfide, as perinatal behavioral toxin, 155
Carbon monoxide, as perinatal behavioral toxin, 155
Cardiac anomalies
  mental retardation with, 100
  and prenatal exposure to antiepileptics, 127
  and progestogen exposure, 123
  ultrasound diagnosis of, 69–70, 77
Cardiac care, neonatal, 418–419
Cardiac pump performance, evaluation of, 419
Cardiovascular system, fetal, 413
Cataract, congenital, ultrasound diagnosis of, 75
Cat eye syndrome, prenatal diagnosis of, 26
Causation, legal definition of, 339–340
Cell transplantation, research on, 458–459
Cellular grafts, 469
Ceramidase deficiency, prenatal diagnosis of, 23
Cerebellum, growth of, correlation with gestational age, 75
Cerebral blood flow, increased, in perinatal asphyxia, 208–209
Cerebral death, 298
Cerebral palsy
  after midforceps delivery, 319
  alcohol-related, 144
Cervical cerclage, 211
  in twin gestation, 254
Cervical incompetence, 211
Cervix, ultrasonographic evaluation of, in pregnancy, 78
Cesarean delivery
  with abdominal wall defects, 333
  with anencephaly, 477
  of anomalous fetus, 332–334
  in breech presentation, 276–278, 284, 287, 332
    elective, 287–289
    preterm, 290
  court-ordered, 6, 235, 236, 435, 444, 526
  in dystocia, 326–328
  elective repeat, recommendations concerning, 329–330
  with fetal distress, 330–332
  in hydrocephalus, 333
  incidence of, changes in, 326–334
  indications for, changes in, 326–334
  and infant mortality, 556
  legal intervention in, 237–238
  for low birth weight infant, 332
  maternal refusal of, 444
  maternal rights in, 13
  maternal risks in, 234
  morbidity with, 234, 318–319
  mortality rate for, 234
  in neural tube defects, 333
  and payment policies, 518
  and presentation, in twin gestation, 258–259
  rate of, 326
    changes in, 559
    at National Maternity Hospital, 326–327
  repeat, 328–330
  start-up time for, 342
  vaginal delivery after, support for, 328–329
  in very low birth weight
    benefit to fetus, 238–239
    ethical considerations in, 233–241
    informed consent in, 239–241
    legal considerations, 234–238
    maternal vs. fetal interests in, 239
    medical considerations in, 238–239
  for very low birth weight infant, 221–222
  vs. midforceps delivery, 324–325
  vs. vaginal delivery, as issue in malpractice suits, 341–342
CHAMPUS, denial of payment for abortion, 515
Charcot-Marie-Tooth disease, prenatal diagnosis of, 26
Chediak-Higashi syndrome, prenatal diagnosis of, 26
Chemical mutagens, reproductive toxicity, 163–166
Child. See also Perfect child
  prenatal rights of, 431–432
  as property, 383–384
Child abuse and neglect
  enforcement of laws, 499
  prenatal, maternal neglect as, 434
  statutes, 530–531
Child Abuse and Neglect Act of 1984, 483, 485–486
Child Abuse Prevention and Treatment Act of 1984, 499
Childbearing
  changing context of, 566–567
  postponed, 560–561
Chimpanzees, as organ sources, 470–471. See also Baby Fae
Chlorambucil, teratogenicity, 117–118
Chloramphenicol
  safety during pregnancy, 119
  toxicity to newborn, 119
Chlordiazepoxide, teratogenicity, 126
Chlorobiphenyls, teratogenicity, 131
Chloroform, as perinatal behavioral toxin, 155
Chloromethyl ether, mutagenicity, 163
Chloroprene, mutagenicity, 163
Chloroquine, teratogenicity, 121
Cholesteryl ester storage disease, prenatal diagnosis of, 23
Cholesteryl-14-methylhexadecanoate, as transplacental carcinogen, 156
Chondrodysplasia punctata, 75
Chorioamnionitis, 217
Chorionic villus sampling, 456–458
  biochemical diagnosis from, 30
  cell culture from, 29–30
  characteristics of patients, 28
  clinical procedure, 20–29
  cytogenetic diagnosis from, 29–30
  evolution of, 185–186
  molecular diagnoses from, 30–32
  for prenatal therapy, 410
  spontaneous abortion after, 27
  technology for, 28

574 Index

Chorionic villus sampling (*continued*)
  timing of, 17
  transabdominal route, 28
  uses of, 17
  vaginosonographic-guided, 74
Choroideremia, prenatal diagnosis of, 26
Choroid plexus, on transvaginal ultrasound, 74–75
Christmas factor deficiency, prenatal diagnosis of, 26
Chromium
  mutagenicity, 163
  reproductive toxicity, 159, 160
Chromosomal abnormalities. *See also* Sex chromosomal abnormalities; Structural chromosomal abnormalities; Translocation
  chemicals inducing, 155
  and congenital heart disease, 418
  detection of, 50–52
  in family, as indication for amniocentesis, 38, 39
  prenatal diagnosis of, 45
  risk of having liveborn child with, by maternal age, 19
  transmission of, from parent to offspring, 94–97
  in twin gestation, 249–250
Chromosomal deletions
  prenatal diagnosis of, 27
  transmission of, from parent to offspring, 96
Chromosomal diagnosis, in preimplantation embryo, 459
Chromosomal disorders, risk factors for, 18–19
Chromosome instability, disorders of, diagnosis of 18–20
Chronic granulomatous disease, prenatal diagnosis of, 26
Chronic vegetative state, 493
Citrullinemia, prenatal diagnosis of, 21
Clavicular fracture, and midforceps delivery, 318
Cleft lip and palate
  disorders associated with, 75
  prenatal diagnosis of, 26
  and prenatal diazepam exposure, 126–127
  and prenatal exposure to antiepileptics, 127
  related disorders, 75
  timing of, in embryogenesis, 155
  ultrasound presentation of, 61, 63, 75
Clomiphene citrate, 79
  in follicle stimulation, for in vitro fertilization, 351
  teratogenicity, 122
Clubfoot, ultrasound presentation of, 69
Coagulopathy
  in fetus, in single twin demise, 247–248
  maternal, in single twin demise, 248
  prenatal diagnosis of, 25–26
Cocaine
  abuse, as prematernal negligence, 528–529
  teratogenicity, 522
Coke production, exposure to toxins in, monitoring using urine analysis, 166
Combination chemotherapy, teratogenicity, 119
Common law, 8
Communicable disease, reporting of, 517
Communication with patient, and risk-management, 343
Computed tomography
  in diagnosis of intraventricular hemorrhage, 208
  pelvimetry, and breech presentation, 282–283
Conceptus. *See* Embryo
Congenital adrenal hyperplasia
  diagnosis of, 20, 404–405
  fetal therapy for, 403–405
  prenatal diagnosis of, 24, 25
Congenital anomalies
  causes of, 522
  and mode of delivery, 332–334
  nontreatment of, 482

observed in breech presentation, 277–278
  perinatal management of, general guidelines for, 334
  prenatal diagnosis of, 220
  survival with, 221
  in twin gestations, 248–249
Congenital enzymopenic methemoglobinemia, prenatal diagnosis of, 26
Congenital erythropoietic porphyria, prenatal diagnosis of, 25
Congenita lethalis, prenatal diagnosis of, 25
Congenital heart disease, 75
  extracardiac anomalies associated with, 417
  risk factors for, 416
  risk of, 77
Congenital hypophosphatasia, prenatal diagnosis of, 25
Congenital malformations. *See* Congenital anomalies
Congestive heart failure, and nonimmune hydrops, 417–418
Congressional Biomedical Ethics Board, 450
Connective tissue disorders, prenatal diagnosis of, 25
Conrad's syndrome, 75
Constitution, fidelity to text of, 541
Constitutional rights. *See also* Privacy, right to
  exercise of, protection of, 539–540
  fundamental, 540–541
  government financial assistance and support for, 537–538
  vs. unprotected government privileges, 538–539
Contagious disease, reportability of, 515
Contraception
  legal issues concerning, 541
  in mental retardation, 107–108
  moral issues in, 364–365
Copper
  metabolic abnormalities, fetal therapy for, 408–409
  reproductive toxicity, 159, 160, 161
Cord blood, ultrasound guided sampling of, 37
Cordocentesis
  risks of, 30
  ultrasonically guided, 30
Cori's disease, type III, prenatal diagnosis of, 21
Coronary heart disease, predictive genetic testing for, 88
Corpus callosum, agenesis of, 400
Corticosteroids, effect on fetal lung maturity, 217
Court(s), role in fetal ethics, 6
Court-ordered actions, 235, 435, 442–443, 444, 493–494, 525–526
Court system, 8–9
Cranial anomalies, ultrasound presentation of, 61, 62
Cretinism, 123–124
Cri du chat syndrome, prenatal diagnosis of, 27
Criminal law, 9
Criminal liability
  in nontreatment, 531
  and nontreatment decisions, 492–493
Crown-rump length, on transvaginal ultrasound, 73
Cryptorchidism, timing of, in embryogenesis, 155
Curlender v. Bio-Science Laboratories, 524
CVS. *See* Chorionic villous sampling
Cyanocobalamin, prenatal treatment with, for methylmalonic acidemia, 406–407
Cycasis, as transplacental carcinogen, 156
Cyclophosphamide
  cytogenetic effects on meiotic chromosomes of oocytes, 164
  reproductive toxicity, 154, 166–167
  teratogenicity, 118
Cyclophosphamide therapy, exposure to toxins in, monitoring using urine analysis, 166
Cystathioninuria, prenatal diagnosis of, 21
Cystic fibrosis, prenatal diagnosis of, 26, 40
Cystic hygromas, fetal, ultrasound presentation of, 62–63, 65

Cystinosis, 410
  prenatal diagnosis of, 26
Cytogenetic abnormality, recurrence risk of, with normal parental karyotypes, 18
Cytogenetic diagnosis
  from CVS, 29–30
  direct technique, 29–30
Cytostatic agents, reproductive toxicity, 167
Cytostatic drug exposure, monitoring using urine analysis, 166
Cytotoxic drugs, teratogenicity, 117–119

D

Dandy-Walker syndrome, 75
DDT
  mutagenicity, 163
  reproductive toxicity of, 154
DDT residues, ratio of concentration in breast milk vs. maternal blood, 158
Dead mother, kept alive during pregnancy, 296–316
Death. *See also* Euthanasia
  definition of, 311, 503
    with anencephaly, 56
  diagnostic criteria for, 315
  hastening, by organ preservation, in anencephalics, 475–476
Defensive medicine, vs. risk management, 344
Delivery options, informed consent regarding, 343
Del Zio case, 378
Dental anesthetics, reproductive toxicity, 167
Department of Health and Human Services
  Ethics Advisory Board. *See* Ethics Advisory Board
  regulation of care of handicapped, 483, 495–499, 517
Depo Provera, for mentally retarded, 107
Developmental delay, in very low birth weight infants, 224
Developmentally disabled. *See also* Mental retardation
  incidence of childbearing in, 102
  parenting skills and training in, 105–106
Dexamethasone, fetal therapy with, in congenital adrenal hyperplasia, 404–405
Diabetes mellitus
  fetal cardiac effects, 417
  maternal serum alpha-fetoprotein levels with, 50
Diagnosis-related groups, 188, 486, 518
Dialkylcarbamoylchloride, mutagenicity, 163
Dialysis, termination of, 492
Diaphragmatic hernia
  congenital
    animal model for, 402
    evaluation of, 401
    fetal surgery for, 397
    incidence of, 401
    management of, 401
    perinatal management of, 333
  timing of, in embryogenesis, 155
  ultrasound presentation of, 66, 68
Diastrophic dwarfism, 75
Diazepam, teratogenicity, 126–127
Diazinon, as perinatal behavioral toxin, 155
Dibenzofurans, reproductive toxicity, 162
Dibromochloropropane
  OSHA standards for exposure to, 152
  reproductive toxicity, 154, 163
Dibutylnitrosamine, as transplacental carcinogen, 156
3,3'-Dichlorobenzidine, as transplacental carcinogen, 156
p,p'-Dichlorodiphenyltrichloroethane, as transplacental carcinogen, 156
Dieldrin, ratio of concentration in breast milk vs. maternal blood, 158

Diet, for mentally retarded, pregnant patient, 103
1,2-Diethylhydrazine, as transplacental carcinogen, 156
Diethylnitrosamine, as transplacental carcinogen, 156
Diethylstilbestrol
  reproductive toxicity, 154
  as transplacental carcinogen, 156, 157
Diethylsulphate, as transplacental carcinogen, 156
Diethyltriazine, as transplacental carcinogen, 156
Dietrich v. Inhabitants of Northampton, 523
Digits, fetal, transvaginal ultrasound of, 75–76
Dihydrobiopterin synthetase deficiency, prenatal diagnosis of, 22
Dihydropteridine reductase deficiency, prenatal diagnosis of, 22
Dihydrostreptomycin, teratogenicity, 120
Dilantin, reproductive toxicity, 154
4-Dimethylaminoazobenzol, as transplacental carcinogen, 157
7,12-Dimethylbenza[a]anthracene, as transplacental carcinogen, 157
7,12-Dimethylbenz[a]anthracene, reproductive toxicity, 162
1,2-Dimethylhydrazine, as transplacental carcinogen, 157
Dimethylnitrosamine, as transplacental carcinogen, 157
Dimethylsulphate, as transplacental carcinogen, 156
Dioxin, reproductive toxicity, 154, 162
Diphenhydramine, teratogenicity, 130
Diphenylhydantoin, teratogenicity, 127–128
Dipropylnitrosamine, as transplacental carcinogen, 157
Diuretics, teratogenicity, 130
DNA, predictive genetic testing using, 85
DNA analysis, for prenatal molecular diagnosis, techniques, 30
DNA hybridization
  for prenatal molecular diagnosis, 30
  technique, 31
Doctor-patient relationship
  confidentiality of, 515
  government intervention in, 513–514
  direct, 517
Dominance, definition of, 439
Dominant approach, definition of, 439
Donor statutes, states that have, 357
Do not resuscitate orders, 493
Doppler ultrasound
  for fetal assessment, in twin gestation, 253
  in fetal heart disease, 419
Double bubble sign, 64, 66
Down syndrome. *See also* Trisomy 21
  congenital anomalies in offspring of parents with, 104
  and congenital heart defect, nontreatment decision with, 494
  and esophageal atresia, nontreatment of, 482–483
  and intestinal atresia, nontreatment of, 488
  and maternal age, 18–19
  parental age as risk factor for, 39
  pregnancy in, 103, 104
  prenatal diagnosis of, 4, 18–19, 52
  sexual abuse in, 103
  transmission of, from parent to offspring, 104
  treatment of, ethical issues in, 56–57, 502
Drug abuse, and intrauterine growth retardation, 204
Drugs
  teratogenic, 116–130
  usage during pregnancy, 116–117
Duchenne muscular dystrophy, prenatal diagnosis of, 25, 27, 39–40
Duodenal atresia
  timing of, in embryogenesis, 155
  ultrasound presentation of, 64, 66
Dysrhythmias, fetal
  detection of, 415–416, 419

Dysrhythmias (*continued*)
  diagnosis of, 70
  management of, 403
Dystocia
  cesarean delivery in, 326–328
    effect on fetal outcome, 327–328
  classification of, 326
  definition of, 326
  management of, unresolved controversy in, 326–327
  with sacrococcygeal teratoma, 333
  vaginal birth with, effect on fetal outcome, 328

E

Ebstein's anomaly, 416
  with prenatal lithium exposure, 126
Echocardiography, 69–70
Echocardiography, fetal
  detection of dysrhythmias, 415–416
  future of, 418
  indications for, 416–418
  principles of, 412–416
  standard views used in, 413, 418
  technique, 413–415
Ectopic pregnancy
  after clomiphene-induced ovulation, 122
  diagnosis of, by transvaginal ultrasound, 72–73
  pseudogestational sac in, 72
  in vitro fertilization and embryo transfer and, 365–366
Edwards, Robert, 349–350, 374
Egg donor, 354, 359, 375, 384
Ehlers-Danlos syndrome, prenatal diagnosis of, 25
Einstadt v. Baird, 385
Electroencephalographic abnormalities, alcohol-related, 143
Electronic fetal monitoring, 330–331
  Dublin trial of, 330–331
  early randomized trials, results of, 330–331
  as issue in malpractice suits, 340–341
Ellis-van Creveld syndrome, 77
Embryo
  cryopreservation of, 350, 353, 358, 368–369
  excess, after in vitro fertilization, disposition of, 366–367, 377
  fate of, upon death of parents, 377
  fertilization, for research alone, ethical issues related to, 369
  implantation and growth, failure of, 388
  moral status of, 366–369
  ownership of, 378
  personhood of, 460
  preimplantation
    chromosomal and genetic diagnosis in, 459
    disposition of, 358
  rights of, 356–357
  sale of, 383
  seen on transvaginal ultrasound, 73–74
  storage of, 368–369
Embryo donation, 384
Embryo flushing, 375
Embryogenesis. *See also* Teratogenesis
  effects of experimental environmental manipulation on, 114–115
  relative timing of malformations in, 155
  toxic effects during, 155
Embryo research, 6, 369, 377, 438, 459, 462
  after in vitro fertilization, questions related to, 366–369
Embryo transfer. *See also* In vitro fertilization and embryo transfer
  research on fertilized embryos not used for, 459
Encephalocele, ultrasound presentation of, 64, 66

Endometrial thickness
  measurement of, 80
  patterns of, 80
Environmental agents, teratogenicity, 131–132
Enzyme deficiency, diagnosis from CVS, 30
Epichlorohydrin
  exposure, monitoring using urine analysis, 166
  mutagenicity, 163
Erb's palsy, and midforceps delivery, 318
Erythromycin, teratogenicity, 119
Esophageal atresia, plus tracheoesophageal fistula, timing of, in embryogenesis, 155
Estimated fetal weight, determination of, 218, 219
Estrogen and progestogen combinations, teratogenicity, 122–123
Estrogens, teratogenicity, 122
Ethambutol, safety in pregnancy, 120–121
Ethanol
  administration, 214
  to arrest labor, 144
  clinical efficacy, 214
  dosage, 214
  mechanism of action, 214
  as perinatal behavioral toxin, 155
  in prevention of preterm delivery, 211–212
  ratio of concentration in breast milk vs. maternal blood, 158
  reproductive toxicity, 154
  side-effects, 214
Ether, reproductive toxicity, 154
Ethical guidance, in reproduction, 6–7
Ethical issues, in management of data from predictive testing, 89–90
Ethical principles, in multiple gestations, 273–275
Ethics
  argument of double effect, 475–476
  descriptive, 4
  fetal, countertrends in, 6
  of fetal therapy, 438–445
  normative, 4
  and reproductive technologies, 4–6
  two-tier approach to, 54
Ethics Advisory Board, 450, 455
  lack of, consequences of, 455–456
  recommendations on control of reproductive technologies, 377
Ethionamide, teratogenicity, 120
Ethoxyethanol, reproductive toxicity, 161–162
Ethylene dibromide, reproductive toxicity, 163
Ethylene oxide
  correlation of genotoxicity with epidemiologic findings, 165
  exposure, and spontaneous abortion, 168
  OSHA standards for exposure to, 152
  reproductive toxicity, 154
Ethylnitrosobiuret, as transplacental carcinogen, 156
Ethylnitrosourea, as transplacental carcinogen, 156
Ethylvinylnitrosamine, as transplacental carcinogen, 157
Eugenic genetic engineering, 430
Eugenics, 380, 381
Euthanasia, decision-making about, historical milestones in, 481–483
Expert testimony, 338–339
  in malpractice suits, 344–345
External cephalic version
  in breech presentation, 279, 283–284
  definition of, 279
External genital masculinization, prevention of, in congenital adrenal hyperplasia, 404–405
Extracorporeal membrane oxygenation, in respiratory failure, 207–208

Index

Extraordinary means. *See* Heroic measures
Eye, fetal, ultrasound examination of, 75

F

Fabry's disease, prenatal diagnosis of, 23
Face, on transvaginal ultrasound, 75
Facial defects, ultrasound presentation of, 61, 62
Facial nerve injury, and midforceps delivery, 318
Facial palsy, and midforceps delivery, 318
Factor IX deficiency, prenatal diagnosis of, 26
Factor X deficiency, prenatal diagnosis of, 26
Factor XIIIA, prenatal diagnosis of, 26
Failure to thrive, alcohol-related, 142–143
Fairness, 6
  in fetal diagnosis, 6
Familial high-density lipoprotein deficiency, prenatal diagnosis of, 23
Familial hypercholesterolemia
  predictive genetic testing for, 85–86
  prenatal diagnosis of, 23
Familial lipoid adrenal hyperplasia, prenatal diagnosis of, 23
Family forms, alternative, 560
Family size, limitation of, 555, 559–560
Fanconi anemia
  diagnosis of, 20
  inheritance of, 20
  prenatal diagnosis of, 26
Fanconi's pancytopenia, 76
Farber's lipogranulomatosis, prenatal diagnosis of, 23
Father
  interests of
    in abortion, 315
    upon brain death of pregnant wife, 315
  rights of
    in abortion, 308–309
    upon brain death of pregnant wife, 308–309
Feminist movement, 561
Fenoterol, in twin gestation, 254–255
Fertilization, failures of, 388
Fetal alcohol effects, 140
Fetal alcohol syndrome, 124, 140, 522
  behavioral abnormalities in, estimating incidence of, 141–142
  cost of, 140
  diagnostic criteria, 140
  genetic contributions to, 141
  incidence of, 140
  partial, 140
  prevention, 144–146
  risk of, problems in assessment of, 140–142
Fetal anomalies. *See also* Congenital anomalies
  management of, 70
  prenatal diagnosis of, 220
  ultrasound detection of, 60–70
Fetal assessment, in higher-order multiple gestations, 261
Fetal biometry, abnormal, ultrasound presentation of, 67–69
Fetal biophysical scoring, 218–220
Fetal blood sampling, technique, 30
Fetal breathing movements
  absence of, 209, 216
  significance of, 218–220
Fetal demise, single, in twin gestation, 246–248
Fetal diagnosis and therapy. *See also* Prenatal diagnosis
  ethics of, 5
  research in, 456–458
Fetal distress
  cesarean delivery with, 330–332
  diagnosis of, 330

  incidence of, 330
  as issue in malpractice suits, 340
Fetal heartbeat, on transvaginal ultrasound, 73
Fetal heart disease
  diagnosis and management of, 412–419
  research on, future of, 419
Fetal heart rate
  antepartum
    testing, 218
    usefulness in monitoring fetus in brain-dead mother, 305
  indications for monitoring, 216
  intrapartum, 206, 221
  monitoring, 340–341
  pathological, 184
  patterns of, physiology of, 183–184
  and respiratory distress syndrome, 220–221
  significance of, 218
Fetal hydantoin syndrome, 127–128
Fetal loss
  causes of, 406
  detection of, 158
Fetal malformations, 521
Fetal-maternal conflicts, 441–442
Fetal motion, abnormalities, on ultrasound, 68–70
Fetal movement, significance of, 218
Fetal phenytoin syndrome, 103
Fetal presentation, in very low birth weight, and obstetric management, 221–222
Fetal protection policies, 151
Fetal research, 433, 516
  controversy about, 449
  equal protection of fetus in, 459–463
  ethical reasoning about, 452–453
  federal regulations for, 449–465
    rationale for, 451–452
  in first trimester, 463
  minimal risk in, 464–465
  objectionable, examples of, 451
  recommendations and restrictions on, 454–455
  states having statutes prohibiting, 358
  substantive and procedural ethical issues, 452–454
Fetal scalp *p*H determination, 331–332
Fetal surgery, 395–402, 433, 438, 530–531. *See also* Fetal therapy
  extrauterine, 436
  malformations that may require, 396
  maternal role in, 13
  research on, need for, 401–402
Fetal therapy, 3, 395–445, 529–530. *See also* Prenatal therapy
  case selection for, 440
  coerced, 441–442
  consent process for, 440
  considerations prior to, 395–396
  by direct access to fetus, 399
  ethical issues in, 438–445
    dominant approach in, 438–439
    guidelines for, 441
  experimental
    early ethical consensus on, 439–445
    ethical issues in, 438–445
    in multiple gestations, 441
    peer or group review, 440
  fetal selection criteria, 395–396
  legal issues in, 431–437
  maternal refusal of, public policy and, 444–445
  medical, 403–411
  nutritional, 410
  pharmacologic, 410
    in congenital adrenal hyperplasia, 404–405
  planning, timing of prenatal diagnosis for, 42

Fetal therapy (continued)
  refusal of, 441–442
  research on, 458
  surgical. See Fetal surgery
Fetal trimethadione syndrome, 128
Fetal valproate syndrome, 128
Fetal wastage
  in autoimmune disease, 391
  in reproductive toxicity, 152–153
Fetoscopy, 36, 220, 455
  risk of, 30
  uses of, 37–38
Fetus
  born, 501–503
  emergent beliefs about, 563–564
  ethical perception of, 442
  humanity of, 461
  legal protection of, 235–236
  legal status of, 235, 307–308, 314, 535
  moral status of, 272–273, 314, 367
  as patient, 13, 314
  as perfect allograft, 387
  rights of, 526, 534
  social value placed on
    long-term trends in, 554–559
    recent trends in, 559–563
  state's interest in protecting, 536–537
  wanted vs. unwanted, 554, 557, 563
First trimester
  abortion in, vs. abortion in second trimester, 17–18
  fetal research in, 463
  laboratory diagnosis in, 29–32
  prenatal diagnosis in, 17–36
5q syndrome, prenatal diagnosis of, 27
Fluorodeoxyuridine, teratogenicity, 120
5-Fluorouracil, teratogenicity, 120
Folic acid antagonists, teratogenicity, 118
Follicle-stimulating hormone, in follicle stimulation, for in vitro fertilization, 351–352
Follicle stimulation, 350
  for in vitro fertilization, 351–352
  monitoring, 352
Follicular measurements, ultrasonographic, 79
Follicular volume, calculation of, 79
Forbes disease, prenatal diagnosis of, 21
Forceps, use with breech presentation, 281
Formaldehyde, reproductive toxicity, 161–162
45,X. See Turner syndrome
46,XX/47,XXX, females, offspring of, chromosomes of, 96
47,XXX, females, offspring of, chromosomes of, 95–96
47,XXY. See Klinefelter syndrome
Fragile X syndrome, 18
  diagnosis of, 18–19, 20, 26
  inheritance of, 20
  transmission of, from parent to offspring, 98–99
Freedom, 6
Fucosidosis, prenatal diagnosis of, 23
Furylfuramide, as transplacental carcinogen, 157

G

Galactokinase deficiency, prenatal diagnosis of, 21
Galactosemia
  prenatal diagnosis of, 21
  prenatal therapy for, 409
Galactose-1-phosphate uridyl transferase deficiency, prenatal therapy for, 409
Galactosylceramide lipidosis, prenatal diagnosis of, 23

Gamete donors, limitations on, 380
Gamma-aminobutyric acid aminotransferase deficiency, prenatal diagnosis of, 21
Gamma globulin, effects on fetal immune system, 176
Gamma-glutamyl synthetase deficiency, prenatal diagnosis of, 21
Gamma-glutamyl transpeptidase deficiency, prenatal diagnosis of, 21
Gangliosidoses, prenatal diagnosis of, 23
Gastroschisis, 221
  fetal surgery for, 396
  perinatal management of, 333
  ultrasound presentation of, 77
Gaucher's disease, prenatal diagnosis of, 23
Gender roles, changes in, 557–558
Gene therapy, 410, 421–430, 567
  expectations for human trials, 425
  germ-line, 427–429
  pediatric
    criteria for successful protocols, 423–425
    delivery, 423–424
    expression, 424
    safety, 424–425
Genetic diagnosis, in preimplantation embryo, 459
Genetic engineering
  enhancement, 429
  eugenic, 430
Genetic screening tests, public policy issues in, 189–190
Genetic therapy, 369
Gentamicin, ototoxicity, 120
Germinal material
  extracorporeal, issues related to, 376
  ownership of, 376–377
Gestational age. See also Appropriate for gestational age infant; Prematurity; Small for gestational age infant
  and neonatal survival, 200–202
Gestational sac
  abnormalities, diagnosis, by transvaginal ultrasound, 73
  double contour, on ultrasound, 72
  earliest ultrasound detection of, 72
Gleitman v. Cosgrove, 376
Glucose-6-phosphate dehydrogenase deficiency, prenatal diagnosis of, 21
Glucose-6-phosphate dehydrogenase deficiency, prenatal therapy for, 410
Glucose phosphate isomerase deficiency, prenatal diagnosis of, 26
Glutaric aciduria, prenatal diagnosis of, 21
Glutathine synthetase, prenatal diagnosis of, 21
Glutathione synthetase deficiency, prenatal therapy for, 410
Glycerol kinase deficiency, prenatal diagnosis of, 21, 27
Glycinemia, ketotic, type I, prenatal diagnosis of, 21
Glycogen storage disease, prenatal diagnosis of, 21
GM_1 gangliosidosis, generalized, prenatal diagnosis of, 23
GM_2 gangliosidosis, adult onset, prenatal diagnosis of, 23
Goiter, neonatal, 123–124
Government
  involvement in health care, 10
  as purchaser of health care, 515
Government interest, legitimate and compelling, 540
Government intervention
  in doctor-patient relationship, 513–514
  in health care, 509–518
    historical overview of, 510–514
    legal aspects of, 514–515
    and political and economic theories, 510–511
  in personal health care, through insurance programs, 517–518
  in practice of medicine, 486–487
  in provision of personal health care, 511–513

Gray syndrome, 119
Great vessels, transposition of, timing of, in embryogenesis, 155
Griswold v. Connecticut, 309
Grodin v. Grodin, 432, 524–525
Growth, effects of alcohol on, 142–143
Growth hormone deficiency, prenatal diagnosis of, 26

H

Habitual abortion
  definition of, 388
  unexplained, 387–388
Hair dyes, correlation of genotoxicity with epidemiologic findings, 165
Halogenated hydrocarbons, reproductive toxicity, 162–163
Haloperidol, teratogenicity, 125, 126
Halothane
  correlation of genotoxicity with epidemiologic findings, 165
  reproductive toxicity, 154, 167
Handicapped
  care of, 486
  definition of, 486
  federal regulation of treatment of, 472, 483
  nontreatment of, 495–496
  treatment of, 494
Handicapped Infant Hotline, 483, 517
Harrison bladder catheter, 399
Harris v. Macrae, 543
Harvard Community Health Plan, coverage of in vitro fertilization costs, controversy about, 191
Head, fetal, on transvaginal ultrasound, 74–75
Health, as public good, 511
Health beliefs, and technology, 13–14
Health care
  constraints on entry of sellers or providers or products in, 513
  consumer information issues in, 513–514
  consumer sovereignty issues in, 513–514
  government intervention in, 10, 509–518
  moral and religious issues in, 11
  payment policies, designed to influence behavior, 518
  political involvement in, 10–11
  postponability of, 514
  self-help movement in, 561–562
  social values in, 514
  supply control in, 515–516
  unevenness of risk in, 514
Health care costs
  control efforts, 188
  future directions in, 190–191
  recent developments in, 188
Health care delivery, recent developments in, 187–189
Health care expenditures, efforts to control, 512–513
Health care financing, 517–518
Health insurance, 517–518
  effects on health care delivery, 188–189
  future directions in, 190–192
Health maintenance organizations, 188, 512, 518
Health Research Extension Act of 1985, 450, 459
Hearing loss, in very low birth weight infants, 224
Heart disease. *See* Congenital heart disease; Congestive heart failure; Dysrhythmias; Fetal heart disease
Heart transplantation, 469
  neonatal, 419
Heavy metals, reproductive toxicity, 159–161
Hemangioma, 333
Heme metabolism disorders, prenatal diagnosis of, 25

Hemoglobin defects, prenatal diagnosis of, 26
Hemophilia, classic, prenatal diagnosis of, 25
Hemophilia A, prenatal diagnosis of, 25
Hemophilia B, prenatal diagnosis of, 26
Heparin, safety in pregnancy, 129
Hepatitis, research, primates used for, 471
Hereditary coproporphyria, prenatal diagnosis of, 25
Hereditary methemoglobinemia, prenatal diagnosis of, 26
Hereditary persistence of fetal hemoglobin, prenatal diagnosis of, 26
Heroic measures. *See also* Treatment, ordinary vs. extraordinary
  demand for research on, 563
  ethical issues in, 313–314, 316
  social value placed on, 554
Heroin, abuse, as prematernal negligence, 528–529
Heterografts. *See also* Baby Fae
Hexachlorophene, reproductive toxicity, 154
Hexamethonium, maternal use of, effect on newborn, 130
Higher-order multiple gestations, 259–261
  antenatal care in, 260–261
  delivery in, 262
  incidence of, 259
Hill-Burton Act of 1968, 511
Histidinemia, prenatal diagnosis of, 21
Histocompatibility antigens, and fetal grafts, 473
HIV. *See* Human immunodeficiency virus
HLA. *See* Human leukocyte antigens
Hoener v. Bertinato, 235
Holoprosencephaly, ultrasound presentation of, 61, 62
Home birth, 562, 564
Homocystinuria, 75
  prenatal diagnosis of, 21
Hormones, teratogenicity, 121–124
Hospital detention, 526
  court-ordered, 444
Human chorionic gonadotropin
  administration after in vitro fertilization and embryo transfer, 354
  beta-subunit, 388
  levels, in pregnancy after in vitro fertilization, 354
Human chorionic gonadotropins, in follicle stimulation, for in vitro fertilization, 351–352
Human experimentation, 516
  immunologic therapy as, 390, 392–393
Human immunodeficiency virus, 517
Human immunodeficiency virus, transfer of, during RhIg administration, 177
Human leukocyte antigens
  in congenital adrenal hyperplasia, 404–405
  in spontaneous abortion, 389–390
Human menopausal gonadotropins, 79
  in follicle stimulation, for in vitro fertilization, 351–352
  in treatment of infertility, multiple gestations with, 269
Hunter syndrome, prenatal diagnosis of, 24
Huntington's disease
  DNA marker for, 87
  linkage analysis in, 31
  predictive genetic testing for, 85, 86–88, 91
  prenatal diagnosis of, 26, 87
  presymptomatic diagnosis, ethical considerations in, 32
  presymptomatic testing for, 40
Hurler syndrome
  diagnosis of, 20
  prenatal diagnosis of, 24
Hyaline membrane disease, 207, 223
Hydantoin, teratogenicity, 75
Hyde Amendment, 536–537
Hydrocephalus, 221
  associated midline CNS malformations, 400

Hydrocephalus (continued)
  cesarean delivery in, 333
  congenital
    evaluation for in utero surgery, 400
    management of, 400–401
  obstructive, fetal surgery for, 396
  ultrasound presentation of, 64, 65
Hydronephrosis, 221. See also Urinary tract obstruction
  obstructive
    animal model for, 402
    fetal surgery for, 396
Hydrops fetalis
  nonimmune, 417–418
  prevention of, 403–404
  ultrasound presentation of, 62–63, 65
4-Hydroxybutyric acidemia, prenatal diagnosis of, 21
21-Hydroxylase deficiency
  diagnosis of, 20
  management of, 403
  prenatal diagnosis of, 24
3-Hydroxy-3-methyl glutaryl CoA lyase deficiency, prenatal diagnosis of, 22
17α-Hydroxyprogesterone, in prevention of preterm delivery, 211
3-Hydroxyxanthine, as transplacental carcinogen, 157
Hyperactivity, alcohol-related, 143–144
Hyperammonemia, postnatal, prevention of, 410
Hypercholesterolemia
  fetal therapy for, 410
  predictive genetic testing for, 85–86
Hyperglycemia, maternal, fetal cardiac effects of, 417
Hyperimidodipeptiduria, prenatal diagnosis of, 22
Hyperlysinemia, persistent form, prenatal diagnosis of, 22
Hyperphenylalanemia
  type I, prenatal diagnosis of, 22
  type IV, prenatal diagnosis of, 22
  type V, prenatal diagnosis of, 22
  type VIII, prenatal diagnosis of, 22
Hypertelorism, 75
  ultrasound presentation of, 68–69
Hypertension. See also Preeclampsia
  and intrauterine growth retardation, 204
Hypervalinemia, prenatal diagnosis of, 22
Hypoglycemic agents, safety in pregnancy, 124
Hypoplastic left heart syndrome, 419, 469
  diagnosis of, 70
  heterograft experiment in, 468. See also Baby Fae
Hypospadias, timing of, in embryogenesis, 155
Hypotelorism, ultrasound presentation of, 68
Hypoxia, fetal, 206

I

I-cell disease, prenatal diagnosis of, 24
Idoxuridine, teratogenicity, 120
IgA deficiency, congenital, and reaction to RhIg administration, 176–177
Immune system, manipulation of, dangers of, 391–392
Immune system disorders, prenatal diagnosis of, 26
Immunologic therapy, 387–393
  approaches to, 390–391
  mouse model for, 390–391
  rationale for, 388–390
  recommendations for, 392–393
Imuran. See Azathioprine
Inborn errors of amino acid metabolism, prenatal diagnosis of, 21–23
Incest, transmission of autosomal recessive disorder in, 98

Inchoate illness
  definition of, 503
  ethical issues concerning, 503–505
  and terminal illness, analogy between, 503–504
Incompetent patient, legal issues concerning, 489, 491, 492, 500
Individual liberty. See Autonomy, principle of
Indomethacin
  administration, 215
  clinical efficacy, 215
  dosage, 215
  mechanism of action, 215
  side-effects, 215
Infant Bioethical Review Boards, 484
Infant Care Review Committees, 496
Infantile gangliosidosis GM_2, prenatal diagnosis of, 23
Infant mortality, decline in, 555–556
Infection, subclinical, and premature delivery, 209, 216
Infertility
  demand for medical services for overcoming, 374
  perceived rates of, as function of postponed childbearing, 560–561
  prevalence of, 374
  transvaginal ultrasound in, 78–82
  unexplained, 387–388
Informed consent, 540
  for cesaraean delivery of very low birth weight infant, 239–241
  from family of brain-dead mother, 305
  for selective trial of labor, in breech presentation, 284
  for sterilization of mentally retarded patient, 111–112
Inhaled anesthetics, occupational exposure to, and pregnancy loss, 129
Inheritance rights
  of fetus, 357
  of offspring of alternative birth technologies, 380
Injury
  legal definition of, 337–338
  prematernally induced, liability for, 524–525
  prenatal, 523–524
Inner ear abnormalities, with pigmentary abnormalities, animal model for, 408
Innovative therapy, vs. research, 440
In re L.H.R., 493
Institute of Medicine, Council on Health Care Technology, 190
Institutional Review Board, 433, 440
Instrumental delivery. See Midforceps delivery
Insulin, safety in pregnancy, 124
Intelligence, long-term, after midforceps delivery, 323
Intrauterine growth retardation, 116, 233. See also Low birth weight; Very low birth weight
  causes of, 202–204
  and congenital anomalies, 205
  fetal anomalies with, 220
  and maternal serum alpha-fetoprotein elevation, 49
  and maternal smoking, 124–125
  and multiple gestation, 244
  and prematurity, 202
  and survival, 202
  in twin gestation, assessment of, 251–253
  type I, 203–205, 233
    prognosis for, 233–234
  type II, 204–205, 234
    prognosis for, 234
Intraventricular hemorrhage
  incidence of, 208
  pathogenesis of, 208
  with perinatal asphyxia, 205

prognosis for, 208, 209
and type of delivery, 222
in very low birth weight infant, 208–209
In utero therapy. *See* Fetal surgery; Fetal therapy
In vitro fertilization and embryo transfer, 3, 78, 349–371, 374, 375
  average age of patients, 351
  clinical and research aspects of, 349–354
  clinical applications of, 349
  cost of, 366
  culture media for, 353
  current methods of, 350–354
  DHHS regulations about, 356
  donor, 354
  embryonic cleavage for, 353
  embryo transfer step, 353–354
  ethical issues in, 361–366
  fertilization for, 353
  follicle stimulation for, 351–352
  gamete preparation for, 353
  government regulation in public interest, 359–360
  history of, 349–350
  indications for, 388
  information on biologic identity of parents, 365
  insurance coverage of costs of, controversy about, 191–192
  legal issues in, 356–360
  local and state regulation of, 356
  miscarriage rate in, 351, 354, 365–366
  moral acceptability
    with donated gametes and embryo research, 365–366
    with donated gametes and embryos, 364–365
    with married couple donors and no research, 363–364
  number of embryos used, 353–354
  oocyte retrieval for, 352–353
  transvaginal ultrasound in, 80–82
  patient selection for, 350–351
  precycle evaluation for, 351
  pregnancy management with, 354
  pregnancy rate per transfer, 354, 366
  preliminary counseling for, 351
  research, 459, 516
  rights and liabilities of physician and hospital, 358–359
  rights of children born consequent to, 365
  rights of embryo in, 356–357
  rights of parents or donor in, 357–358
  success rates for, 351
  as unnatural act, 361–363
Iodides, inorganic, teratogenicity, 124
Iodine
  radioactive, teratogenicity, 124
  teratogenicity, 123
Ionizing radiation, mutagenicity, 164–165
IQ, at age 4
  effect of type of delivery and socioeconomic status on, 321–322
  effect of type of delivery on, 319–321
  prenatal and delivery variables affecting, 319–320
  relationship between type of delivery and socioeconomic status and, 321–322
Iron, excess, as perinatal behavioral toxin, 155
Isoniazid, safety in pregnancy, 120
Isopropyl-a-2-methylhydrazine-p-tolumid, as transplacental carcinogen, 157
Isotretinoin, teratogenicity, 417
Isovalinic acidemia, prenatal diagnosis of, 22
Isoxsuprine, in prevention of preterm delivery, 212

J

Jefferson v. Griffin Spalding County Hospital Authority, 236–238, 435–436, 525–526, 530
Justice
  in fetal diagnosis, 6
  principle of, 5, 274, 379, 511

K

Kaiser, coverage of costs of in vitro fertilization, 191–192
Kanamycin, ototoxicity, 120
Karyotypes, parental, normal, and risk of cytogenetic abnormality, 18
Karyotyping
  from CVS cell culture, 29–30
  obtaining fetal tissue for, 37
Kepone, reproductive toxicity, 154, 162, 163
3-Ketothiolase deficiency, prenatal diagnosis of, 22
Ketotic hyperglycinemia, prenatal diagnosis of, 22
Keynes, John Maynard, 510
Kidney
  normal, ultrasound presentation of, 61, 63
  polycystic, ultrasound diagnosis of, 68, 77
Kidney circumference–abdominal circumference ratio, on ultrasound, significance of, 68
Kielland's forceps, outcome for infants delivered by, 318–319
Klinefelter syndrome, prenatal diagnosis of, 42
Krabbe's disease, prenatal diagnosis of, 23
Kristellar pressure, 281

L

Labor and delivery. *See also* Cesarean delivery; Delivery options; Midforceps delivery; Preterm delivery; Vaginal delivery
  active management of, 327
  with breech presentation, 278–283
  difficulties of, anticipated in mentally retarded patient, 104
  and fetal hypoxia, 206
  in higher-order multiple gestations, 262
  hypoxia in, 206
  intermittent auscultation during, 330–331
    vs. unmonitored labor, 330–331
  in twin gestation, 256
  variables in, effects on long-term intellectual development, 319–322
  with very low birth weight, 220–223
Labor trial, after previous cesarean section, 328–329
Lactation, reproductive toxins excreted during, 157–158
Lactosyl ceramidosis, prenatal diagnosis of, 23
Laparoscopy, for oocyte retrieval, 352
Lawsuits. *See* Malpractice suits
Lead
  detection of toxic effects, 158
  mutagenicity, 163
  OSHA standards for exposure to, 152
  as perinatal behavioral toxin, 155
  ratio of concentration in breast milk vs. maternal blood, 158
  reproductive toxicity, 154, 159–161
Lead plus cadmium, mutagenicity, 163
Legal analysis, 8–9
Legal issues, in human reproduction, 372–385
Legal methodology, 9
Legal system, American, 8–9
Legislatures, 8–9
Legitimacy, of child conceived by artificial insemination, 357–358, 365, 378

582 Index

Lens dislocation, disorders associated with, 75
Lesch-Nyhan syndrome, prenatal diagnosis of, 25
Leukocyte immunization, for treatment of habitual abortion and infertility, 390–393
Life, society's interest in preserving, 460–461, 490–491, 525
Limb defects, unilateral vs. bilateral, 76
Limbs, fetal, transvaginal ultrasound of, 75–76
Lindane, reproductive toxicity of, 154
Linkage analysis
  for prenatal molecular diagnosis, 30
  technique, 31–32
Lipid metabolism disorders, prenatal diagnosis of, 23
Lipomyelomeningocele, 333
Lips, on transvaginal ultrasound, 75
Literature, and risk management, 344
Lithium
  ratio of concentration in breast milk vs. maternal blood, 158
  reproductive toxicity, 159, 160
  teratogenicity, 125, 126, 416–417
Liver phosphorylase deficiency, type VIII, prenatal diagnosis of, 21
Liver transplantation, 469
Lövsett maneuver, 280
Low birth weight. *See also* Very low birth weight
  alcohol-related, 142
  and maternal occupational exposure to anesthetics, 167–168
Low birth weight infant
  breech presentation of, 332
    management of, 289–291
  cesarean section for, 332
  ethical issues concerning, 502–505
LSD, teratogenicity, 125
LSD-25, cytogenetic effects on meiotic chromosomes of oocytes, 164
Lung maturity, fetal
  amniotic fluid phospholipids as indicators of, 216, 218
  assessment, in twin gestation, 256
  effect of corticosteroids on, 217–218
  in higher-order multiple gestations, 262
Lupus anticoagulant, 391
Lysosomal storage disease
  fetal therapy for, 410
  prenatal diagnosis of, 23–24

M

Magnesium sulfate
  administration, 214
  clinical efficacy, 214
  dosage, 214
  mechanism of action, 214
  in prevention of preterm delivery, 212
  side-effects, 214
Maher v. Roe, 536
Major histocompatibility complex, in rodent reproduction, 388–390
Malahoff case, 378, 382
Malpractice, and standard of care, 193–194, 196–197
Malpractice suits, 337, 515
  damages awarded in, 337
  defense of, key issues in, 340–345
  and risk-management, 342–344
Managed care insurance, 188
Manganese, metabolic abnormalities, fetal therapy for, 407–408
Mannosidosis, prenatal diagnosis of, 23
Maple syrup urine disease, prenatal diagnosis of, 22
Marfan syndrome, 75
  prenatal diagnosis of, 25

Marijuana, teratogenicity, 125
Maroteaux-Larriy syndrome, prenatal diagnosis of, 24
Masculinization, fetal, and prenatal androgen exposure, 121–122
Maternal age
  as indication for amniocentesis, 38, 39
  and risk of congenital heart disease, 77
  and risk of fetal cytogenetic disorders, 18–19
Maternal serum AFP. *See* Alpha-fetoprotein, maternal serum
Maternal weight, and maternal serum alpha-fetoprotein level, 49
Matter of Hofbauer, 494, 497
Matter of Storar, 500–501
Mauriceau-Smellie-Veit maneuver, 280–281, 287
Meclizine, safety in pregnancy, 129
Meconium aspiration
  intrauterine, 406
  prevention of, 223
Medicaid, 511–513, 518
  abortion funding, state regulation of, 543
  compensation for expenses of pregnancy and childbirth, 538, 540
    vs. denial of compensation for abortion, 540
  denial of payment for abortion, 515, 536
Medical feasibility, legal definition of, 489–490
Medical records, legal issues concerning, 343–344
Medicare, 511–513, 518
Medicare Prospective Payment System, 188, 191
Medicolegal issues, and emerging technology, 192–193
Medium-chain acyl CoE-A dehydrogenase deficiency, prenatal diagnosis of, 24
Mendelian disorders
  prenatal diagnosis of, 19–20
  risk factors for, 19–20
  risk of, as indication for amniocentesis, 38
  transmission of, from parent to offspring, 97–100
Meningomyelocele
  nontreatment of, 494
  timing of, in embryogenesis, 155
  ultrasound presentation of, 64, 67
Menkes' disease, prenatal diagnosis of, 25
Menkes' kinky hair syndrome, prenatal therapy for, 408
Menopause, onset of, and smoking, 162
Mentally retarded
  contraception for, 106–107
  sterilization of, 106–107
    American College of Obstetricians and Gynecologists Ethics Committee statement on, 108, 110–113
Mental retardation
  after midforceps delivery, 319
  alcohol-related, 144
  in fetal alcohol syndrome, 141–142
  in fragile X syndrome, 18
  idiopathic
    recurrence risk, 99–100
    transmission of, from parent to offspring, 99–100
  incidence of childbearing in, 102
  labor and delivery in, 104
  management of reproductive health in, principles of, 102–103
  medical concerns of prenatal care in, 103
  normalization, 106–107
  pregnancy in, management of, 101–108
  pregnancy termination in, 104–105
  reproductive health concerns in, 101
  sex education and counseling in, 106–107
  sexual abuse prevention in, 107
  transmission of, from parent to offspring, 104

transmission of genetic disorders from parent to offspring in, 94–100
Meprobamate
　cytogenetic effects on meiotic chromosomes of oocytes, 164
　teratogenicity, 126
6-Mercaptopurine, teratogenic risk of, 118
Mercury
　cytogenetic effects on meiotic chromosomes of oocytes, 164
　mutagenicity, 163
　organic, teratogenicity, 131
　ratio of concentration in breast milk vs. maternal blood, 158
　reproductive toxicity, 159, 160, 161
Metabolic acidosis, with fetal hypoxia, 206
Metabolic defects, genetically determined, medical management of, 404–405
Metachromatic leukodystrophy, prenatal diagnosis of, 24
Metal metabolism disorders, prenatal diagnosis of, 25
Methadone, ratio of concentration in breast milk vs. maternal blood, 158
Methimazole, teratogenicity, 123
Methotrexate
　cytogenetic effects on meiotic chromosomes of oocytes, 164
　teratogenicity, 118
Methylazoxymethanol
　as perinatal behavioral toxin, 155
　as transplacental carcinogen, 156
1-Methyl-2-benzylhydrazine, as transplacental carcinogen, 157
Methylbutylnitrosamine, as transplacental carcinogen, 157
3-Methylcholanthrene
　reproductive toxicity, 162
　as transplacental carcinogen, 157
3-Methylcrotinyl glycinuria, prenatal diagnosis of, 22
Methylene tetrahydrofolate reductase deficiency, prenatal diagnosis of, 22
Methylmalonic acidemia
　fetal therapy for, 406–407
　prenatal diagnosis of, 22
Methyl mercury, as perinatal behavioral toxin, 155
Methylmethane sulfonate
　cytogenetic effects on meiotic chromosomes of oocytes, 164
　as transplacental carcinogen, 156
Methylnitrosourea, as transplacental carcinogen, 156
Methylnitrosourethane, as transplacental carcinogen, 156
Methylphenidate, for treatment of hyperactivity associated with FAS, 143–144
Methyltetrahydrofolate methyl transferase deficiency, prenatal diagnosis of, 22
Metronidazole, teratogenicity, 120
Metronidazole therapy, exposure to toxins in, monitoring using urine analysis, 166
Microcephaly, diagnosis of, 67
Microwaves, as perinatal behavioral toxin, 155
Midforceps delivery, 317–325
　associated risk factors, 317–323
　controversy about, 317
　immediate outcome with, 318–319
　indications for, 323–325
　legal issues in, 342
　long-term intellectual development after, 323
　long-term minimal brain dysfunction after, 322
　long-term neurobehavioral outcome with, 319–322
　maternal morbidity with, 318
　neonatal morbidity with, 318–319
　role of, in obstetric care, 324–325
　studies of, 317, 321–322
　　assessment of, 323–325
　vs. cesarean delivery, 324–325
Midline fusion disorder. See also Cleft lip and palate
Mill, John Stuart, 510

Mineral metabolism, abnormalities, fetal therapy for, 407–409
Minimal brain dysfunction, long-term, after midforceps delivery, 322
Minimal risk, 450, 451
　definition of, 455, 464–465
Minors, time limits for filing lawsuits, Illinois statute on, 337
Missed abortion, diagnosis, by transvaginal ultrasound, 73
Mitomycin C, teratogenicity, 120
Mixed lymphocyte culture, hyporesponsiveness, 390–391
Molar pregnancy, after clomiphene-induced ovulation, 122
Molecular disorders, diagnosis from CVS, 30–32
Monosodium glutamate, as perinatal behavioral toxin, 155
Moral codes, 510
Morality, and health care, 11
Morquio syndrome, prenatal diagnosis of, 24
Mosaicism
　parental, and risk to fetus, 18
　parental germinal, 95
Mother. See also Dead mother
　legal protection of, 236–237
　rights of, vs. fetus's rights, 431
MSAFP. See Alpha-fetoprotein, maternal serum
Mucolipidoses
　type I, prenatal diagnosis of, 24
　type II, prenatal diagnosis of, 24
　type III, prenatal diagnosis of, 24
　type IV, prenatal diagnosis of, 24
Mucopolysaccharidoses
　prenatal diagnosis of, 24
　type I, prenatal diagnosis of, 24
　type II, prenatal diagnosis of, 24
　type III, prenatal diagnosis of, 24
　type IV, prenatal diagnosis of, 24
　type VI, prenatal diagnosis of, 24
　type VII, prenatal diagnosis of, 24
Multiple carboxylase deficiency
　biotin-responsive, 406
　fetal therapy for, 405–406
　prenatal diagnosis of, 22
Multiple gestation, 242–261. See also Higher-order multiple gestations; Twin gestation
　bed rest in, 213
　early diagnosis of, 243
　ethical issues in, 269–271
　experimental fetal therapy in, 441
　and intrauterine growth retardation, 204, 244
　and prematurity, 243–244
　screening tests for, 243
　selective termination in, 269–271
　　and abortion rights, 272–273
Multiple sulfatase deficiency, prenatal diagnosis of, 24
Murder, of fetus, legal definition of, 357
Muscle disorders, prenatal diagnosis of, 25
Musculoskeletal disorders, pregnancy in, 103
Mutagenic compounds, 163–166
Mutagenicity, 163–166. See also Teratogenesis
Myelomeningocele, 333
　nontreatment of, criteria for, 482
Myotonic dystrophy
　linkage analysis in, 32
　prenatal diagnosis of, 25, 32

N

Naphthalene, teratogenicity, 131
Narcotics
　maternal use of, and obstetrical complications, 125
　neonatal withdrawal from, 125

National Center for Health Care Technology, 189–190
National Collaborative Perinatal Project, 319–322
National Commission for the Protection of Human Subjects of Biomedical and Behavioral Research, 449, 451–452
Naujoks maneuver, 280
Needle aspiration, ultrasound-guided, 37–38
Neglect, medical, 499
Negligence
  legal definition of, 339–340
  prematernal, 527–528
    liability for, 529
  prenatal, 434
  professional, 193, 196–197
Neomort, 312
Neomycin, ototoxicity, 120
Neonatal intensive care
  costs of, 486
  ethical issues concerning, 502
  infants admitted to, categories of, 483
Neonatal mortality
  and prematurity, 200–202
  and very low birth weight, 200–202
Neonatal survival, conditions with very low chance of, 221
Neonatologists, decision making about neonatal intensive care, 486–487
Neural tissue transplants, 469
Neural tube defects
  cesarean delivery in, 333
  early diagnosis of, 29
  embryology of, 64
  failure to screen for, medicolegal risks of, 52
  incidence of, 44–45
  moral status of fetus or newborn afflicted with, 55–56
  prenatal diagnosis of, 44, 45
  previous, as indication for amniocentesis, 38
  recurrence of, 45
  treatment of, ethical issues in, 56–57
  ultrasound presentation of, 64–68
Neurologic damage, risk of, and delivery options, 341–342
Neurologic disorders
  alcohol-related, 143–144
  in very low birth weight infants, 224
Newborn, needs and rights of, 489
Nickel, reproductive toxicity, 159, 160
Niemann-Pick disease, prenatal diagnosis of, 24
Nifedipine
  administration, 215
  clinical efficacy, 215
  dosage, 215
  mechanism of action, 215
  in prevention of premature delivery, 212
  side-effects, 215
Niridazole exposure, monitoring using urine analysis, 166
Nitrofen, teratogenicity, 158
Nitrogen mustard, teratogenicity, 118
4-Nitroquinoline 1-oxide, as transplacental carcinogen, 157
Nitrosohexamethyleneimine, as transplacental carcinogen, 157
Nitrosopiperidine, as transplacental carcinogen, 157
Nitrous oxide
  correlation of genotoxicity with epidemiologic findings, 165
  reproductive toxicity, 167
No discernible risk, 450
Non-ketotic hyperglycinemia, prenatal diagnosis of, 22
Non-maleficence, 378
  principle of, 5, 274
Nonstress test, 216, 218
  in twin gestation, 253
Nontreatment, 500. See also Euthanasia
  case law concerning, 489–495

consent issues in, 493–494, 498
criminal liability in, 531
decision making in
  aids for, 483–484
  historical milestones in, 481–485
  medical aspects of, 483–485
  neonatologist's viewpoint of, 486–487
  problems in, 485–486
  process of, 484–485
ethical issues in, 488–501, 501–505
medical issues in, 481–487
Nont's syndrome, and intestinal atresia, nontreatment of, 488
Norethindrone, reproductive toxicity, 167
Norrie disease, prenatal diagnosis of, 27
19-Nortestosterone, teratogenicity, 121–122
Nucleoside phosphorylase deficiency with immunodeficiency, prenatal diagnosis of, 25
Nutrition, artificial, 499–500

O

Obstetric complications, medical vs. legal view of, 336–337
Obstetric practice, standard of care in, 194–197
Occupational exposures
  data on, 150
  and female reproduction, 149–168
Occupational hazards
  assessment of, 150–152
  and employer health policies, 151–152
  and legal standards, 152
  paternal risk factors, 150–151
Occupational Safety and Health Act, 152
Occupational Safety and Health Administration, 152
Ocular albinism, 408
Oligohydramnios, 220, 221
  with urinary tract obstruction, 397
Omphalocele, 221
  fetal surgery for, 396
  perinatal management of, 333
  timing of, in embryogenesis, 155
  ultrasound presentation of, 66, 67, 77
Oocyte retrieval
  for in vitro fertilization, 352–353
  history of, 350
  for in vitro fertilization and embryo transfer, 80–82
  perurethral technique, 352
  by vaginal ultrasound, 352–353
Oral contraceptives
  cytogenetic effects on meiotic chromosomes of oocytes, 164
  for mentally retarded, 107
  teratogenicity, 121–122, 122–123
Orbital distance. See also Hypertelorism; Hypotelorism
  on ultrasound, significance of, 68–69
Organ donation, preservation of cadaver for, 312
Organochlorine insecticides, reproductive toxicity of, 157–158
Organophosphates, mutagenicity, 163
Organ procurement, 475–476
  consent of parents in, 476
  ethical issues in, 476–477
Organ transplantation
  ethical issues in, 476–477
  as fetal therapy, 411
  need for, for dying children, 469
  pediatric, 468–469
    using organs from anencephalics, 472–473
  research on, 458–459
  supply of organs for, 468–469
Ornithine-alpha-ketoacid transaminase deficiency, prenatal diagnosis of, 22

Ornithine transcarbamylase deficiency, prenatal diagnosis of, 22
Orofacial digital syndrome, 77
Orotic aciduria, prenatal diagnosis of, 25
Orphans, intentional creation of, 380
Orthoaminoazotoluene, as transplacental carcinogen, 157
Orthotoluidine, as transplacental carcinogen, 157
Osteogenesis imperfecta
  prenatal diagnosis of, 25
  type I, prenatal diagnosis of, 25
  type IV, prenatal diagnosis of, 25
Ovulation, induction of, ultrasonographic monitoring of, 78–80
Ovulation induction, chromosomal abnormalities seen after, 122
Oxidizing agents, teratogenicity, 131
5-Oxoprolinuria, prenatal diagnosis of, 22
Oxytocin
  in labor, 327, 328
    with breech presentation, 286–287
  teratogenicity, 121
Oxytocin challenge test
  controversy about, 184–185
  evolution of, as diagnostic test, 183–186
  medical applications of, 183–184
  medicolegal issues surrounding, 194–197
  in twin gestation, 253

P

Para-aminosalicylic acid, safety in pregnancy, 120
Para-aortic nodes, importance of, in rodent reproduction, 389
Parenthood
  issues concerning, 377–379
  right to, 563
Parenthood by choice, 559–560
Parenting
  instruction, for mentally retarded, 105–106
  by mentally retarded, 105–106
Parents
  prenatal rights and duties of, 432–437
  right to refuse treatment, 493–494
  role in decision making about neonatal intensive care, 484–485
Parkland Maternity Hospital, Dallas, obstetric practice at, and perinatal outcome, 327
Parturition. *See also* Labor and delivery
  factors initiating, 202
  mechanisms of, 202
Paternal age, as indication for amniocentesis, 39
Paternity, presumption of, 382
Patient's rights, 488
PCBs, reproductive toxicity, 154
PCR. *See* Polymerase chain reaction
Peer review, 518
Pelvimetry
  and breech presentation, 282–283
  x-ray, and breech presentation, 282–283
D-Penicillamine, teratogenicity, 131
Penicillin, safety during pregnancy, 119
Perchloroethylene, as perinatal behavioral toxin, 155
Perfect child, desire for, 556–557, 563
Perfectionism, parental trend toward, and legal actions, 6
Pergonal, multiple gestations with, 269
Pericardial effusion, fetal, ultrasound presentation of, 63, 65
Periventricular hemorrhage, and type of delivery, 222
Persistent vegetative state, 298
Personal health care, public support of, 511
Personhood, legal and ethical definition of, 474

Phenobarbital
  ratio of concentration in breast milk vs. maternal blood, 158
  teratogenicity, 128
Phenothiazine derivatives, teratogenicity, 125–127
1-Phenyl-3,3-diethyltriazine, as transplacental carcinogen, 157
1-Phenyl-3,3-dimethyltriazine, as transplacental carcinogen, 157
Phenylketonuria
  maternal, 116, 417, 529–530
    fetal therapy for, 404
  prenatal diagnosis of, 22
Phenytoin
  effect on fetus, 103
  reproductive toxicity, 154
  teratogenicity, 417
Phillip B case, 494
Phleomycin, cytogenetic effects on meiotic chromosomes of oocytes, 164
Phosphate, as transplacental carcinogen, 156
Phospholipids, amniotic fluid, in twin gestation, 256
o-Phthalodinitrile, mutagenicity, 163
Physical anomalies, alcohol-related, 142
Physician
  duty to unborn, 437
  prenatal rights and duties of, 432–437
  protection from liability, in nontreatment decisions, 492–493
Phytanic acid storage, prenatal diagnosis of, 23
Piazzi case, 307–310
Pierre Robin syndrome, 75
Piper forceps, use with breech presentation, 281
Pituitary steroids, teratogenicity, 121
Placenta
  monochorionic, vascular anastomoses in, 244, 246
  transfer across, 116
  ultrasound examination of, 78
Placental insufficiency, evaluation of, 183–184
Placental sulfatase deficiency, prenatal diagnosis of, 25
Placenta previa, management of, 213
Placentocentesis, in fetal heart disease, 419
Plasmapheresis, risks of, 177–178
Plutonium, reproductive toxicity, 159
Poland syndrome, 76–77
Political involvement, in health care, 10–11
Polybrominated biphenyls
  ratio of concentration in breast milk vs. maternal blood, 158
  reproductive toxicity, 162–163
Polychlorinated biphenyls
  as perinatal behavioral toxin, 155
  ratio of concentration in breast milk vs. maternal blood, 158
  reproductive toxicity, 162
Polycyclic aromatic hydrocarbons, reproductive toxicity, 154, 162–163
Polycystic kidney disease, autosomal dominant form, prenatal diagnosis of, 26
Polycystic kidney disease, late-onset, presymptomatic testing for, 40
Polydactyly, prenatal diagnosis of, 76–77
Polygenic, multifactorial disorders
  recurrence risk
    for first-degree relatives, 100
    for second-degree relatives, 100
  transmission of, from parent to offspring, 99–100
Polyhydramnios, 220
Polymerase chain reaction
  for prenatal molecular diagnosis, 30–31
  technique, 32–33
Pompe's disease, type II, prenatal diagnosis of, 21
Population, protection of, 515

Porphyria
    hepato-erythropoietic, prenatal diagnosis of, 25
    prenatal diagnosis of, 25
Porphyrin metabolism disorders, prenatal diagnosis of, 25
Positional deformities of fetus, 217
Prader-Willi syndrome, prenatal diagnosis of, 27
Prague maneuver, modified, 281
Predictive genetic testing
    definition of, 84
    of fetus, 91
    for frequent disorders, 88–90
Predictive genetic testing (continued)
    protection of data obtained in, 89–90
    protection of tested person's rights in, 90–91
    for simply inherited disorders, 85–88
    technologies for, 84–85
Preeclampsia
    and intrauterine growth retardation, 204
    management of, 213–216
Preferred provider organizations, 188, 518
Pregnancy. See also under Prematernal
    anthropological perspective on, 12–14
    combined intra- and extrauterine, incidence of, 72
    drug usage during, 116–117
    immune response in, 388–389
    legal issues in, 520–532
    management of, in mentally handicapped, 101–108
    social and cultural significance of, 12
    standard of care for, 527–528
    termination, with fetal malformation, 33–34
    in trisomy, 94–95
    ultrasonographic evaluation of cervix in, 78
Pregnancy complications, and health beliefs, 13
Pregnancy outcome, adverse, alcohol-related, 142–143
Pregnancy termination. See also Abortion
    psychological effects of, 17
Prematernal behavior, reasonable, 528–529
Prematernal duty, 431, 437, 442–445
    implications of, 529–532
    legal background for, 523–524
    nature and scope of, 526–529
    and primary prevention of poor pregnancy outcome, 527
    recognition of, 525
Prematernal influences, 521–523
Prematernal liability, 520–532
Premature infant
    as born fetus, 501
    small, ethical issues concerning, 502–505
Premature rupture of membranes, management of, 216–217
Prematurity, 233
    management of, critical questions in, 199–200
    and multiple gestation, 243–244
    prediction of, 209–211
    prevention program, 209–211
    risk factors for, 202–204
    and single twin demise, 247
    survival rates with, 200–202
    and twin gestation, 243–244
Prenatal care
    and health beliefs, 14
    maternal responsibility in, 13
Prenatal diagnosis, 529
    access to, 58
    after age of viability, 41–42
    ethics of, 6, 34
    in first trimester, 17–36
    freedom and coercion issues related to, 59
    future of, 564
    informing patients about options for, 59
    legal issues in, 33–34
    research in, 454, 456–457
    resource allocation for, 58
    in second and third trimester, 36–42
Prenatal injury, liability for, 432
Prenatal therapy. See also Fetal therapy
    coerced, 435–436
    established procedures, duty to employ, 434
    experimental, 432–433
        discretion to employ procedures, 433
        duty to employ procedures, 432–433
    refusal of, resolving conflicts over, 437
Preterm delivery
    and maternal serum alpha-fetoprotein elevation, 49
    pharmacologic therapy to prevent, 211–212
    prevention of, 209
Prevention, 527, 529–530
    of prematernally induced injury, 531
Primates, as organ sources, 469–471
Prince v. Commonwealth of Massachusetts, 235
Privacy
    of family life, 309, 310–311
    right to, 379, 384–385, 490–491, 515, 517, 525, 526, 528, 535, 541–544, 567
Private sphere of social existence, 6
Procarbazine
    teratogenicity, 119
    as transplacental carcinogen, 157
Procreative liberty, 384–385
Professional Standards Review Organizations, 512
Progestational agents, teratogenicity, 122–123
Progesterone
    administration after in vitro fertilization and embryo transfer, 354
    in prevention of preterm delivery, 211
Progestins
    administration after in vitro fertilization and embryo transfer, 354
    teratogenicity, 416–417
Progestogens, teratogenicity, 122–123
Prolidase deficiency, prenatal diagnosis of, 22
PROM. See Premature rupture of membranes
Propane sulfone, as transplacental carcinogen, 156
Propionic acidemia, prenatal diagnosis of, 21, 22
Proportionality, principle of, 274
Propoxyphene, neonatal withdrawal from, 125
Propranolol, maternal use of, effect on newborn, 130
n-Propylnitrosourea, as transplacental carcinogen, 156
Prostaglandin synthetase inhibitors, in prevention of premature delivery, 212
Proximate cause, legal definition of, 339–340
Prune belly syndrome, prenatal diagnosis of, 77
Pseudogestational sac, in ectopic pregnancy, 72
Psychotropic drugs, teratogenicity, 125–127
Public health, 511
Pulmonary hypoplasia, 77
    in fetus, 217
Purine metabolism disorders, prenatal diagnosis of, 25
Purine nucleoside phosphorylase deficiency, prenatal diagnosis of, 25
1-(3-Pyridyl)-3,3-diethyltriazine, as transplacental carcinogen, 157
1-(3-Pyridyl)-3,3-dimethyltriazine, as transplacental carcinogen, 157
Pyrimethamine
    folic acid supplementation with, 121
    safety in pregnancy, 121
Pyrimidine metabolism disorders, prenatal diagnosis of, 25
Pyruvate carboxylase deficiency, prenatal diagnosis of, 21

Pyruvate decarboxylase deficiency, prenatal diagnosis of, 21
Pyruvate dehydrogenase complex deficiency, prenatal diagnosis of, 21

Q

Quality of life issues, 486, 489–490, 491, 492, 501, 527
Quickening, moral and legal significance of, 534, 356
Quinacrine hydrochloride, teratogenicity, 121
Quinine
  as abortifacient, 121
  safety in pregnancy, 121
Quinlan case, 490–491, 500

R

Race, and maternal serum alpha-fetoprotein level, 49–50
Radiation. *See also* Ionizing radiation; X-irradiation
Radiation exposure, and fetal cytogenetic abnormalities, 19
Radius, aplasia of, timing of, in embryogenesis, 155
Raleigh Fitkin-Paul Morgan Memorial Hospital v. Anderson, 235, 237–238, 435–436, 525, 530
Rectal atresia, with fistula, timing of, in embryogenesis, 155
Refsum's disease, prenatal diagnosis of, 23
Rehabilitation Act of 1973, Section 504, 483, 495–499
Religion, and health care, 11
Renal agenesis, ultrasound presentation of, 61, 63
Renslow v. Mennonite Hospital, 524–525
Reproduction
  changing issues concerning, 566–567
  ethical guidance and, 6–7
  increased medical intervention in, 558–559
  sociologic issues related to, 11–12
Reproductive health, monitoring of, 158–159
Reproductive outcome, paternal risk factors, 150–151
Reproductive possibilities, 372–375
Reproductive system
  postnatal development of, 154
  prenatal development of, 153–154
Reproductive technology. *See also* Biomedical technology
  anthropological perspective on, 12–14
  control issues, 376–377
  injury from, 376
  and interests of child, 377–379
  issues related to, 376–380
  and parenthood issues, 377–379
  safety of, 376
Reproductive toxicity
  in female, 153
  postnatal, 154–158
  prenatal, 153–154
  types of, 152–158
  xenobiotics associated with, 153, 154
Reproductive toxins, 159–168
  detection of toxic effects, 158–159
Research
  funded by DHHS, regulations governing, 449–450
  vs. innovative therapy, 440
  medical and clinical, ethical principles in, 274–275
  nontherapeutic, public policy on, 461–462
  resources for, allocation of, 516
Reserpine, maternal use of, effect on newborn, 130
Respiratory distress syndrome
  and fetal heart rate patterns, 220–221
  incidence of, 206
  with perinatal asphyxia, 205
  prevention of, by corticosteroid administration, 217
  and very low birth weight, 206–208

Restriction endonuclease analysis
  for prenatal molecular diagnosis, 30
  technique, 31
Restriction fragment length polymorphisms, 31–32
  linkage analysis with, limitations of, 40
Resuscitation, 493
  in delivery room, of very low birth weight infant, 222–223
  of newborn, code system for, 223
Retinitis pigmentosa, prenatal diagnosis of, 26
Retinoblastoma, prenatal diagnosis of, 26, 27
Retinoic acid, teratogenicity, 130
Retroviral vector systems, for gene therapy, 423–424
RFLPs. *See* Restriction fragment length polymorphisms
Rhesus antigen, prenatal diagnosis of, 26
Rh immune globulin prophylaxis
  adverse reaction to, 176–177
  alternatives to, 178–179
  controversy about, 173, 174–178
  cost-benefit ratios, 178
  dosage and administration recommendations, 173
  efficacy of, 174–176
  historical background, 172–173
  informed consent for, 179
  production and supply problems in, 177–178
  programs for, 173
  rationale for, 173–174
  recommendations about, 179
  risks to fetus, 176
  risks to mother, 176–177
  in third trimester, 173
  and transfer of HIV, 177
  trials of, data from, 174, 175
Rh isoimmunization
  antenatal
    incidence of, 173
    mechanism of, 173–174
  fetal therapy for, 404
  grandmother theory of, 173–174
  irreducible rate for, 179
  pregnancies at risk for, identification of, 178–179
  prevention of. *See also* Rh immune globulin prophylaxis
    failure of, reasons for, 172
RhoGAM therapy, 404
Rifampin, safety in pregnancy, 120–121
Right to life, 535
  of fetus in brain-dead mother, 308
Right to refuse treatment, 490–491, 492
Ring chromosomes, transmission of, from parent to offspring, 96–97
Risk factors
  for chromosomal disorders, 18–19
  for Mendelian disorders, 19–20
Risk management, legal issues in, 342–344
Ritodrine
  administration, 214
  clinical efficacy, 214
  dosage, 214
  mechanism of action, 214
  in prevention of preterm delivery, 212
  side-effects, 214
  in twin gestation, 254–255
Robertsonian translocation, and risk of cytogenetic abnormality in fetus, 18
Roe v. Wade, 235–236, 310–311, 377, 431–432, 434, 436, 477, 525, 526, 528, 532, 535–537, 540–542, 544
  application to life support for brain-dead mother, 307–308
Rubber manufacturing, exposure to toxins in, monitoring using urine analysis, 166

Rubella
  and intrauterine growth retardation, 204
  maternal, 114
Rubella immunization, teratogenicity, 131

S

Saccharopinuria, prenatal diagnosis of, 22
Sacrococcygeal teratoma, 333
Salbutamol, in prevention of preterm delivery, 212
Salicylates
  ratio of concentration in breast milk vs. maternal blood, 158
  teratogenicity, 129
Sandhoff disease, prenatal diagnosis of, 23
Sanfilippo A disease, prenatal diagnosis of, 24
Sanfilippo B disease, prenatal diagnosis of, 24
Sanfilippo C disease, prenatal diagnosis of, 24
Sanfilippo syndrome, prenatal diagnosis of, 24
SAX vector, for gene therapy, 425
Scheie syndrome, prenatal diagnosis of, 24
Screening, definition of, 84
Second trimester
  prenatal diagnosis in, 36–42
  RhIg administration in, effects on pregnancy outcome, 176–177
  steroid concentrations in amniotic fluid in, 405
Seizure disorder, maternal, prenatal care with, 103
Seizures, neonatal, in very low birth weight infants, 224
Selenium, reproductive toxicity, 159, 160
Self-help, medical, 561–562
Semen donor, legal protection of, 379
Sepsis, fetal, 217
Septo-optic dysplasia, 400
Septum pellucidum, absence of, 400
Serial amniocentesis, in twin-to-twin transfusion, 246
Serum-blocking factors, 389
Severe combined immunodeficiency disease, prenatal diagnosis of, 25
Sex, fetal, determination by transvaginal ultrasound, 77
Sex chromosomal abnormalities, transmission of, from parent to offspring, 95–96
Sex discrimination, in employment, 151–152
Sex hormones, synthetic, reproductive toxicity, 154
Sex selection
  amniocentesis for, 40–41
  ethical issues in, 269
Sex steroids
  synthetic, reproductive toxicity, 167
  teratogenicity, 417
Sexual abuse, prevention, in mental retardation, 107
Sexuality
  changing issues concerning, 566–567
  education and counseling about, for mentally retarded, 106–107
Shoulder dystocia, and midforceps delivery, 318
Sialic acid storage disease, infantile, prenatal diagnosis of, 24
Sialidosis, prenatal diagnosis of, 24
Sickle cell anemia
  and fetal hypoxia, 206
  and intrauterine growth retardation, 204
  prenatal diagnosis of, 26, 30, 31
Single parenthood, 560
Sirenomelus, timing of, in embryogenesis, 155
Sister chromatid exchange, and chemical mutagens, 163, 165
Skeletal dysplasia, diagnosis of, 67–68
Skull fracture, with midforceps delivery, 318
Sleep problems, alcohol-related, 143
Sly syndrome, prenatal diagnosis of, 24
Small bowel obstruction, fetal, ultrasound presentation of, 64, 66
Small for gestational age infant
  and preeclampsia, 213
  preterm, congenital anomalies in, 205
  prognosis for, 224
  survival of, 202
Smith, Adam, 510
Smoking
  correlation of genotoxicity with epidemiologic findings, 165
  exposure to toxins in, monitoring using urine analysis, 166
  and fetal hypoxia, 206
  and intrauterine growth retardation, 204
  and onset of menopause, 162
  during pregnancy, as prematernal negligence, 529
  teratogenicity, 124–125
Socially used drugs, teratogenicity, 124–125
Social Security Amendments of 1972, 512
Social Security Amendments of 1983, 513
Sociologic issues, in reproduction, 11–12
Sodium fluoride, cytogenetic effects on meiotic chromosomes of oocytes, 164
Sodium valproate, reproductive toxicity, 154
Solvents, reproductive toxicity, 161–162
Somatic cell gene therapy, 421
  in-utero, potential uses for, 425–430
  pediatric, 422–425
    candidates for clinical trials, 422–423
Speciesism, 367
Sperm donor, 354, 375
  identity of, issues concerning, 378
Spina bifida
  mental retardation with, 100
  open, maternal serum alpha-fetoprotein in, 48
  perinatal management of, 333
  recurrence risk, 100
  treatment, ethical issues concerning, 502
  ultrasound presentation of, 64, 67
Spontaneous abortion. *See also* Fetal wastage
  after clomiphene-induced ovulation, 122
  alcohol-related, 142
  and ethylene oxide exposure, 168
  human leukocyte antigens in, 389–390
  incidence of
    and chromosomal abnormality, 18
    in normal pregnancies, 18
  in vitro fertilization and embryo transfer and, 365–366
  normal pregnancies prior to, 392
  and occupational exposure to solvents, 161–162
  rate
    in dental workers, 167
    and employment, 150
    in women pharmaceutical workers, 167
  risk of
    with amniocentesis, 27
    with chorionic villous sampling, 27
    and vinyl chloride, 163–164
Spray adhesives, mutagenicity, 163
Standard of care, 193–194
  legal definition of, 338
  locality rule, 193, 338
  in obstetric practice, 194–197
  for pregnancy, 527–528
Standards for Obstetric-Gynecologic Services, as guidelines only, 339
Standards of the American College of Obstetricians and Gynecologists
  recommendation on fetal monitoring, 340
  recommendation on start-up time for cesarean section, 342
Steptoe, Patrick, 349–350, 374

Sterilization, 541
  of mentally retarded patient, 107–108
    alternatives to, 112
    American College of Obstetricians and Gynecologists
      Ethics Committee statement on, 108, 110–113
    best interests of patient in, 112–113
    ethical considerations, 111
    informed consent issues in, 111–112
    legal considerations in, 113
    proxy consent in, 112
Steroid concentrations, in amniotic fluid, in second trimester, 405
Steroid metabolism disorders, prenatal diagnosis of, 24–25
Steroids
  in higher-order multiple gestations, 261–262
  therapy for infertility, 388
Stilbesterol, teratogenicity, 122
Stillbirth
  alcohol-related, 142
  and maternal smoking, 124–125
Stiver case, 378
Streptomycin
  ototoxicity, 120
  teratogenicity, 120
Streptonigrin, cytogenetic effects on meiotic chromosomes of oocytes, 164
Structural chromosomal abnormalities, transmission of, from parent to offspring, 95–96
Styrene, reproductive toxicity, 154, 161–162
Styrene exposure, monitoring using urine analysis, 166
Styrene oxide, mutagenicity, 163
Substitute father, 375
Sulfite oxidase deficiency, prenatal diagnosis of, 26
Sulfocysteinuria, prenatal diagnosis of, 26
Sulfonamides, teratogenicity, 119–120
Sulfonylureas, safety in pregnancy, 124
Sulfur dioxide, cytogenetic effects on meiotic chromosomes of oocytes, 164
Superintendent of Belchertown State School v. Saikewicz, 491–492
Surfactant
  artificial, 207
  in newborn lung, 206–207
Surrogate motherhood, 6
  commercial, prohibition of, 383–384
  contracts, 381–382
    legal status of, 359–360
  definition of, 375
  discouragement of, constitutional objections to, 384–385
  interests of child in, 377–378
  legal issues in, 372–385
  legislation governing, 380
    goals of, 381
  payment for, 382–383
  presumption of paternity in, 382
  protection of offspring of, 379–380
  public policy goals for, 379–380
  screening of participants, 381
  self-help in, 562
  standards of fitness of couples for, 381
  statute forbidding, 360
  unpaid, 384
Susceptibility genes, and risk of disease, 88–89
Syndactyly
  prenatal diagnosis of, 76–77
  severe, timing of, in embryogenesis, 155
Syntocinon stress testing. *See also* Oxytocin challenge test
  historical background, 183–184
Systemic lupus erythematosus, 391

T

2,4,5-T, reproductive toxicity, 154
Tamoxifen, in follicle stimulation, for in vitro fertilization, 351–352
Tangier disease, prenatal diagnosis of, 23
Tay-Sachs disease
  diagnosis of, 20
  prenatal diagnosis of, 23
Technologic imperative, 315, 439
Technology
  advancements in, costs of, 187
  changing, implications of, 566–567
  effect on moral status of fetus, 442
  emerging
    coverage of costs of, 192
    and liability, 192–197
  ethical issues concerning, 504
  high, preferred over basic technology, 558–559
  new, 488
    evolution of, 183, 185–186
Technology assessment, 185–186
  future directions in, 190–192
  public policy issues in, 189–190
  and reimbursement, 187–192
Tegretol. *See* Carbamazepine
TEM. *See* Triethylenemelamine
Teratogenesis, 4. *See also* Mutagenicity
  contributing factors, 115–116
  critical periods in, 115
  underlying mechanisms, 115–116
Teratogens, 116–130
  cardiac, 416–417
  dosage, differential effects of, 116
Teratology, 114
Teratomas, fetal, ultrasound presentation of, 61–62, 64
Terbutaline
  administration, 214
  clinical efficacy, 214
  dosage, 214
  mechanism of action, 214
  side-effects, 214
  in twin gestation, 254–255
Terminal illness, vs. inchoate illness, 504–505
Termination of treatment, 493
  case law concerning, 489–495, 490–491
2,3,7,8-Tetrachlorodibenzo-p-dioxin, reproductive toxicity, 162
Tetrachloroethylene, ratio of concentration in breast milk vs. maternal blood, 158
Tetracyclines, teratogenicity, 120
Thalidomide, 114, 115, 521
  reproductive toxicity, 154
  teratogenicity, 125, 417
Thanatophoric dwarfism, 77
Theobromine, ratio of concentration in breast milk vs. maternal blood, 158
Theophylline, ratio of concentration in breast milk vs. maternal blood, 158
Thiazide diuretics, safety in pregnancy, 130
Thio-TEPA. *See* Triethylenethiophosphoramide
Thiourea agents, teratogenicity, 123
Third trimester
  abortion in, for anencephaly, 472
  prenatal diagnosis in, 36–42
  termination of pregnancy in, for anencephaly, 476–477
Thoracic circumference-abdominal circumference ratio, 77
Thoracic measurements, fetal, on ultrasound, 77
Threatened abortion, progestogen therapy for, teratogenic risk of, 123

Thrombocytopenia-absent radius syndrome, 76
Thymic cell infusion, as fetal therapy, 411
Thyroid and related drugs, teratogenicity, 123–124
Tissue transplantation, research on, 458–459
Tocolysis, in twin gestation, 254–255
Tocolytic agents
 comparison of, 214–215
 in higher-order multiple gestations, 261–262
 in prevention of preterm delivery, 211–212
Toluene
 mutagenicity, 163
 reproductive toxicity, 161
TORCH infections, and intrauterine growth retardation, 204–205
TORCH screening, 220
Tort immunity, intrafamilial, demise of, 434, 523–524, 529
Tort law, 9
 and in vitro fertilization, 358–359
Torts
 preconception, 524
 prenatal, third-party liability for, 523–524
Tourette syndrome, prenatal diagnosis of, 27
Toxins, occupational exposures to, 149–150
 assessment of hazards, 150–152
 demographics of, 149–150
Tracheoesophageal fistula, 221
Tranquilizers, teratogenicity, 125–127
Transcobalamin 2 deficiency, prenatal diagnosis of, 23
Transfusion, of fetus, 37
Translocation. *See also* Robertsonian translocation
 balanced reciprocal, and risk of cytogenetic abnormality in fetus, 18
 in family, and risk of fetal abnormality, 39
 risk of, 18, 20
 transmission of, from parent to offspring, 97
Transport disorders, prenatal diagnosis of, 26
Treatment
 appropriate, legal issues concerning, 499–500
 ordinary vs. extraordinary, 500
Triaziquone, cytogenetic effects on meiotic chromosomes of oocytes, 164
1,1,1-Trichloroethane, reproductive toxicity, 161–162
Trichloroethylene
 mutagenicity, 163
 reproductive toxicity, 161–162
Tricyclic antidepressants, teratogenicity, 127
Triethylenemelamine
 cytogenetic effects on meiotic chromosomes of oocytes, 164
 teratogenic risk of, 118
Triethylenethiophosphoramide, teratogenic risk of, 118
Trimethadione, teratogenicity, 128, 417
Trimethoprim–sulfamethoxazole, teratogenicity, 119
Triose phosphate isomerase deficiency, prenatal diagnosis of, 26
Trisomy
 autosomal, transmission of, from parent to offspring, 94–95
 maternal serum alpha-fetoprotien in prediction of, 40
 nontreatment with, 482
 plant studies of, application to humans, 95
 in previous pregnancy, and risk of fetal abnormality, 39
Trisomy 8, 94–95
Trisomy 9, 94–95
Trisomy 13, 75, 77, 94, 472
 and maternal age, 18
Trisomy 18, 42, 75, 94, 472
 and intrauterine growth retardation, 204
 and maternal age, 18
Trisomy 21, 75. *See also* Down syndrome
 after clomiphene-induced ovulation, 122
 pregnancy in, 95
 prevalence of, 18
 sterility of males in, 95
 transmission of, from parent to offspring, 95
Trisomy 22, 94–95
Trophoblast-lymphocyte cross-reactive antigen system, 390–391
Trophoblast-specific antigen, 389
Tumor, ability to escape immune surveillance, 392
Turner syndrome
 and intrauterine growth retardation, 204
 prenatal diagnosis of, 42
 in previous pregnancy, and risk of fetal abnormality, 39
Twin gestation. *See also* Multiple gestation
 acardia in, 248–249
 antenatal care in, 250–253
 antenatal concerns, 243–250
 biparietal diameter in, 250–253
 chromosomal abnormalities in, 249–250
 congenital malformations in, 248–249
 discordant growth in, 251–253
 early diagnosis of, 243
 ethical issues in, 266–269
 experimental fetal therapy in, 441
 fetal assessments in, 253
 fetal lung maturity in, assessment of, 256
 growth rates in
  discordancy in, 244
  and IQ, 244
  incidence of abnormalities in, 267
 intrapartum risks in, 257–258
 and intrauterine growth retardation, 244
 intrauterine growth retardation in, assessment of, 251–253
 in vitro fertilization and embryo transfer and, 366
 labor and delivery in, 256
  elective timing of, 257
  interlocking of twins in, 258
  mechanical twin-to-twin interaction in, 258
  route of delivery, 258–259
 labor management in, 257
 maternal serum alpha-fetoprotein levels with, 50
 with one abnormal fetus, ethical issue in, 266–269
 and prematurity, 243–244
 prophylactic therapy in, 253–256
 risks of, 242–243
 selective termination in, ethical issues in, 267–269
 single fetal demise in, 246–248
 specialized outpatient clinic for, 255
 ultrasound examinations in, 250–253
Twin-to-twin transfusion, 244–246
 and acardia, 249
 diagnosis of, 245–246
 management of, 246
 mortality with, 246
 sequelae of, 245
 serial amniocentesis in, 246
 ultrasonic diagnosis of, 250–251
Tyrosinemia, prenatal diagnosis of, 22

U

Ultrasound. *See also* Echocardiography, fetal
 abnormal fetal biometry seen on, 67–69
 absence of normally presented structure on, 61–63
 cardiac, 412
 detection of fetal anomalies with, 60–70
  diagnostic methods, 60
 detection of neural tube defects with, 333
 in diagnosis of intraventricular hemorrhage, 208

in diagnosis of urinary tract obstruction, 397–398
dilatation behind an obstruction presented on, 64–66
early diagnosis of multiple gestation with, 243
evaluation of hydrocephalus, 400
examinations, in twin gestation, 250–253
fetal, 412
fetal motion seen on, abnormal or absent, 68–70
fetal weight estimation by, 218, 219
herniations through structural defects seen on, 64–68
in higher-order multiple gestations, 261
for oocyte retrieval, 352–353
presence of additional structure distorting normal contour on, 61–65
suspicious cardiac findings on, 418
transvaginal, 71–82
   advantages of, 71
   in early pregnancy, 72–78
   evaluation of cervix with, in pregnancy, 78
   in infertility, 78–82
   in monitoring of ovulation induction, 78–80
   scanner and probe for, 71–72
   transducer for, 71–72
uses of, 36–37
Ultrasound needle aspiration procedures, 37–38
Umbilical cord
   catheterization, for prenatal therapy, 410
   compression, 216
      in breech delivery, 279
   prolapse, 216
      in breech delivery, 279
   prolapse of, and fetal size, 406
Unborn
   legal rights of, 356–358
   moral status of, 367
   prenatal rights and duties of mother and physician to, 431–437
   rights of, 377, 526, 527
Unemployment, health hazards of, 150
Uniform Anatomical Gift Act, 458, 473
United Steelworkers of America v. Marshall, 152
Ureteral dilatation, ultrasound presentation of, 64, 66
Urethane, as transplacental carcinogen, 157
Urinary tract obstruction
   fetal, ultrasound presentation of, 64, 66
   fetal surgery for, 397
      evaluation for, 397
      management options, 397–400
   prenatal diagnosis of, 397
Urine analysis, for monitoring exposure to mutagenic substances, 166
Urine electrolytes, as indicator of fetal renal function, 398
Usual customary and reasonable, 518
Uterine contractions
   monitoring, at home, 255
   in predicition of preterm labor, 255
   in twin gestations, 255–256
Uteroplacental insufficiency
   evaluation of, 183–184
   and intrauterine growth retardation, 204
Uterus
   bicornuate, timing of, in embryogenesis, 155
   borrowing or rental of, 375
Utilization review, 518

V

VACTERL anomalies, association with congenital heart disease, 77
VACTERL complex, and oral contraceptive exposure, 123

Vacuum extraction, 324
Vaginal delivery, for very low birth weight infant, 221–222
Valproic acid
   effects on fetus, 103
   teratogenicity, 128, 417
Vanishing twin, 246
Varigate porphyria, prenatal diagnosis of, 25
Ventricular septal defect, timing of, in embryogenesis, 155
Ventriculomegaly. *See* Hydrocephalus
Very low birth weight
   antepartum management of, special issues in, 212–220
   causes of, 202–205, 233
   cesarean delivery in
      ethical considerations in, 233–241
      legal considerations, 234–238
   cesarean section vs. vaginal delivery in, 221–222
   and congenital anomalies, 205
   definition of, 199
   fetal evaluation in, 218–220
   intrapartum fetal evaluation with, 220–221
   labor and delivery with, 220–223
   long-term follow-up in, 223–224
   maternal transfer to tertiary care center in, 220
   morbidity and mortality, 233
   neonatal complications with, 205–209
   and neurological deficits, 223–224
   obstetric management of
      critical questions in, 199–200
      ethical considerations in, 233–241
      medical considerations in, 199–224
      patient involvement in decision-making about, 222, 240–241
   preterm delivery with, prevention of, 209
   prognosis in, 223–224
   resuscitation of infant in delivery room, 222–223
   risk factors for, 202–204
   risks to fetus, 200
   survival rates, 200–202, 221
   treatment team, 200
Very low birth weight infant, ethical issues concerning, 502–505
Viability
   and abortion, 309–310
   and life-support of brain-dead mother, 309, 316
   moral and legal implications of, 220, 356–357, 461, 535, 563
Vinblastine, teratogenicity, 119
Vincristine, teratogenicity, 119
Vinyl chloride
   mutagenicity, 163
   reproductive toxicity, 154
   and spontaneous abortion, 163–164
Vitamin B$_1$2 metabolic defect, prenatal diagnosis of, 23
Vitamin E, prenatal therapy with, 409–410
Vitamins
   prenatal therapy with, 409–410
   teratogenicity, 130
Von Gierke's disease, type I, prenatal diagnosis of, 21
Von Willebrand's disease, prenatal diagnosis of, 26

W

Warfarin
   reproductive toxicity, 154
   teratogenicity, 75
Warfarin derivatives, teratogenicity, 128–129
Wigand-Martin maneuver, 287
Wigand-Martin-Winkle maneuver, 281
Williams' syndrome, 130
Wilms' tumor, 161
   prenatal diagnosis of, 27

Wilson disease
  fetal therapy for, 410
  prenatal diagnosis of, 25
Withholding of treatment, 499. *See also* Nontreatment
Wolfe-Hirschhorn syndrome, prenatal diagnosis of, 27
Wolman's disease, prenatal diagnosis of, 23
Womack v. Buchhorn, 524–525
Women
  employment of
    changing patterns in, 557–558
    restrictions on, 531
  social roles of, 12–13
Wright v. Olin Corp., 531
Wrongful birth, 359
Wrongful life, 358–359, 376, 530

X

Xenografts, 470. *See also* Baby Fae
Xeroderma pigmentosum
  diagnosis of, 20
  inheritance of, 20
X-irradiation, as perinatal behavioral toxin, 155
X-linked disorders
  diagnosis of, 77
  prenatal diagnosis of, 39
  recessive, transmission of, from parent to offspring, 99
X-ray pelvimetry, 282–283

Y

Yolk sac abnormalities, diagnosis, by transvaginal ultrasound, 73–74

Z

Zellweger syndrome, prenatal diagnosis of, 27
Zineb, mutagenicity, 163
Ziram, mutagenicity, 163